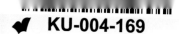
WinkingSkull.com *PLUS*

<u>Your</u> study aid for must-know anatomy

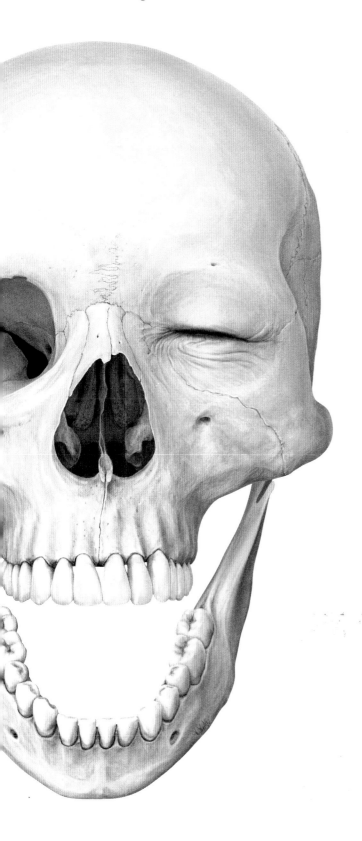

Register for WinkingSkull.com *PLUS* – master human anatomy with this unique interactive online learning tool.

Use the access code below to register for **WinkingSkull.com** *PLUS* and view over 1,900 full-color illustrations and radiographs from the book. After studying this invaluable image bank, you can quiz yourself on key body structures and get your score instantly to check your progress or to compare with other users' results.

WinkingSkull.com *PLUS* has everything you need for course study and exam prep:

- More than 1,900 full-color anatomy illustrations
- Intuitive design that simplifies navigation
- "Labels-on, labels-off" function that makes studying easy and fun
- Timed self-tests–with instant results

Simply visit WinkingSkull.com and follow these instructions to get started today.

If you do not already have a free WinkingSkull.com account, visit www.winkingskull.com, click on "Register" and complete the registration form. Enter the scratch-off code below.

If you already have a WinkingSkull.com account, go to the "Manage Account" page and click on the "Register a Code" link. Enter the scratch-off code below.

This product cannot be returned if the access code panel is scratched off.

Some functionalities on WinkingSkull.com require support for advanced web technologies. A major browser (IE, Chrome, Firefox, Safari) within the last three major versions is suggested for use on the site.

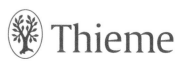

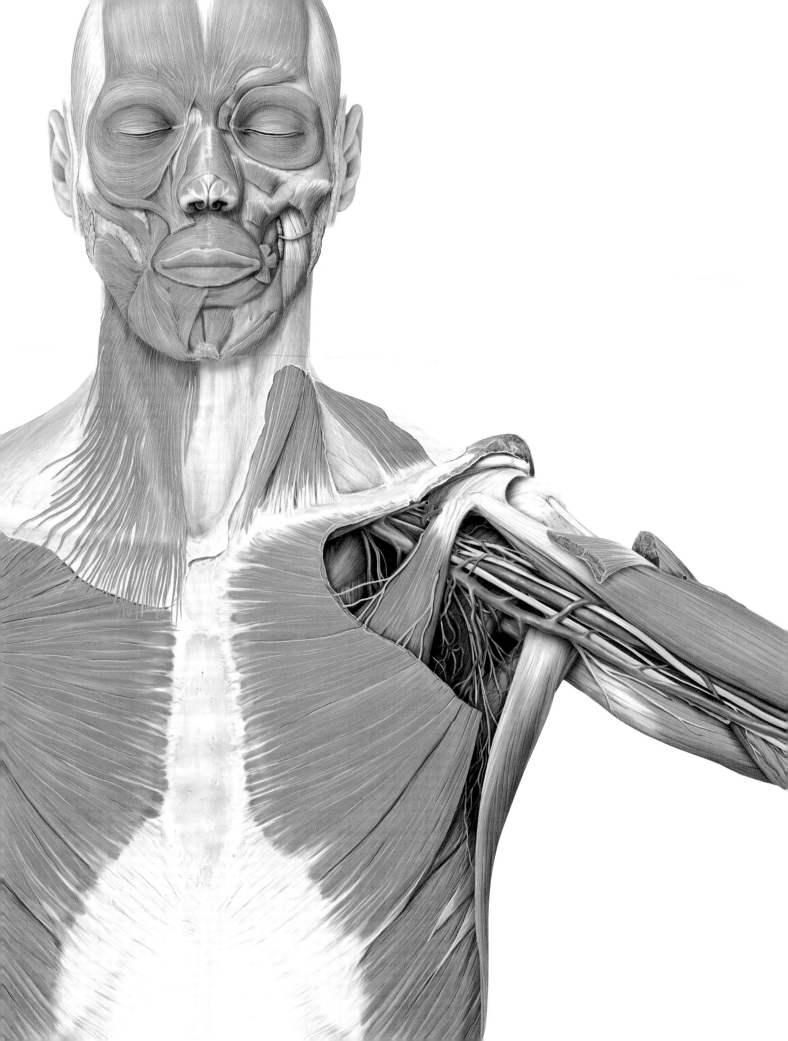

Atlas of Anatomy

Third Edition

Edited by

Anne M. Gilroy, MA
Associate Professor
Department of Radiology
University of Massachusetts Medical School
Worcester, Massachusetts

Brian R. MacPherson, PhD
Professor and Vice-Chair
Department of Anatomy and Neurobiology
University of Kentucky College of Medicine
Lexington, Kentucky

Based on the work of

Michael Schuenke, MD, PhD
Institute of Anatomy
Christian Albrecht University Kiel
Kiel, Germany

Erik Schulte, MD
Department of Functional and Clinical Anatomy
University Medicine
Johannes Gutenberg University
Mainz, Germany

Udo Schumacher, MD, FRCPath, CBiol, FSB, DSc
Institute of Anatomy and Experimental Morphology
Center for Experimental Medicine
University Cancer Center
University Medical Center Hamburg-Eppendorf
Hamburg, Germany

Illustrations by
Markus Voll
Karl Wesker

1935 illustrations

Thieme

New York · Stuttgart · Delhi · Rio de Janeiro

Editorial Director, Educational Products: Anne M. Sydor
Developmental Editor: Julie O'Meara
Editorial Assistant: Tony Paese
Director, Editorial Services: Mary Jo Casey
International Production Director: Andreas Schabert
Vice President, Editorial and E-Product Development: Vera Spillner
International Marketing Director: Fiona Henderson
International Sales Director: Louisa Turrell
Director of Sales, North America: Mike Roseman
Senior Vice President and Chief Operating Officer: Sarah Vanderbilt
President: Brian D. Scanlan
Illustrations: Markus Voll and Karl Wesker
Production Editor: Barbara Chernow
Compositor: Carol Pierson, Chernow Editorial Services, Inc.

Library of Congress Cataloging-in-Publication Data

Names: Gilroy, Anne M., editor. | MacPherson, Brian R., editor. | Voll,
    Markus M., illustrator. | Wesker, Karl, illustrator. | Schuenke, Michael.
    Thieme atlas of anatomy. Based on (work):
Title: Atlas of anatomy / edited by Anne M. Gilroy, Brian R. MacPherson ;
    based on the work of Michael Schuenke, Erik Schulte, Udo Schumacher ;
    illustrations by Markus Voll, Karl Wesker.
Other titles: Atlas of Anatomy (Gilroy)
Description: Third edition. | New York : Thieme, [2016] | Includes index.
Identifiers: LCCN 2015051118 (print) | LCCN 2016001057 (ebook) |
    ISBN 9781626232525 | ISBN 9781626232532 (eISBN) | ISBN
    9781626232532 ()
Subjects: | MESH: Anatomy | Atlases
Classification: LCC QM25 (print) | LCC QM25 (ebook) | NLM QS 17 | DDC
    611.0022/2--dc23
LC record available at http://lccn.loc.gov/2015051118

Copyright ©2016 by Thieme Medical Publishers, Inc.
Thieme Publishers New York
333 Seventh Avenue, New York, NY 10001 USA
+1 800 782 3488, customerservice@thieme.com

Thieme Publishers Stuttgart
Rüdigerstrasse 14, 70469 Stuttgart, Germany
+49 [0]711 8931 421, customerservice@thieme.de

Thieme Publishers Delhi
A-12, Second Floor, Sector-2, Noida-201301
Uttar Pradesh, India
+91 120 45 566 00, customerservice@thieme.in

Thieme Publishers Rio de Janeiro, Thieme Publicações Ltda.
Edifício Rodolpho de Paoli, 25º andar
Av. Nilo Peçanha, 50 – Sala 2508
Rio de Janeiro 20020-906 Brasil
+55 21 3172 2297

Printed in Canada by Transcontinental, Quebec   5 4 3 2 1

ISBN 978-1-62623-252-5

Also available as an e-book:
eISBN 978-1-62623-253-2

Important note: Medicine is an ever-changing science undergoing continual development. Research and clinical experience are continually expanding our knowledge, in particular our knowledge of proper treatment and drug therapy. Insofar as this book mentions any dosage or application, readers may rest assured that the authors, editors, and publishers have made every effort to ensure that such references are in accordance with **the state of knowledge at the time of production of the book.**

Nevertheless, this does not involve, imply, or express any guarantee or responsibility on the part of the publishers in respect to any dosage instructions and forms of applications stated in the book. **Every user is requested to examine carefully** the manufacturers' leaflets accompanying each drug and to check, if necessary in consultation with a physician or specialist, whether the dosage schedules mentioned therein or the contraindications stated by the manufacturers differ from the statements made in the present book. Such examination is particularly important with drugs that are either rarely used or have been newly released on the market. Every dosage schedule or every form of application used is entirely at the user's own risk and responsibility. The authors and publishers request every user to report to the publishers any discrepancies or inaccuracies noticed. If errors in this work are found after publication, errata will be posted at www.thieme.com on the product description page.

Some of the product names, patents, and registered designs referred to in this book are in fact registered trademarks or proprietary names even though specific reference to this fact is not always made in the text. Therefore, the appearance of a name without designation as proprietary is not to be construed as a representation by the publisher that it is in the public domain.

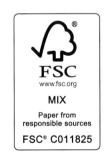

Dedication

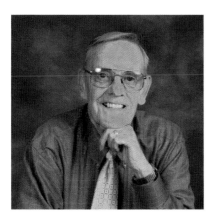

We dedicate this third edition of the *Atlas of Anatomy* to the memory of Lawrence ("Larry") McIvor Ross, 1938–2015. Larry was an outstanding anatomist and cherished mentor and colleague. He started his academic career in 1968 as a faculty member in the Department of Anatomy at UTMB – Galveston. After six years he accepted an appointment in the Department of Anatomy at Michigan State University (MSU) and remained there until he retired in 2000. Larry was passionate about making a difference in the lives of his students, however, and continued to teach as a visiting professor at St. George's University on Grenada in the West Indies for nine years and as an adjunct professor in the Department of Neurobiology and Anatomy at the University of Texas Medical School – Houston until 2014. Fellow anatomists admired his dedication as a member of the American Association of Clinical Anatomists where he served the association in every position on the Executive Council. In 2015 he was honored for his service to the association with the *R. Benton Adkins Jr. Distinguished Service Award*.

As an academician, Larry was a true multidisciplinary anatomist, teaching histology, neuroanatomy, gross anatomy, and embryology to thousands of medical and graduate students as well as numerous non-medical groups. As an author, he will be remembered best for his work with Thieme Publishers. From 2005 to 2007 he co-edited the English translation of all three volumes of *Prometheus: Atlas of Anatomy*. Following the critical success of the three-volume atlas in English-speaking countries, he was instrumental in helping Thieme create the concept for the single-volume *Atlas of Anatomy*. This atlas, now in its third edition, is highly acclaimed in its own right and is distributed worldwide and translated in over 14 languages. As his co-authors, we are most grateful to Larry for his mentorship. He was responsible for bringing us onto the project and into the world of medical publications. We feel personally indebted for all he did for us, and will fondly remember him as a great mentor, friend, and colleague.

Anne and Brian

Table of Contents

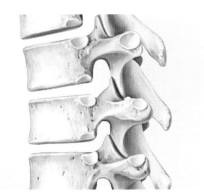

Back

1 Surface Anatomy

2 Bones, Ligaments & Joints

3 Muscles

4 Neurovasculature

5 Sectional & Radiographic Anatomy

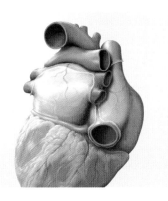

Thorax

6 Surface Anatomy

7 Thoracic Wall

8 Thoracic Cavity

Abdomen

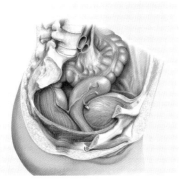

Pelvis & Perineum

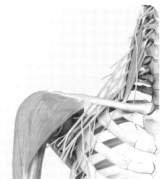

Upper Limb

28 Neurovasculature

29 Sectional & Radiographic Anatomy

Lower Limb

30 Surface Anatomy

31 Hip & Thigh

32 Knee & Leg

33 Ankle & Foot

34 Neurovasculature

35 Sectional & Radiographic Anatomy

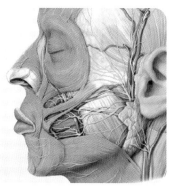

Head & Neck

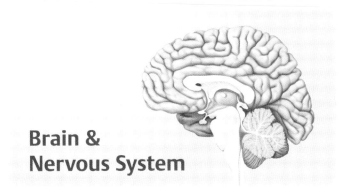

Brain & Nervous System

47 Brain

48 Blood Vessels of the Brain

49 Functional Systems

50 Autonomic Nervous System

51 Sectional & Radiographic Anatomy

Acknowledgments

We would like to thank the authors of the original award-winning *Thieme Atlas of Anatomy* three-volume series, Michael Schuenke, Erik Schulte, and Udo Schumacher, and the illustrators, Karl Wesker and Marcus Voll, for their work over the course of many years.

We thank the many instructors and students who have pointed out to us what we have done well and brought to our attention errors, ambiguities, and new information, or have suggested how we could present a topic more effectively. This input, combined with our experience teaching with the Atlas, have guided our work on this edition.

We again cordially thank the members of the first edition Advisory Board for their contributions:

- Bruce M. Carlson, MD, PhD
  University of Michigan
  Ann Arbor, Michigan

- Derek Bryant (Class of 2011)
  University of Toronto Medical School
  Burlington, Ontario

- Peter Cole, MD
  Glamorum Healing Centre
  Orangeville, Ontario

- Michael Droller, MD
  The Mount Sinai Medical Center
  New York, New York

- Anthony Firth, PhD
  Imperial College London
  London

- Mark H. Hankin, PhD
  University of Virginia, School of Medicine
  Charlottesville, Virginia

- Katharine Hudson (Class of 2010)
  McGill Medical School
  Montreal, Quebec

- Christopher Lee (Class of 2010)
  Harvard Medical School
  Cambridge, Massachusetts

- Francis Liuzzi, PhD
  Lake Erie College of Osteopathic Medicine
  Bradenton, Florida

- Graham Louw, PhD
  University of Cape Town Medical School
  University of Cape Town

- Estomih Mtui, MD
  Weill Cornell Medical College
  New York, New York

- Srinivas Murthy, MD
  Harvard Medical School
  Boston, Massachusetts

- Jeff Rihn, MD
  The Rothman Institute
  Philadelphia, Pennsylvania

- Lawrence Rizzolo, PhD
  Yale University
  New Haven, Connecticut

- Mikel Snow, PhD
  University of Southern California
  Los Angeles, California

- Kelly Wright (Class of 2010)
  Wayne State University School of Medicine
  Detroit, Michigan

Foreword

This *Atlas of Anatomy*, in my opinion, is the finest single-volume atlas of human anatomy that has ever been created. Two factors make it so: the images and the way they have been organized.

The artists, Markus Voll and Karl Wesker, have created a new standard of excellence in anatomical art. Their graceful use of transparency and their sensitive representation of light and shadow give the reader an accurate three-dimensional understanding of every structure.

The authors have organized the images so that they give just the flow of information a student needs to build up a clear mental image of the human body. Each two-page spread is a self-contained lesson that unobtrusively shows the hand of an experienced and thoughtful teacher. I wish I could have held this book in my hands when I was a student; I envy any student who does so now.

Robert D. Acland, 1941–2016
Louisville, Kentucky   December 2015

Preface

It is with a mix of pride and humility that we offer our 3rd edition of the *Atlas of Anatomy*. As with the previous editions, we have tried to respond to the requests, comments, and criticisms of our readers. Although this edition was prepared without the contributions of our friend and co-author, Lawrence Ross, who passed away in 2015, we have tried to maintain the same quality of excellence and attention to detail that he helped bring to the previous editions.

In this latest edition we focused our attention on three major tasks. The first reflects an understanding that anatomy is a changing science. Our readers understand that it is a dynamic part of clinical medicine, itself a science undergoing constant evolution. Concepts and terminology change accordingly and we feel a responsibility to pass on to our readers the most accurate and current information available.

Our second task was to add additional examples of sectional and radiographic images to help students apply their knowledge of anatomic structure and relationships to comparable clinical representations. While radiology as a clinical discipline is a specialty that requires expertise in diagnoses and treatment (and as such is not addressed here), the topographic interpretation of radiographic images is a natural companion to the study of anatomy. To this end, we have moved some images that were previously integrated into earlier chapters and added many new images to create a new *Sectional and Radiographic Anatomy* chapter in each unit.

Finally, we have expanded areas that deserved greater attention. A newly titled *Brain and Nervous System* unit replaces the former Neuro-anatomy unit. Here, the reader will find a greater focus on the gross anatomy of the brain and peripheral nervous system. We've also added new spreads on the autonomic nervous system, a topic that needed to be expanded. In the *Pelvis and Perineum* unit, some images were removed and others revised to illustrate current anatomic theory. In addition, new art that better demonstrates the complex pelvic anatomy has been added throughout the unit.

As always, we thank reviewers, colleagues, and students who commented on previous editions and have suggested appropriate corrections.

We recognize that our efforts, though important, are just one part of the process that brings this textbook to your desk. Support from the entire Thieme Publishers team has been essential in creating the third edition. We are especially grateful to Julie O'Meara, Developmental Editor; Tony Paese, Editorial Assistant; Anne M. Sydor, PhD, Editorial Director, Educational Products; Barbara Chernow, PhD, Production Manager; and Carol Pierson, compositor, for excellence in their individual areas of expertise and their unwavering confidence in our ability to produce a quality manuscript.

Anne M. Gilroy
Worcester, Massachusetts

Brian R. MacPherson
Lexington, Kentucky

December 2015

Preface to the First Edition

Each of the authors was amazed and impressed with the extraordinary detail, accuracy, and beauty of the illustrations that were created for the *Thieme Atlas of Anatomy*. We feel these images are one of the most significant additions to anatomical education in the past 50 years. It was our intent to use these exceptional illustrations as the cornerstone of our effort in creating a concise single volume *Atlas of Anatomy* for the curious and eager health science student.

Our challenge was first to select from this extensive collection those images that are most instructive and illustrative of current dissection approaches. Along the way, however, we realized that creating a single-volume atlas was much more than choosing images: each image has to convey a significant amount of detail while the appeal and labeling need to be clean and soothing to the eye. Therefore, hundreds of illustrations were drawn new or modified to fit the approach of this new atlas. In addition, key schematic diagrams and simplified summary-form tables were added wherever needed. Dozens of applicable radiographic images and important clinical correlates have been added where appropriate. Additionally, surface anatomy illustrations are accompanied by questions designed to direct the student's attention to anatomic detail that is most relevant in conducting the physical exam. Elements from each of these features are arranged in a regional format to facilitate common dissection approaches. Within each region, the various components are examined systemically, followed by topographical images to tie the systems together within the region. In all of this, a clinical perspective on the anatomical structures is taken. The unique two facing pages "spread" format focuses the user to the area/topic being explored.

We hope these efforts — the results of close to 100 combined years experience teaching the discipline of anatomy to bright, enthusiastic students — has resulted in a comprehensive, easy-to-use resource and reference.

We would like to thank our colleagues at Thieme Publishers who so professionally facilitated this effort. We cannot thank enough Cathrin E. Schulz, MD, Editorial Director, Educational Products, who so graciously reminded us of deadlines, while always being available to "trouble shoot" problems. More importantly, she encouraged, helped, and complimented our efforts.

We also wish to extend very special thanks and appreciation to Bridget Queenan, Developmental Editor, who edited and developed the manuscript with an outstanding talent for visualization and intuitive flow of information. We are very grateful to her for catching many details along the way while always patiently responding to requests for artwork and labeling changes.

Cordial thanks to Elsie Starbecker, Senior Production Editor, who with great care and speed produced this atlas with its over 2,200 illustrations. Finally, thanks to Rebecca McTavish, Developmental Editor, for joining the team in the correction phase. So very much of their hard work has made the *Atlas of Anatomy* a reality.

Anne M. Gilroy
Worcester, Massachusetts

Brian R. MacPherson
Lexington, Kentucky

Lawrence M. Ross
Houston, Texas

March 2008

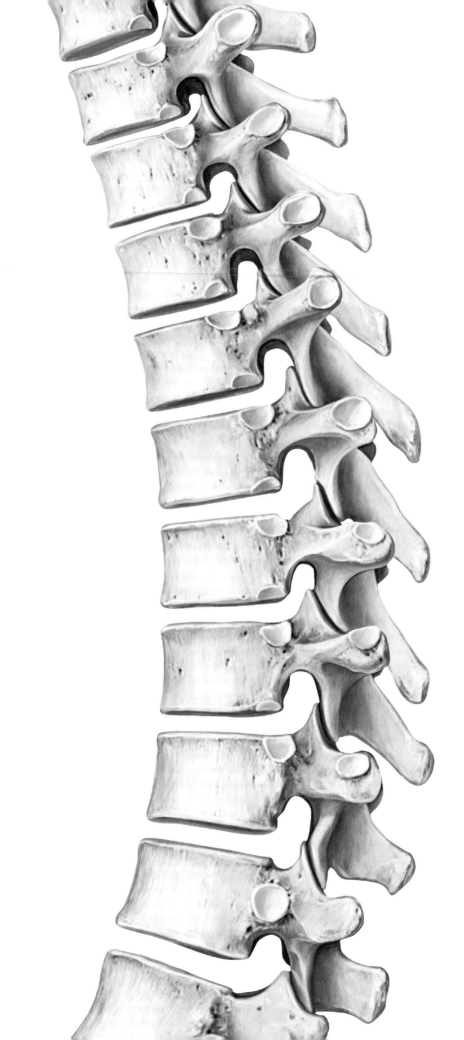

Back

Surface Anatomy

Fig. 1.1 Palpable structures of the back
Posterior view.

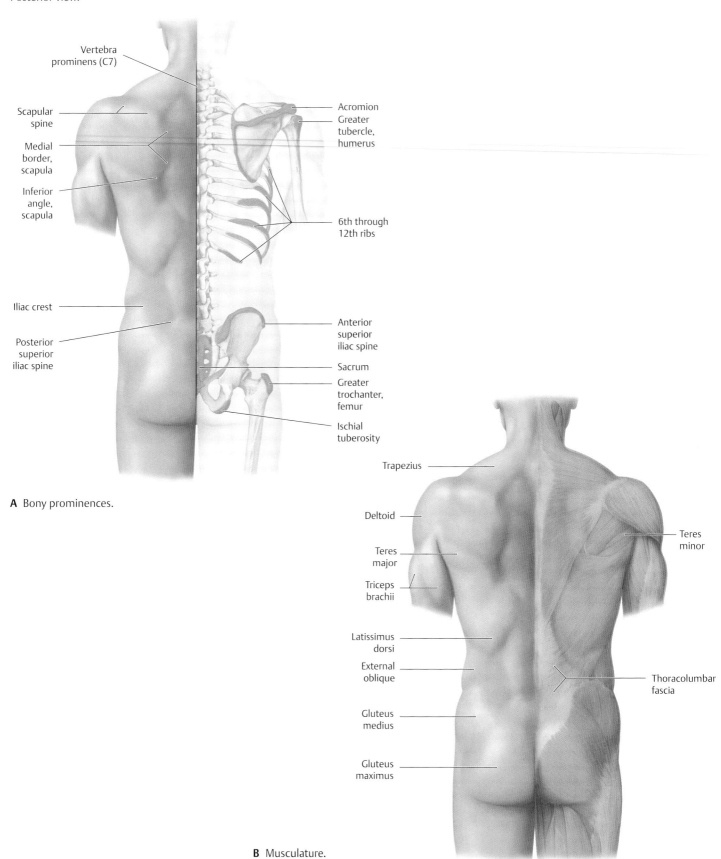

Vertebra prominens (C7)

Scapular spine

Medial border, scapula

Inferior angle, scapula

Iliac crest

Posterior superior iliac spine

Acromion

Greater tubercle, humerus

6th through 12th ribs

Anterior superior iliac spine

Sacrum

Greater trochanter, femur

Ischial tuberosity

A Bony prominences.

Trapezius

Deltoid

Teres major

Triceps brachii

Latissimus dorsi

External oblique

Gluteus medius

Gluteus maximus

Teres minor

Thoracolumbar fascia

B Musculature.

Fig. 1.2 Regions of the back and buttocks
Posterior view.

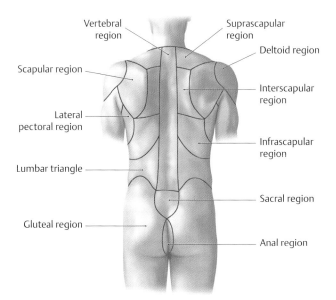

Vertebral region
Suprascapular region
Deltoid region
Scapular region
Interscapular region
Lateral pectoral region
Infrascapular region
Lumbar triangle
Sacral region
Gluteal region
Anal region

Fig. 1.3 Spinous processes and landmarks of the back
Posterior view.

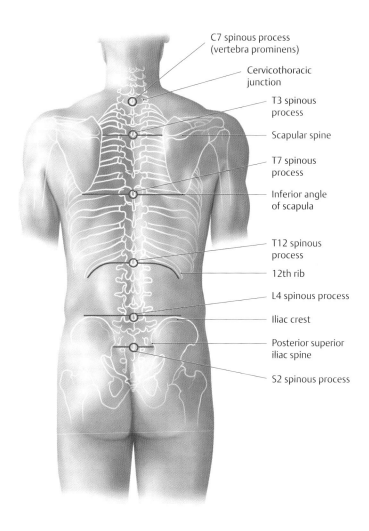

C7 spinous process (vertebra prominens)
Cervicothoracic junction
T3 spinous process
Scapular spine
T7 spinous process
Inferior angle of scapula
T12 spinous process
12th rib
L4 spinous process
Iliac crest
Posterior superior iliac spine
S2 spinous process

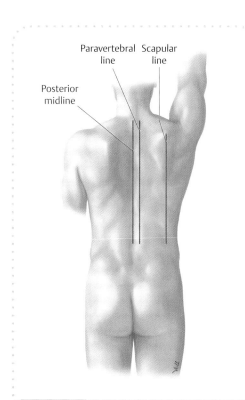

Paravertebral line
Scapular line
Posterior midline

Table 1.1	Reference lines of the back
Posterior midline	Posterior trunk midline at the level of the spinous processes
Paravertebral line	Line at the level of the transverse processes
Scapular line	Line through the inferior angle of the scapula

Table 1.2	Spinous processes that provide useful posterior landmarks
Vertebral spinous process	**Posterior landmark**
C7	Vertebra prominens (the projecting spinous process of C7 is clearly visible and palpable)
T3	The scapular spine
T7	The inferior angle of the scapula
T12	Just below the 12th rib
L4	The summit of the iliac crest
S2	The posterior superior iliac spine (recognized by small skin depressions directly over the iliac spines)

Vertebral Column: Overview

The vertebral column (spine) is divided into four regions: the cervical, thoracic, lumbar, and sacral spines. Both the cervical and lumbar spines demonstrate lordosis (inward curvature); the thoracic and sacral spines demonstrate kyphosis (outward curvature).

Fig. 2.1 **Vertebral column**
Left lateral view.

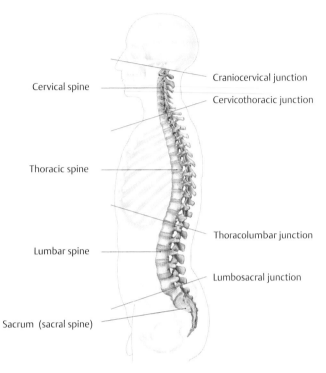

Cervical spine — Craniocervical junction
Cervicothoracic junction
Thoracic spine
Thoracolumbar junction
Lumbar spine — Lumbosacral junction
Sacrum (sacral spine)

A Regions of the spine.

Clinical box 2.1

Spinal development

The characteristic curvatures of the adult spine appear over the course of postnatal development, being only partially present in a newborn. The newborn has a "kyphotic" spinal curvature (**A**); lumbar lordosis develops later and becomes stable at puberty (**C**).

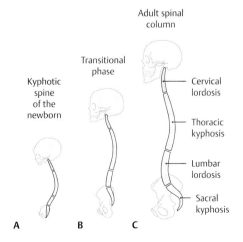

Adult spinal column

Transitional phase

Kyphotic spine of the newborn

Cervical lordosis
Thoracic kyphosis
Lumbar lordosis
Sacral kyphosis

A   **B**   **C**

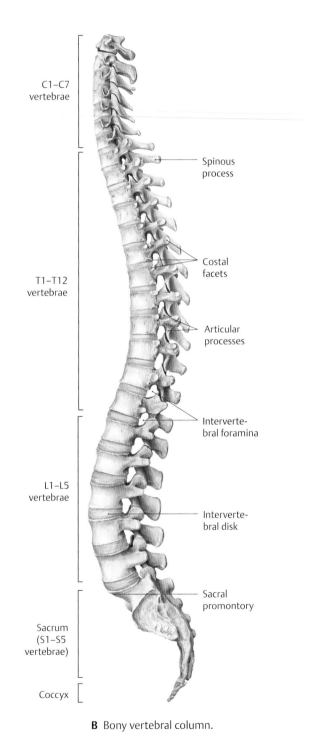

C1–C7 vertebrae

Spinous process

Costal facets

T1–T12 vertebrae

Articular processes

Intervertebral foramina

L1–L5 vertebrae

Intervertebral disk

Sacrum (S1–S5 vertebrae)

Sacral promontory

Coccyx

B Bony vertebral column.

Fig. 2.2 Normal anatomical position of the spine

Left lateral view.

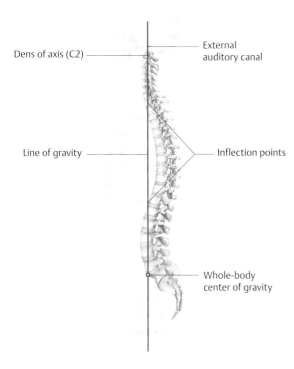

A Line of gravity. The line of gravity passes through certain anatomical landmarks, including the inflection points at the cervicothoracic and thoracolumbar junctions. It continues through the center of gravity (anterior to the sacral promontory) before passing through the hip joint, knee, and ankle.

Dens of axis (C2)

Line of gravity

External auditory canal

Inflection points

Whole-body center of gravity

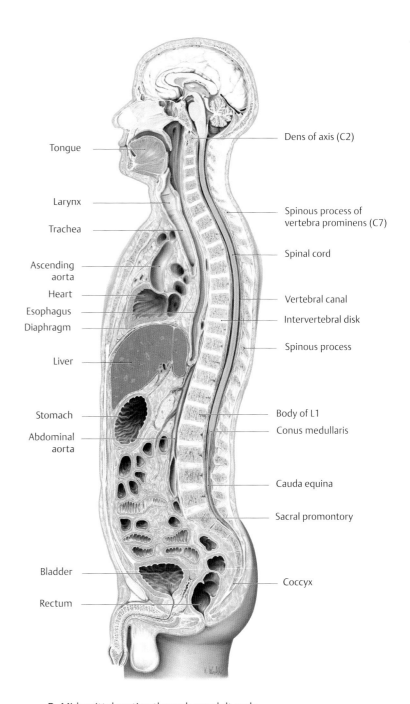

Tongue

Larynx

Trachea

Ascending aorta

Heart

Esophagus

Diaphragm

Liver

Stomach

Abdominal aorta

Bladder

Rectum

Dens of axis (C2)

Spinous process of vertebra prominens (C7)

Spinal cord

Vertebral canal

Intervertebral disk

Spinous process

Body of L1

Conus medullaris

Cauda equina

Sacral promontory

Coccyx

B Midsagittal section through an adult male.

Vertebral Column: Elements

***Fig. 2.3* Bones of the vertebral column**
The transverse processes of the lumbar vertebrae are originally rib rudiments and so are named costal processes.

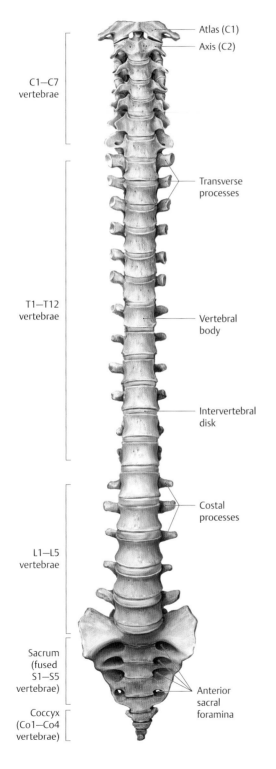

C1–C7 vertebrae

T1–T12 vertebrae

L1–L5 vertebrae

Sacrum (fused S1–S5 vertebrae)

Coccyx (Co1–Co4 vertebrae)

Atlas (C1)
Axis (C2)
Transverse processes
Vertebral body
Intervertebral disk
Costal processes
Anterior sacral foramina

A Anterior view.

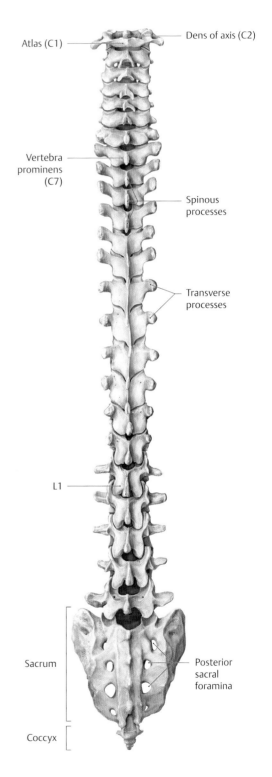

Atlas (C1)
Vertebra prominens (C7)
L1
Sacrum
Coccyx

Dens of axis (C2)
Spinous processes
Transverse processes
Posterior sacral foramina

B Posterior view.

Fig. 2.4 Structural elements of a vertebra

Left posterosuperior view. With the exception of the atlas (C1) and axis (C2), all vertebrae consist of the same structural elements.

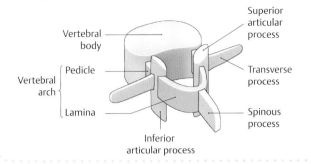

Fig. 2.5 Typical vertebrae

Superior view.

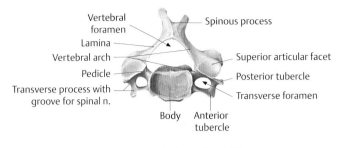

A Cervical vertebra (C4).

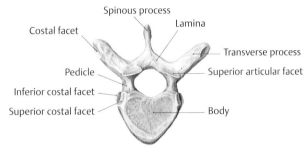

B Thoracic vertebra (T6).

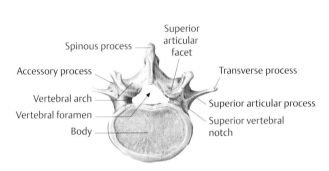

C Lumbar vertebra (L4).

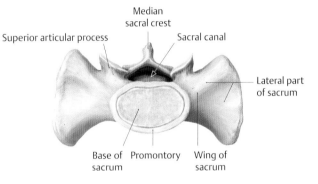

D Sacrum.

Table 2.1	Structural elements of vertebrae				
Vertebrae	Body	Vertebral foramen	Transverse processes	Articular processes	Spinous process
Cervical vertebrae C3*–C7	Small (kidney-shaped)	Large (triangular)	Small (may be absent on C7); anterior and posterior tubercles enclose transverse foramen	Superoposteriorly and inferoanteriorly; oblique facets: most nearly horizontal	Short (C3–C5); bifid (C3–C6); long (C7)
Thoracic vertebrae T1–T12	Medium (heart-shaped); includes costal facets	Small (circular)	Large and strong; length decreases T1–T12; costal facets (T1–T10)	Posteriorly (slightly laterally) and anteriorly (slightly medially); facets in coronal plane	Long, sloping postero-inferiorly; tip extends to level of vertebral body below
Lumbar vertebrae L1–L5	Large (kidney-shaped)	Medium (triangular)	Called costal processes, long and slender; accessory process on posterior surface	Posteromedially (or medially) and anterolaterally (or laterally); facets nearly in sagittal plane; mammillary process on posterior surface of each superior articular process	Short and broad
Sacral vertebrae (sacrum) S1–S5 (fused)	Decreases from base to apex	Sacral canal	Fused to rudimentary rib (ribs, see **pp. 56–59**)	Superoposteriorly (SI) superior surface of lateral sacrum-auricular surface	Median sacral crest

*C1 (atlas) and C2 (axis) are considered atypical (see **pp. 8–9**).

Cervical Vertebrae

 The seven vertebrae of the cervical spine differ most conspicuously from the common vertebral morphology. They are specialized to bear the weight of the head and allow the neck to move in all directions. C1 and C2 are known as the atlas and axis, respectively. C7 is called the vertebra prominens for its long, palpable spinous process.

Fig. 2.6 Cervical spine
Left lateral view.

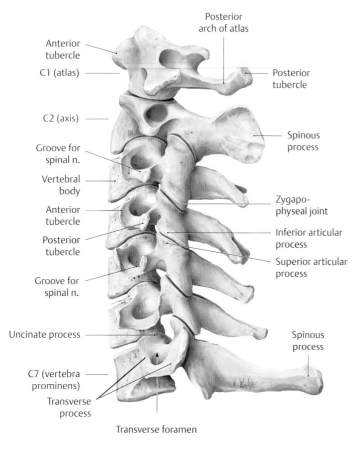

Anterior tubercle
C1 (atlas)
Posterior arch of atlas
Posterior tubercle
C2 (axis)
Spinous process
Groove for spinal n.
Vertebral body
Anterior tubercle
Zygapophyseal joint
Posterior tubercle
Inferior articular process
Groove for spinal n.
Superior articular process
Uncinate process
Spinous process
C7 (vertebra prominens)
Transverse process
Transverse foramen

A Bones of the cervical spine, left lateral view.

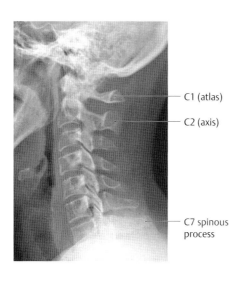

C1 (atlas)
C2 (axis)
C7 spinous process

B Radiograph of the cervical spine, left lateral view.

Fig. 2.7 Atlas (C1)

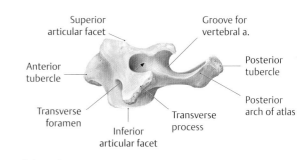

Superior articular facet
Groove for vertebral a.
Anterior tubercle
Posterior tubercle
Transverse foramen
Posterior arch of atlas
Inferior articular facet
Transverse process

A Left lateral view.

Fig. 2.8 Axis (C2)

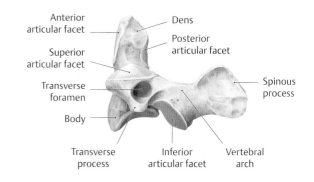

Anterior articular facet
Dens
Superior articular facet
Posterior articular facet
Transverse foramen
Spinous process
Body
Transverse process
Inferior articular facet
Vertebral arch

A Left lateral view.

Fig. 2.9 Typical cervical vertebra (C4)

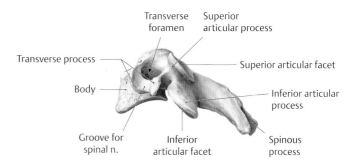

Transverse foramen
Superior articular process
Transverse process
Superior articular facet
Body
Inferior articular process
Groove for spinal n.
Inferior articular facet
Spinous process

A Left lateral view.

⚕ Clinical box 2.2

Injuries in the cervical spine

The cervical spine is prone to hyperextension injuries, such as "whiplash," which can occur when the head extends back much farther than it normally would. The most common injuries of the cervical spine are fractures of the dens of the axis, traumatic spondylolisthesis (anterior slippage of a vertebral body), and atlas fractures. Patient prognosis is largely dependent on the spinal level of the injuries (see **p. 42**).

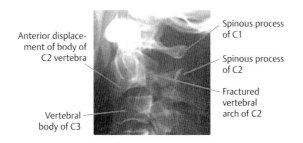

This patient hit the dashboard of his car while not wearing a seat belt. The resulting hyperextension caused the traumatic spondylolisthesis of C2 (axis) with fracture of the vertebral arch of C2, as well as tearing of the ligaments between C2 and C3. This injury is often referred to as "hangman's fracture."

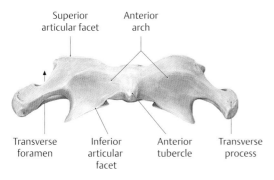

B Anterior view.

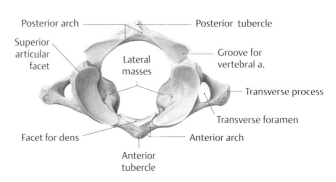

C Superior view.

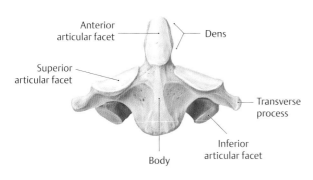

B Anterior view.

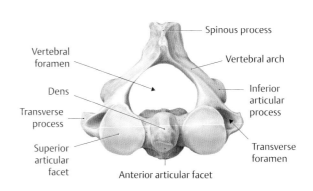

C Superior view.

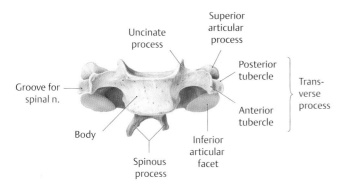

B Anterior view.

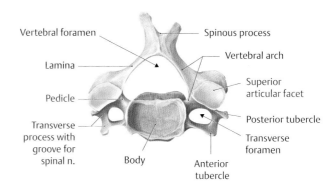

C Superior view.

Thoracic & Lumbar Vertebrae

Fig. 2.10 Thoracic spine
Left lateral view.

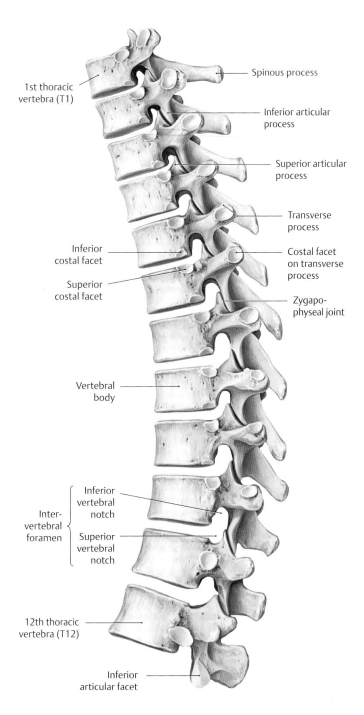

1st thoracic vertebra (T1)

Spinous process

Inferior articular process

Superior articular process

Transverse process

Inferior costal facet

Costal facet on transverse process

Superior costal facet

Zygapophyseal joint

Vertebral body

Inferior vertebral notch

Intervertebral foramen

Superior vertebral notch

12th thoracic vertebra (T12)

Inferior articular facet

Fig. 2.11 Typical thoracic vertebra (T6)

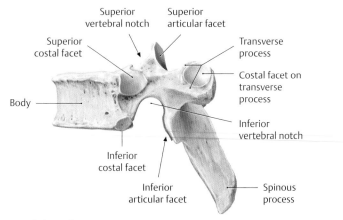

Superior vertebral notch

Superior articular facet

Superior costal facet

Transverse process

Body

Costal facet on transverse process

Inferior costal facet

Inferior vertebral notch

Inferior articular facet

Spinous process

A Left lateral view.

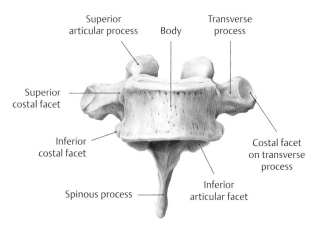

Superior articular process

Body

Transverse process

Superior costal facet

Inferior costal facet

Costal facet on transverse process

Spinous process

Inferior articular facet

B Anterior view.

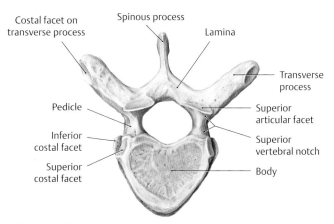

Costal facet on transverse process

Spinous process

Lamina

Transverse process

Pedicle

Superior articular facet

Inferior costal facet

Superior vertebral notch

Superior costal facet

Body

C Superior view.

Fig. 2.12 Lumbar spine
Left lateral view.

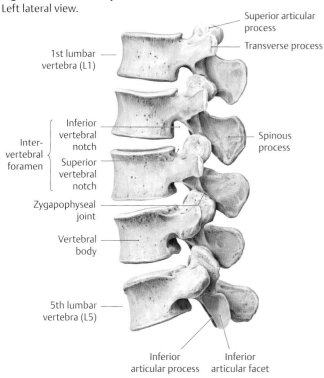

Fig. 2.13 Typical lumbar vertebra (L4)

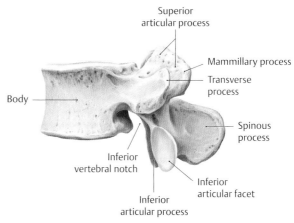

A Left lateral view.

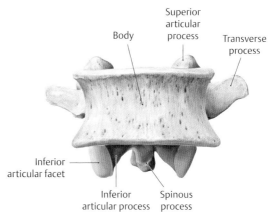

B Anterior view.

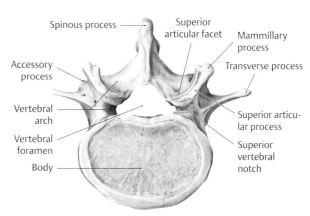

C Superior view.

⚕ Clinical box 2.3

Osteoporosis
The spine is the structure most affected by degenerative diseases of the skeleton, such as arthrosis and osteoporosis. In osteoporosis, more bone material gets reabsorbed than built up, resulting in a loss of bone mass. Symptoms include compression fractures and resulting back pain.

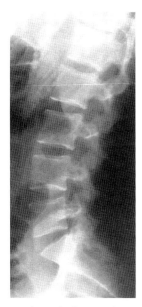

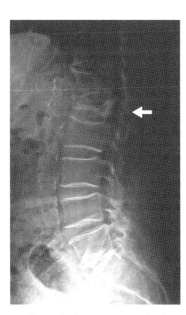

A Radiograph of a normal lumbar spine, left lateral view.

B Radiograph of an osteoporotic lumbar spine with a compression fracture at L1 (*arrow*). Note that the vertebral bodies are decreased in density, and the internal trabecular structure is coarse.

Sacrum & Coccyx

 The sacrum is formed from five postnatally fused sacral vertebrae. The base of the sacrum articulates with the 5th lumbar vertebra, and the apex articulates with the coccyx, a series of three or four rudimentary vertebrae. See **Fig. 19.1, p. 228.**

Fig. 2.14 Sacrum and coccyx

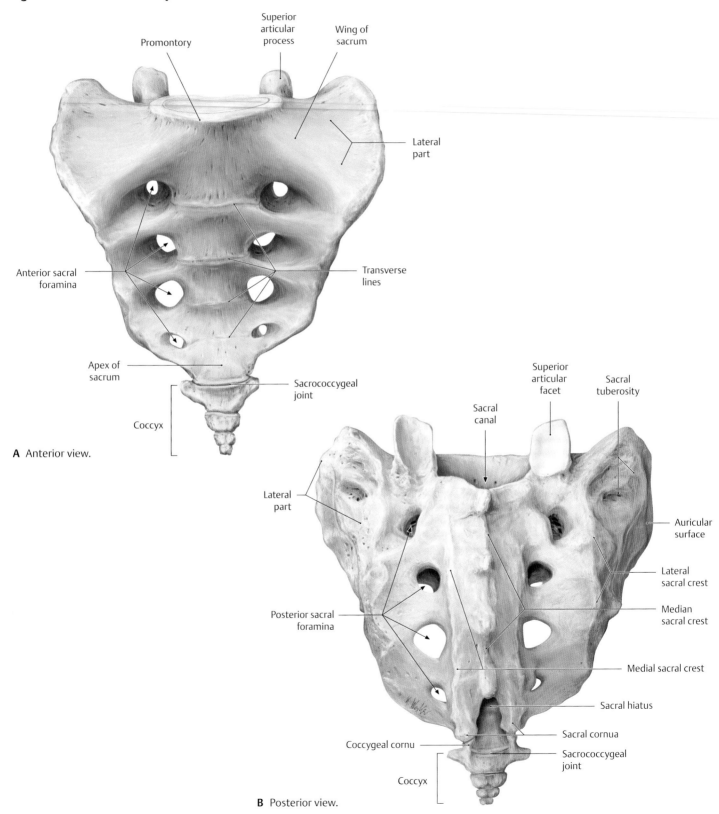

A Anterior view.

B Posterior view.

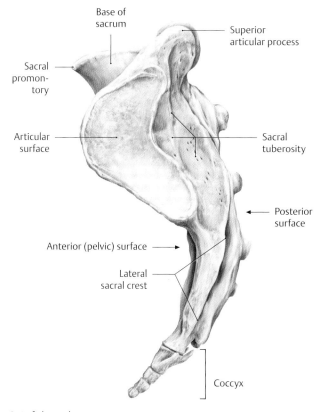

C Left lateral view.

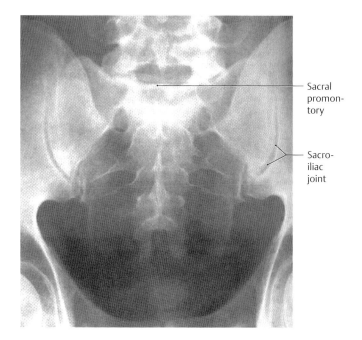

D Radiograph of sacrum, anteroposterior view.

Fig. 2.15 **Sacrum**
Superior view.

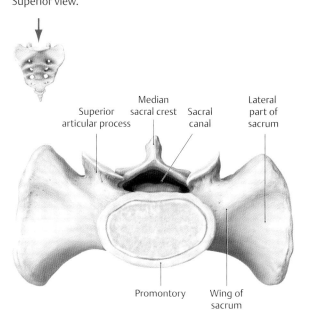

A Base of sacrum, superior view.

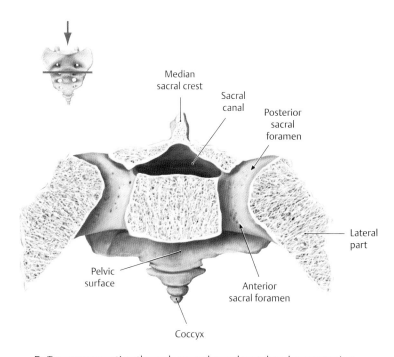

B Transverse section through second sacral vertebra demonstrating anterior and posterior sacral foramina, superior view.

Intervertebral Disks

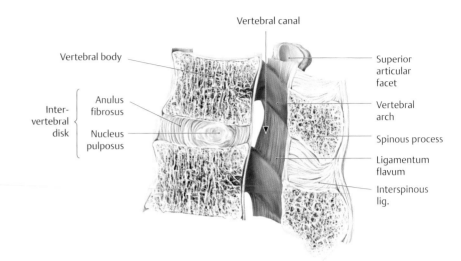

Fig. 2.16 Intervertebral disk in the vertebral column
Midsagittal section of T11–T12, left lateral view. The intervertebral disks occupy the spaces between vertebrae (intervertebral joints, see **p. 16**).

Vertebral canal

Vertebral body

Anulus fibrosus

Inter-vertebral disk

Nucleus pulposus

Superior articular facet

Vertebral arch

Spinous process

Ligamentum flavum

Interspinous lig.

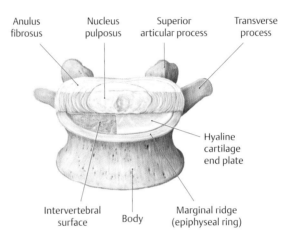

Fig. 2.17 Structure of intervertebral disk
Anterosuperior view with the anterior half of the disk and the right half of the end plate removed. The intervertebral disk consists of an external fibrous ring (anulus fibrosus) and a gelatinous core (nucleus pulposus).

Anulus fibrosus

Nucleus pulposus

Superior articular process

Transverse process

Hyaline cartilage end plate

Intervertebral surface

Body

Marginal ridge (epiphyseal ring)

Fig. 2.18 Relation of intervertebral disk to vertebral canal
Fourth lumbar vertebra, superior view.

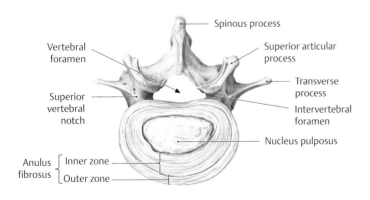

Spinous process

Vertebral foramen

Superior articular process

Transverse process

Intervertebral foramen

Superior vertebral notch

Nucleus pulposus

Anulus fibrosus — Inner zone / Outer zone

Fig. 2.19 Outer zone of the annulus fibrosus
Anterior view of L3–L4 with intervertebral disk.

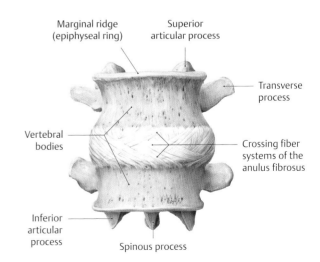

Marginal ridge (epiphyseal ring)

Superior articular process

Transverse process

Vertebral bodies

Crossing fiber systems of the anulus fibrosus

Inferior articular process

Spinous process

14

Back

Fig. 2.21 Uncovertebral joints

Anterior view. Uncovertebral joints form during childhood between the uncinate processes of C3–C7 and the vertebral bodies immediately superior. The joints may result from fissures in the cartilage of the disks that assume an articular character. If the fissures become complete tears, the risk of nucleus pulposus herniation is increased (see **p. 15**).

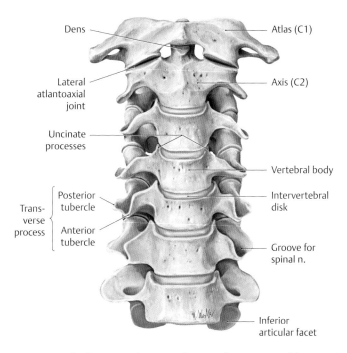

A Uncovertebral joints in the cervical spine of an 18-year-old man, anterior view.

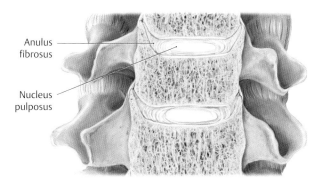

B Uncovertebral joint (enlarged), anterior view of coronal section.

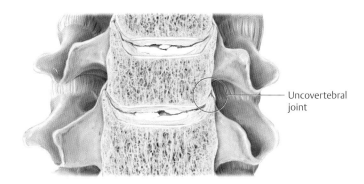

C Uncovertebral joints, split intervertebral disks, anterior view of coronal section.

✚ Clinical box 2.5

Proximity of the spinal nerve and vertebral artery to the uncinate process

The spinal nerve and vertebral artery pass through the intervertebral and transverse foramina, respectively. Bony outgrowths (osteophytes) on the uncinate process resulting from uncovertebral arthrosis (degeneration) may compress both the nerve and the artery and can lead to chronic pain in the cervical region.

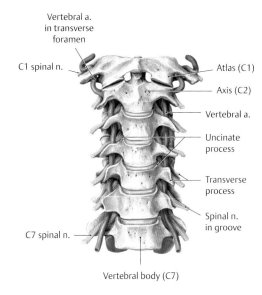

A Cervical spine, anterior view.

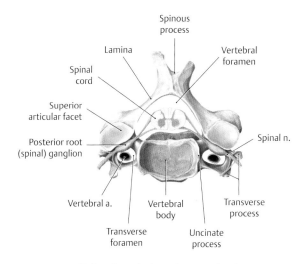

B Fourth cervical vertebra, superior view.

Joints of the Vertebral Column: Craniovertebral Region

Fig. 2.22 **Craniovertebral joints**

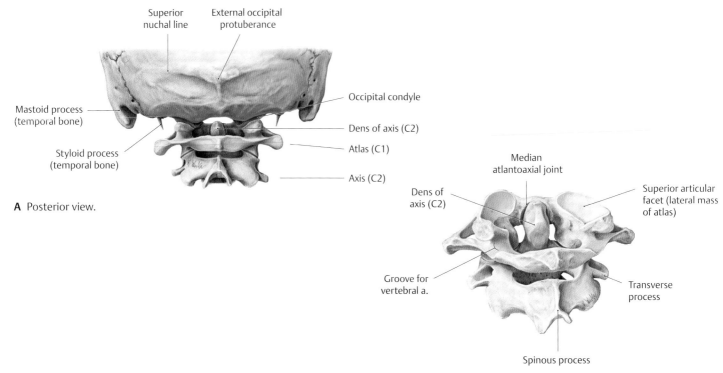

Superior nuchal line
External occipital protuberance
Mastoid process (temporal bone)
Occipital condyle
Dens of axis (C2)
Atlas (C1)
Styloid process (temporal bone)
Axis (C2)

A Posterior view.

Median atlantoaxial joint
Dens of axis (C2)
Superior articular facet (lateral mass of atlas)
Groove for vertebral a.
Transverse process
Spinous process

B Atlas and axis, posterosuperior view.

Fig. 2.23 **Ligaments of the craniovertebral joints**

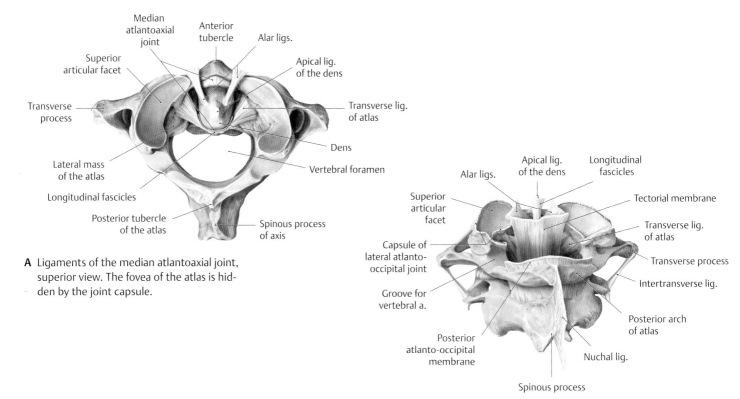

Median atlantoaxial joint
Anterior tubercle
Alar ligs.
Superior articular facet
Apical lig. of the dens
Transverse process
Transverse lig. of atlas
Lateral mass of the atlas
Dens
Longitudinal fascicles
Vertebral foramen
Posterior tubercle of the atlas
Spinous process of axis

A Ligaments of the median atlantoaxial joint, superior view. The fovea of the atlas is hidden by the joint capsule.

Apical lig. of the dens
Longitudinal fascicles
Alar ligs.
Tectorial membrane
Superior articular facet
Transverse lig. of atlas
Capsule of lateral atlanto-occipital joint
Transverse process
Intertransverse lig.
Groove for vertebral a.
Posterior arch of atlas
Posterior atlanto-occipital membrane
Nuchal lig.
Spinous process

B Ligaments of the craniovertebral joints, posterosuperior view. The dens of the axis is hidden by the tectorial membrane.

The atlanto-occipital joints are the two articulations between the convex occipital condyles of the occipital bone and the slightly concave superior articular facets of the atlas (C1). The atlanto-axial joints are the two lateral and one medial articulations between the atlas (C1) and axis (C2).

Fig. 2.24 Dissection of the craniovertebral joint ligaments

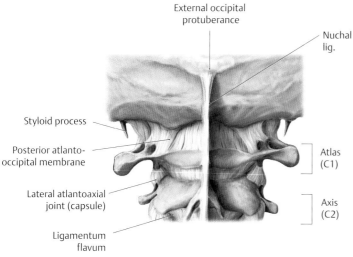

A Nuchal ligament and posterior atlanto-occipital membrane.

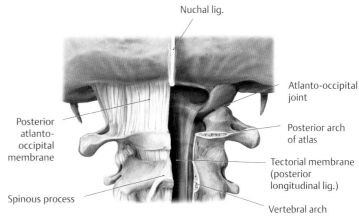

B Posterior longitudinal ligament. *Removed:* Spinal cord; vertebral canal windowed.

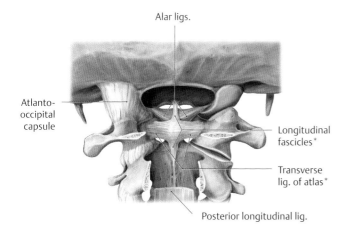

C Cruciform ligament of atlas (*). *Removed:* Tectorial membrane, posterior atlanto-occipital membrane, and vertebral arches.

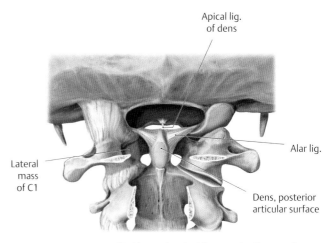

D Alar and apical ligaments. *Removed:* Transverse ligament of atlas.

Vertebral Ligaments: Overview & Cervical Spine

The ligaments of the spinal column bind the vertebrae and enable the spine to withstand high mechanical loads and shearing stresses and limit the range of motion. The ligaments are subdivided into vertebral body ligaments and vertebral arch ligaments.

Fig. 2.25 Vertebral ligaments

Viewed obliquely from the left posterior view.

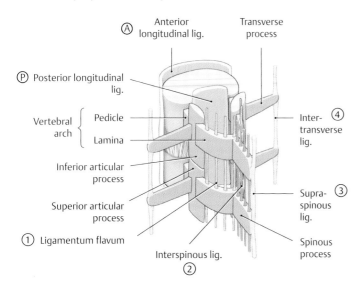

Table 2.3	Vertebral ligaments	
Ligament		**Location**
Vertebral body ligaments		
Ⓐ	Anterior longitudinal lig.	Along anterior surface of vertebral body
Ⓟ	Posterior longitudinal lig.	Along posterior surface of vertebral body
Vertebral arch ligaments		
①	Ligamentum flavum	Between laminae
②	Interspinous lig.	Between spinous process
③	Supraspinous lig.	Along posterior ridge of spinous processes
④	Intertransverse lig.	Between transverse processes
	Nuchal lig.*	Between external occipital protuberance and spinous process of C7

*Corresponds to a supraspinous ligament that is broadened superiorly.

Fig. 2.26 Anterior longitudinal ligament

Anterior view with base of skull removed.

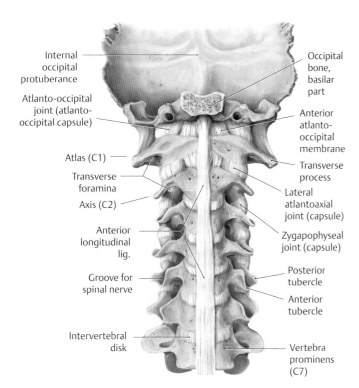

Fig. 2.27 Posterior longitudinal ligament

Posterior view with vertebral canal opened via laminectomy and spinal cord removed. The tectorial membrane is a broadened expansion of the posterior longitudinal ligament.

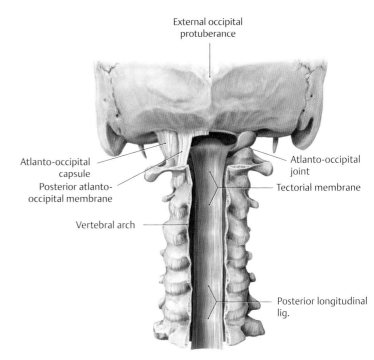

Fig. 2.28 Ligaments of the cervical spine

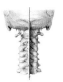

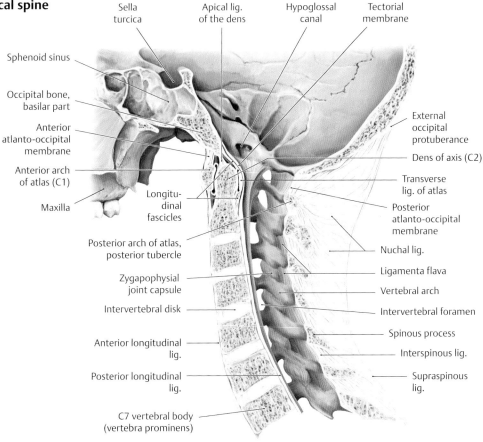

Sella turcica

Apical lig. of the dens

Hypoglossal canal

Tectorial membrane

Sphenoid sinus

Occipital bone, basilar part

Anterior atlanto-occipital membrane

Anterior arch of atlas (C1)

Maxilla

Longitudinal fascicles

Posterior arch of atlas, posterior tubercle

Zygapophysial joint capsule

Intervertebral disk

Anterior longitudinal lig.

Posterior longitudinal lig.

C7 vertebral body (vertebra prominens)

External occipital protuberance

Dens of axis (C2)

Transverse lig. of atlas

Posterior atlanto-occipital membrane

Nuchal lig.

Ligamenta flava

Vertebral arch

Intervertebral foramen

Spinous process

Interspinous lig.

Supraspinous lig.

A Midsagittal section, left lateral view. The nuchal ligament is the broadened, sagittally oriented part of the supraspinous ligament that extends from the vertebra prominens (C7) to the external occipital protuberance.

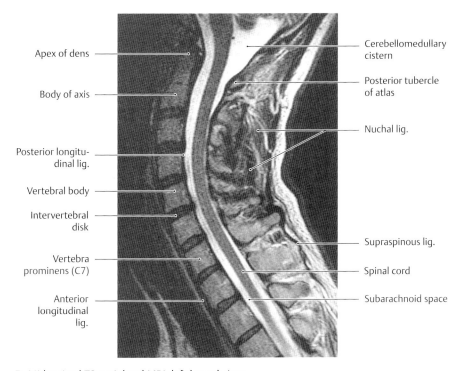

Apex of dens

Body of axis

Posterior longitudinal lig.

Vertebral body

Intervertebral disk

Vertebra prominens (C7)

Anterior longitudinal lig.

Cerebellomedullary cistern

Posterior tubercle of atlas

Nuchal lig.

Supraspinous lig.

Spinal cord

Subarachnoid space

B Midsagittal T2-weighted MRI, left lateral view.

Vertebral Ligaments: Thoracolumbar Spine

Fig. 2.29 Ligaments of the vertebral column: Thoracolumbar junction
Left lateral view of T11–L3, with T11–T12 sectioned in the midsagittal plane.

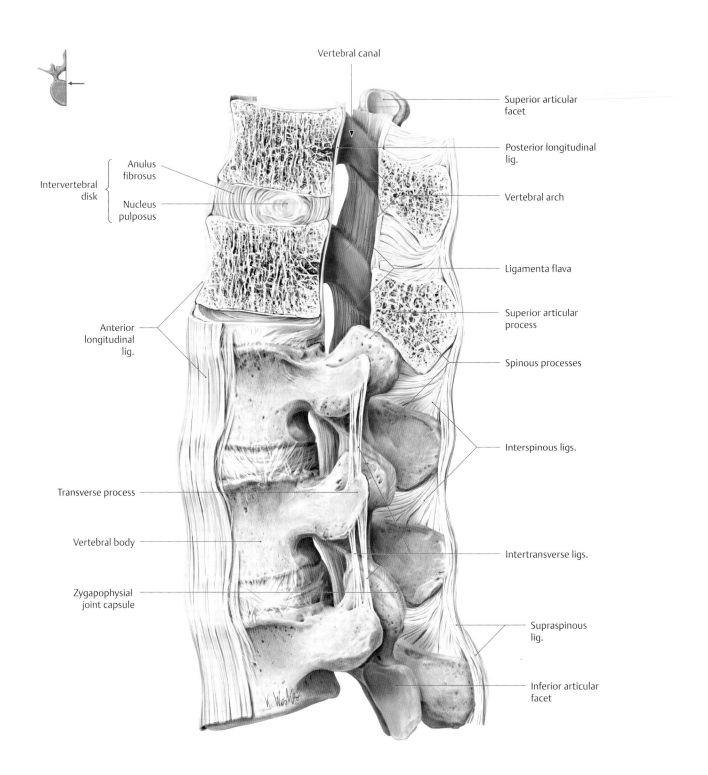

Vertebral canal

Superior articular facet

Posterior longitudinal lig.

Intervertebral disk
- Anulus fibrosus
- Nucleus pulposus

Vertebral arch

Ligamenta flava

Superior articular process

Anterior longitudinal lig.

Spinous processes

Interspinous ligs.

Transverse process

Intertransverse ligs.

Vertebral body

Zygapophysial joint capsule

Supraspinous lig.

Inferior articular facet

Fig. 2.30 Anterior longitudinal ligament

Anterior view of L3–L5.

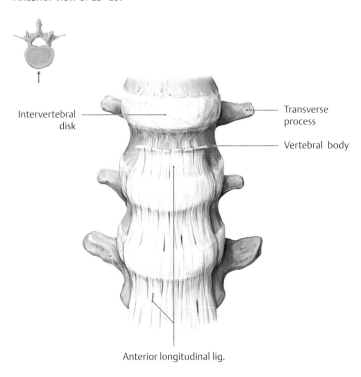

Intervertebral disk

Transverse process

Vertebral body

Anterior longitudinal lig.

Fig. 2.31 Ligamenta flava and intertransverse ligaments

Anterior view of opened vertebral canal at level of L2–L5.
Removed: L2–L4 vertebral bodies.

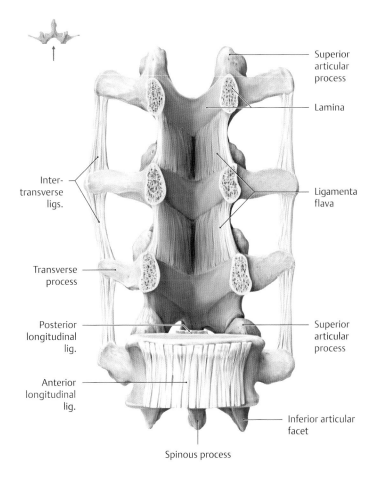

Superior articular process

Lamina

Inter-transverse ligs.

Ligamenta flava

Transverse process

Posterior longitudinal lig.

Superior articular process

Anterior longitudinal lig.

Inferior articular facet

Spinous process

Fig. 2.32 Posterior longitudinal ligament

Posterior view of opened vertebral canal at level of L2–L5.
Removed: L2–L4 vertebral arches at pedicular level.

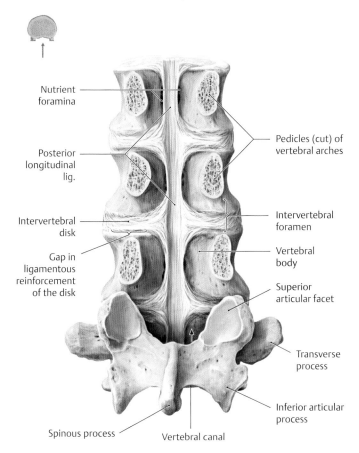

Nutrient foramina

Posterior longitudinal lig.

Pedicles (cut) of vertebral arches

Intervertebral disk

Gap in ligamentous reinforcement of the disk

Intervertebral foramen

Vertebral body

Superior articular facet

Transverse process

Spinous process

Vertebral canal

Inferior articular process

Muscles of the Back: Overview

 The muscles of the back are divided into two groups, the extrinsic and the intrinsic muscles, which are separated by the posterior layer of the thoracolumbar fascia. The superficial extrinsic muscles are considered muscles of the upper limb that have migrated to the back; these muscles are discussed in the Upper Limb, **pp. 312–317.**

Fig. 3.1 **Superficial extrinsic muscles of the back**
Posterior view. *Removed:* Trapezius and latissimus dorsi (right). *Revealed:* Thoracolumbar fascia. *Note:* The posterior layer of the thoracolumbar fascia is reinforced by the aponeurotic origin of the latissimus dorsi.

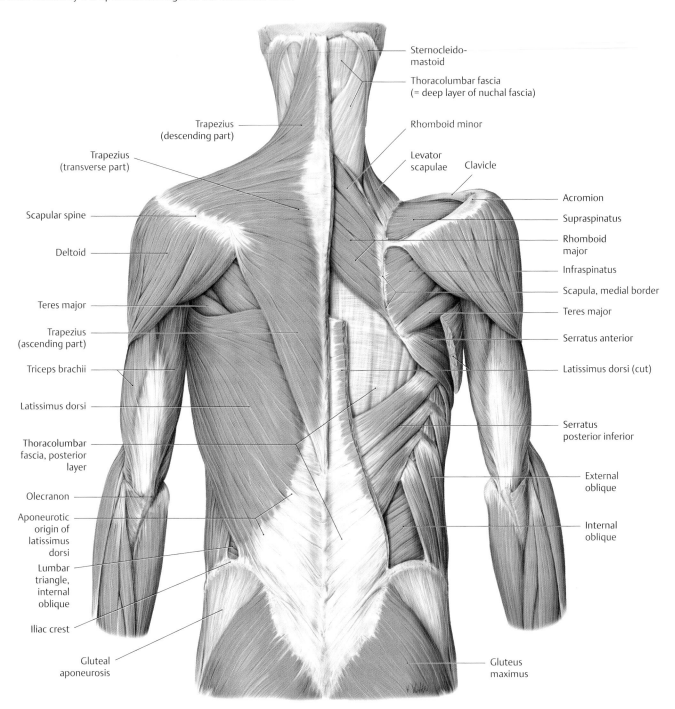

Fig. 3.2 Thoracolumbar fascia

Transverse section, superior view. The intrinsic back muscles are sequestered in an osseofibrous canal, formed by the thoracolumbar fascia, the vertebral arches, and the spinous and transverse processes of associated vertebrae. The thoracolumbar fascia consists of a posterior and middle layer that unite at the lateral margin of the intrinsic back muscles. In the neck, the posterior layer blends with the nuchal fascia (deep layer), becoming continuous with the deep cervical fascia (prevertebral layer).

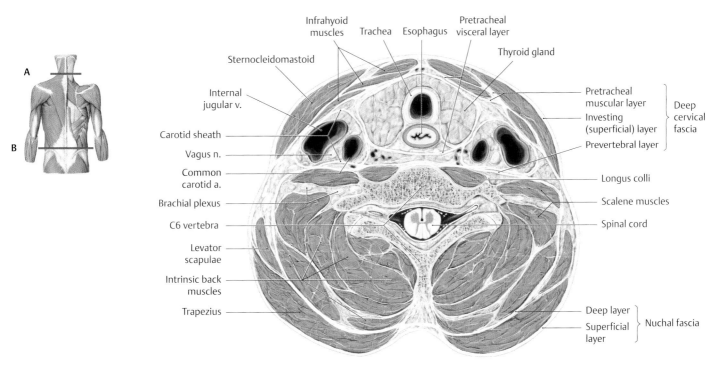

A Transverse section at level of C6 vertebra, superior view.

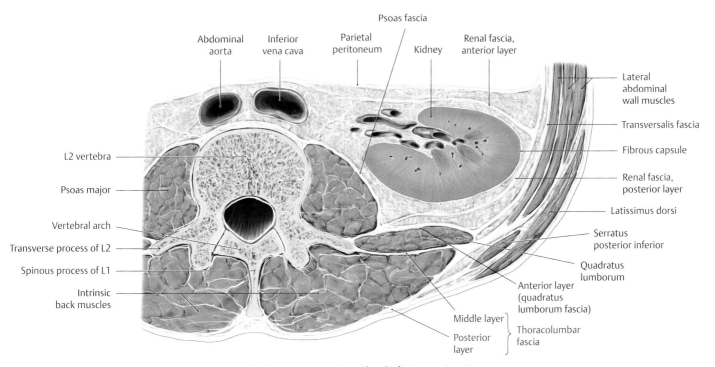

B Transverse section at level of L2, superior view.
Removed: Cauda equina and anterior trunk wall.

Intrinsic Muscles of the Cervical Spine

***Fig. 3.3* Muscles in the nuchal region**

Posterior view. *Removed:* Trapezius, sternocleidomastoid, splenius, and semispinalis muscles (right). *Revealed:* Nuchal muscles (right).

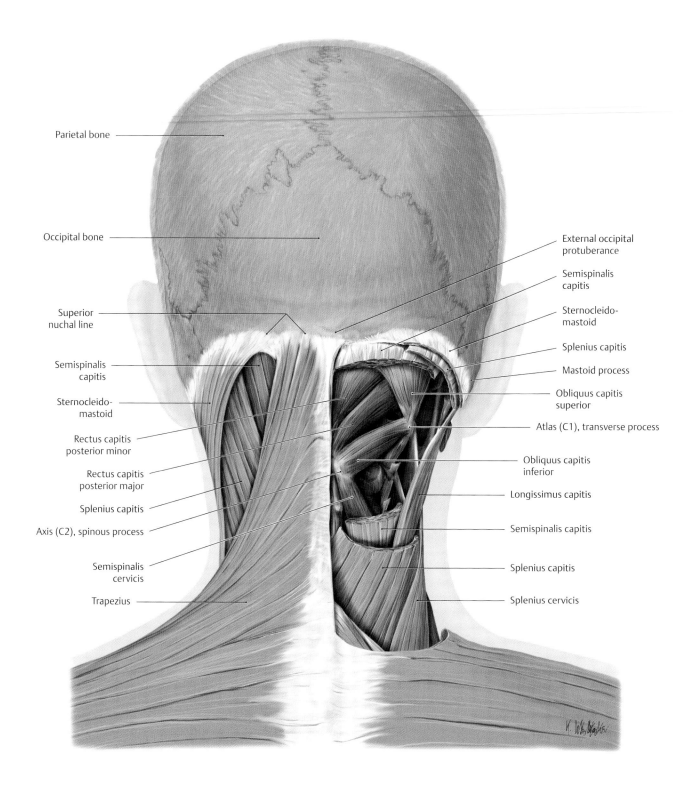

Parietal bone

Occipital bone

Superior nuchal line

Semispinalis capitis

Sternocleido-mastoid

Rectus capitis posterior minor

Rectus capitis posterior major

Splenius capitis

Axis (C2), spinous process

Semispinalis cervicis

Trapezius

External occipital protuberance

Semispinalis capitis

Sternocleido-mastoid

Splenius capitis

Mastoid process

Obliquus capitis superior

Atlas (C1), transverse process

Obliquus capitis inferior

Longissimus capitis

Semispinalis capitis

Splenius capitis

Splenius cervicis

Fig. 3.4 **Short nuchal muscles**

Posterior view. See **Fig. 3.6.**
Three of the short nuchal muscles (obliquus capitis inferior, obliquus capitis superior and the rectus capitis posterior major) form the boundaries of the suboccipital triangle (region).

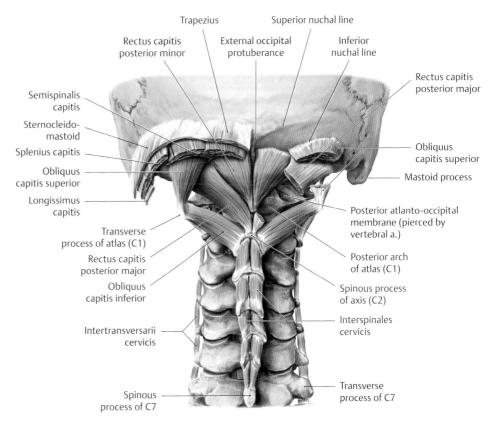

A Course of the short nuchal muscles.

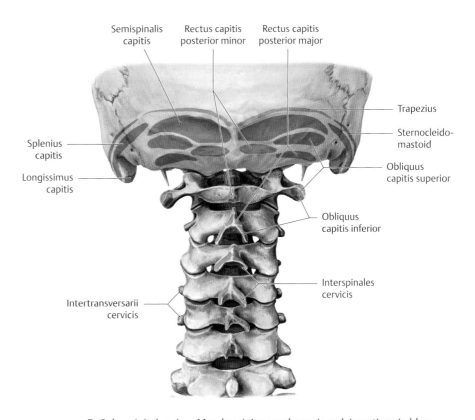

B Suboccipital region. Muscle origins are shown in red, insertions in blue.

Intrinsic Muscles of the Back

 The extrinsic muscles of the back (trapezius, latissimus dorsi, levator scapulae, and rhomboids) are discussed in the Upper Limb, **pp. 316–317.**

The serratus posterior, considered an intermediate extrinsic back muscle, has been included with the superficial intrinsic muscles in this unit.

Fig. 3.5 **Intrinsic muscles of the back**

Posterior view. Sequential dissection of the thoracolumbar fascia, superficial intrinsic muscles, intermediate intrinsic muscles, and deep intrinsic muscles of the back.

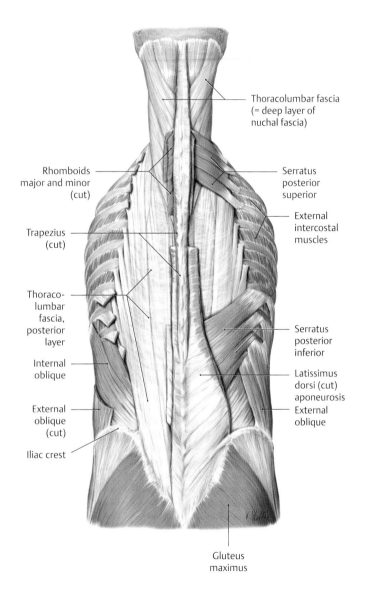

A Thoracolumbar fascia. *Removed:* Shoulder girdles and extrinsic back muscles (except serratus posterior and aponeurotic origin of latissimus dorsi). *Revealed:* Posterior layer of thoracolumbar fascia.

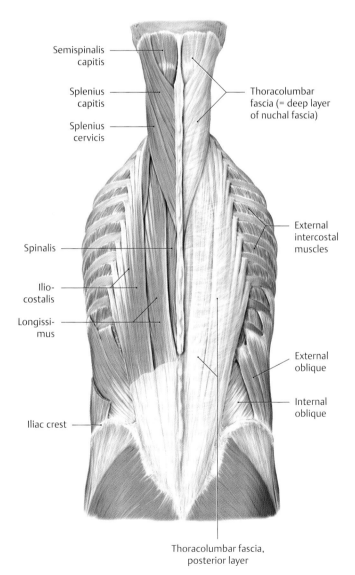

B Superficial and intermediate intrinsic back muscles. *Removed:* Thoracolumbar fascia, posterior layer (left). *Revealed:* Erector spinae and splenius muscles.

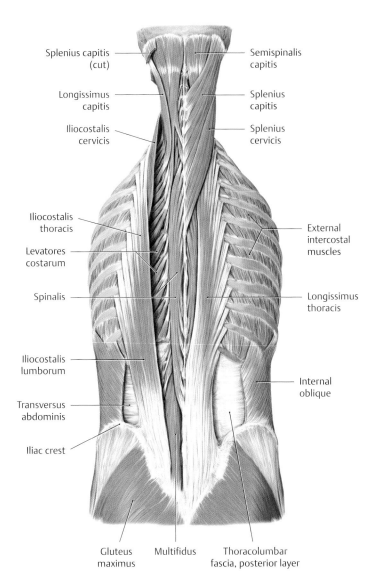

Splenius capitis (cut)
Semispinalis capitis
Longissimus capitis
Splenius capitis
Iliocostalis cervicis
Splenius cervicis
Iliocostalis thoracis
External intercostal muscles
Levatores costarum
Spinalis
Longissimus thoracis
Iliocostalis lumborum
Internal oblique
Transversus abdominis
Iliac crest
Gluteus maximus
Multifidus
Thoracolumbar fascia, posterior layer

C Intermediate and deep intrinsic back muscles. *Removed:* Longissimus thoracis and cervicis, splenius muscles (left); iliocostalis (right).
Note: The posterior layer of the thoracolumbar fascia gives origin to the internal oblique and transversus abdominus. *Revealed:* Deep muscles of the back.

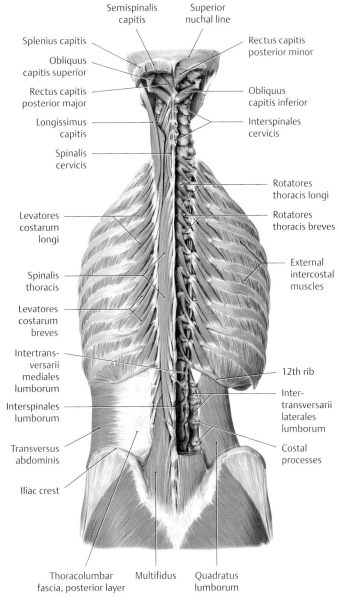

Semispinalis capitis
Superior nuchal line
Splenius capitis
Rectus capitis posterior minor
Obliquus capitis superior
Rectus capitis posterior major
Obliquus capitis inferior
Longissimus capitis
Interspinales cervicis
Spinalis cervicis
Rotatores thoracis longi
Levatores costarum longi
Rotatores thoracis breves
Spinalis thoracis
External intercostal muscles
Levatores costarum breves
Intertransversarii mediales lumborum
12th rib
Interspinales lumborum
Intertransversarii laterales lumborum
Transversus abdominis
Costal processes
Iliac crest
Thoracolumbar fascia, posterior layer
Multifidus
Quadratus lumborum

D Deep intrinsic back muscles. *Removed:* Superficial and intermediate intrinsic back muscles (all); deep fascial layer and multifidus (right). *Revealed:* Intertransversarii and quadratus lumborum (right).

29

Muscle Facts (I)

Fig. 3.6 **Short nuchal and craniovertebral joint muscles**

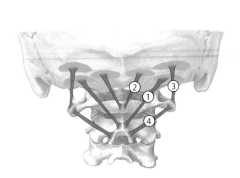

A Posterior view, schematic.

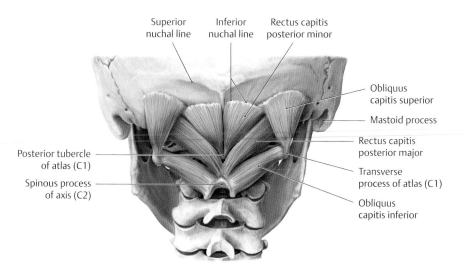

B Suboccipital muscles, posterior view.

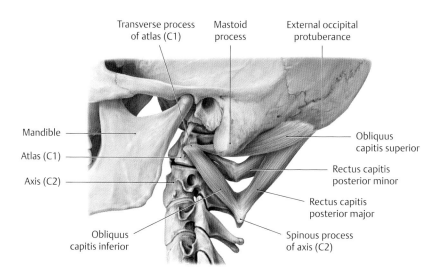

C Suboccipital muscles, left lateral view.

Table 3.1		Short nuchal and craniovertebral joint muscles				
Muscle			**Origin**	**Insertion**	**Innervation**	**Action**
Rectus capitis posterior	① Rectus capitis posterior major		C2 (spinous process)	Occipital bone (inferior nuchal line, middle third)	C1 (posterior ramus = suboccipital n.)	*Bilateral:* Extends head *Unilateral:* Rotates head to same side
	② Rectus capitis posterior minor		C1 (posterior tubercle)	Occipital bone (inferior nuchal line, inner third)		
Obliquus capitis	③ Obliquus capitis superior		C1 (transverse process)	Occipital bone (inferior nuchal line, middle third; above rectus capitis posterior major)		*Bilateral:* Extends head *Unilateral:* Tilts head to same side; rotates to opposite side
	④ Obliquus capitis inferior		C2 (spinous process)	C1 (transverse process)		*Bilateral:* Extends head *Unilateral:* Rotates head to same side

Fig. 3.7 Prevertebral muscles

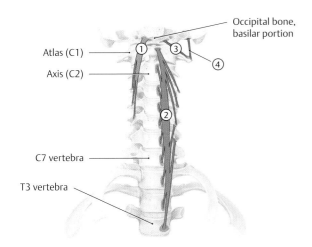

Atlas (C1)
Axis (C2)
Occipital bone, basilar portion
C7 vertebra
T3 vertebra

A Anterior view, schematic.

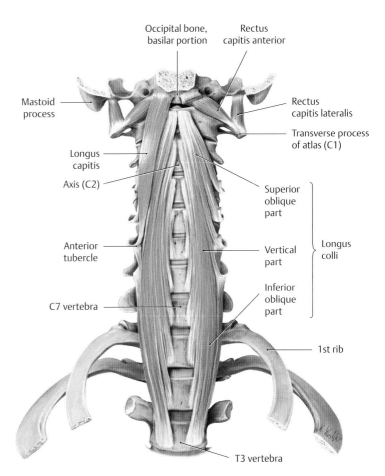

Occipital bone, basilar portion
Rectus capitis anterior
Mastoid process
Rectus capitis lateralis
Longus capitis
Transverse process of atlas (C1)
Axis (C2)
Superior oblique part
Anterior tubercle
Vertical part
Longus colli
Inferior oblique part
C7 vertebra
1st rib
T3 vertebra

B Prevertebral muscles, anterior view.
Removed: Longus capitis (left); cervical viscera.

Table 3.2		Prevertebral muscles			
Muscle		**Origin**	**Insertion**	**Innervation**	**Action**
① Longus capitis		C3–C6 (transverse processes, anterior tubercles)	Occipital bone (basilar part)	Direct branches from cervical plexus (C1–C3)	*Bilateral:* Flexes head *Unilateral:* Tilts and slightly rotates head to same side
② Longus colli (cervicis)	Vertical (medial) part	C5–T3 (anterior sides of vertebral bodies)	C2–C4 (anterior sides of vertebral bodies)	Direct branches from cervical plexus (C2–C6)	*Bilateral:* Flexes cervical spine *Unilateral:* Tilts and rotates cervical spine to same side
	Superior oblique part	C3–C5 (transverse processes, anterior tubercles)	C1 (transverse process, anterior tubercle)		
	Inferior oblique part	T1–T3 (anterior sides of vertebral bodies)	C5–C6 (transverse processes, anterior tubercles)		
③ Rectus capitis anterior		C1 (lateral mass)	Occipital bone (basilar part)	C1 (anterior ramus)	*Bilateral:* Flexion at atlanto-occipital joint *Unilateral:* Lateral flexion at atlanto-occipital joint
④ Rectus capitis lateralis		C1 (transverse process)	Occipital bone (basilar part, lateral to occipital condyles)		

Muscle Facts (II)

The intrinsic back muscles are divided into superficial, intermediate, and deep layers. The serratus posterior muscles are extrinsic back muscles, innervated by the anterior rami of intercostal nerves, not the posterior rami, which innervate the intrinsic back muscles. They are included here as they are encountered in dissection of the back musculature.

Table 3.3	**Superficial intrinsic back muscles**				
Muscle		**Origin**	**Insertion**	**Innervation**	**Action**
Serratus posterior	① Serratus posterior superior	Nuchal lig.; C7–T3 (spinous processes)	2nd–4th ribs (superior borders)	Spinal nn. T2–T5 (anterior rami)	Elevates ribs
	② Serratus posterior inferior	T11–L2 (spinous processes)	8th–12th ribs (inferior borders, near angles)	Spinal nn. T9–T12 (anterior rami)	Depresses ribs
Splenius	③ Splenius capitis	Nuchal lig.; C7–T3 or T4 (spinous processes)	Lateral 1/3 nuchal line (occipital bone); mastoid process (temporal bone)	Spinal nn. C1–C6 (posterior rami, lateral branches)	*Bilateral:* Extends cervical spine and head *Unilateral:* Flexes and rotates head to the same side
	④ Splenius cervicis	T3–T6 or T7 (spinous processes)	C1–C3/4 (transverse processes)		

Fig. 3.8 Superficial intrinsic back muscles, schematic
Right side, posterior view.

Fig. 3.9 Intermediate intrinsic back muscles, schematic
Right side, posterior view. These muscles are collectively known as the erector spinae.

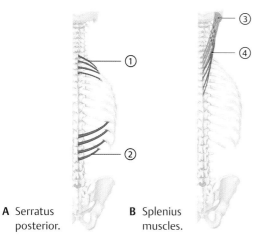

A Serratus posterior.

B Splenius muscles.

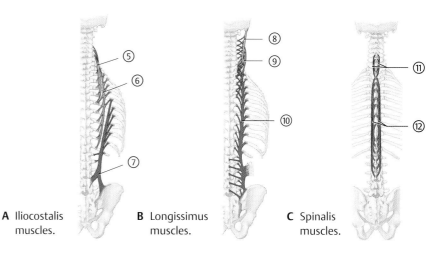

A Iliocostalis muscles.

B Longissimus muscles.

C Spinalis muscles.

Table 3.4	**Intermediate intrinsic back muscles (erector spinae)**				
Muscle		**Origin**	**Insertion**	**Innervation**	**Action**
Iliocostalis	⑤ Iliocostalis cervicis	3rd–7th ribs	C4–C6 (transverse processes)	Spinal nn. C8–L1 (posterior rami, lateral branches)	*Bilateral:* Extends spine *Unilateral:* Bends spine laterally to same side
	⑥ Iliocostalis thoracis	7th–12th ribs	1st–6th ribs		
	⑦ Iliocostalis lumborum	Sacrum; iliac crest; thoracolumbar fascia (posterior layer)	6th–12th ribs; thoracolumbar fascia (posterior layer); upper lumbar vertebrae (transverse processes)		
Longissimus	⑧ Longissimus capitis	T1–T3 (transverse processes); C4–C7 (transverse and articular processes)	Temporal bone (mastoid process)	Spinal nn. C1–L5 (posterior rami, lateral branches)	*Bilateral:* Extends head *Unilateral:* Flexes and rotates head to same side
	⑨ Longissimus cervicis	T1–T6 (transverse processes)	C2–C5 (transverse processes)		*Bilateral:* Extends spine *Unilateral:* Bends spine laterally to same side
	⑩ Longissimus thoracis	Sacrum; iliac crest; lumbar vertebrae (spinous processes); lower thoracic vertebrae (transverse processes)	2nd–12th ribs; thoracic and lumbar vertebrae (transverse processes)		
Spinalis	⑪ Spinalis cervicis	C5–T2 (spinous processes)	C2–C5 (spinous processes)	Spinal nn. (posterior rami)	*Bilateral:* Extends cervical and thoracic spine *Unilateral:* Bends cervical and thoracic spine to same side
	⑫ Spinalis thoracis	T10–L3 (spinous processes, lateral surfaces)	T2–T8 (spinous processes, lateral surfaces)		

Fig. 3.10 **Superficial and intermediate intrinsic back muscles**
Posterior view.

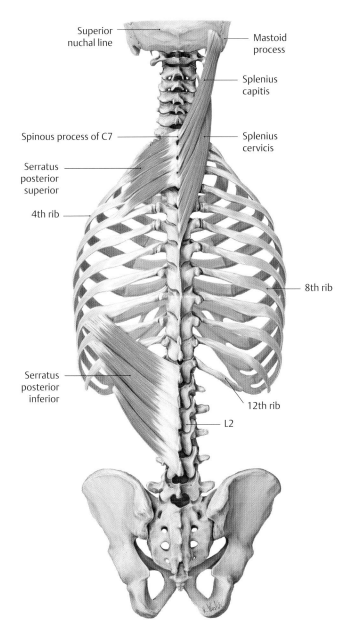

Superior
nuchal line

Mastoid
process

Splenius
capitis

Splenius
cervicis

Spinous process of C7

Serratus
posterior
superior

4th rib

8th rib

Serratus
posterior
inferior

12th rib

L2

A Superficial back muscles:
Splenius and serratus posterior muscles.

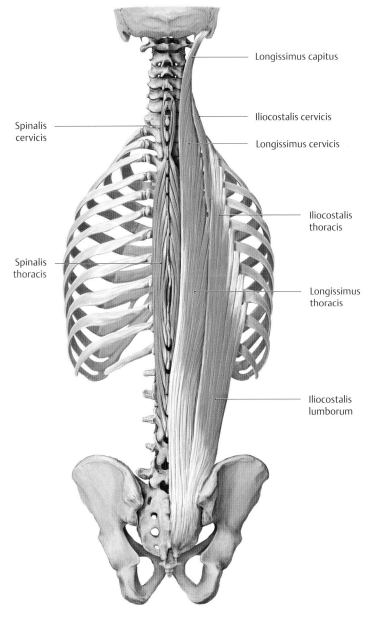

Longissimus capitus

Spinalis
cervicis

Iliocostalis cervicis

Longissimus cervicis

Iliocostalis
thoracis

Spinalis
thoracis

Longissimus
thoracis

Iliocostalis
lumborum

B Intermediate intrinsic back muscles (erector spinae): Iliocostalis,
longissimus, and spinalis muscles.

Muscle Facts (III)

 The deep intrinsic back muscles are divided into two groups: transversospinalis and deep segmental muscles. The transverso-spinalis muscles pass between the transverse and spinous processes of the vertebrae.

Table 3.5		Transversospinalis muscles			
Muscle		**Origin**	**Insertion**	**Innervation**	**Action**
Rotatores	① Rotatores breves	T1–T12 (between transverse and spinous processes of adjacent vertebrae)			*Bilateral:* Extends thoracic spine *Unilateral:* Rotates thoracic spine to opposite side
	② Rotatores longi	T1–T12 (between transverse and spinous processes, skipping one vertebra)			
Multifidus ③		Sacrum, ilium, mamillary processes of L1–L5, transverse and articular processes of T1–T4, C4–C7	Superomedially to spinous processes, skipping two to four vertebrae	Spinal nn. (posterior rami)	*Bilateral:* Extends spine *Unilateral:* Flexes spine to same side, rotates it to opposite side
Semispinalis	④ Semispinalis capitis	C4–T7 (transverse and articular processes)	Occipital bone (between superior and inferior nuchal lines)		*Bilateral:* Extends thoracic and cervical spines and head (stabilizes craniovertebral joints)
	⑤ Semispinalis cervicis	T1–T6 (transverse processes)	C2–C5 (spinous processes)		*Unilateral:* Bends head, cervical and thoracic spines to same side, rotates to opposite side
	⑥ Semispinalis thoracis	T6–T12 (transverse processes)	C6–T4 (spinous processes)		

Fig. 3.11 Transversospinalis muscles
Posterior view, schematic.

Fig. 3.12 Deep segmental muscles
Posterior view, schematic.

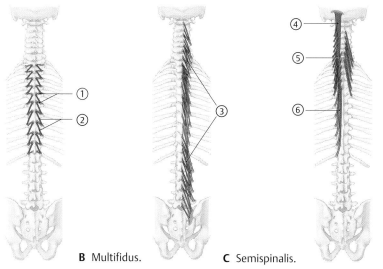

A Rotatores muscles.

B Multifidus.

C Semispinalis.

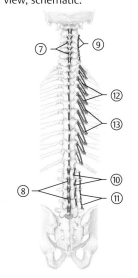

Table 3.6		Deep segmental back muscles			
Muscle		**Origin**	**Insertion**	**Innervation**	**Action**
Interspinales*	⑦ Interspinales cervicis	C1–C7 (between spinous processes of adjacent vertebrae)		Spinal nn. (posterior rami)	Extends cervical and lumbar spines
	⑧ Interspinales lumborum	L1–L5 (between spinous processes of adjacent vertebrae)			
Inter-transversarii*	Intertransversarii anteriores cervicis	C2–C7 (between anterior tubercles of adjacent vertebrae)		Spinal nn. (anterior rami)	*Bilateral:* Stabilizes and extends the cervical and lumbar spines *Unilateral:* Bends the cervical and lumbar spines laterally to same side
	⑨ Intertransversarii posteriores cervicis	C2–C7 (between posterior tubercles of adjacent vertebrae)		Spinal nn. (posterior rami)	
	⑩ Intertransversarii mediales lumborum	L1–L5 (between mamillary processes of adjacent vertebrae)			
	⑪ Intertransversarii laterales lumborum	L1–L5 (between transverse processes of adjacent vertebrae)		Spinal nn. (anterior rami)	
Levatores costarum	⑫ Levatores costarum breves	C7–T11 (transverse processes)	Costal angle of next lower rib	Spinal nn. (posterior rami)	*Bilateral:* Extends thoracic spine *Unilateral:* Bends thoracic spine to same side, rotates to opposite side
	⑬ Levatores costarum longi		Costal angle of rib two vertebrae below		

*Both the interspinales and intertransversarii muscles traverse the entire spine; only their clinically relevant components have been included.

Fig. 3.13 Deep intrinsic back muscles
Posterior view.

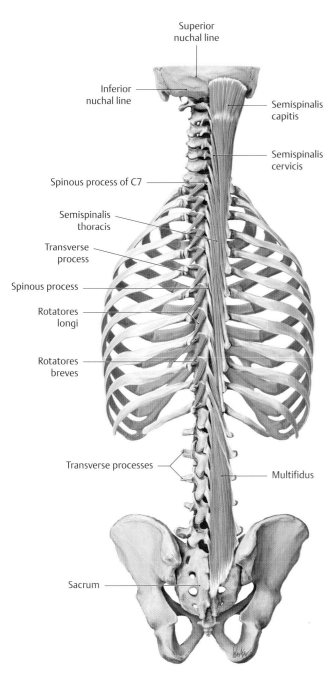

A Transversospinalis muscles: Rotatores, multifidus, and semispinalis.

Superior nuchal line

Inferior nuchal line

Semispinalis capitis

Semispinalis cervicis

Spinous process of C7

Semispinalis thoracis

Transverse process

Spinous process

Rotatores longi

Rotatores breves

Transverse processes

Multifidus

Sacrum

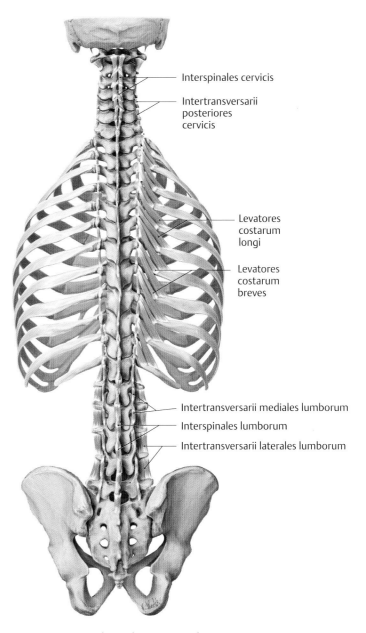

B Deep segmental muscles: Interspinales, intertransversarii, and levatores costarum.

Interspinales cervicis

Intertransversarii posteriores cervicis

Levatores costarum longi

Levatores costarum breves

Intertransversarii mediales lumborum

Interspinales lumborum

Intertransversarii laterales lumborum

Arteries & Veins of the Back

Fig. 4.1 Arteries of the back

The structures of the back are supplied by branches of the posterior intercostal arteries, which arise from the thoracic aorta or from the subclavian artery.

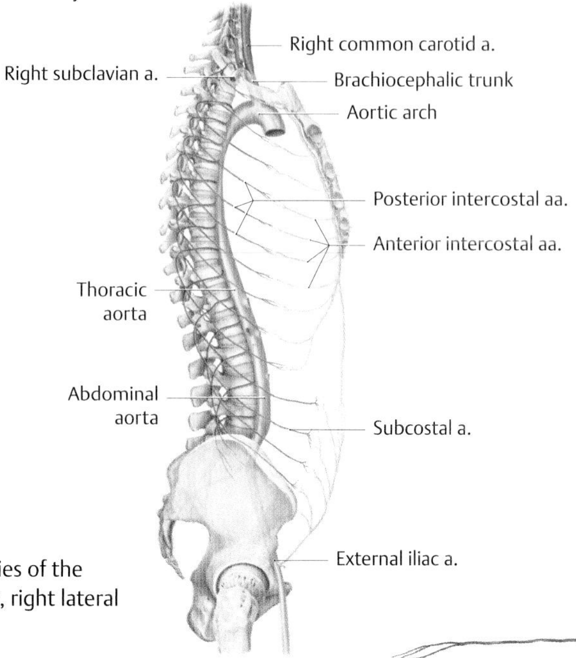

A Arteries of the trunk, right lateral view.

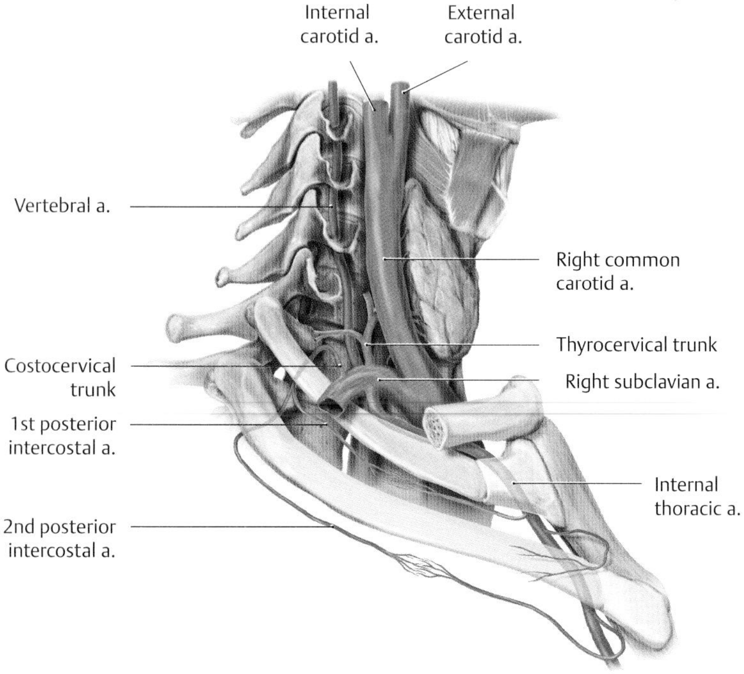

B Vascular supply to the nuchal region, posterolateral view. *Note:* The first and second posterior intercostal arteries arise from the costocervical trunk, a branch of the subclavian artery.

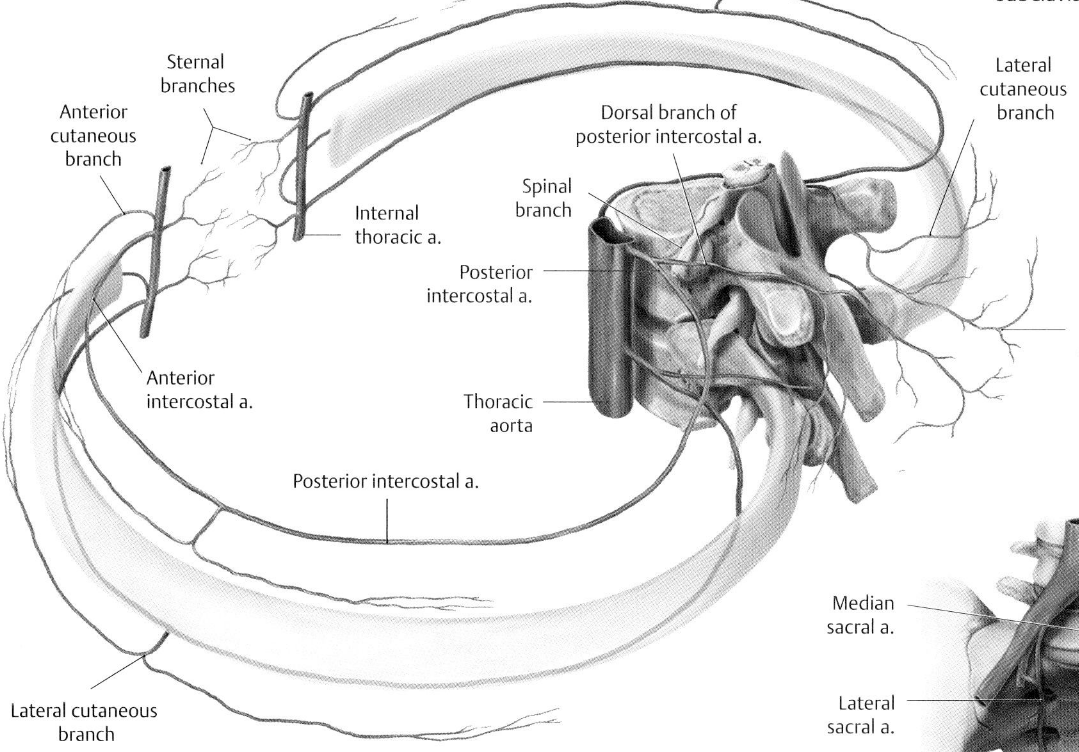

C Posterior intercostal arteries, oblique posterosuperior view. The posterior intercostal arteries give rise to cutaneous and muscular branches, as well as spinal branches that supply the spinal cord.

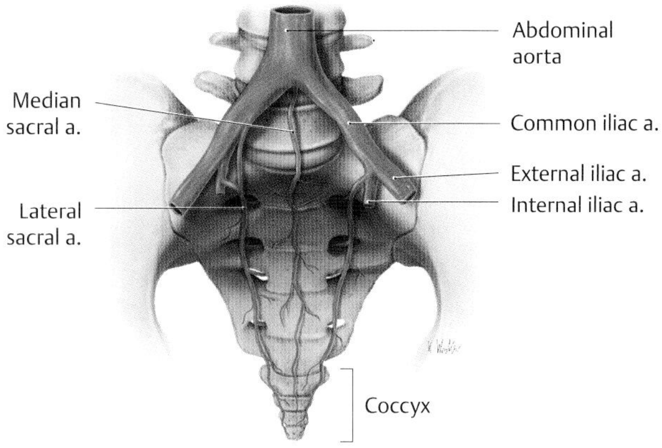

D Vascular supply to the sacrum, anterior view.

Fig. 4.2 Veins of the back

The veins of the back drain into the azygos vein via the posterior intercostal veins, hemiazygos vein, and ascending lumbar veins. The interior of the spinal column is drained by the vertebral venous plexus that runs the length of the spine.

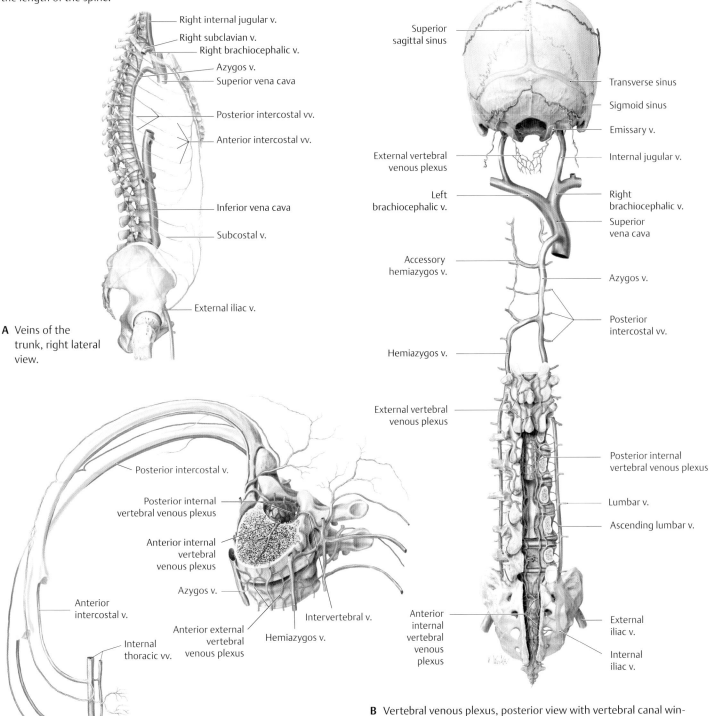

A Veins of the trunk, right lateral view.

Right internal jugular v.
Right subclavian v.
Right brachiocephalic v.
Azygos v.
Superior vena cava
Posterior intercostal vv.
Anterior intercostal vv.
Inferior vena cava
Subcostal v.
External iliac v.

Superior sagittal sinus
Transverse sinus
Sigmoid sinus
Emissary v.
External vertebral venous plexus
Internal jugular v.
Left brachiocephalic v.
Right brachiocephalic v.
Superior vena cava
Accessory hemiazygos v.
Azygos v.
Posterior intercostal vv.
Hemiazygos v.
External vertebral venous plexus
Posterior internal vertebral venous plexus
Lumbar v.
Ascending lumbar v.
Anterior internal vertebral venous plexus
External iliac v.
Internal iliac v.

B Vertebral venous plexus, posterior view with vertebral canal windowed in the lumbar and sacral spine. The external vertebral venous plexus communicates with the sigmoid sinus through emissary veins in the skull. The *external* vertebral venous plexus is divided into an anterior and a posterior portion that run along the exterior of the vertebral column. The anterior and posterior *internal* vertebral venous plexus run in the vertebral foramen and drain the spinal cord.

Posterior intercostal v.
Posterior internal vertebral venous plexus
Anterior internal vertebral venous plexus
Azygos v.
Anterior intercostal v.
Intervertebral v.
Anterior external vertebral venous plexus
Hemiazygos v.
Internal thoracic vv.

C Intercostal veins and anterior vertebral venous plexus, anterosuperior view. The intercostal veins follow a similar course to the intercostal nerves and arteries (see **pp. 36, 38**). *Note:* The anterior external vertebral venous plexus can be seen communicating with the azygos vein.

Nerves of the Back

 The back receives its innervation from branches of the spinal nerves. The *posterior (dorsal) rami* of the spinal nerves supply most of the intrinsic muscles of the back. The extrinsic muscles of the back are supplied by the *anterior (ventral) rami* of the spinal nerves.

Fig. 4.3 Nerves of the back
Cross section of the vertebral column and spinal cord with surrounding musculature, superior view.

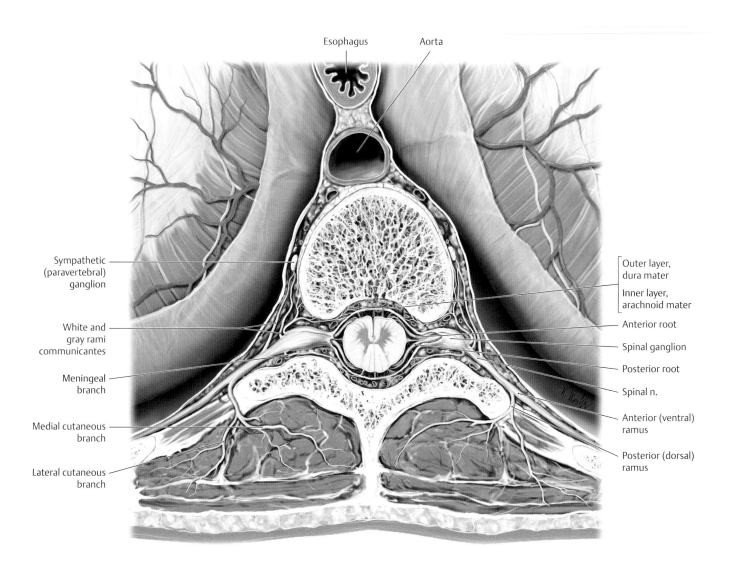

Fig. 4.4 Nerves of the nuchal region

Right side, posterior view. Like the back, the nuchal region receives most of its motor and sensory innervation from the *posterior* rami of the spinal nerves. The posterior rami of C1–C3 have specific names: suboccipital nerve (C1), greater occipital nerve (C2), and third occipital nerve (C3). The lesser occipital and great auricular nerves arise from the *anterior* rami of the C1–C4 spinal nerves (cervical plexus) and innervate the skin of the anterolateral head and neck. The anterior rami of C1–C4 also give rise to the *ansa cervicalis,* which innervates the infrahyoid muscles (see **p. 620**).

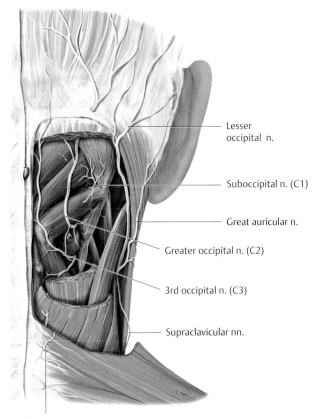

Lesser occipital n.

Suboccipital n. (C1)

Great auricular n.

Greater occipital n. (C2)

3rd occipital n. (C3)

Supraclavicular nn.

C5 spinal n., posterior ramus

Fig. 4.5 Cutaneous innervation of the back

Color denotes the skin areas innervated by (**A**) particular peripheral nerves or (**B**) particular pairs of segmental spinal nerves. Patterns of loss of cutaneous sensation can be helpful in diagnosis of nerve lesions.

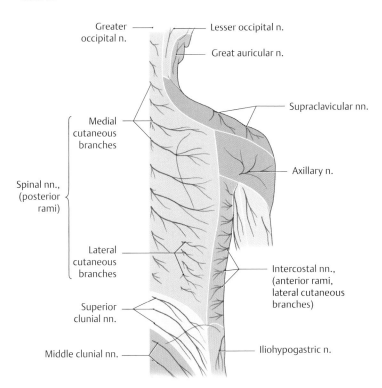

Greater occipital n.

Lesser occipital n.

Great auricular n.

Medial cutaneous branches

Supraclavicular nn.

Spinal nn., (posterior rami)

Axillary n.

Lateral cutaneous branches

Intercostal nn., (anterior rami, lateral cutaneous branches)

Superior clunial nn.

Middle clunial nn.

Iliohypogastric n.

A Cutaneous innervation patterns of specific peripheral nerves.

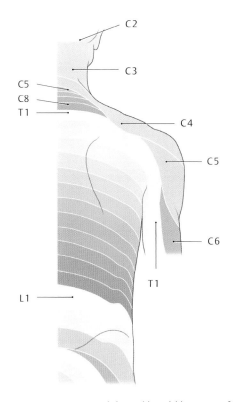

C2

C3

C5
C8
T1

C4

C5

C6

T1

L1

B Dermatomes: Dermatomes are bilateral band-like areas of skin receiving innervation from a single pair of spinal nerves (from a single segment of the spinal cord). *Note:* Spinal nerve C1 is purely motor; consequently there is no C1 dermatome.

Spinal Cord

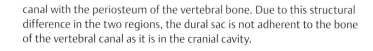 The dura mater of the cranial cavity is composed of two layers, the periosteal and meningeal. Only the meningeal layer extends into the vertebral canal with the spinal cord. The periosteal layer of dura terminates at the foramen magnum and is replaced in the vertebral canal with the periosteum of the vertebral bone. Due to this structural difference in the two regions, the dural sac is not adherent to the bone of the vertebral canal as it is in the cranial cavity.

Fig. 4.6 Spinal cord in situ
Posterior view with vertebral canal windowed.

Fig. 4.7 Spinal cord and its meningeal layers
Posterior view. The dura mater is opened and the arachnoid is sectioned. The detailed anatomy of the spinal cord can be found on **pp. 678–679.**

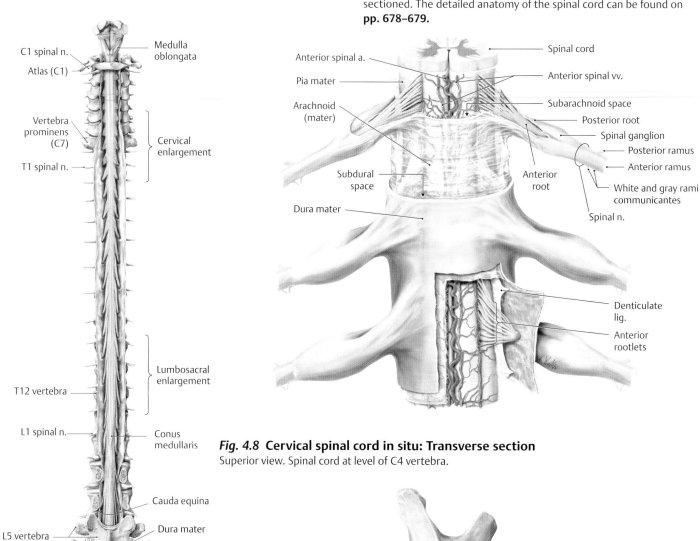

Fig. 4.8 Cervical spinal cord in situ: Transverse section
Superior view. Spinal cord at level of C4 vertebra.

Fig. 4.9 Cauda equina in the vertebral canal

Posterior view. The lamina and posterior surface of the sacrum have been partially removed.

Fig. 4.10 Cauda equina in situ: Transverse section

Superior view. Cauda equina at level of L2 vertebra.

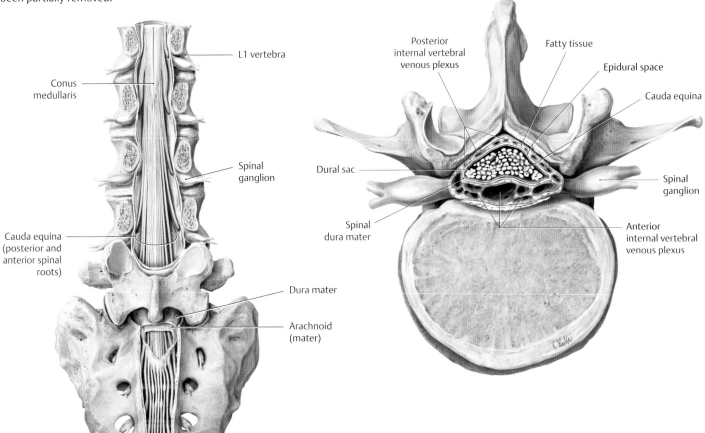

L1 vertebra
Conus medullaris
Spinal ganglion
Cauda equina (posterior and anterior spinal roots)
Dura mater
Arachnoid (mater)
Sacral hiatus
Filum terminale

Posterior internal vertebral venous plexus
Fatty tissue
Epidural space
Cauda equina
Dural sac
Spinal ganglion
Spinal dura mater
Anterior internal vertebral venous plexus

Fig. 4.11 Spinal cord, dural sac, and vertebral column at different ages.

Anterior view. Longitudinal growth of the spinal cord lags behind that of the vertebral column. At birth, the distal end of the spinal cord, the conus medullaris, is at the level of the L3 vertebral body, but in the average adult it extends to the level of L1/L2. The dural sac always extends into the upper sacrum.

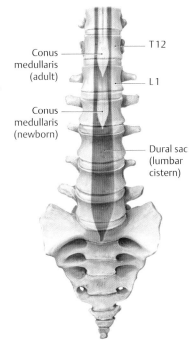

Conus medullaris (adult)
Conus medullaris (newborn)
T 12
L 1
Dural sac (lumbar cistern)

Clinical box 4.1

Lumbar puncture

A needle introduced into the dural sac (lumbar cistern) generally slips past the spinal nerve roots without injuring the spinal cord or spinal nerves. Cerebrospinal fluid (CSF) samples are therefore taken between the L3 and L4 vertebrae (2), once the patient has leaned forward to separate the spinous processes of the lumbar spine.

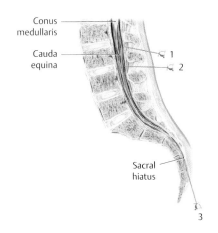

Conus medullaris
Cauda equina
1
2
Sacral hiatus
3

Anesthesia

Lumbar anesthesia may be administered in a similar fashion (2). Epidural anesthesia is administered by placing a catheter in the epidural space without penetrating the dural sac (1). This may also be done by passing a needle through the sacral hiatus (3).

Spinal Cord Segments & Spinal Nerves

Fig. 4.12 Spinal cord segment

The spinal cord consists of 31 segments, each innervating a specific area of the skin (a dermatome) of the head, trunk, or limbs. Afferent (sensory) posterior rootlets and efferent (motor) anterior rootlets form the posterior and anterior roots of the spinal nerve for that segment. The two roots fuse to form a mixed (motor and sensory) spinal nerve that exits the intervertebral foramen and immediately thereafter divides into an anterior and posterior ramus.

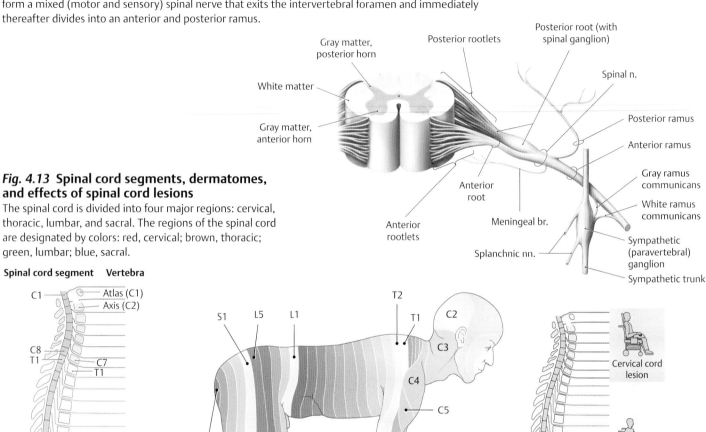

Fig. 4.13 Spinal cord segments, dermatomes, and effects of spinal cord lesions

The spinal cord is divided into four major regions: cervical, thoracic, lumbar, and sacral. The regions of the spinal cord are designated by colors: red, cervical; brown, thoracic; green, lumbar; blue, sacral.

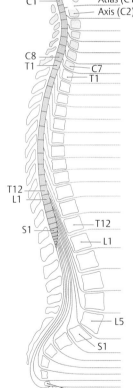

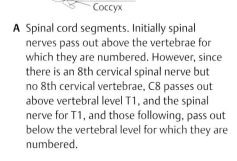

A Spinal cord segments. Initially spinal nerves pass out above the vertebrae for which they are numbered. However, since there is an 8th cervical spinal nerve but no 8th cervical vertebrae, C8 passes out above vertebral level T1, and the spinal nerve for T1, and those following, pass out below the vertebral level for which they are numbered.

B Dermatomes, band-like areas of skin receiving sensory innervation from a single pair of spinal nerves (from a single segment of the spinal cord). *Note:* Spinal nerve C1 is purely motor; consequently there is no C1 dermatome.

C Effects of lesions in each region of the spinal cord.

Fig. 4.14 Spinal nerve branches

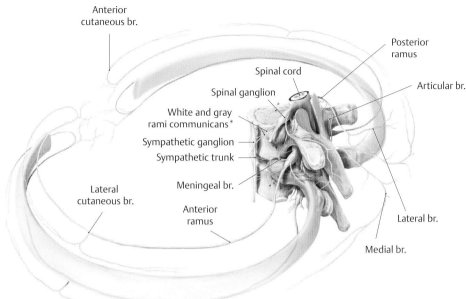

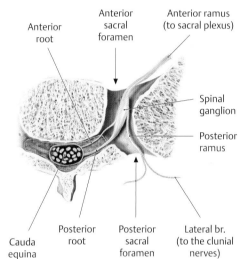

A Superolateral view of a thoracic spinal nerve. The *posterior (dorsal) rami* of the spinal nerves give rise to muscular and cutaneous branches, as well as articular branches to the zygapophyseal joints. The *anterior (ventral) rami* of the spinal nerves form the cervical plexus (C1–C4), the brachial plexus (C5–T1), the lumbar plexus (T12–L4), and the sacral plexus (L4–S3). The anterior rami of spinal nerves T1–T11 produce the intercostal nerves (T12 produces the subcostal nerve).

B Spinal nerve branches in the sacral foramina. Superior view of transverse section through right half of sacrum.

Table 4.1	Branches of a spinal nerve		
Branches			**Territory**
Meningeal br.			Spinal meninges; ligaments of spinal column
Posterior (dorsal) ramus	Medial brs.	Articular br.	Zygapophyseal joints
		Muscular br.	Intrinsic back muscles
		Cutaneous br.	Skin of posterior head, neck, back, and buttocks
	Lateral brs.	Cutaneous br.	
		Muscular br.	Intrinsic back muscles
Anterior (ventral) ramus	Lateral cutaneous brs.		Skin of lateral chest wall
	Anterior cutaneous brs.		Skin of anterior chest wall
*The white and gray rami communicans carry pre- and postganglionic fibers between the sympathetic trunk and spinal n.			

Arteries & Veins of the Spinal Cord

 Like the spinal cord itself, the arteries and veins of the spinal cord consist of multiple horizontal systems (blood vessels of the spinal cord segments) that are integrated into a vertical system.

Fig. 4.15 Arteries of the spinal cord

The unpaired anterior and paired posterior spinal arteries typically arise from the vertebral arteries. As they descend within the vertebral canal, the spinal arteries are reinforced by anterior and posterior segmental medullary arteries. Depending on the spinal level, these reinforcing branches may arise from the vertebral, ascending or deep cervical, posterior intercostal, lumbar, or lateral sacral arteries.

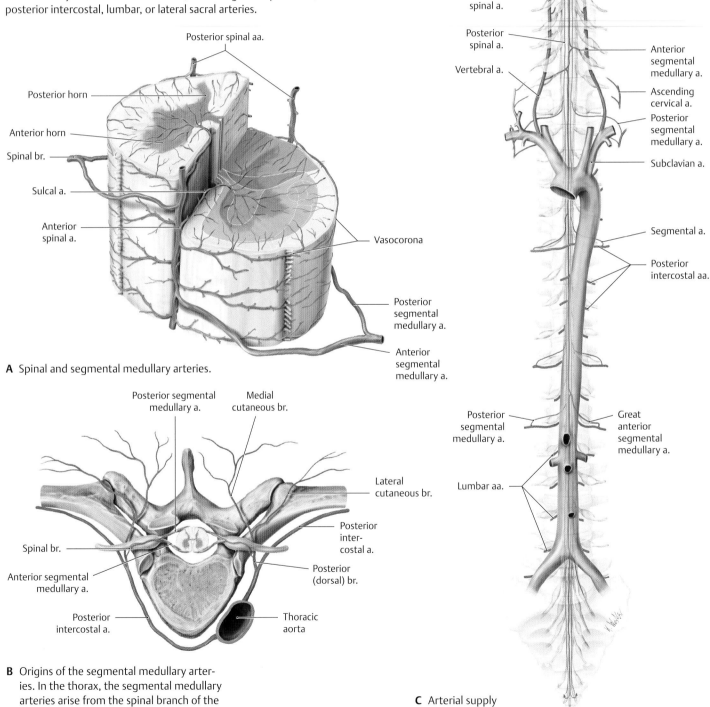

A Spinal and segmental medullary arteries.

B Origins of the segmental medullary arteries. In the thorax, the segmental medullary arteries arise from the spinal branch of the posterior intercostal arteries (see **p. 36**).

C Arterial supply system.

44

Fig. 4.16 Veins of the spinal cord

The interior of the spinal cord drains via venous plexuses into an anterior and a posterior spinal vein. The radicular and spinal veins connect the veins of the spinal cord with the internal vertebral venous plexus. The intervertebral and basivertebral veins connect the internal and external venous plexuses, which drain into the azygos system.

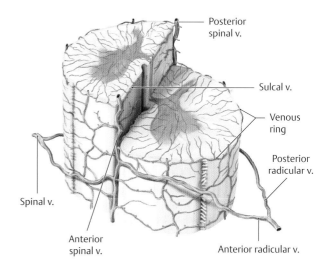

B Spinal and radicular veins.

Posterior spinal v.
Sulcal v.
Venous ring
Posterior radicular v.
Spinal v.
Anterior spinal v.
Anterior radicular v.

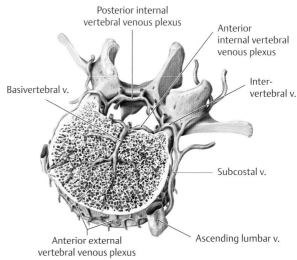

C Vertebral venous plexuses.

Posterior internal vertebral venous plexus
Anterior internal vertebral venous plexus
Basivertebral v.
Inter-vertebral v.
Subcostal v.
Anterior external vertebral venous plexus
Ascending lumbar v.

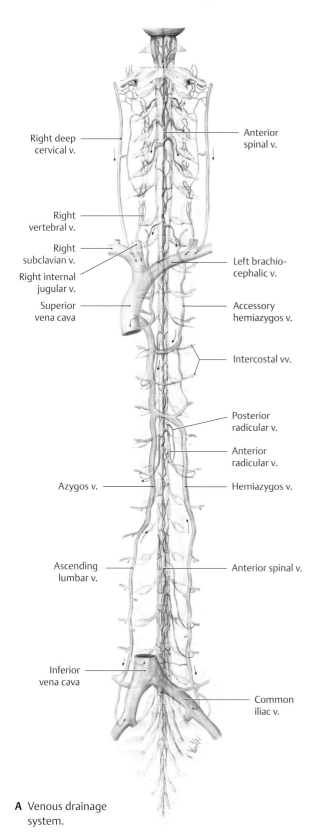

A Venous drainage system.

Right deep cervical v.
Anterior spinal v.
Right vertebral v.
Right subclavian v.
Right internal jugular v.
Left brachio-cephalic v.
Superior vena cava
Accessory hemiazygos v.
Intercostal vv.
Posterior radicular v.
Anterior radicular v.
Azygos v.
Hemiazygos v.
Ascending lumbar v.
Anterior spinal v.
Inferior vena cava
Common iliac v.

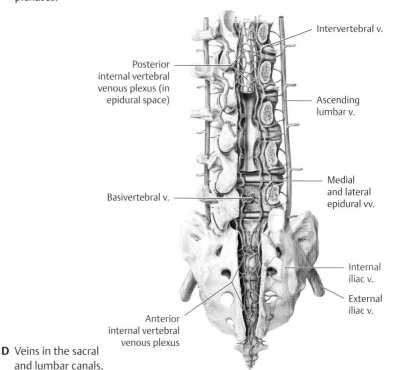

D Veins in the sacral and lumbar canals.

Intervertebral v.
Posterior internal vertebral venous plexus (in epidural space)
Ascending lumbar v.
Basivertebral v.
Medial and lateral epidural vv.
Internal iliac v.
External iliac v.
Anterior internal vertebral venous plexus

Neurovascular Topography of the Back

Fig. 4.17 Neurovasculature of the nuchal region

Posterior view. *Removed:* Trapezius, sterno-cleidomastoid, and semispinalis capitis.
Revealed: Suboccipital region.

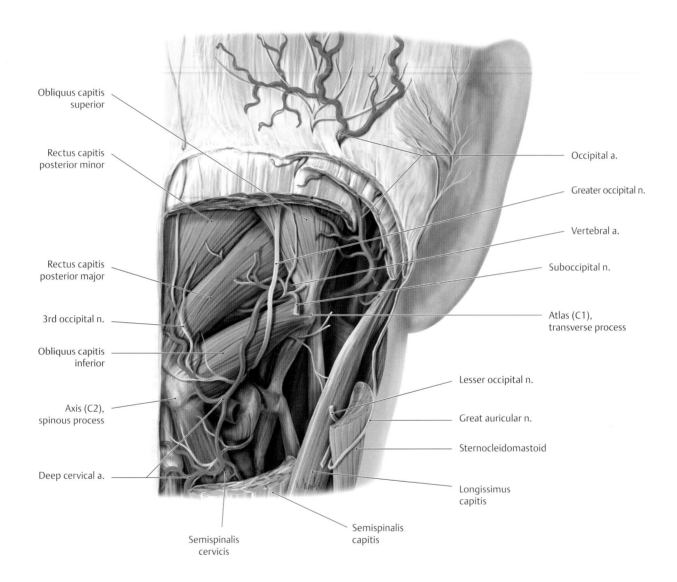

Obliquus capitis superior

Rectus capitis posterior minor

Rectus capitis posterior major

3rd occipital n.

Obliquus capitis inferior

Axis (C2), spinous process

Deep cervical a.

Occipital a.

Greater occipital n.

Vertebral a.

Suboccipital n.

Atlas (C1), transverse process

Lesser occipital n.

Great auricular n.

Sternocleidomastoid

Longissimus capitis

Semispinalis cervicis

Semispinalis capitis

Fig. 4.18 Neurovasculature of the back

Posterior view. *Removed:* Muscle fascia (except posterior layer of thoracolumbar fascia); latissimus dorsi (right). *Reflected:* Trapezius (right). *Revealed:* Transverse cervical artery in the deep scapular region. See **p. 72** for the course of the intercostal vessels.

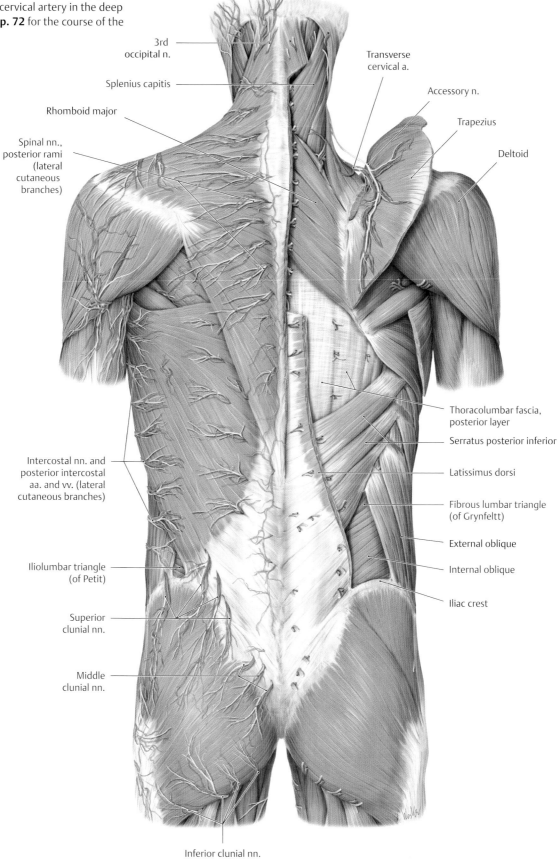

3rd occipital n.

Splenius capitis

Rhomboid major

Spinal nn., posterior rami (lateral cutaneous branches)

Transverse cervical a.

Accessory n.

Trapezius

Deltoid

Thoracolumbar fascia, posterior layer

Serratus posterior inferior

Latissimus dorsi

Fibrous lumbar triangle (of Grynfeltt)

External oblique

Internal oblique

Iliac crest

Intercostal nn. and posterior intercostal aa. and vv. (lateral cutaneous branches)

Iliolumbar triangle (of Petit)

Superior clunial nn.

Middle clunial nn.

Inferior clunial nn.

47

Radiographic Anatomy of the Back (I)

***Fig. 5.1* MRI of the spine**
Sagittal view.

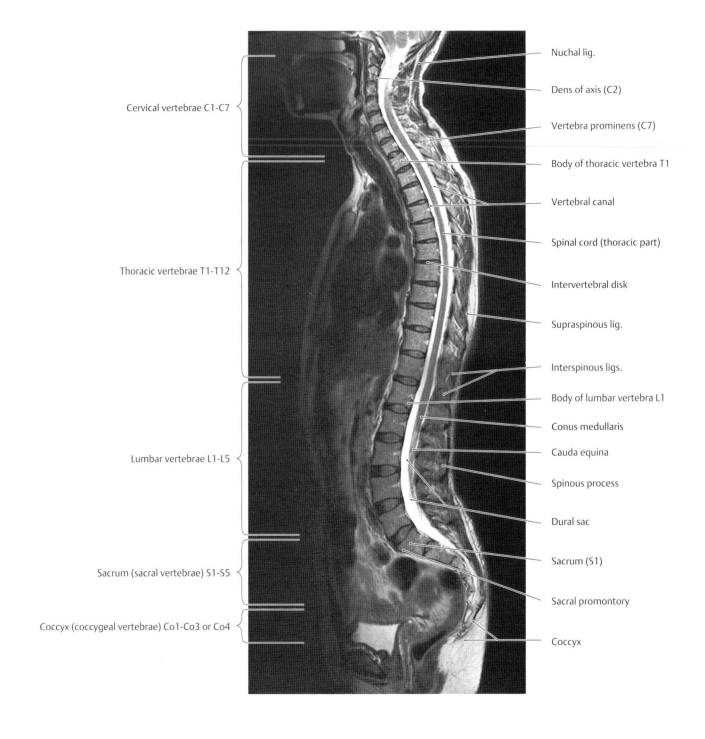

Cervical vertebrae C1–C7

Thoracic vertebrae T1–T12

Lumbar vertebrae L1–L5

Sacrum (sacral vertebrae) S1–S5

Coccyx (coccygeal vertebrae) Co1–Co3 or Co4

Nuchal lig.

Dens of axis (C2)

Vertebra prominens (C7)

Body of thoracic vertebra T1

Vertebral canal

Spinal cord (thoracic part)

Intervertebral disk

Supraspinous lig.

Interspinous ligs.

Body of lumbar vertebra L1

Conus medullaris

Cauda equina

Spinous process

Dural sac

Sacrum (S1)

Sacral promontory

Coccyx

Fig. 5.2 **Radiograph of the cervical spine**
Oblique view.

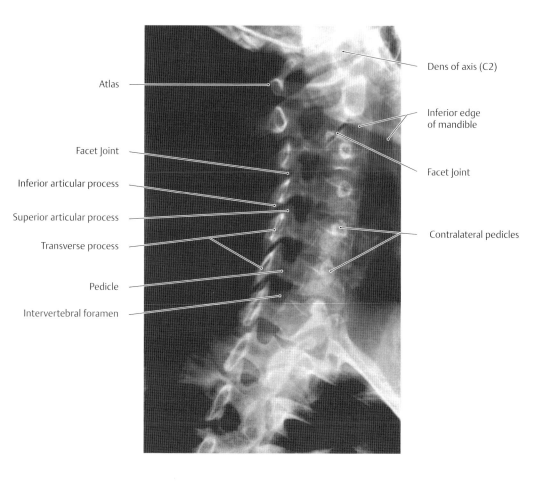

Dens of axis (C2)

Atlas

Inferior edge
of mandible

Facet Joint

Inferior articular process

Facet Joint

Superior articular process

Transverse process

Contralateral pedicles

Pedicle

Intervertebral foramen

Fig. 5.3 **Radiograph of the thoracic spine**
Anteroposterior view. Lower thoracic region.

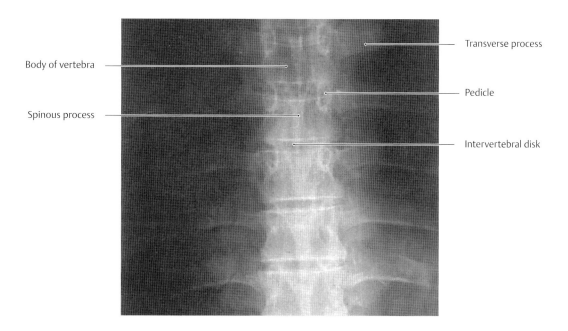

Body of vertebra

Transverse process

Pedicle

Spinous process

Intervertebral disk

Radiographic Anatomy of the Back (II)

Fig. 5.4 **Radiograph of the lumbar spine**
Lateral view.

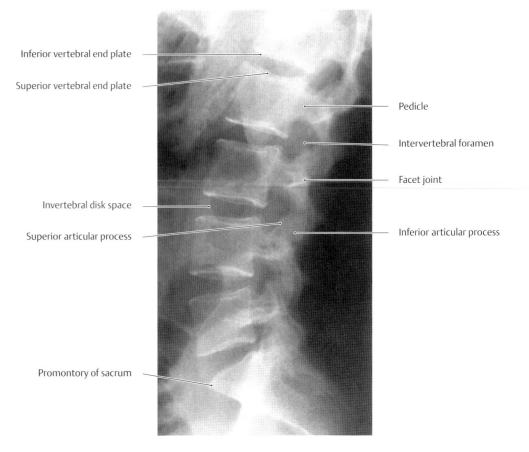

Inferior vertebral end plate

Superior vertebral end plate

Pedicle

Intervertebral foramen

Facet joint

Invertebral disk space

Superior articular process

Inferior articular process

Promontory of sacrum

Fig. 5.5 **MRI of the lumbar spine**
Parasagittal view.

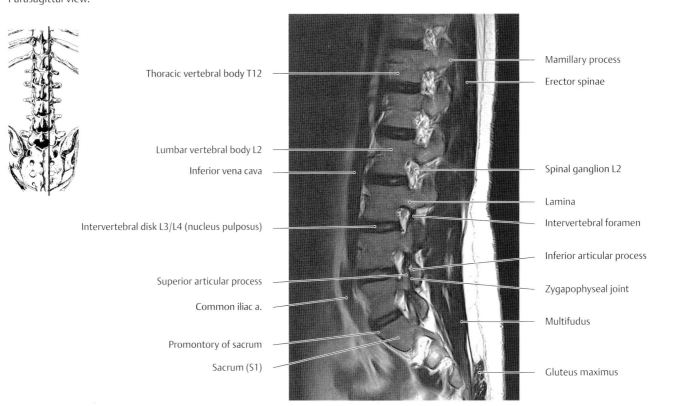

Thoracic vertebral body T12

Mamillary process

Erector spinae

Lumbar vertebral body L2

Inferior vena cava

Spinal ganglion L2

Lamina

Intervertebral foramen

Intervertebral disk L3/L4 (nucleus pulposus)

Inferior articular process

Superior articular process

Zygapophyseal joint

Common iliac a.

Multifudus

Promontory of sacrum

Sacrum (S1)

Gluteus maximus

Fig. 5.6 MRI of the sacrum I
Oblique view.

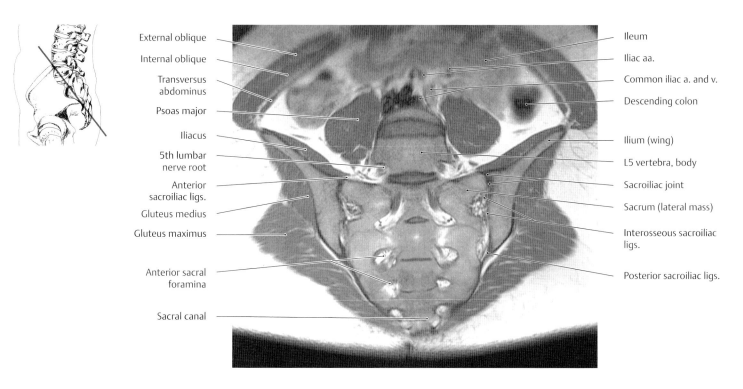

External oblique — Ileum
Internal oblique — Iliac aa.
Transversus abdominus — Common iliac a. and v.
Psoas major — Descending colon
Iliacus
5th lumbar nerve root — Ilium (wing)
Anterior sacroiliac ligs. — L5 vertebra, body
Gluteus medius — Sacroiliac joint
Gluteus maximus — Sacrum (lateral mass)
Anterior sacral foramina — Interosseous sacroiliac ligs.
Sacral canal — Posterior sacroiliac ligs.

Fig. 5.7 MRI of the sacrum II
Oblique view.

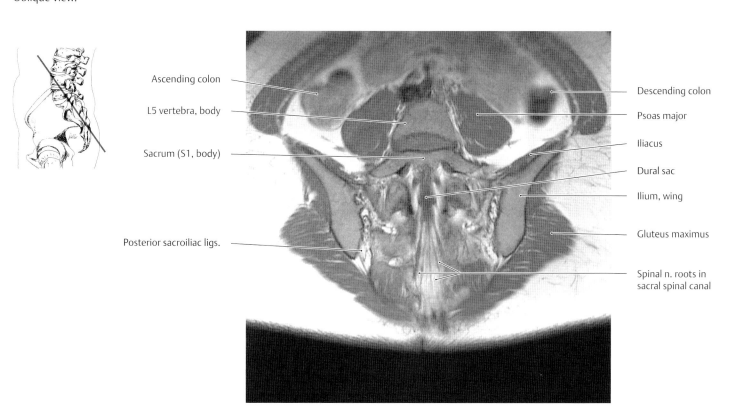

Ascending colon — Descending colon
L5 vertebra, body — Psoas major
Sacrum (S1, body) — Iliacus
— Dural sac
— Ilium, wing
Posterior sacroiliac ligs. — Gluteus maximus
— Spinal n. roots in sacral spinal canal

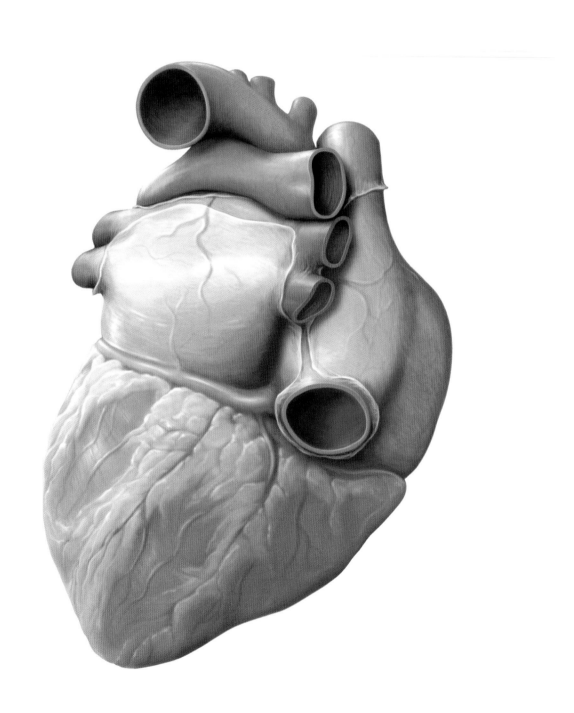

Thorax

Surface Anatomy

***Fig. 6.1* Regions of the thorax**
Anterior view.

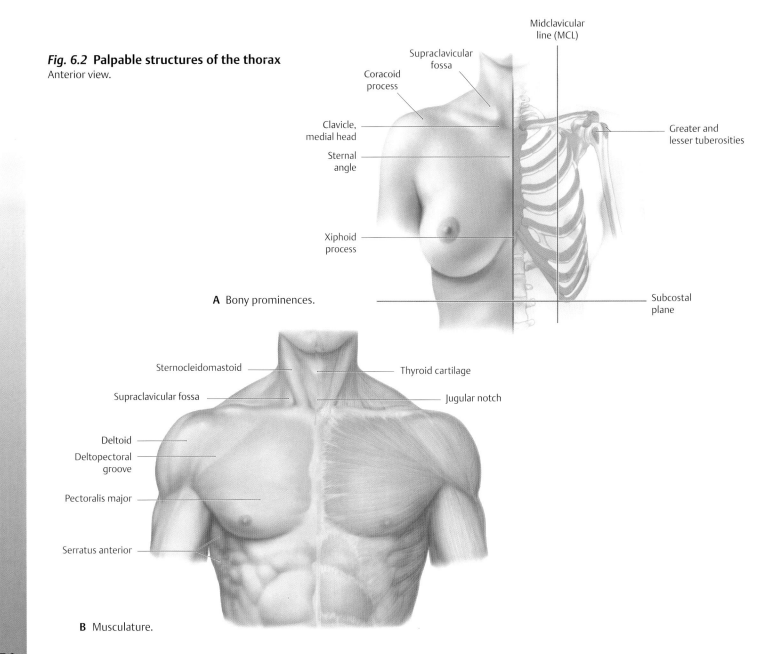

Presternal region

Infraclavicular fossa

Clavipectoral triangle

Deltoid region

Axillary region

Pectoral region

Inframammary region

Lateral pectoral region

Hypochondriac region

Epigastric region (epigastrium)

***Fig. 6.2* Palpable structures of the thorax**
Anterior view.

Midclavicular line (MCL)

Supraclavicular fossa

Coracoid process

Clavicle, medial head

Sternal angle

Greater and lesser tuberosities

Xiphoid process

Subcostal plane

A Bony prominences.

Sternocleidomastoid

Thyroid cartilage

Supraclavicular fossa

Jugular notch

Deltoid

Deltopectoral groove

Pectoralis major

Serratus anterior

B Musculature.

Fig. 6.3 Vertical reference lines of the thorax

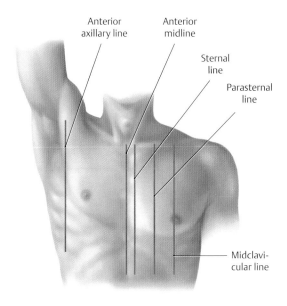

Anterior
axillary line

Anterior
midline

Sternal
line

Parasternal
line

Midclavi-
cular line

A Anterior view.

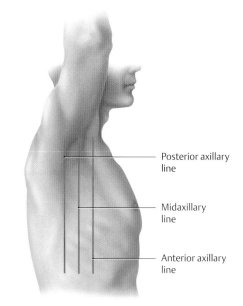

Posterior axillary
line

Midaxillary
line

Anterior axillary
line

B Right lateral view.

Fig. 6.4 Pleural cavities and lungs projected onto the thoracic skeleton

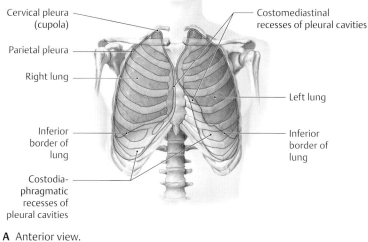

Cervical pleura
(cupola)

Parietal pleura

Right lung

Costomediastinal
recesses of pleural cavities

Left lung

Inferior
border of
lung

Inferior
border of
lung

Costodia-
phragmatic
recesses
of pleural cavities

A Anterior view.

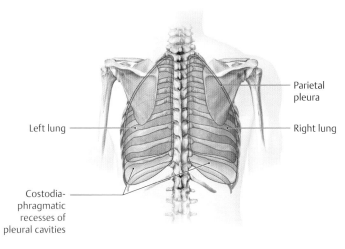

Left lung

Parietal
pleura

Right lung

Costodia-
phragmatic
recesses of
pleural cavities

B Posterior view.

Thoracic Skeleton

 The thoracic skeleton consists of 12 thoracic vertebrae (**p. 10**), 12 pairs of ribs with costal cartilages, and the sternum. In addition to participating in respiratory movements, it provides a measure of protection to vital organs. The female thorax is generally narrower and shorter than the male equivalent.

Fig. 7.1 Thoracic skeleton

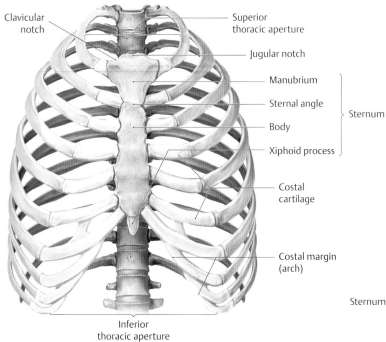

Clavicular notch
Superior thoracic aperture
Jugular notch
Manubrium
Sternal angle
Body
Xiphoid process
Sternum
Costal cartilage
Costal margin (arch)
Inferior thoracic aperture

A Anterior view.

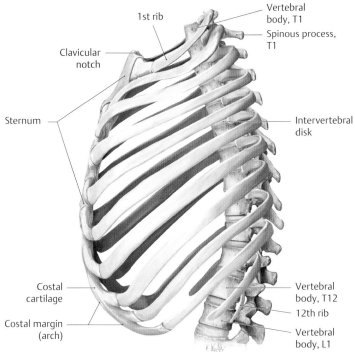

1st rib
Vertebral body, T1
Spinous process, T1
Clavicular notch
Sternum
Intervertebral disk
Costal cartilage
Costal margin (arch)
Vertebral body, T12
12th rib
Vertebral body, L1

B Left lateral view.

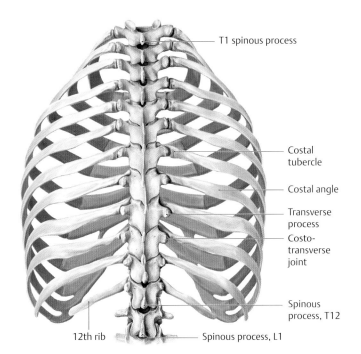

T1 spinous process
Costal tubercle
Costal angle
Transverse process
Costo-transverse joint
Spinous process, T12
12th rib
Spinous process, L1

C Posterior view.

Fig. 7.2 Structure of a thoracic segment
Superior view of 6th rib pair.

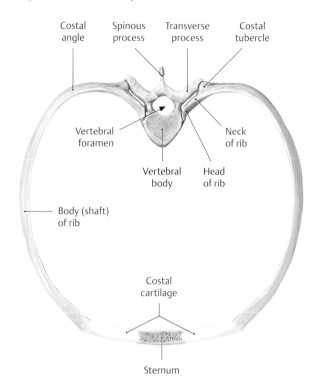

Table 7.1	Elements of a thoracic segment		
Vertebra			
Rib	Bony part (costal bone)	Head	
		Neck	
		Costal tubercle	
		Body (including costal angle)	
	Costal part (costal cartilage)		
Sternum (articulates with costal cartilage of true ribs only; see **Fig. 7.3**)			

Fig. 7.3 Types of ribs
Left lateral view.

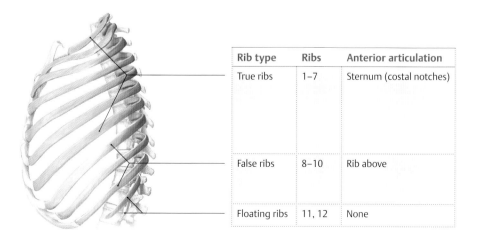

Rib type	Ribs	Anterior articulation
True ribs	1–7	Sternum (costal notches)
False ribs	8–10	Rib above
Floating ribs	11, 12	None

Sternum & Ribs

Fig. 7.4 **Sternum**

The sternum is a blade-like bone consisting of the manubrium, body, and xiphoid process. The junction of the manubrium and body (the sternal angle) is typically elevated and marks the articulation of the second rib. The sternal angle is an important landmark for internal structures.

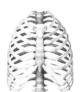

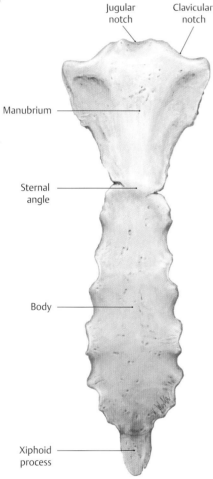

Jugular notch

Clavicular notch

Manubrium

Sternal angle

Body

Xiphoid process

A Anterior view.

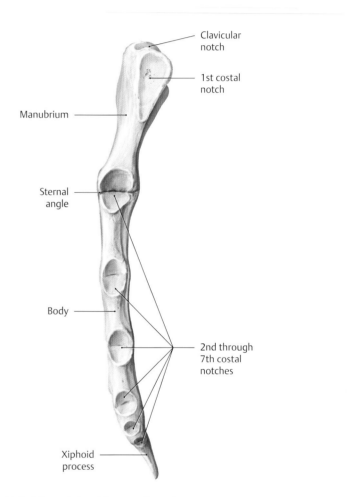

Clavicular notch

1st costal notch

Manubrium

Sternal angle

Body

2nd through 7th costal notches

Xiphoid process

B Left lateral view. The costal notches are sites of articulation with the costal cartilage of the true ribs (see **Fig. 7.3**).

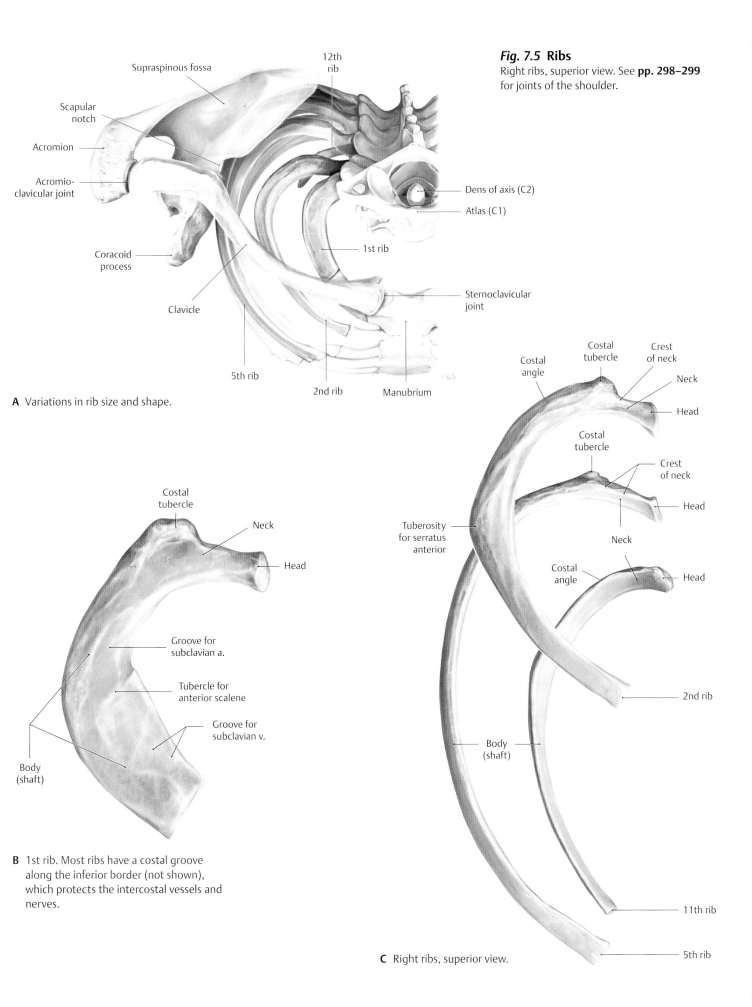

Supraspinous fossa

12th rib

Fig. 7.5 **Ribs**
Right ribs, superior view. See **pp. 298–299** for joints of the shoulder.

Scapular notch

Acromion

Acromio-clavicular joint

Dens of axis (C2)

Atlas (C1)

Coracoid process

1st rib

Sternoclavicular joint

Clavicle

5th rib

2nd rib

Manubrium

A Variations in rib size and shape.

Costal angle

Costal tubercle

Crest of neck

Neck

Head

Costal tubercle

Costal tubercle

Neck

Head

Crest of neck

Head

Tuberosity for serratus anterior

Neck

Groove for subclavian a.

Costal angle

Head

Tubercle for anterior scalene

Groove for subclavian v.

Body (shaft)

2nd rib

Body (shaft)

B 1st rib. Most ribs have a costal groove along the inferior border (not shown), which protects the intercostal vessels and nerves.

11th rib

5th rib

C Right ribs, superior view.

Joints of the Thoracic Cage

 The diaphragm is the chief muscle for quiet respiration (see **p. 64**). The muscles of the thoracic wall (see **p. 62**) contribute to deep (forced) inspiration.

Fig. 7.6 Rib cage movement

Full inspiration (red); full expiration (blue). In deep inspiration, there is an increase in transverse and anteroposterior (AP) dimensions, as well as the infrasternal angle. The descent of the diaphragm further increases the volume of the thoracic cavity.

Inspiration

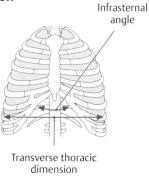

Infrasternal angle

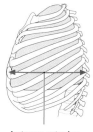

Transverse thoracic dimension

Anteroposterior (AP) dimension

Expiration

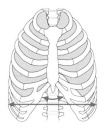

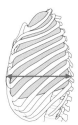

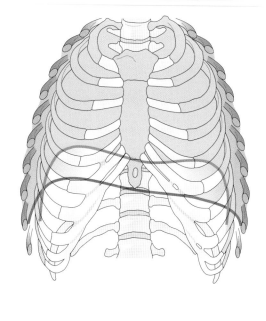

A Anterior view.

B Left lateral view.

C Position of diaphragm during respiration.

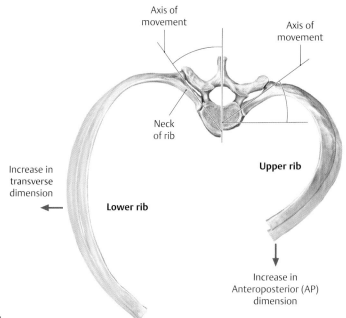

Axis of movement

Axis of movement

Neck of rib

Upper rib

Increase in transverse dimension

Lower rib

Increase in Anteroposterior (AP) dimension

D Axes of rib movement, superior view.

Fig. 7.7 Sternocostal joints

Anterior view with right half of sternum sectioned frontally. True joints are generally found only at ribs 2 to 5; ribs 1, 6, and 7 attach to the sternum by synchondroses.

Fig. 7.8 Costovertebral joints

Two synovial joints make up the costovertebral articulation of each rib. The costal tubercle of each rib articulates with the costal facet of its accompanying vertebra (**A**). The head of most ribs articulates with the vertebra of its own number and the vertebra immediately superior. Ribs 1, 11, and 12 typically articulate only with their own vertebrae.

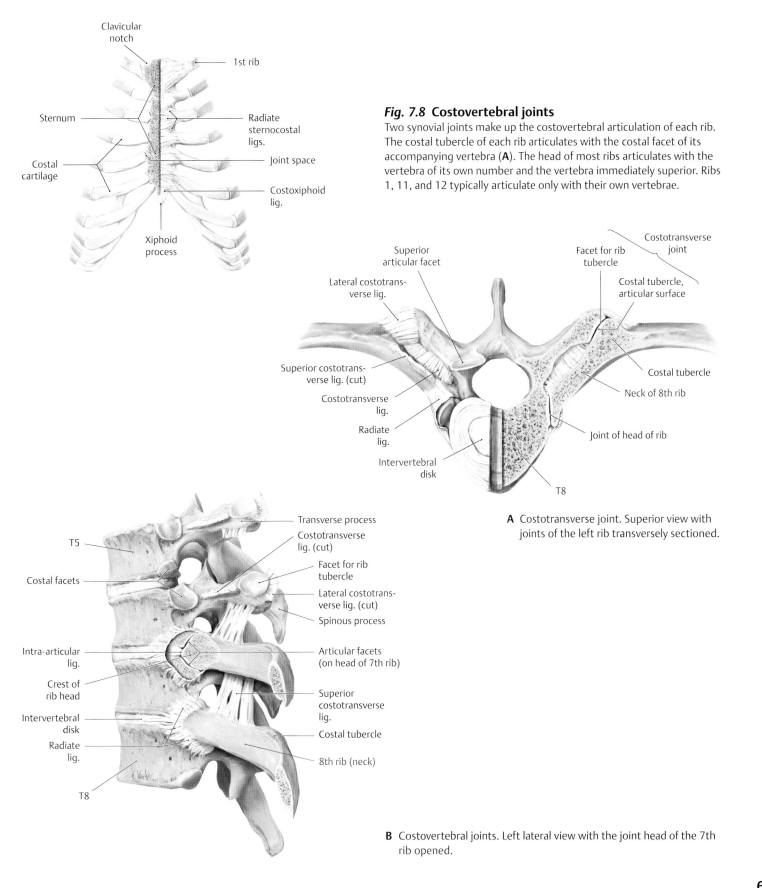

A Costotransverse joint. Superior view with joints of the left rib transversely sectioned.

B Costovertebral joints. Left lateral view with the joint head of the 7th rib opened.

61

Thoracic Wall Muscle Facts

The muscles of the thoracic wall are primarily responsible for chest respiration, although other muscles aid in *deep* inspiration: the pectoralis major and serratus anterior are discussed with the shoulder (see **pp. 314–315**), and the serratus posterior is discussed with the back (see **p. 32**).

Fig. 7.9 **Muscles of the thoracic wall**

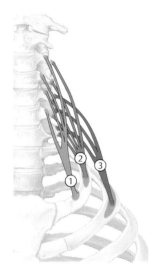

A Scalene muscles, anterior view.

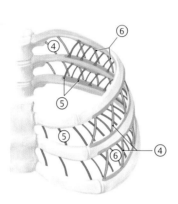

B Intercostal muscles, anterior view.

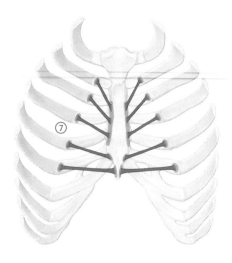

C Transversus thoracis, posterior view.

Table 7.2	Muscles of the thoracic wall				
Muscle		**Origin**	**Insertion**	**Innervation**	**Action**
Scalene mm.	① Anterior scalene m.	C3–C6 (transverse processes, anterior tubercles)	1st rib (anterior scalene tubercle)	Anterior rami of C4–C6 spinal nn.	*With ribs mobile*: Raises upper ribs (inspiration) *With ribs fixed*: Bends cervical spine to same side (unilateral); flexes neck (bilateral)
	② Middle scalene m.	C3–C7 (transverse processes, posterior tubercles)	1st rib (posterior to groove for subclavian a.)	Anterior rami of C3–C8 spinal nn.	
	③ Posterior scalene m.	C5–C7 (transverse processes, posterior tubercles)	2nd rib (outer surface)	Anterior rami of C67–C8 spinal nn.	
Intercostal mm.	④ External intercostal mm.	Lower margin of rib to upper margin of next lower rib (courses obliquely forward and downward from costal tubercle to chondro-osseous junction)		1st to 11th intercostal nn.	Raises ribs (inspiration); supports intercostal spaces; stabilizes chest wall
	⑤ Internal intercostal mm.	Lower margin of rib to upper margin of next lower rib (courses obliquely forward and upward from costal angle to sternum)			Lowers ribs (expiration); supports intercostal spaces, stabilizes chest wall
	⑥ Innermost intercostal mm.				
Subcostal mm.		Lower margin of lower ribs to inner surface of ribs two to three ribs below		Adjacent intercostal nn.	Lowers ribs (expiration)
⑦ Transversus thoracis m.		Sternum and xiphoid process (inner surface)	2nd to 6th ribs (costal cartilage, inner surface)	2nd to 6th intercostal nn.	Weakly lowers ribs (expiration)

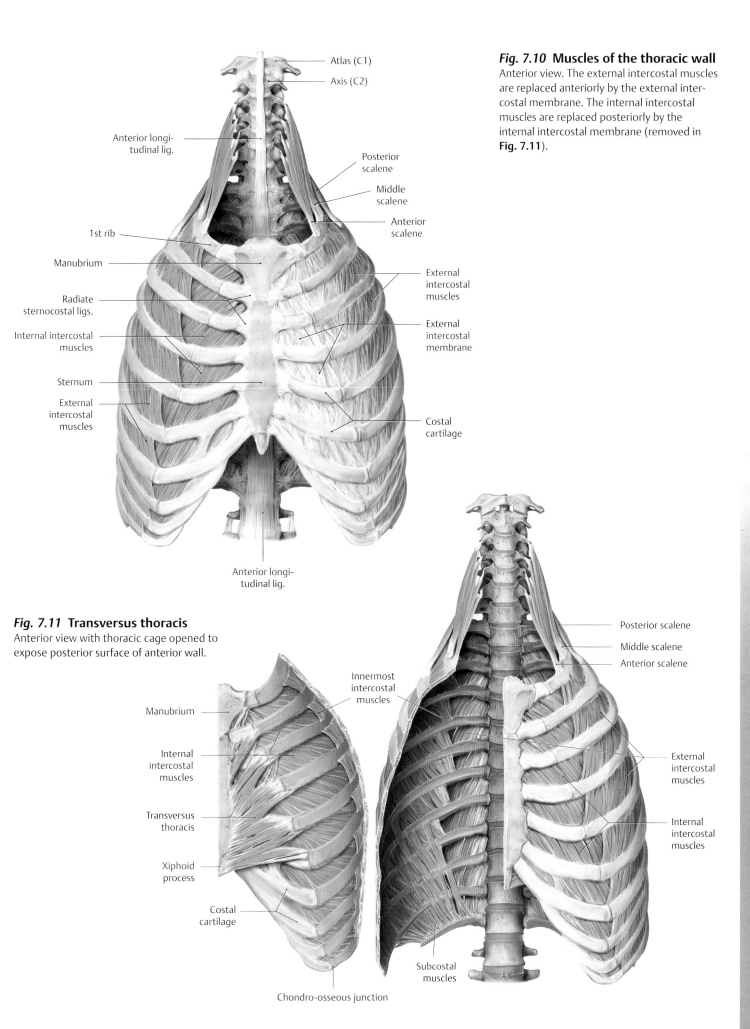

Atlas (C1)

Axis (C2)

Anterior longi-
tudinal lig.

Posterior
scalene

Middle
scalene

Anterior
scalene

1st rib

Manubrium

External
intercostal
muscles

Radiate
sternocostal ligs.

External
intercostal
membrane

Internal intercostal
muscles

Sternum

External
intercostal
muscles

Costal
cartilage

Anterior longi-
tudinal lig.

Fig. 7.10 Muscles of the thoracic wall

Anterior view. The external intercostal muscles are replaced anteriorly by the external intercostal membrane. The internal intercostal muscles are replaced posteriorly by the internal intercostal membrane (removed in **Fig. 7.11**).

Fig. 7.11 Transversus thoracis

Anterior view with thoracic cage opened to expose posterior surface of anterior wall.

Manubrium

Internal
intercostal
muscles

Innermost
intercostal
muscles

Transversus
thoracis

Xiphoid
process

Costal
cartilage

Chondro-osseous junction

Posterior scalene

Middle scalene

Anterior scalene

External
intercostal
muscles

Internal
intercostal
muscles

Subcostal
muscles

Diaphragm

Fig. 7.12 **Diaphragm**
The diaphragm, which separates the thorax from the abdomen, has two asymmetric domes and three apertures (for the aorta, vena cava, and esophagus; see **Fig. 7.13C**).

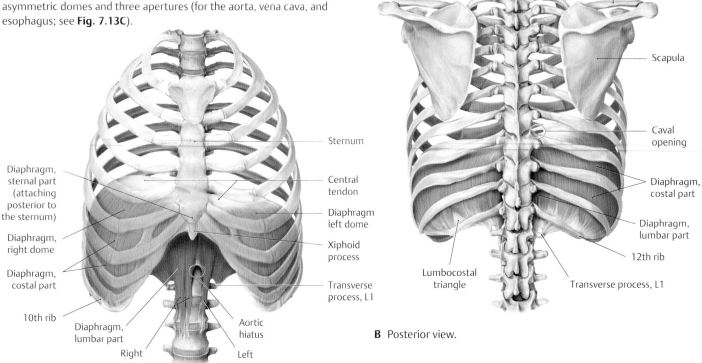

Sternum

Central tendon

Diaphragm, sternal part (attaching posterior to the sternum)

Diaphragm, right dome

Diaphragm, costal part

Diaphragm left dome

Xiphoid process

Transverse process, L1

10th rib

Diaphragm, lumbar part

Aortic hiatus

Right crus

Left crus

A Anterior view.

Clavicle

Scapula

Caval opening

Diaphragm, costal part

Diaphragm, lumbar part

12th rib

Lumbocostal triangle

Transverse process, L1

B Posterior view.

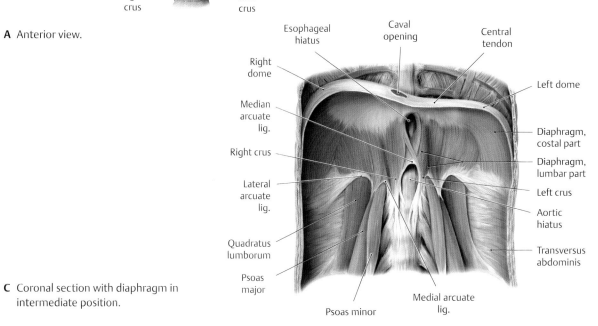

Esophageal hiatus

Caval opening

Central tendon

Right dome

Left dome

Median arcuate lig.

Diaphragm, costal part

Right crus

Diaphragm, lumbar part

Lateral arcuate lig.

Left crus

Aortic hiatus

Quadratus lumborum

Transversus abdominis

Psoas major

Medial arcuate lig.

Psoas minor

C Coronal section with diaphragm in intermediate position.

Table 7.3	Diaphragm				
Muscle		**Origin**	**Insertion**	**Innervation**	**Action**
Diaphragm	Costal part	7th to 12th ribs (inner surface; lower margin of costal arch)	Central tendon	Phrenic n. (C3–C5, cervical plexus)	Principal muscle of respiration (diaphragmatic and thoracic breathing); aids in compressing abdominal viscera (abdominal press)
	Lumbar part	Medial part: L1–L3 vertebral bodies, intervertebral disks, and anterior longitudinal lig. as right and left crura			
		Lateral parts: lateral and medial arcuate ligs.			
	Sternal part	Xiphoid process (posterior surface)			

Fig. 7.13 **Diaphragm in situ**

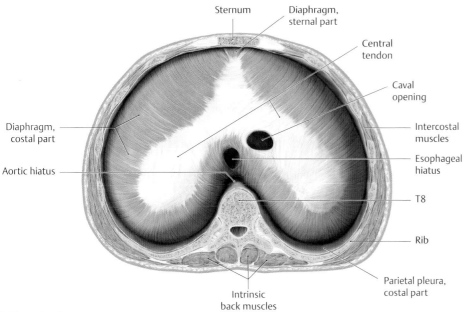

Sternum

Diaphragm, sternal part

Central tendon

Caval opening

Diaphragm, costal part

Intercostal muscles

Esophageal hiatus

Aortic hiatus

T8

Rib

Parietal pleura, costal part

Intrinsic back muscles

A Superior view.

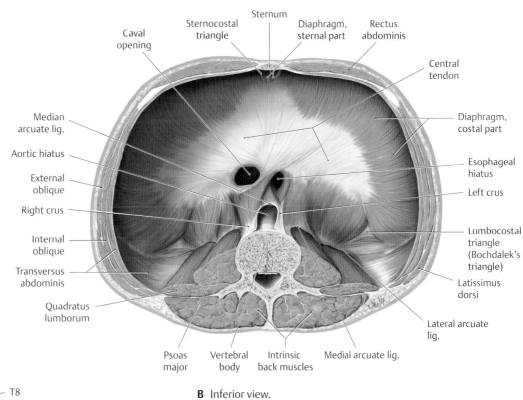

Caval opening

Sternocostal triangle

Sternum

Diaphragm, sternal part

Rectus abdominis

Central tendon

Median arcuate lig.

Aortic hiatus

External oblique

Right crus

Internal oblique

Transversus abdominis

Quadratus lumborum

Psoas major

Vertebral body

Intrinsic back muscles

Medial arcuate lig.

Diaphragm, costal part

Esophageal hiatus

Left crus

Lumbocostal triangle (Bochdalek's triangle)

Latissimus dorsi

Lateral arcuate lig.

B Inferior view.

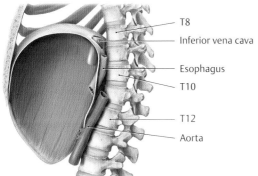

T8

Inferior vena cava

Esophagus

T10

T12

Aorta

C Diaphragmatic apertures, left lateral view.

Neurovasculature of the Diaphragm

Fig. 7.14 Neurovasculature of the diaphragm
Anterior view of opened thoracic cage.

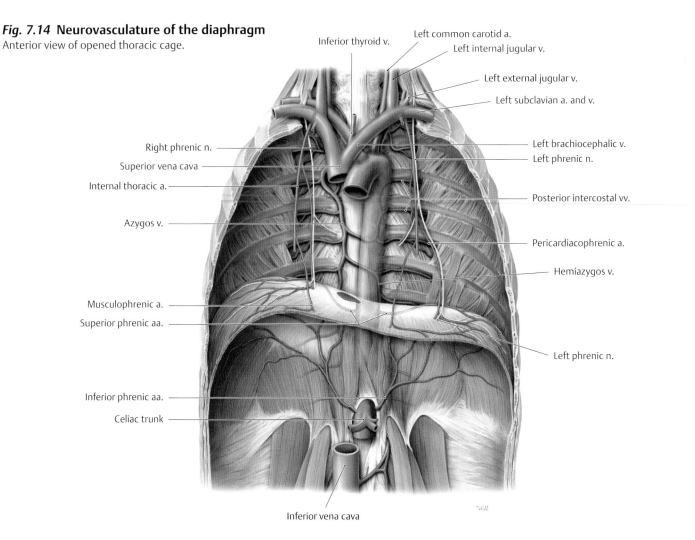

- Inferior thyroid v.
- Left common carotid a.
- Left internal jugular v.
- Left external jugular v.
- Left subclavian a. and v.
- Right phrenic n.
- Superior vena cava
- Internal thoracic a.
- Azygos v.
- Left brachiocephalic v.
- Left phrenic n.
- Posterior intercostal vv.
- Pericardiacophrenic a.
- Hemiazygos v.
- Musculophrenic a.
- Superior phrenic aa.
- Left phrenic n.
- Inferior phrenic aa.
- Celiac trunk
- Inferior vena cava

Fig. 7.15 Innervation of the diaphragm
Anterior view. The phrenic nerves lie on the lateral surfaces of the fibrous pericardium together with the pericardiacophrenic arteries and veins. *Note*: The phrenic nerves also innervate the pericardium.

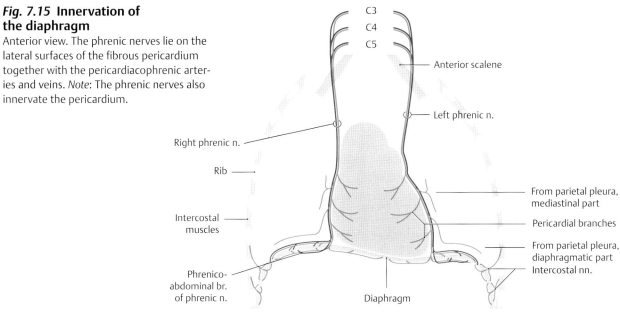

- C3
- C4
- C5
- Anterior scalene
- Left phrenic n.
- Right phrenic n.
- Rib
- From parietal pleura, mediastinal part
- Pericardial branches
- From parietal pleura, diaphragmatic part
- Intercostal nn.
- Intercostal muscles
- Phrenico-abdominal br. of phrenic n.
- Diaphragm

—— Efferent fibers —— Afferent fibers

Table 7.4	Blood vessels of the diaphragm		
Artery	**Origin**	**Vein**	**Drainage**
Inferior phrenic aa. (chief blood supply)	Abdominal aorta; occasionally from celiac trunk	Inferior phrenic vv.	Inferior vena cava
Superior phrenic aa.	Thoracic aorta	Superior phrenic vv.	Azygos v. (right side), hemiazygos v. (left side)
Pericardiacophrenic aa.	Internal thoracic aa.	Pericardiacophrenic vv.	Internal thoracic vv. or brachiocephalic vv.
Musculophrenic aa.		Musculophrenic vv.	Internal thoracic vv.

Fig. 7.16 Arteries and nerves of the diaphragm

Note: The margins of the diaphragm receive sensory innervation from the lowest intercostal nerves.

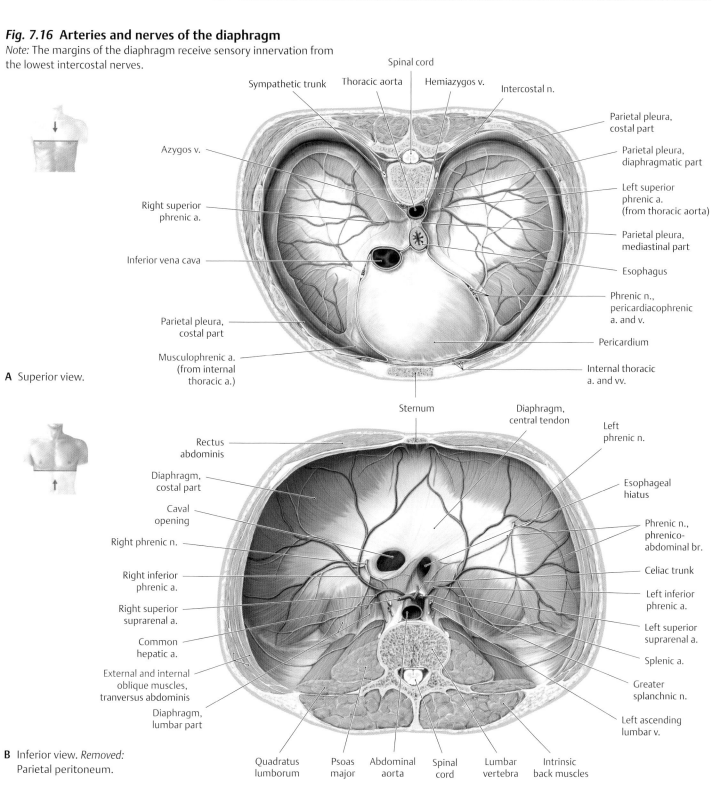

A Superior view.

B Inferior view. *Removed:* Parietal peritoneum.

Arteries & Veins of the Thoracic Wall

 The posterior intercostal arteries anastomose with the anterior intercostal arteries to supply the structures of the thoracic wall. The posterior intercostal arteries branch from the thoracic aorta, with the exception of the 1st and 2nd, which arise from the superior intercostal artery (a branch of the costocervical trunk).

Fig. 7.17 Arteries of the thoracic wall
Anterior view.

Table 7.5	Arteries of the thoracic wall
Origin	**Branch**
Axillary a.	Lateral thoracic a.
	Thoracoacromial a.
Subclavian a.	Posterior intercostal aa. (1st and 2nd; see **Fig. 4.1, p. 36**)
	Superior thoracic a.
Thoracic aorta	Posterior intercostal aa. (3rd through 12th)
Internal thoracic a.	Anterior intercostal aa.
	Musculophrenic a.
	Superior epigastric a.

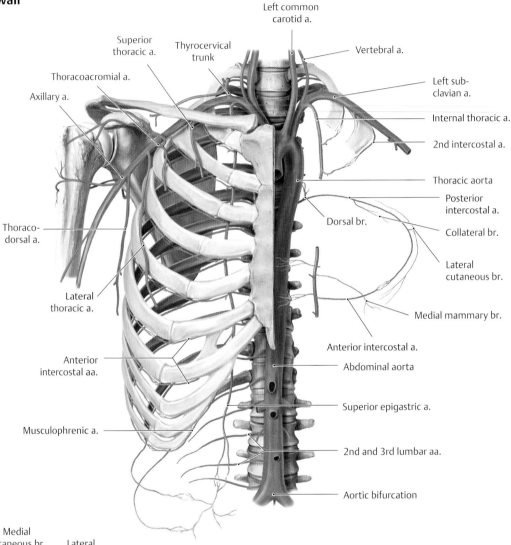

Fig. 7.18 Branches of the posterior intercostal arteries
Superior view.

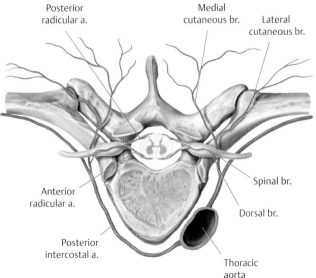

Table 7.6	Branches of the intercostal arteries		
Artery	**Branches**		**Supplies**
Posterior intercostal aa.	Dorsal br.	Spinal br.	Spinal cord
		Medial cutaneous br.	Posterior thoracic wall
		Lateral cutaneous br.	
	Collateral br.		Lateral thoracic wall
Anterior intercostal aa.	Lateral cutaneous br.*		Anterior thoracic wall

*The lateral mammary br. from the lateral cutaneous br. supplies the breast along with the medial mammary br. from the internal thoracic artery.

The intercostal veins drain primarily into the azygos system, but also into the internal thoracic vein. This blood ultimately returns to the heart via the superior vena cava. The intercostal veins follow a similar course to their arterial counterparts. However, the veins of the vertebral column form an external vertebral venous plexus that traverses the entire length of the spine (see **p. 36**).

Fig. 7.19 **Veins of the thoracic wall**

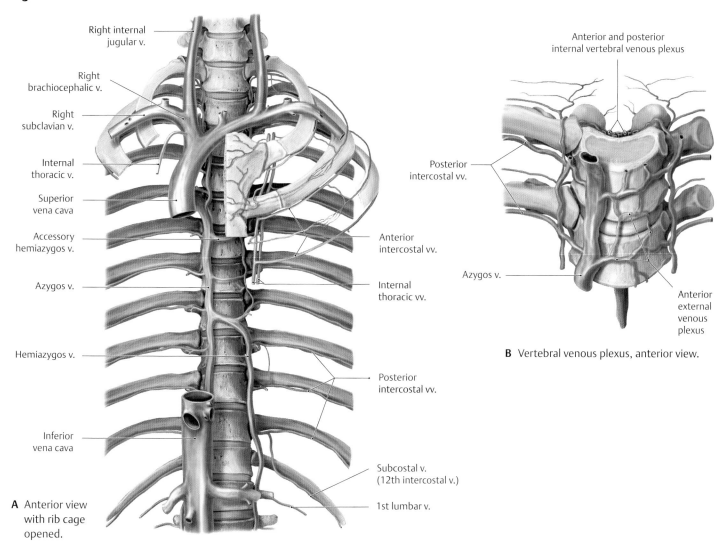

A Anterior view with rib cage opened.

Right internal jugular v.
Right brachiocephalic v.
Right subclavian v.
Internal thoracic v.
Superior vena cava
Accessory hemiazygos v.
Azygos v.
Hemiazygos v.
Inferior vena cava

Anterior intercostal vv.
Internal thoracic vv.
Posterior intercostal vv.
Subcostal v. (12th intercostal v.)
1st lumbar v.

Anterior and posterior internal vertebral venous plexus
Posterior intercostal vv.
Azygos v.
Anterior external venous plexus

B Vertebral venous plexus, anterior view.

Fig. 7.20 **Superficial veins**

Anterior view. The thoracoepigastric veins are a potential superficial collateral venous drainage route in the event of superior or inferior vena cava obstruction.

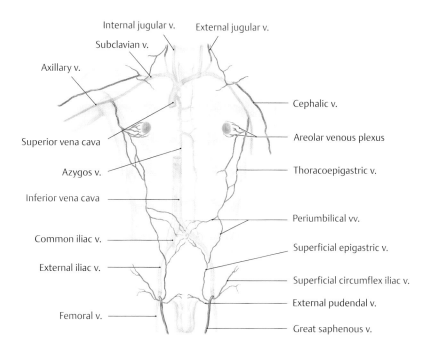

Internal jugular v.
External jugular v.
Subclavian v.
Axillary v.
Superior vena cava
Azygos v.
Inferior vena cava
Common iliac v.
External iliac v.
Femoral v.

Cephalic v.
Areolar venous plexus
Thoracoepigastric v.
Periumbilical vv.
Superficial epigastric v.
Superficial circumflex iliac v.
External pudendal v.
Great saphenous v.

Nerves of the Thoracic Wall

Fig. 7.21 Intercostal nerves

Anterior view. The 1st rib has been removed
to reveal the 1st and 2nd intercostal nerves.

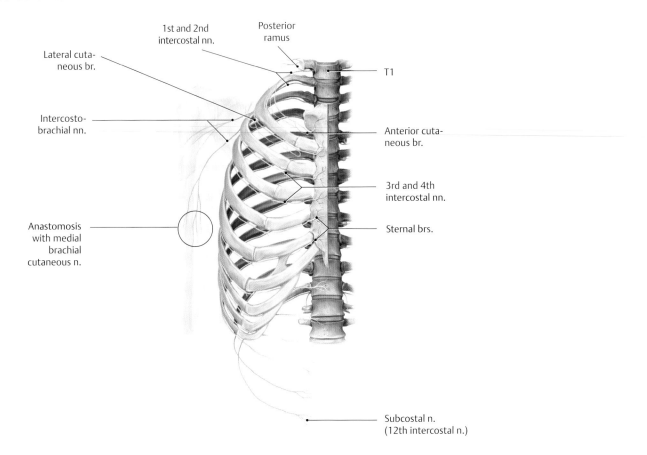

Fig. 7.22 Cutaneous innervation of the thoracic wall

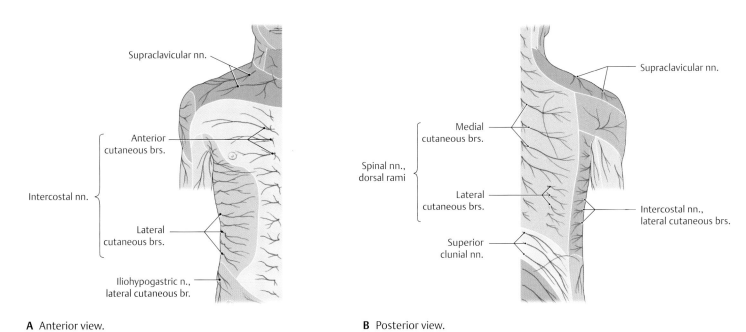

A Anterior view.

B Posterior view.

Fig. 7.23 Spinal nerve branches

Superior view. The spinal nerve is formed by the union of posterior (dorsal) and anterior (ventral) roots. The posterior root contains sensory fibers and the anterior root contains motor fibers. The spinal nerve and all its subsequent branches are mixed nerves, containing both motor and sensory fibers. The spinal nerve exits the vertebral canal via the intervertebral foramen. Its posterior ramus innervates the skin and intrinsic muscles of the back; its anterior ramus forms the cervical, brachial, lumbar, and sacral plexuses, and the intercostal nerves. See **p. 38** for more details.

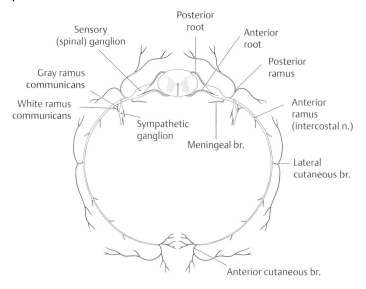

Fig. 7.24 Course of the intercostal nerves

Coronal section, anterior view.

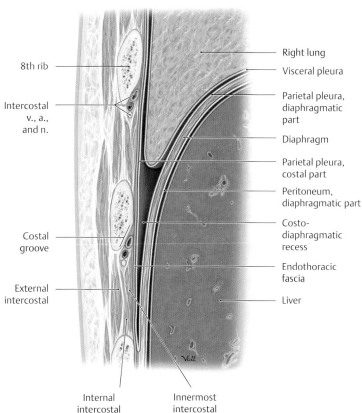

Fig. 7.25 Dermatomes of the thoracic wall

Landmarks: T4 generally includes the nipple; T6 innervates the skin over the xiphoid.

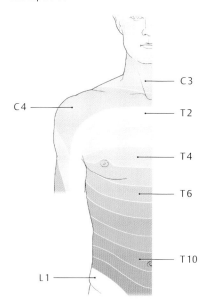

A Anterior view.

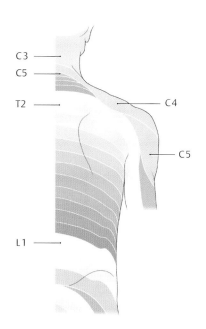

B Posterior view.

Neurovascular Topography of the Thoracic Wall

Fig. 7.26 Anterior structures
Anterior view (see Chapter 4 for neurovasculature of the back).

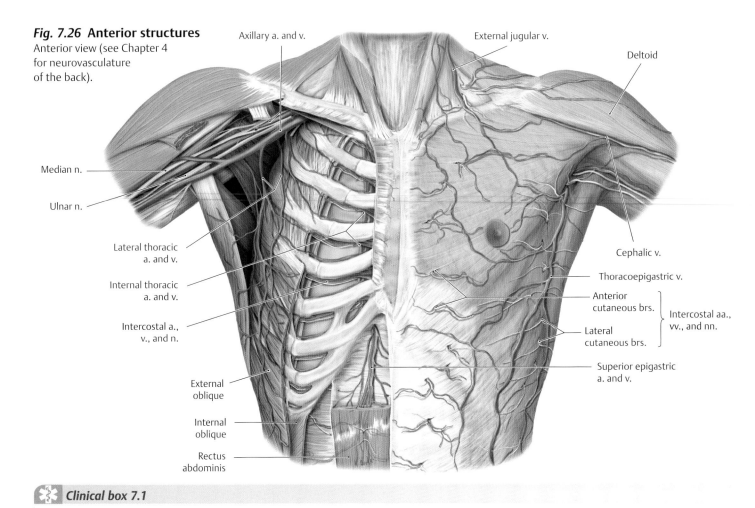

Labels on figure:
- Axillary a. and v.
- External jugular v.
- Deltoid
- Median n.
- Ulnar n.
- Lateral thoracic a. and v.
- Internal thoracic a. and v.
- Intercostal a., v., and n.
- External oblique
- Internal oblique
- Rectus abdominis
- Cephalic v.
- Thoracoepigastric v.
- Anterior cutaneous brs.
- Lateral cutaneous brs.
- Intercostal aa., vv., and nn.
- Superior epigastric a. and v.

✚ Clinical box 7.1

Insertion of a chest tube

Abnormal fluid collection in the pleural space (e.g., pleural effusion due to bronchial carcinoma) may necessitate the insertion of a chest tube. Generally, the optimal puncture site in a sitting patient is at the level of the 7th or 8th intercostal space on the posterior axillary line. The drain should always be introduced at the upper margin of a rib to avoid injuring the intercostal vein, artery, and nerve. See **p. 123** for details on collapsed lungs.

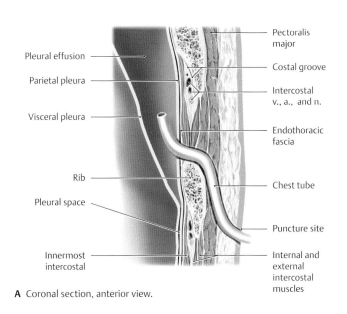

Labels:
- Pleural effusion
- Parietal pleura
- Visceral pleura
- Rib
- Pleural space
- Innermost intercostal
- Pectoralis major
- Costal groove
- Intercostal v., a., and n.
- Endothoracic fascia
- Chest tube
- Puncture site
- Internal and external intercostal muscles

A Coronal section, anterior view.

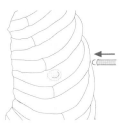

B Drainage tube is inserted perpendicular to chest wall.

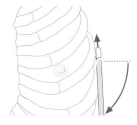

C At ribs, the tube is angled and advanced parallel to the chest wall in the subcutaneous plane.

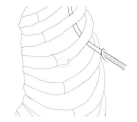

D At the superior margin of the rib, the tube is passed through the intercostal muscles and advanced into the pleural cavity.

Fig. 7.27 **Intercostal structures in cross section**

Transverse section, anterosuperior view. The relationship of the intercostal vessels in the costal groove, from superior to inferior, is vein,
artery, and nerve (see clinical box, **p. 72**).

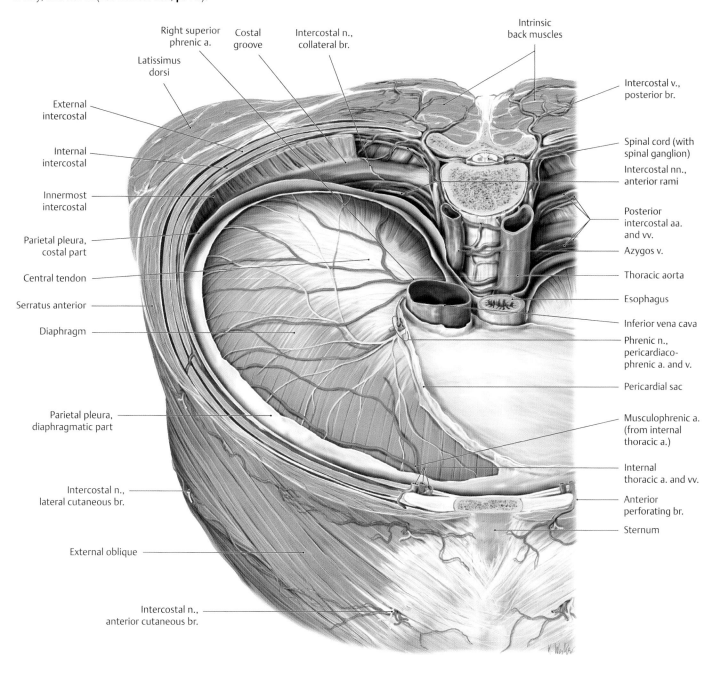

Female Breast

 The female breast, a modified sweat gland in the subcutaneous tissue layer, consists of glandular tissue, fibrous stroma, and fat. The breast extends from the 2nd to the 6th rib and is loosely attached to the pectoral, axillary, and superficial abdominal fascia by connective tissue. The breast is additionally supported by suspensory ligaments. An extension of the breast tissue into the axilla, the axillary tail, is often present.

Fig. 7.28 Female breast
Right breast, anterior view.

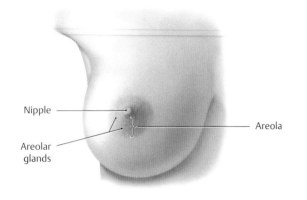

Nipple

Areolar glands

Areola

Fig. 7.29 Mammary ridges
Rudimentary mammary glands form in both sexes along the mammary ridges. Occasionally, these may persist in humans to form accessory nipples (*polythelia*), although only the thoracic pair normally remains.

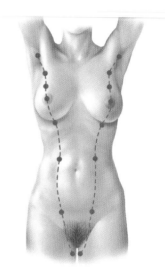

Fig. 7.30 Blood supply to the breast

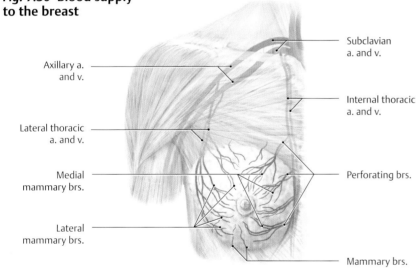

Axillary a. and v.

Lateral thoracic a. and v.

Medial mammary brs.

Lateral mammary brs.

Subclavian a. and v.

Internal thoracic a. and v.

Perforating brs.

Mammary brs.

Fig. 7.31 Sensory innervation of the breast

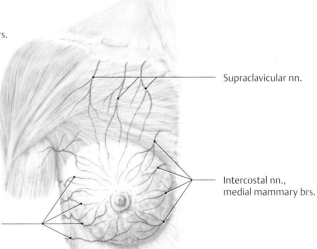

Supraclavicular nn.

Intercostal nn., medial mammary brs.

Intercostal nn., lateral mammary brs.

The glandular tissue is composed of 10 to 20 individual lobes, each with its own lactiferous duct. The gland ducts open on the elevated nipple at the center of the pigmented areola. Just proximal to the duct opening is a dilated portion called the lactiferous sinus. Areolar elevations are the openings of the areolar glands (sebaceous). The glands and lactiferous ducts are surrounded by firm, fibrofatty tissue with a rich blood supply.

Fig. 7.32 **Structures of the breast**

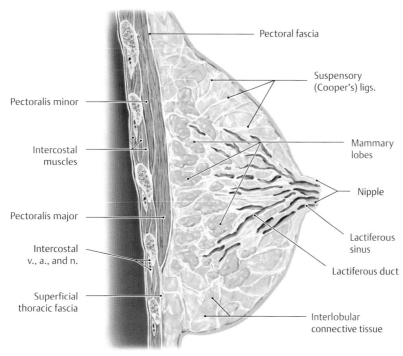

Pectoral fascia

Suspensory (Cooper's) ligs.

Pectoralis minor

Intercostal muscles

Mammary lobes

Nipple

Pectoralis major

Lactiferous sinus

Intercostal v., a., and n.

Lactiferous duct

Superficial thoracic fascia

Interlobular connective tissue

A Sagittal section along midclavicular line.

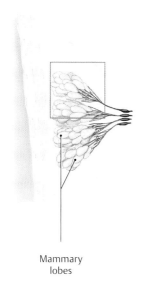

Mammary lobes

B Duct system and portions of a lobe, sagittal section. In the nonlactating breast (shown here), the lobules contain clusters of rudimentary acini.

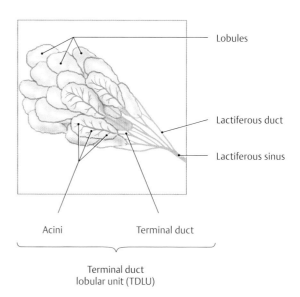

Lobules

Lactiferous duct

Lactiferous sinus

Acini

Terminal duct

Terminal duct lobular unit (TDLU)

C Terminal duct lobular unit (TDLU). The clustered acini composing the lobule empty into a terminal ductule; these structures are collectively known as the TDLU.

Lymphatics of the Female Breast

 The lymphatic vessels of the breast (not shown) are divided into three systems: superficial, subcutaneous, and deep. These drain primarily into the axillary lymph nodes, which are classified based on their relationship to the pectoralis minor (**Table 7.7**). The medial portion of the breast is drained by the parasternal lymph nodes, which are associated with the internal thoracic vessels.

Fig. 7.33 **Axillary lymph nodes**

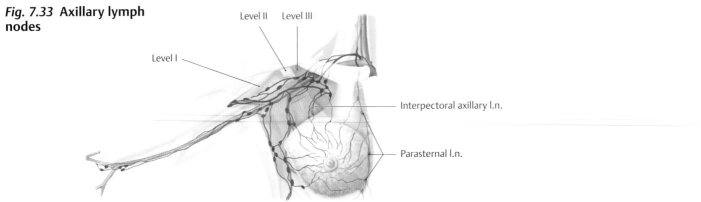

A Lymphatic drainage of the breast. See **Table 7.7** for explanation of level I, II, and III.

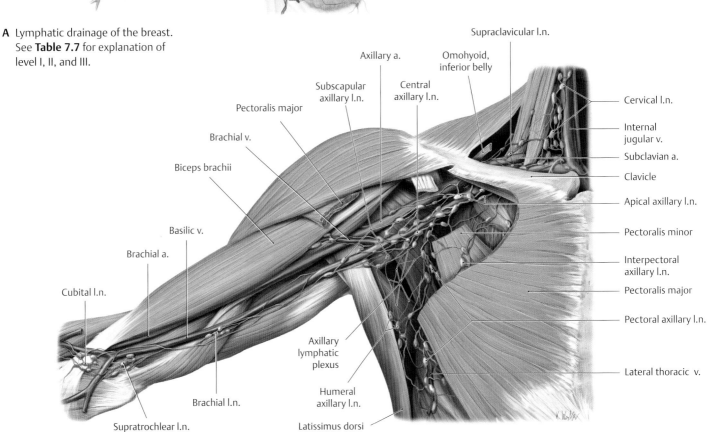

B Anterior view.

Table 7.7	Levels of axillary lymph nodes		
Level		**Position**	**Lymph nodes (l.n.)**
I	Lower axillary group	Lateral to pectoralis minor	Pectoral axillary l.n.
			Subscapular axillary l.n.
			Humeral axillary l.n.
II	Middle axillary group	Along pectoralis minor	Central axillary l.n.
			Interpectoral axillary l.n.
III	Upper infraclavicular group	Medial to pectoralis minor	Apical axillary l.n.

Clinical box 7.2

Breast cancer

Stem cells in the intralobular connective tissue give rise to tremendous cell growth, necessary for duct system proliferation and acini differentiation. This makes the terminal duct lobular unit (TDLU) the most common site of origin of malignant breast tumors.

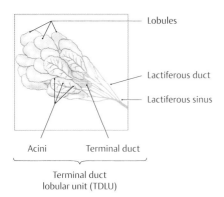

A Terminal duct lobular unit.

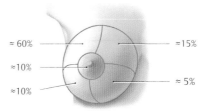

B Origin of malignant tumors by quadrant.

Tumors originating in the breast spread via the lymphatic vessels. The deep system of lymphatic drainage (level III) is of particular importance, although the parasternal lymph nodes provide a route by which tumor cells may spread across the midline. The survival rate in breast cancer correlates most strongly with the number of lymph nodes involved at the axillary nodal level. Metastatic involvement is gauged through scintigraphic mapping with radiolabeled colloids (technetium [Tc] 99m sulfur microcolloid). The downstream sentinel node is the first to receive lymphatic drainage from the tumor and is therefore the first to be visualized with radiolabeling. Once identified, it can then be removed (via *sentinel lymphadenectomy*) and histologically examined for tumor cells. This method is 98% accurate in predicting the level of axillary nodal involvement.

Metastatic involvement	5-year survival rate
Level I	65%
Level II	31%
Level III	~0%

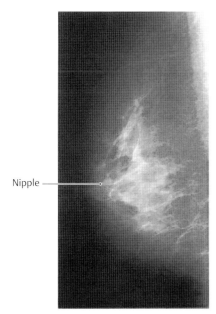

C Normal mammogram.

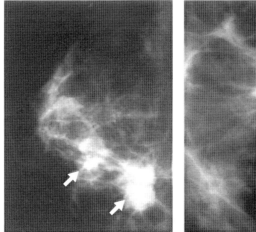

D Mammogram of invasive ductal carcinoma (irregular white areas, *arrows*). The large lesion has changed the architecture of the neighboring breast tissue.

Divisions of the Thoracic Cavity

 The thoracic cavity is divided into three large spaces: the mediastinum (**p. 90**) and the two pleural cavities (**p. 112**).

***Fig. 8.1* Thoracic cavity**
Coronal section, anterior view.

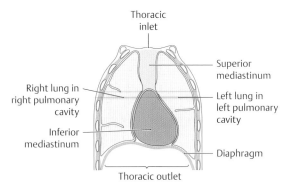

A Divisions of the thoracic cavity.

Table 8.1	Major structures of the thoracic cavity		
Mediastinum	Superior mediastinum		Thymus, great vessels, trachea, esophagus, and thoracic duct
	Inferior mediastinum	Anterior	Thymus (especially in children)
		Middle	Heart, pericardium, and roots of great vessels
		Posterior	Thoracic aorta, thoracic duct, esophagus, and azygos venous system
Pulmonary cavities	Right pulmonary cavity		Right lung
	Left pulmonary cavity		Left lung

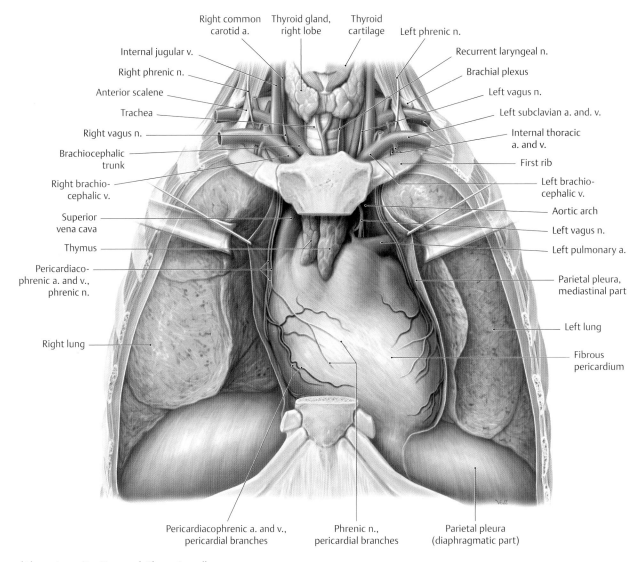

B Opened thoracic cavity. *Removed:* Thoracic wall; connective tissue of anterior mediastinum.

Fig. 8.2 Divisions of the mediastinum

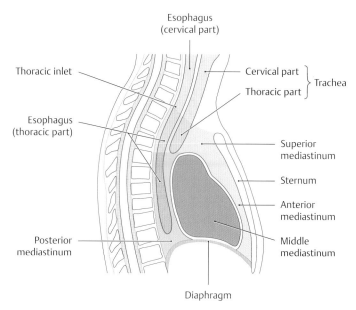

Esophagus (cervical part)

Thoracic inlet

Cervical part ⎱ Trachea
Thoracic part ⎰

Esophagus (thoracic part)

Superior mediastinum

Sternum

Anterior mediastinum

Middle mediastinum

Posterior mediastinum

Diaphragm

A Midsagittal section, lateral view.

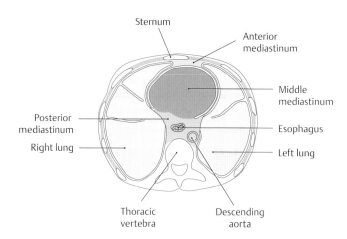

Sternum

Anterior mediastinum

Middle mediastinum

Posterior mediastinum

Esophagus

Right lung

Left lung

Thoracic vertebra

Descending aorta

B Transverse section, inferior view.

Fig. 8.3 Transverse sections of the thorax

Computed tomography (CT) scan of thorax, inferior view.

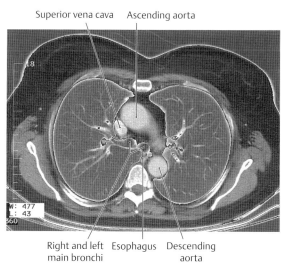

Superior vena cava   Ascending aorta

Right and left main bronchi   Esophagus   Descending aorta

A Superior mediastinum.

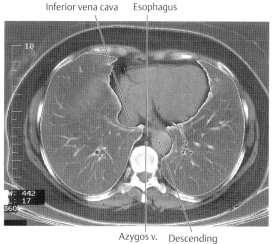

Inferior vena cava   Esophagus

Azygos v.   Descending aorta

B Inferior mediastinum.

Arteries of the Thoracic Cavity

 The arch of the aorta has three major branches: the brachio-cephalic trunk, left common carotid artery, and left subclavian artery. After the aortic arch, the aorta begins its descent, becoming the thoracic aorta at the level of the sternal angle and the abdominal aorta once it passes through the aortic hiatus in the diaphragm.

Fig. 8.4 **Thoracic aorta**

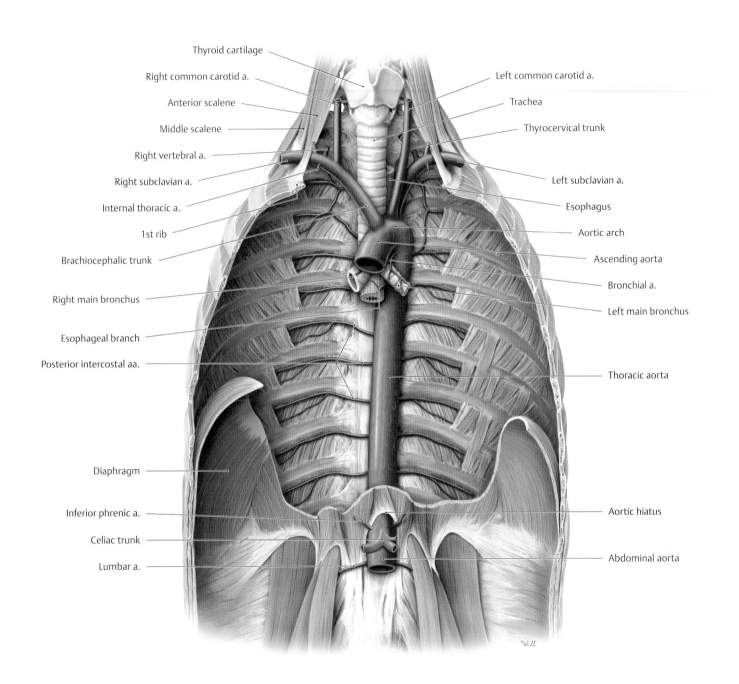

A Thoracic aorta in situ, anterior view. *Removed:* Heart, lungs, portions of diaphragm.

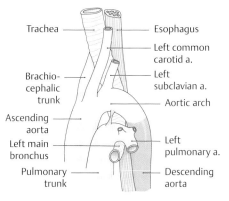

Trachea
Esophagus
Left common carotid a.
Brachio-cephalic trunk
Left subclavian a.
Aortic arch
Ascending aorta
Left main bronchus
Left pulmonary a.
Pulmonary trunk
Descending aorta

B Parts of the aorta, left lateral view. *Note:* The aortic arch begins and ends at the level of the sternal angle (see **p. 58**).

Table 8.2   Branches of the thoracic aorta

The thoracic organs are supplied by direct branches from the thoracic aorta, as well as indirect branches from the subclavian arteries.

Branches			Region supplied
Brachiocephalic trunk	Right subclavian a.		See left subclavian a.
	Right common carotid a.		Head and neck
Left common carotid a.			Head and neck
Left subclavian a.	Vertebral a.		
	Internal thoracic a.	Anterior intercostal aa.	Anterior chest wall
		Thymic branches	Thymus
		Mediastinal branches	Posterior mediastinum
		Pericardiacophrenic a.	Pericardium, diaphragm
	Thyrocervical trunk	Inferior thyroid a.	Esophagus, trachea, thyroid gland
	Costocervical trunk	Superior intercostal a.	Chest wall
Descending thoracic aorta	Visceral brs.		Bronchi, trachea, esophagus
	Parietal brs.	Posterior intercostal aa.	Posterior chest wall
		Superior phrenic aa.	Diaphragm
Ascending aorta	Right and left coronary aa.		Heart

✚ *Clinical box 8.1*

Aortic dissection

A tear in the inner wall (intima) of the aorta allows blood to separate the layers of the aortic wall, creating a "false lumen" and potentially resulting in life-threatening aortic rupture. Symptoms are dyspnea (shortness of breath) and sudden onset of excruciating pain. Acute aortic dissections occur most often in the ascending aorta and generally require surgery. More distal aortic dissections may be treated conservatively, provided there are no complications (e.g., obstruction of blood supply to the organs, in which case a stent may be inserted to restore perfusion). Aortic dissections occurring at the base of a coronary artery may cause myocardial infarction.

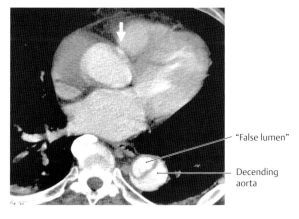

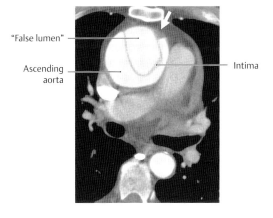

"False lumen"
Ascending aorta
Intima

A Aortic dissection. Parts of the intima are still attached to the connective tissue in the wall of the aorta (*arrow*).

B The flow in the coronary arteries is intact (*arrow*).

Veins of the Thoracic Cavity

The superior vena cava is formed by the union of the two brachiocephalic veins at the level of the T2–T3 junction. It receives blood drained by the azygos system (the inferior vena cava has no tributaries in the thorax).

Fig. 8.5 **Superior vena cava and azygos system**

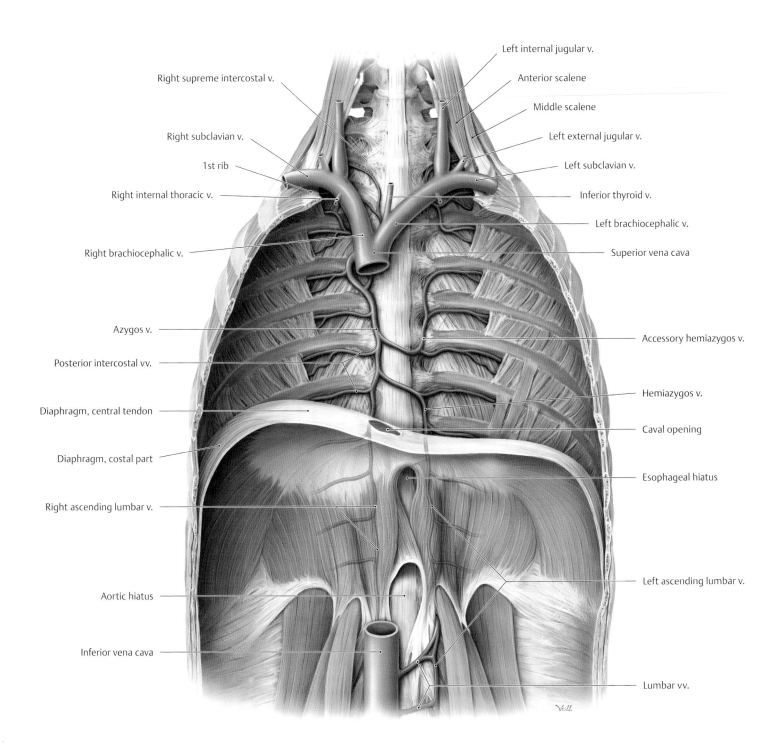

A Veins of the thoracic cavity, anterior view of opened thorax.

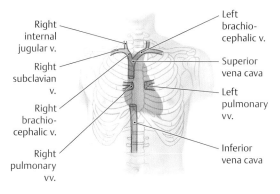

B Projection of venae cavae onto chest, anterior view.

Table 8.3		Thoracic tributaries of the superior vena cava		
Major vein	**Tributaries**			**Region drained**
Brachiocephalic vv.	Inferior thyroid v.			Esophagus, trachea, thyroid gland
	Internal jugular vv.			Head, neck, upper limb
	External jugular vv.			
	Subclavian vv.			
	Supreme intercostal vv.			
	Pericardial vv.			
	Left superior intercostal v.			
Azygos system (left side: accessory hemiazygos v.; right side: azygos v.)	Visceral brs.			Trachea, bronchi, esophagus
	Parietal brs.		Posterior intercostal vv.	Inner chest wall and diaphragm
			Superior phrenic vv.	
			Right superior intercostal v.	
Internal thoracic v.	Thymic vv.			Thymus
	Mediastinal tributaries			Posterior mediastinum
	Anterior intercostal vv.			Anterior chest wall
	Pericardiacophrenic v.			Pericardium
	Musculophrenic v.			Diaphragm

Note: Structures of the superior mediastinum may also drain directly to the brachiocephalic veins via the tracheal, esophageal, and mediastinal veins.

Fig. 8.6 Azygos system
Anterior view.

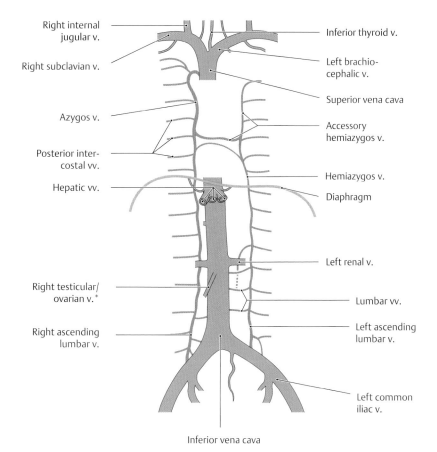

*The left testicular/ovarian vein arises from the left renal vein.

Lymphatics of the Thoracic Cavity

 The body's chief lymph vessel is the thoracic duct. Beginning in the abdomen at the level of L1 as the *cisterna chyli*, the thoracic duct empties into the junction of the left internal jugular and subclavian veins. The right lymphatic duct drains to the right junction of the internal jugular and subclavian veins.

***Fig. 8.7* Lymphatic trunks in the thorax**
Anterior view of opened thorax.

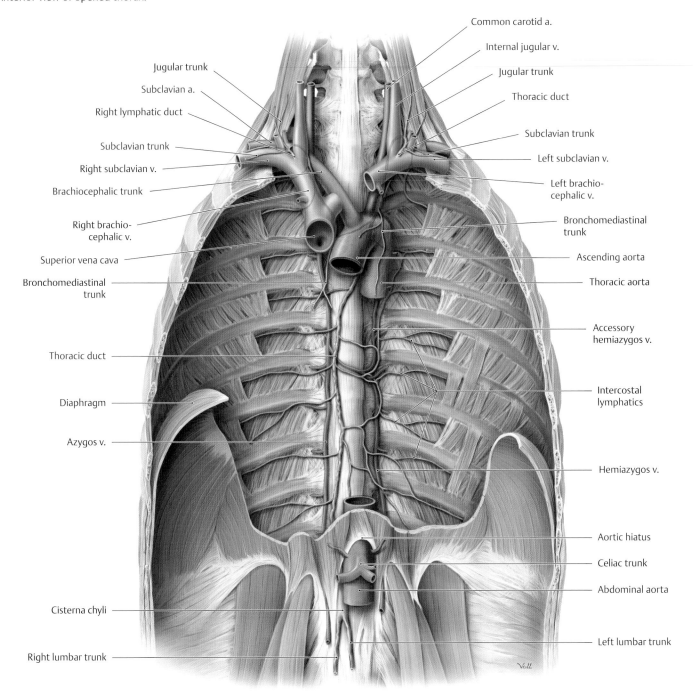

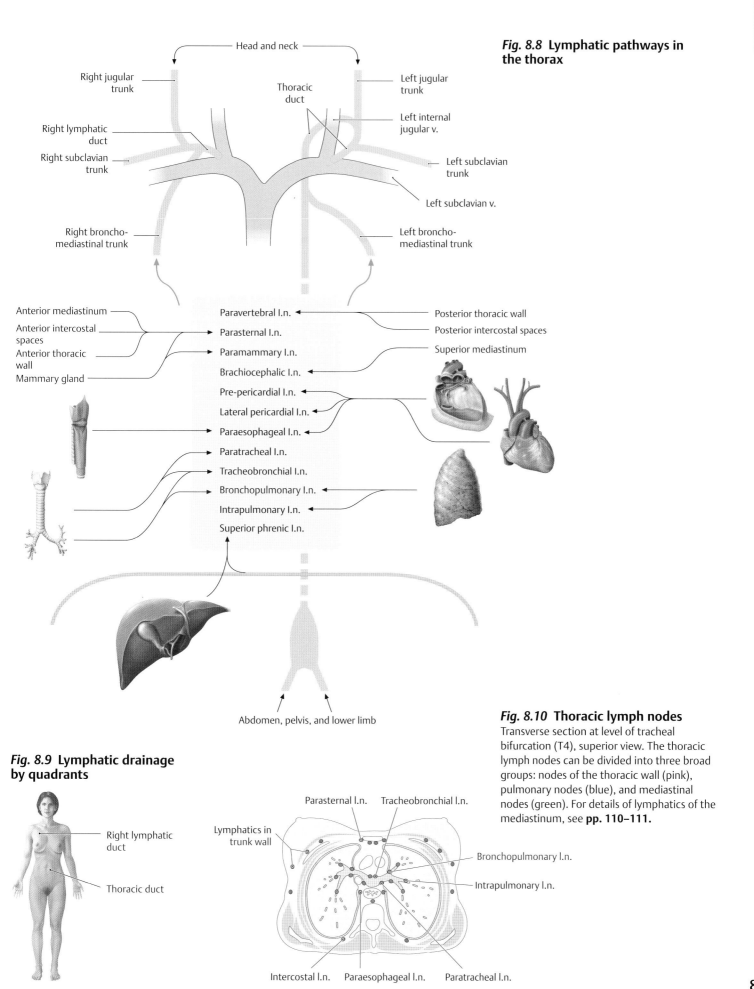

Head and neck

Right jugular
trunk

Thoracic
duct

Left jugular
trunk

Right lymphatic
duct

Left internal
jugular v.

Right subclavian
trunk

Left subclavian
trunk

Left subclavian v.

Right broncho-
mediastinal trunk

Left broncho-
mediastinal trunk

Fig. 8.8 **Lymphatic pathways in the thorax**

Anterior mediastinum

Paravertebral l.n.

Posterior thoracic wall

Anterior intercostal
spaces

Parasternal l.n.

Posterior intercostal spaces

Anterior thoracic
wall

Paramammary l.n.

Superior mediastinum

Mammary gland

Brachiocephalic l.n.

Pre-pericardial l.n.

Lateral pericardial l.n.

Paraesophageal l.n.

Paratracheal l.n.

Tracheobronchial l.n.

Bronchopulmonary l.n.

Intrapulmonary l.n.

Superior phrenic l.n.

Abdomen, pelvis, and lower limb

Fig. 8.9 **Lymphatic drainage by quadrants**

Right lymphatic
duct

Thoracic duct

Fig. 8.10 **Thoracic lymph nodes**
Transverse section at level of tracheal bifurcation (T4), superior view. The thoracic lymph nodes can be divided into three broad groups: nodes of the thoracic wall (pink), pulmonary nodes (blue), and mediastinal nodes (green). For details of lymphatics of the mediastinum, see **pp. 110–111.**

Parasternal l.n.

Tracheobronchial l.n.

Lymphatics in
trunk wall

Bronchopulmonary l.n.

Intrapulmonary l.n.

Intercostal l.n.

Paraesophageal l.n.

Paratracheal l.n.

Nerves of the Thoracic Cavity

 Thoracic innervation is mostly autonomic, arising from the paravertebral sympathetic trunks and parasympathetic vagus nerves. There are two exceptions: the phrenic nerves innervate the pericardium and diaphragm (**p. 66**) and the intercostal nerves innervate the thoracic wall (**p. 70**).

Fig. 8.11 **Nerves in the thorax**
Anterior view of opened thorax.

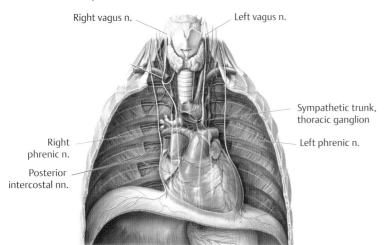

Right vagus n.

Left vagus n.

Sympathetic trunk, thoracic ganglion

Right phrenic n.

Left phrenic n.

Posterior intercostal nn.

A Thoracic innervation.

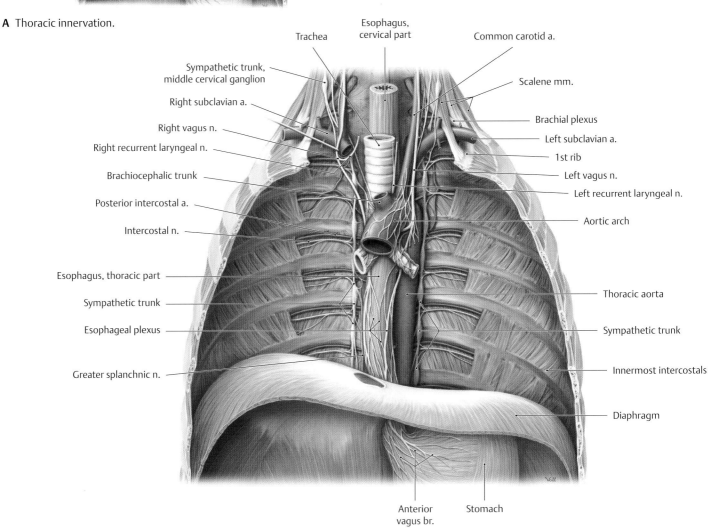

Trachea

Esophagus, cervical part

Common carotid a.

Sympathetic trunk, middle cervical ganglion

Scalene mm.

Right subclavian a.

Brachial plexus

Right vagus n.

Left subclavian a.

Right recurrent laryngeal n.

1st rib

Brachiocephalic trunk

Left vagus n.

Posterior intercostal a.

Left recurrent laryngeal n.

Intercostal n.

Aortic arch

Esophagus, thoracic part

Thoracic aorta

Sympathetic trunk

Sympathetic trunk

Esophageal plexus

Innermost intercostals

Greater splanchnic n.

Diaphragm

Anterior vagus br.

Stomach

B Nerves of the thorax in situ. *Note:* The recurrent laryngeal nerves have been slightly anteriorly retracted; normally, they occupy the groove between the trachea and the esophagus, making them vulnerable during thyroid gland surgery.

The autonomic nervous system innervates smooth muscle, cardiac muscle, and glands. It is subdivided into the sympathetic (red) and parasympathetic (blue) nervous systems, which together regulate blood flow, secretions, and organ function.

Fig. 8.12 Sympathetic and parasympathetic nervous systems in the thorax

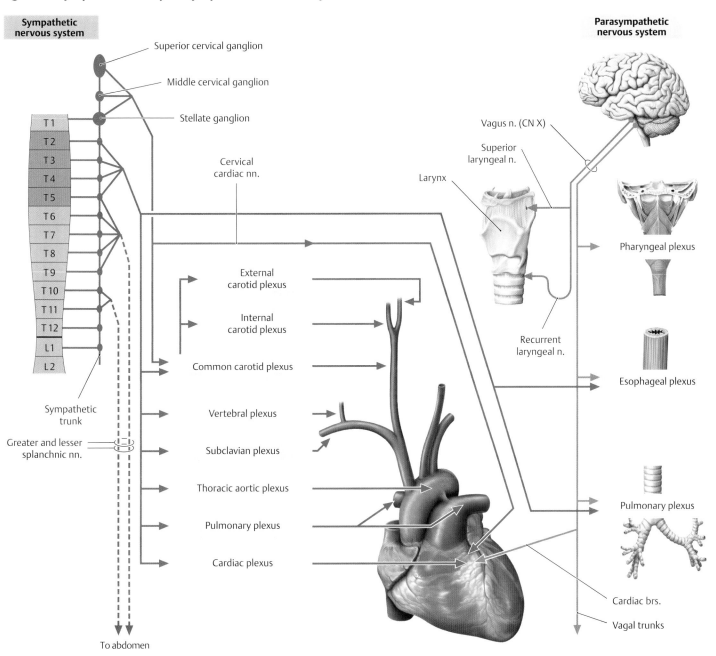

Table 8.4	**Peripheral sympathetic nervous system**		
Origin of pre-ganglionic fibers[*]	**Ganglion cells**	**Course of post-ganglionic fibers**	**Target**
Spinal cord	Sympathetic trunk	Follow intercostal nn.	Blood vessels and glands in chest wall
		Accompany intrathoracic aa.	Visceral targets
		Gather in greater and lesser splanchnic nn.	Abdomen

[*]The axons of preganglionic neurons exit the spinal cord via the anterior roots and synapse with *post*ganglionic neurons in the sympathetic ganglia.

Table 8.5	**Peripheral parasympathetic nervous system**		
Origin of pre-ganglionic fibers	**Course of preganglionic motor axons**[*]		**Target**
Brainstem	Vagus n. (CN X)	Cardiac brs.	Cardiac plexus
		Esophageal brs.	Esophageal plexus
		Tracheal brs.	Trachea
		Bronchial brs.	Pulmonary plexus (bronchi, pulmonary vessels)

[*]The ganglion cells of the parasympathetic nervous system are scattered in microscopic groups in their target organs. The vagus n. thus carries the *pre*ganglionic motor axons to these targets.
CN, cranial n.

Mediastinum: Overview

Thorax

 The mediastinum is the space in the thorax between the pleural sacs of the lungs. It is divided into two parts: superior and inferior.

The inferior mediastinum is further divided into anterior, middle, and posterior portions.

Fig. 9.1 Divisions of the mediastinum

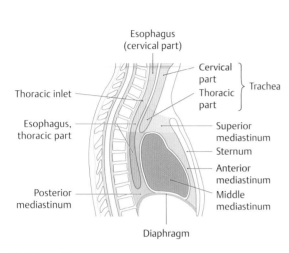

Esophagus (cervical part)

Thoracic inlet

Esophagus, thoracic part

Posterior mediastinum

Cervical part
Thoracic part
} Trachea

Superior mediastinum

Sternum

Anterior mediastinum

Middle mediastinum

Diaphragm

A Schematic.

Table 9.1	Contents of the mediastinum			
	○ Superior mediastinum	Inferior mediastinum		
		○ Anterior	● Middle	○ Posterior
Organs	• Thymus • Trachea • Esophagus	• Thymus, inferior aspects (especially in children)	• Heart • Pericardium	• Esophagus
Arteries	• Aortic arch • Brachiocephalic trunk • Left common carotid a. • Left subclavian a.	• Smaller vessels	• Ascending aorta • Pulmonary trunk and brs. • Pericardiacophrenic aa.	• Thoracic aorta and branches
Veins and lymph vessels	• Superior vena cava • Brachiocephalic vv. • Thoracic duct and right lymphatic duct	• Smaller vessels, lymphatics, and l.n.	• Superior vena cava • Azygos v. • Pulmonary vv. • Pericardiacophrenic vv.	• Azygos v. • Accessory hemiazygous and hemiazygous vv. • Thoracic duct
Nerves	• Vagus nn. • Left recurrent laryngeal n. • Cardiac nn. • Phrenic nn.	• None	• Phrenic nn.	• Vagus nn.

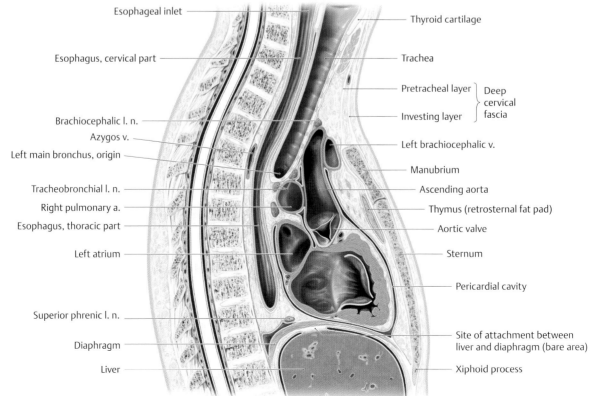

Esophageal inlet

Esophagus, cervical part

Brachiocephalic l. n.

Azygos v.

Left main bronchus, origin

Tracheobronchial l. n.

Right pulmonary a.

Esophagus, thoracic part

Left atrium

Superior phrenic l. n.

Diaphragm

Liver

Thyroid cartilage

Trachea

Pretracheal layer
Investing layer
} Deep cervical fascia

Left brachiocephalic v.

Manubrium

Ascending aorta

Thymus (retrosternal fat pad)

Aortic valve

Sternum

Pericardial cavity

Site of attachment between liver and diaphragm (bare area)

Xiphoid process

B Midsagittal section, right lateral view.

Fig. 9.2 Contents of the mediastinum

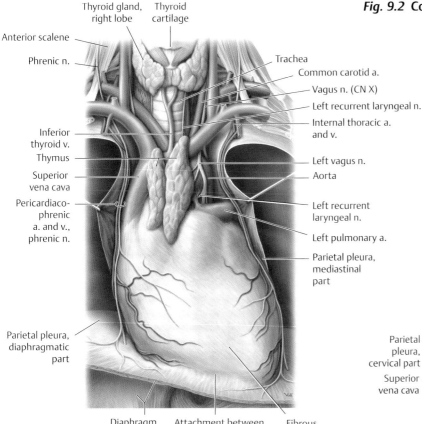

Thyroid gland, right lobe — Thyroid cartilage — Anterior scalene — Phrenic n. — Trachea — Common carotid a. — Vagus n. (CN X) — Left recurrent laryngeal n. — Internal thoracic a. and v. — Inferior thyroid v. — Thymus — Left vagus n. — Aorta — Superior vena cava — Left recurrent laryngeal n. — Pericardiaco-phrenic a. and v., phrenic n. — Left pulmonary a. — Parietal pleura, mediastinal part — Parietal pleura, diaphragmatic part — Diaphragm — Attachment between fibrous pericardium and central tendon of the diaphragm — Fibrous pericardium

A Anterior view. The thymus extends into the anterior division of the inferior mediastinum and grows throughout childhood. At puberty, high levels of circulating sex hormones cause the thymus to atrophy leaving indistinguishable pieces embedded in the fat that now occupies the anterior mediastinum.

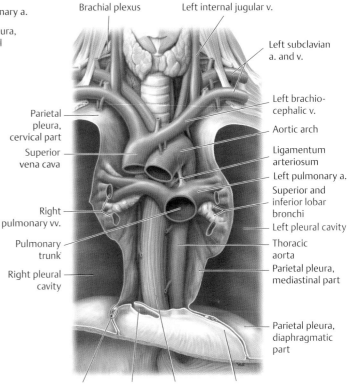

Brachial plexus — Left internal jugular v. — Left subclavian a. and v. — Parietal pleura, cervical part — Superior vena cava — Left brachio-cephalic v. — Aortic arch — Ligamentum arteriosum — Left pulmonary a. — Superior and inferior lobar bronchi — Left pleural cavity — Right pulmonary vv. — Pulmonary trunk — Right pleural cavity — Thoracic aorta — Parietal pleura, mediastinal part — Parietal pleura, diaphragmatic part — Pericardiacophrenic a. and v., phrenic n. — Caval opening — Esophagus, thoracic part — Fibrous pericardium

B Anterior view with heart, pericardium, and thymus removed.

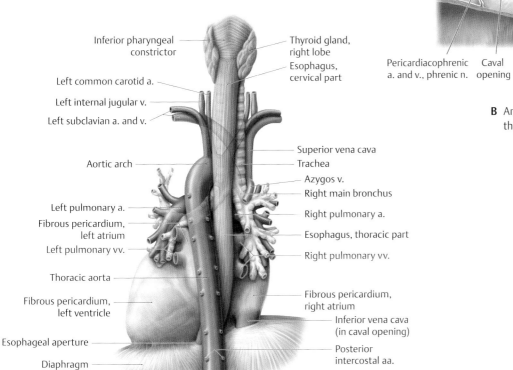

Inferior pharyngeal constrictor — Thyroid gland, right lobe — Esophagus, cervical part — Left common carotid a. — Left internal jugular v. — Left subclavian a. and v. — Aortic arch — Superior vena cava — Trachea — Azygos v. — Right main bronchus — Left pulmonary a. — Right pulmonary a. — Fibrous pericardium, left atrium — Left pulmonary vv. — Esophagus, thoracic part — Right pulmonary vv. — Thoracic aorta — Fibrous pericardium, left ventricle — Fibrous pericardium, right atrium — Inferior vena cava (in caval opening) — Esophageal aperture — Posterior intercostal aa. — Diaphragm

C Posterior view.

Mediastinum: Structures

Fig. 9.3 **Mediastinum**

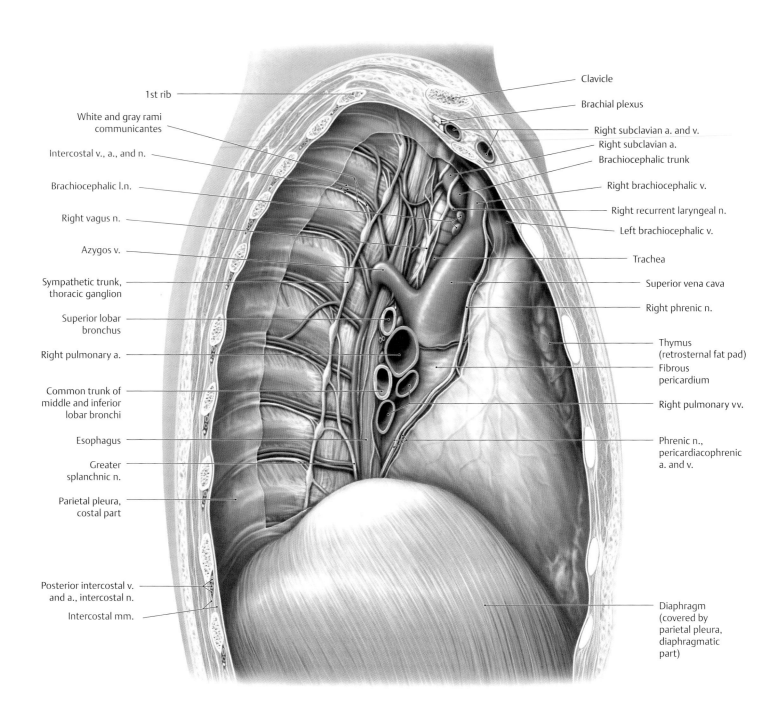

Clavicle
Brachial plexus
Right subclavian a. and v.
Right subclavian a.
Brachiocephalic trunk
Right brachiocephalic v.
Right recurrent laryngeal n.
Left brachiocephalic v.
Trachea
Superior vena cava
Right phrenic n.
Thymus (retrosternal fat pad)
Fibrous pericardium
Right pulmonary vv.
Phrenic n., pericardiacophrenic a. and v.
Diaphragm (covered by parietal pleura, diaphragmatic part)

1st rib
White and gray rami communicantes
Intercostal v., a., and n.
Brachiocephalic l.n.
Right vagus n.
Azygos v.
Sympathetic trunk, thoracic ganglion
Superior lobar bronchus
Right pulmonary a.
Common trunk of middle and inferior lobar bronchi
Esophagus
Greater splanchnic n.
Parietal pleura, costal part
Posterior intercostal v. and a., intercostal n.
Intercostal mm.

A Right lateral view, parasagittal section. Note the many structures passing between the superior and inferior (middle and posterior) mediastinum.

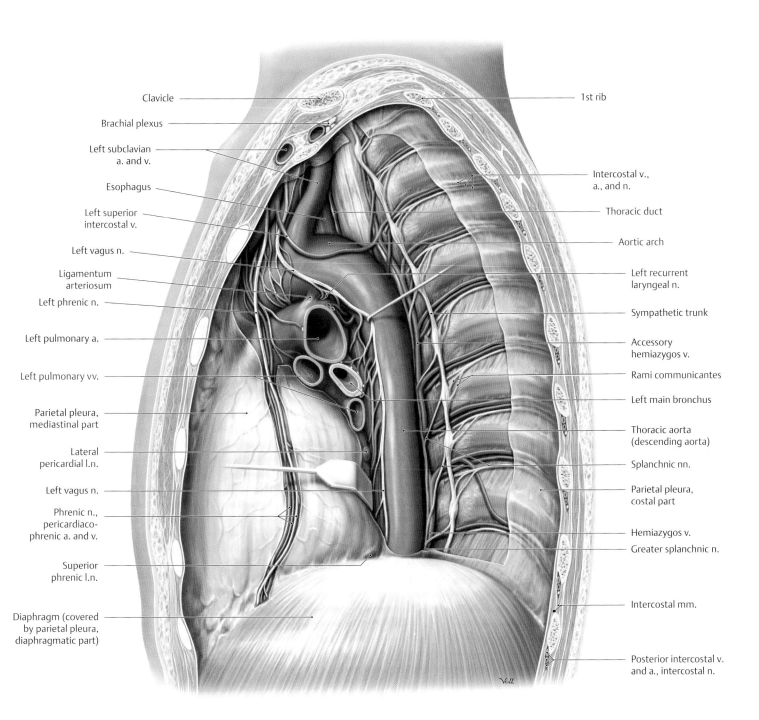

Clavicle

Brachial plexus

Left subclavian a. and v.

Esophagus

Left superior intercostal v.

Left vagus n.

Ligamentum arteriosum

Left phrenic n.

Left pulmonary a.

Left pulmonary vv.

Parietal pleura, mediastinal part

Lateral pericardial l.n.

Left vagus n.

Phrenic n., pericardiaco-phrenic a. and v.

Superior phrenic l.n.

Diaphragm (covered by parietal pleura, diaphragmatic part)

1st rib

Intercostal v., a., and n.

Thoracic duct

Aortic arch

Left recurrent laryngeal n.

Sympathetic trunk

Accessory hemiazygos v.

Rami communicantes

Left main bronchus

Thoracic aorta (descending aorta)

Splanchnic nn.

Parietal pleura, costal part

Hemiazygos v.

Greater splanchnic n.

Intercostal mm.

Posterior intercostal v. and a., intercostal n.

B Left lateral view, parasagittal section. *Removed:* Left lung and parietal pleura. *Revealed:* Posterior mediastinal structures.

Heart: Functions and Relations

 The heart pumps the blood: unoxygenated blood to the lungs and oxygenated blood throughout the body. It is located posterior to the sternum in the middle portion of the mediastinum in the pericardial cavity, located between the right and left pleural cavities containing the lungs. The cone-shaped heart points anteriorly and to the left in the thoracic cavity.

Fig. 9.4 Circulation
Oxygenated blood is shown in red; deoxygenated blood in blue. See **p. 104** for prenatal circulation.

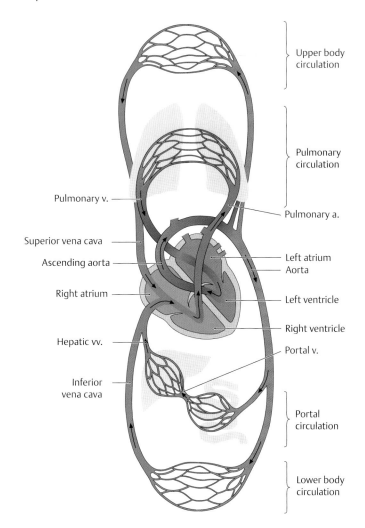

Fig. 9.5 Topographical relations of the heart

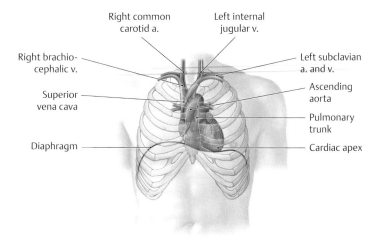

A Projection of the heart and great vessels onto chest, anterior view.

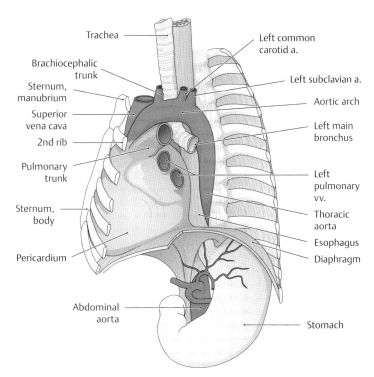

B Left lateral view. *Removed:* Left thoracic wall and left lung.

Fig. 9.6 Heart in situ

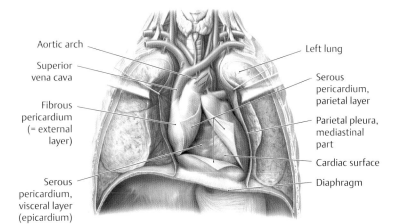

A Anterior view of the opened thorax with the thymus removed and flaps of the anterior pericardium reflected to reveal the heart.

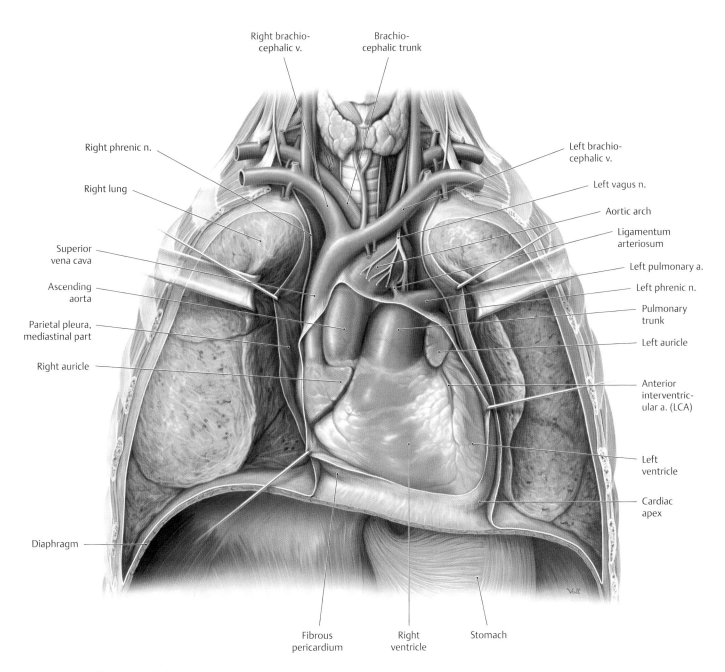

B Anterior view of the opened thorax with thymus and anterior pericardium removed to reveal the heart.

Pericardium

Fig. 9.7 Posterior pericardial cavity

Anterior view of opened thorax with the anterior pericardium removed. The heart has been partially elevated to reveal the posterior pericardial cavity and the oblique pericardial sinus.

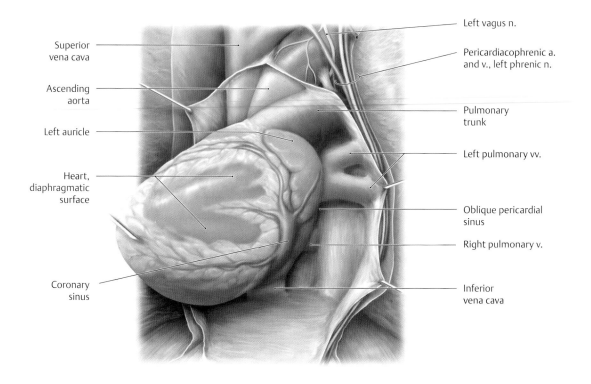

Superior vena cava — Left vagus n. — Pericardiacophrenic a. and v., left phrenic n. — Ascending aorta — Pulmonary trunk — Left auricle — Left pulmonary vv. — Heart, diaphragmatic surface — Oblique pericardial sinus — Right pulmonary v. — Coronary sinus — Inferior vena cava

Fig. 9.8 Posterior pericardium

Anterior view of the opened thorax with the anterior pericardium and heart removed to reveal the posterior pericardium and the oblique pericardial sinus. The transverse pericardial sinus is the passage between the reflections of the serous layer of the pericardium around the arterial and venous great vessels of the heart.

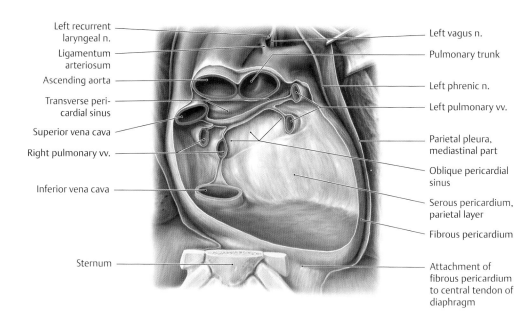

Left recurrent laryngeal n. — Left vagus n. — Ligamentum arteriosum — Pulmonary trunk — Ascending aorta — Left phrenic n. — Transverse pericardial sinus — Superior vena cava — Left pulmonary vv. — Right pulmonary vv. — Parietal pleura, mediastinal part — Inferior vena cava — Oblique pericardial sinus — Serous pericardium, parietal layer — Fibrous pericardium — Sternum — Attachment of fibrous pericardium to central tendon of diaphragm

Fig. 9.9 **Posterior relations of the heart**

Anterior view of the opened thorax with the anterior pericardium and heart removed and a window cut in the posterior pericardium to reveal the structures immediately posterior to the heart. This shows the close relationship of the esophagus to the heart, which is used in the trans-esophageal sonogram to assess the left atrium of the heart.

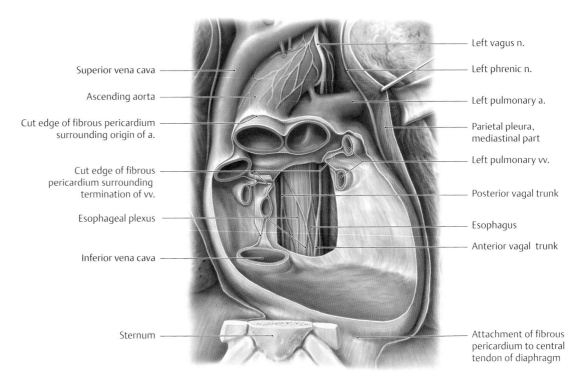

Superior vena cava

Ascending aorta

Cut edge of fibrous pericardium surrounding origin of a.

Cut edge of fibrous pericardium surrounding termination of vv.

Esophageal plexus

Inferior vena cava

Sternum

Left vagus n.

Left phrenic n.

Left pulmonary a.

Parietal pleura, mediastinal part

Left pulmonary vv.

Posterior vagal trunk

Esophagus

Anterior vagal trunk

Attachment of fibrous pericardium to central tendon of diaphragm

Fig. 9.10 **Pericardium, pericardial cavity, and transverse pericardial sinus**

Sagittal section through the mediastinum. The fibrous pericardium is attached to the central tendon of the diaphragm and is continuous with the outer layer of the great vessels. The parietal layer of serous pericardium lines the inner surface of the fibrous pericardium and the visceral layer adheres to the heart. The pericardial cavity, the space between the parietal and visceral layers of serous pericardium around the heart, is filled with a thin layer of serous fluid that allows for frictionless movement. Where the parietal and visceral layers of serous pericardium reach and reflect around the great vessels, they are continuous with one another. The passage between the arterial and venous reflections of the serous pericardium is the transverse pericardial sinus.

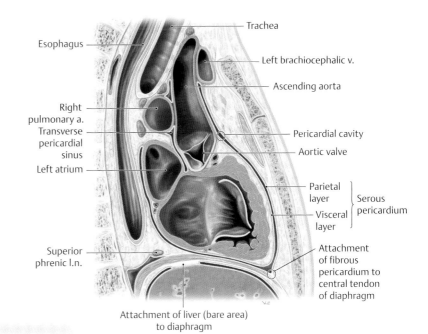

Esophagus

Right pulmonary a.
Transverse pericardial sinus
Left atrium

Superior phrenic l.n.

Trachea

Left brachiocephalic v.

Ascending aorta

Pericardial cavity

Aortic valve

Parietal layer } Serous
Visceral layer } pericardium

Attachment of fibrous pericardium to central tendon of diaphragm

Attachment of liver (bare area) to diaphragm

 Clinical box 9.1

Cardiac Tamponade

Rapid increases of fluid or blood within the pericardial sac inhibits full expansion of the heart, reducing cardiac blood return, thus decreasing cardiac output. This condition, cardiac tamponade (compression), is potentially fatal, unless relieved. The fluid or blood must first be removed to restore cardiac function and then the cause of the fluid or blood accumulation corrected.

Heart: Surfaces & Chambers

 Note the reflection of visceral serous pericardium to become parietal serous pericardium.

Fig. 9.11 Surfaces of the heart

The heart has three surfaces: anterior (sternocostal), posterior (base), and inferior (diaphragmatic).

Left subclavian a.

Left common carotid a.

Aortic arch

Ligamentum arteriosum

Brachio-cephalic trunk

Left pulmonary a.

Right pulmonary a.

Left pulmonary vv.

Superior vena cava

Pulmonary trunk

Ascending aorta

Left auricle

Right auricle

Fibrous pericardium (cut edge)

Right atrium

Anterior inter-ventricular sulcus

Coronary (right atrioventricular) sulcus

Left ventricle

Right ventricle

Inferior vena cava

Cardiac apex

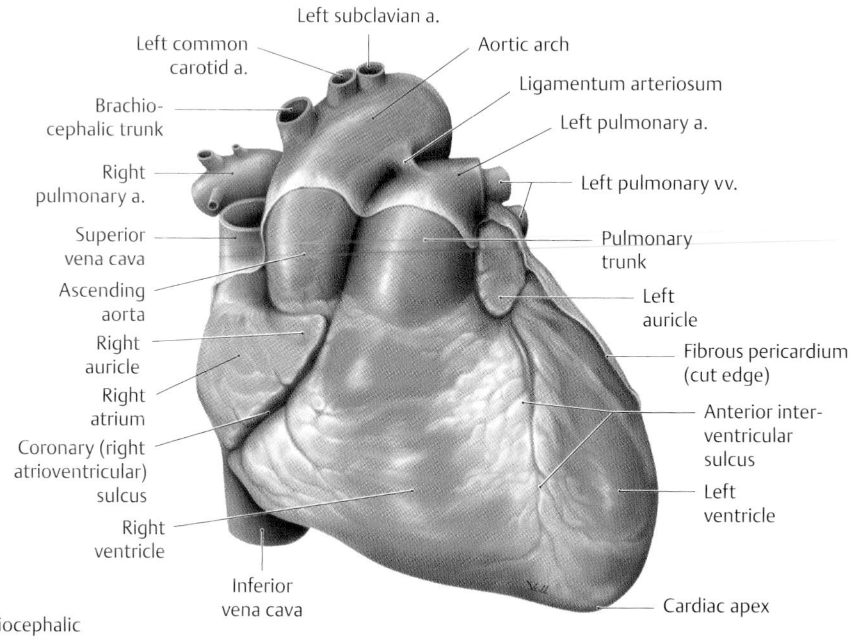

A Anterior (sternocostal) surface.

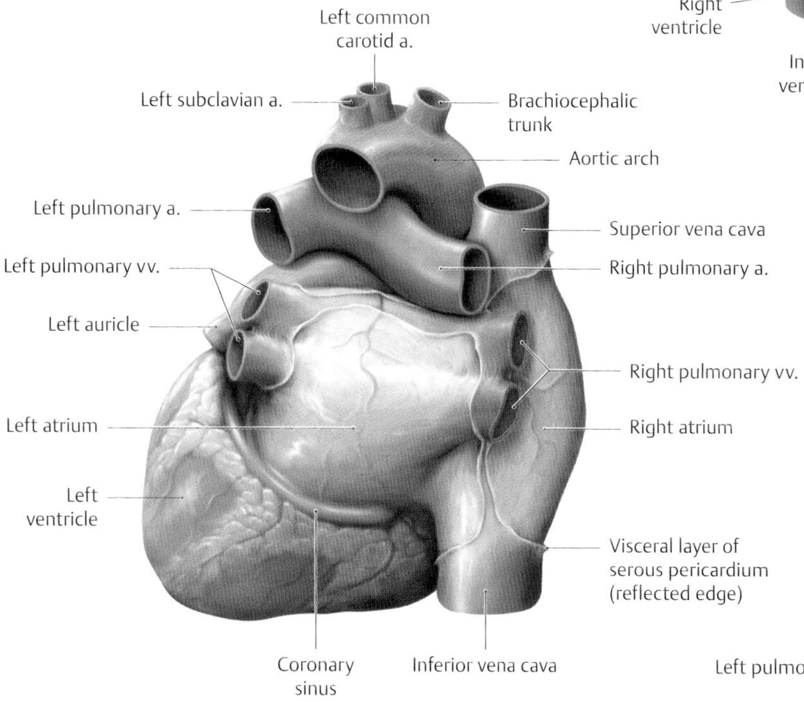

Left common carotid a.

Left subclavian a.

Brachiocephalic trunk

Aortic arch

Left pulmonary a.

Superior vena cava

Left pulmonary vv.

Right pulmonary a.

Left auricle

Left atrium

Right pulmonary vv.

Right atrium

Left ventricle

Coronary sinus

Inferior vena cava

Visceral layer of serous pericardium (reflected edge)

B Posterior surface (base).

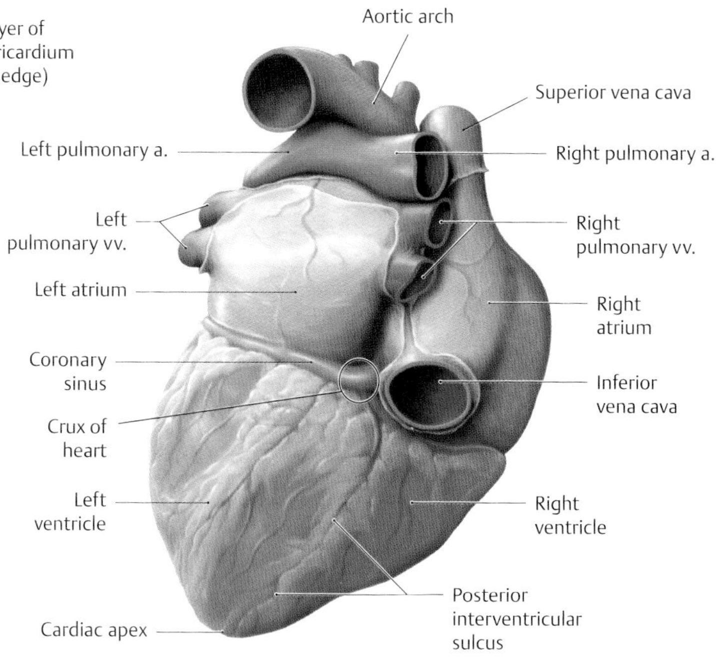

Aortic arch

Superior vena cava

Left pulmonary a.

Right pulmonary a.

Left pulmonary vv.

Right pulmonary vv.

Left atrium

Right atrium

Coronary sinus

Inferior vena cava

Crux of heart

Left ventricle

Right ventricle

Posterior interventricular sulcus

Cardiac apex

C Inferior (diaphragmatic) surface.

Fig. 9.12 **Chambers of the heart**

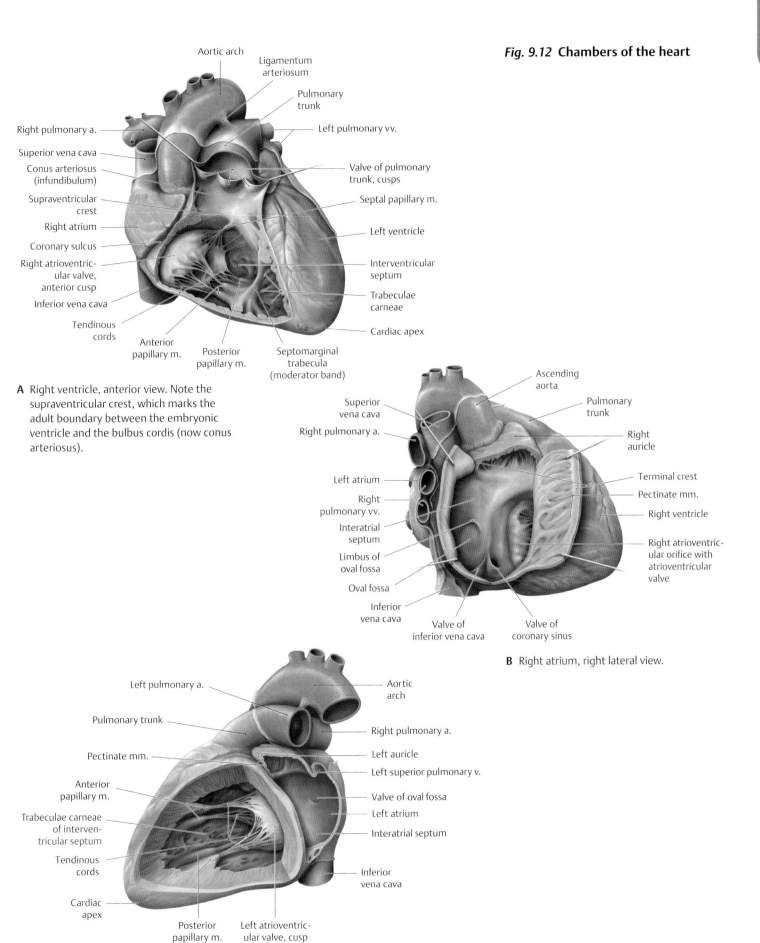

A Right ventricle, anterior view. Note the supraventricular crest, which marks the adult boundary between the embryonic ventricle and the bulbus cordis (now conus arteriosus).

B Right atrium, right lateral view.

C Left atrium and ventricle, left lateral view. Note the irregular trabeculae carneae characteristic of the ventricular wall.

97

Heart: Valves

 The cardiac valves are divided into two groups: semilunar and atrioventricular. The two semilunar valves (aortic and pulmonary) located at the base of the two great arteries of the heart regulate passage of blood from the ventricles to the aorta and pulmonary trunk. The two atrioventricular valves (left and right) lie at the interface between the atria and ventricles.

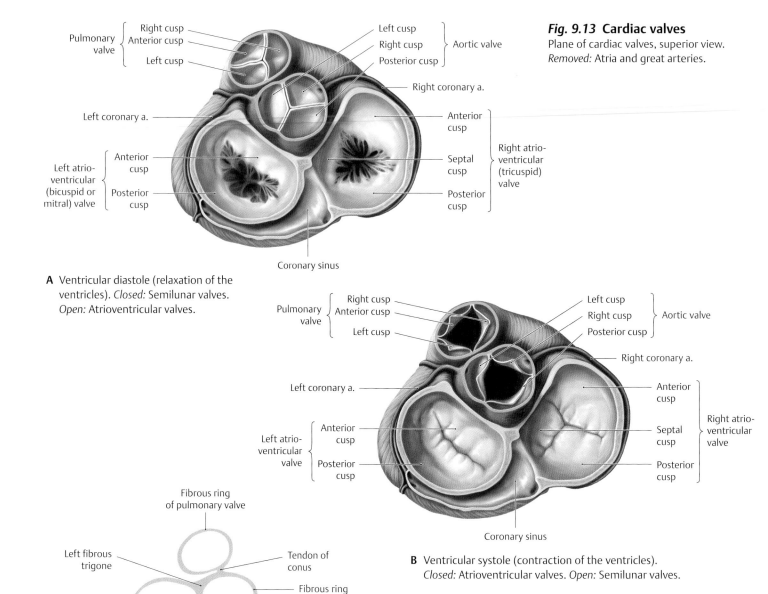

Fig. 9.13 Cardiac valves
Plane of cardiac valves, superior view. *Removed:* Atria and great arteries.

A Ventricular diastole (relaxation of the ventricles). *Closed:* Semilunar valves. *Open:* Atrioventricular valves.

B Ventricular systole (contraction of the ventricles). *Closed:* Atrioventricular valves. *Open:* Semilunar valves.

C Cardiac skeleton, superior view. The cardiac skeleton is formed by dense fibrous connective tissue. The fibrous anuli (rings) and intervening trigones separate the atria from the ventricles. This provides mechanical stability, electrical insulation (see **p. 102** for cardiac conduction system), and an attachment point for the cardiac muscles and valve cusps.

Table 9.2	Position and auscultation sites of cardiac valves	
Valve	**Anatomical projection**	**Auscultation site**
Aortic valve	Left sternal border (at level of 3rd rib)	Right 2nd intercostal space (at sternal margin)
Pulmonary valve	Left sternal border (at level of 3rd costal cartilage)	Left 2nd intercostal space (at sternal margin)
Left atrioventricular valve	Left 4th/5th costal cartilage	Left 5th intercostal space (at midclavicular line) or cardiac apex
Right atrioventricular valve	Sternum (at level of 5th costal cartilage)	Left 5th intercostal space (at sternal margin)

Fig. 9.14 Semilunar valves

Valves have been longitudinally sectioned and opened.

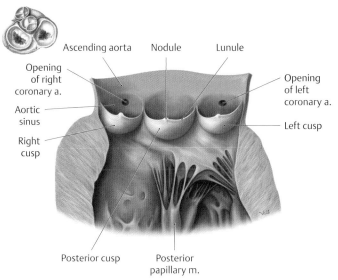

A Aortic valve.

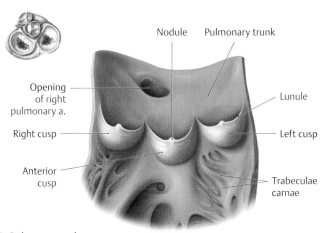

B Pulmonary valve.

Fig. 9.15 Atrioventricular valves

Anterior view during ventricular systole.

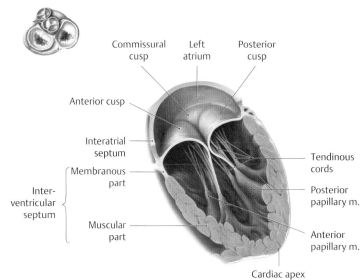

A Left atrioventricular valve.

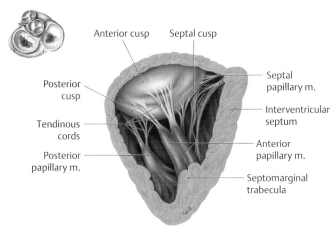

B Right atrioventricular valve.

Clinical box 9.2

Auscultation of the cardiac valves

Heart sounds, produced by closure of the semilunar and atrioventricular valves, are carried by the blood flowing through the valve. The resulting sounds are therefore best heard "downstream," at defined auscultation sites (dark circles on diagram). Valvular heart disease causes turbulent blood flow through the valve; this produces a murmur that may be detected in the region of ascultation.

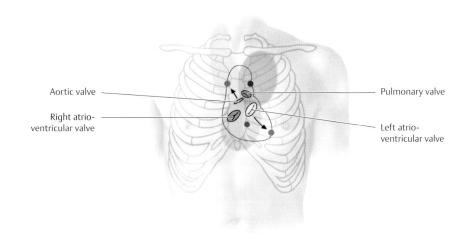

Arteries & Veins of the Heart

Fig. 9.16 **Coronary arteries and cardiac veins**

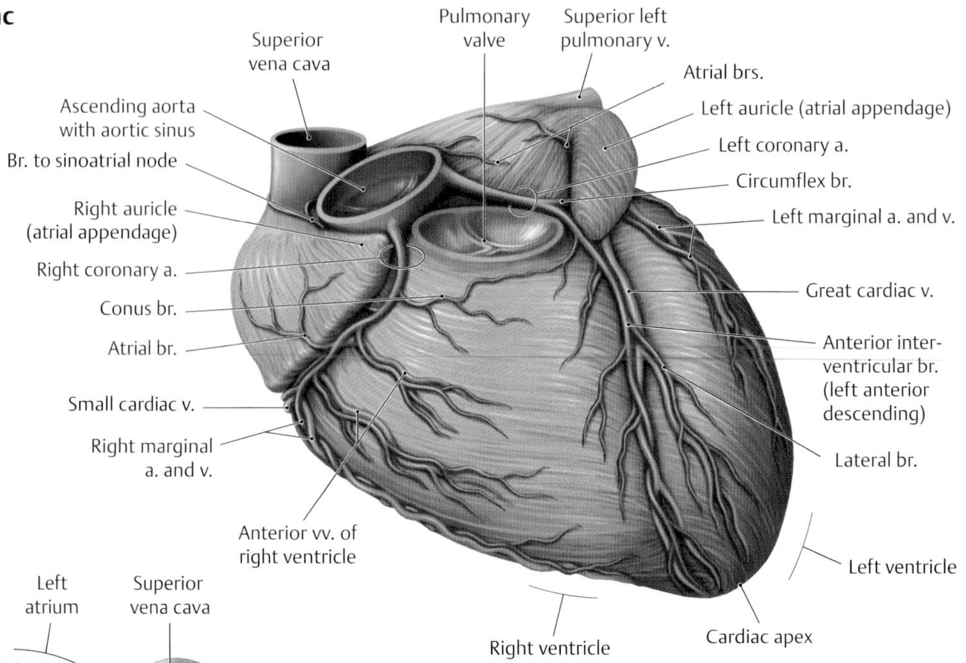

Pulmonary valve
Superior left pulmonary v.
Superior vena cava
Ascending aorta with aortic sinus
Br. to sinoatrial node
Right auricle (atrial appendage)
Right coronary a.
Conus br.
Atrial br.
Small cardiac v.
Right marginal a. and v.
Anterior vv. of right ventricle
Atrial brs.
Left auricle (atrial appendage)
Left coronary a.
Circumflex br.
Left marginal a. and v.
Great cardiac v.
Anterior inter-ventricular br. (left anterior descending)
Lateral br.
Left ventricle
Cardiac apex
Right ventricle

A Anterior view.

Oblique v. of left atrium
Atrial brs.
Left atrium
Superior vena cava
Left pulmonary vv.
Circumflex br.
Great cardiac v.
Left marginal v.
Br. to sinoatrial node
Right pulmonary vv.
Right atrium
Coronary sinus
Inferior vena cava
Right coronary a.
Small cardiac v.
Right ventricle
Left posterior ventricular v.
Right posterolateral a.
Left ventricle
Posterior interventricular a. (posterior descending a.)
Middle cardiac v.

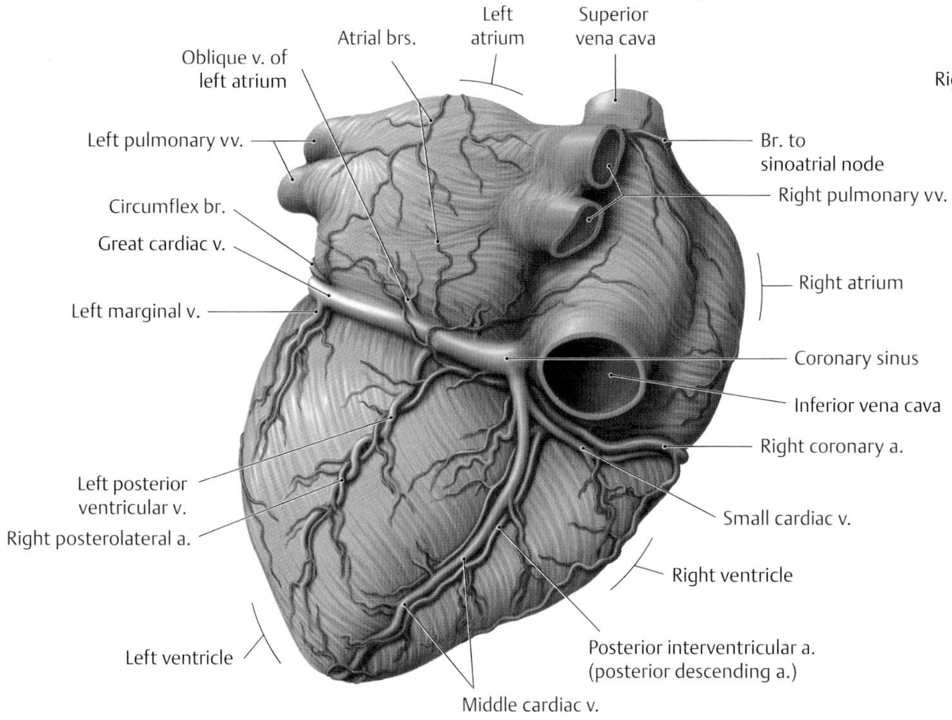

B Posteroinferior view. *Note*: The right and left coronary arteries typically anastomose posteriorly at the left atrium and ventricle.

Table 9.3	Branches of the coronary arteries
Left coronary artery	**Right coronary artery**
Circumflex br. • Atrial br. • Left marginal a. • Posterior left ventricular br.	Br. to SA node
	Conus br.
	Atrial br.
	Right marginal a.
Anterior interventricular br. (left anterior descending) • Conus br. • Lateral br. • Interventricular septal brs.	Posterior interventricular br. (posterior descending) • Interventricular septal brs.
	Br. to AV node
	Right posterolateral a.
AV, atrioventricular; SA, sinoatrial.	

Table 9.4	Divisions of the cardiac veins	
Vein	**Tributaries**	**Drainage to**
Anterior cardiac vv. (not shown)		Right atrium
Great cardiac v.	Anterior interventricular v.	Coronary sinus
	Left marginal v.	
	Oblique v. of left atrium	
Left posterior ventricular v.		
Middle cardiac v. (posterior interventricular v.)		
Small cardiac v.	Anterior vv. of right ventricle	
	Right marginal v.	

Fig. 9.17 Distribution of the coronary arteries

Anterior and posterior views of the heart, with superior views of transverse sections through the ventricles. The "distribution" of the coronary arteries refers to the area of the myocardium supplied by each artery, as seen in the transverse views, but the term "dominance" refers to the artery that gives rise to the posterior interventricular artery, as seen in the anterior and posterior views. Right coronary artery and branches (green); left coronary artery and branches (red).

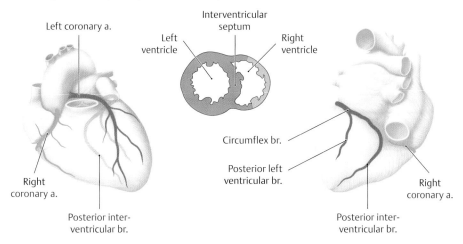

A Left coronary dominance (15–17%).

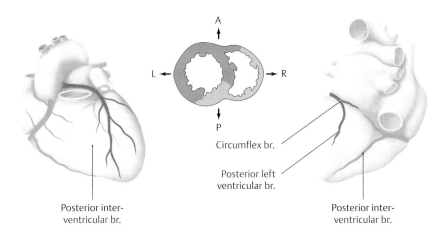

B Balanced distribution, right coronary artery dominance (67–70%).

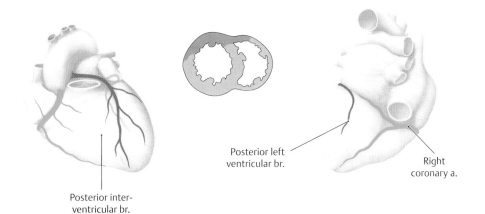

C Right coronary dominance (~15%).

Clinical box 9.3

Disturbed coronary blood flow

Although the coronary arteries are connected by structural anastomoses, they are end arteries from a functional standpoint. The most frequent cause of deficient blood flow is *atherosclerosis*, a narrowing of the coronary lumen due to plaque-like deposits on the vessel wall. When the decrease in luminal size (stenosis) reaches a critical point, coronary blood flow is restricted, causing chest pain (*angina pectoris*). Initially, this pain is induced by physical effort, but eventually it persists at rest, often radiating to characteristic sites (e.g., medial side of left upper limb, left side of head and neck). A myocardial infarction occurs when deficient blood supply causes myocardial tissue to die (necrosis). The location and extent of the infarction depends on the stenosed vessel (see **A–E**, after Heinecker).

A Supra-apical anterior infarction.

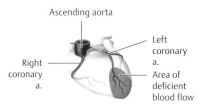

B Apical anterior infarction.

C Anterior lateral infarction.

D Posterior lateral infarction.

E Posterior infarction.

Conduction & Innervation of the Heart

Contraction of cardiac muscle is modulated by the cardiac conduction system. This system of specialized myocardial cells (Purkinje fibers) generates and conducts excitatory impulses in the heart. The conduction system contains two nodes, both located in the right atrium: the sinoatrial (SA) node, known as the pacemaker, and the atrioventricular (AV) node.

Fig. 9.18 Cardiac conduction system

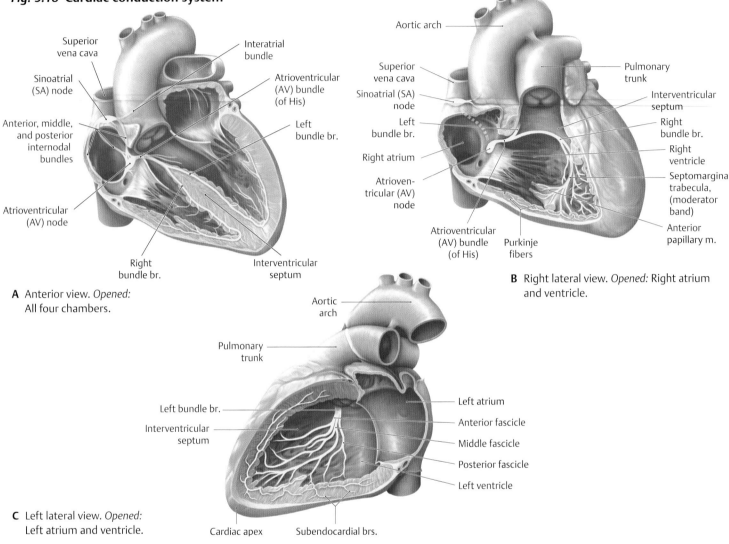

A Anterior view. *Opened:* All four chambers.

Superior vena cava
Sinoatrial (SA) node
Anterior, middle, and posterior internodal bundles
Atrioventricular (AV) node
Interatrial bundle
Atrioventricular (AV) bundle (of His)
Left bundle br.
Right bundle br.
Interventricular septum

B Right lateral view. *Opened:* Right atrium and ventricle.

Aortic arch
Superior vena cava
Sinoatrial (SA) node
Left bundle br.
Right atrium
Atrioventricular (AV) node
Atrioventricular (AV) bundle (of His)
Purkinje fibers
Pulmonary trunk
Interventricular septum
Right bundle br.
Right ventricle
Septomargina trabecula, (moderator band)
Anterior papillary m.

C Left lateral view. *Opened:* Left atrium and ventricle.

Aortic arch
Pulmonary trunk
Left bundle br.
Interventricular septum
Cardiac apex
Subendocardial brs.
Left atrium
Anterior fascicle
Middle fascicle
Posterior fascicle
Left ventricle

 Clinical box 9.4

Electrocardiogram (ECG)

The cardiac impulse (a physical dipole) travels across the heart and may be detected with electrodes. The use of three electrodes that separately record electrical activity of the heart along three axes or vectors (Einthoven limb leads) generates an electrocardiogram (ECG). The ECG graphs the cardiac cycle ("heartbeat"), reducing it to a series of waves, segments, and intervals. These ECG components can be used to determine whether cardiac impulses are normal or abnormal (e.g., myocardial infarction, chamber enlargement). *Note:* Although only three leads are required, a standard ECG examination includes at least two others (Goldberger, Wilson leads).

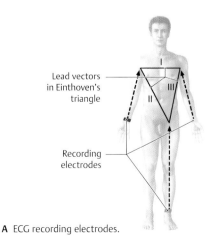

A ECG recording electrodes.

Lead vectors in Einthoven's triangle
Recording electrodes

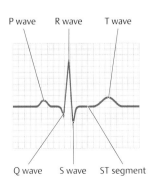

B ECG.

P wave   R wave   T wave
Q wave   S wave   ST segment

Sympathetic innervation: Preganglionic neurons from T1 to T6 spinal cord segments send fibers to synapse on postganglionic neurons in the cervical and upper thoracic sympathetic ganglia. The three cervical cardiac nerves and thoracic cardiac branches contribute to the cardiac plexus. Parasympathetic innervation: Preganglionic neurons and fibers reach the heart via cardiac branches, some of which also arise in the cervical region. They synapse on postganglionic neurons near the SA node and along the coronary arteries.

Fig. 9.19 **Autonomic innervation of the heart**

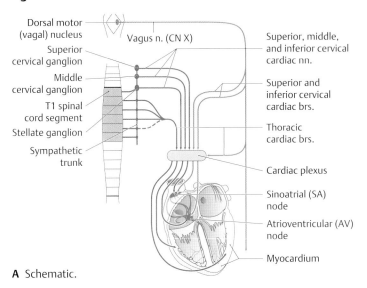

A Schematic.

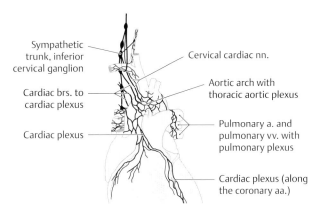

B Autonomic plexuses of the heart, right lateral view. Note the continuity between the cardiac, aortic, and pulmonary plexuses.

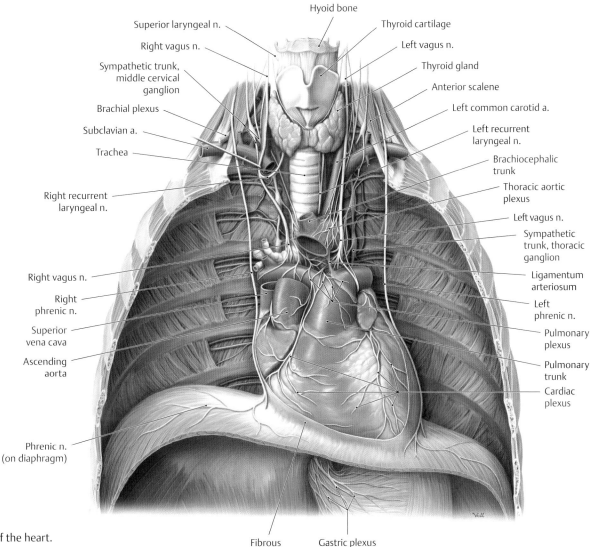

C Autonomic nerves of the heart.
Anterior view of opened thorax.

Pre- & Postnatal Circulation

Fig. 9.20 **Prenatal circulation**
After Fritsch and Kühnel.

① Oxygenated and nutrient-rich fetal blood from the placenta passes to the fetus via the umbilical *vein*.

② Approximately half of this blood bypasses the liver (via the ductus venosus) and enters the inferior vena cava. The remainder enters the portal vein to supply the liver with nutrients and oxygen.

③ Blood entering the right atrium from the inferior vena cava bypasses the right ventricle (as the lungs are not yet functioning) to enter the left atrium via the oval foramen, a right-to-left shunt.

④ Blood from the superior vena cava enters the right atrium, passes to the right ventricle, and moves into the pulmonary trunk. Most of this blood enters the aorta via the ductus arteriosus, a right-to-left shunt.

⑤ The partially oxygenated blood in the aorta returns to the placenta via the paired umbilical arteries that arise from the internal iliac arteries.

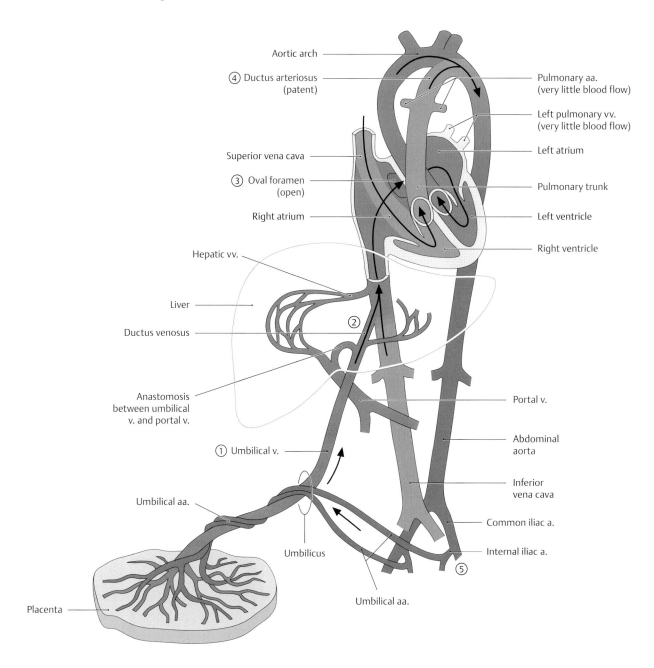

① As pulmonary respiration begins at birth, pulmonary blood pressure falls, causing blood from the right pulmonary trunk to enter the pulmonary arteries.

② The foramen ovale and ductus arteriosus close, eliminating the fetal right-to-left shunts. The pulmonary and systemic circulations in the heart are now separate.

③ As the infant is separated from the placenta, the umbilical arteries occlude (except for the proximal portions), along with the umbilical vein and ductus venosus.

④ Blood to be metabolized now passes through the liver.

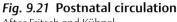

Fig. 9.21 Postnatal circulation
After Fritsch and Kühnel.

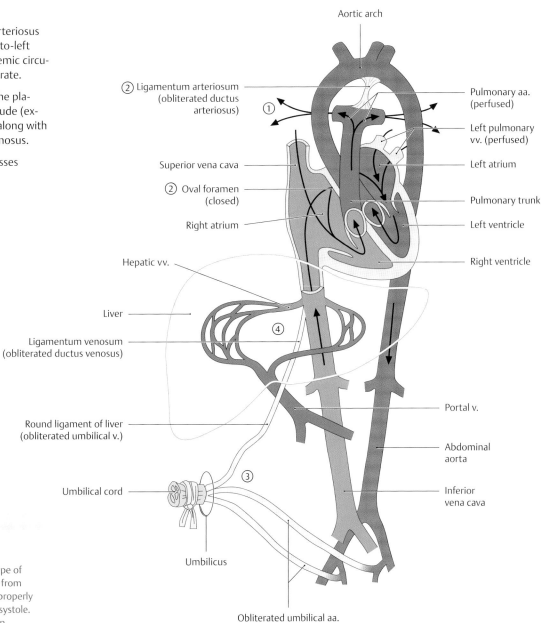

Aortic arch

② Ligamentum arteriosum (obliterated ductus arteriosus)
①

Pulmonary aa. (perfused)

Left pulmonary vv. (perfused)

Superior vena cava

Left atrium

② Oval foramen (closed)

Pulmonary trunk

Right atrium

Left ventricle

Hepatic vv.

Right ventricle

Liver

Ligamentum venosum (obliterated ductus venosus)

④

Round ligament of liver (obliterated umbilical v.)

Portal v.

Abdominal aorta

Umbilical cord

③

Inferior vena cava

Umbilicus

Obliterated umbilical aa. (medial umbilical ligaments)

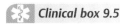 **Clinical box 9.5**

Septal defects
Septal defects, the most common type of congenital heart defect, allow blood from the left chambers of the heart to improperly pass into the right chambers during systole. Ventricular septal defect (VSD, shown below) is a defect in either the membranous or muscular portion of the ventricular septum—most commonly the membranous portion. Patent foramen ovale, the most prevalent form of *atrial* septal defect (ASD), results from improper closure of the fetal shunt. LV, left ventricle; RV, right ventricle.

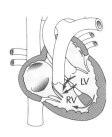

Table 9.5	Derivatives of fetal circulatory structures
Fetal structure	**Adult remnant**
Ductus arteriosus	Ligamentum arteriosum
Foramen ovale	Oval fossa
Ductus venosus	Ligamentum venosum
Umbilical v.	Round lig. of the liver (ligamentum teres)
Umbilical a.	Medial umbilical lig.

Esophagus

 The esophagus is divided into three parts: cervical (C6–T1), thoracic (T1 to the esophageal hiatus of the diaphragm), and abdominal (the diaphragm to the cardiac orifice of the stomach).

It descends slightly to the right of the thoracic aorta and pierces the diaphragm slightly to the left, just below the xiphoid process of the sternum.

Fig. 9.22 Esophagus: Location and constrictions

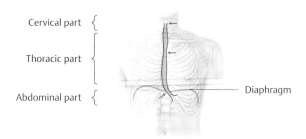

Cervical part

Thoracic part

Abdominal part

Diaphragm

A Projection of esophagus onto chest wall. Esophageal constrictions are indicated with arrows.

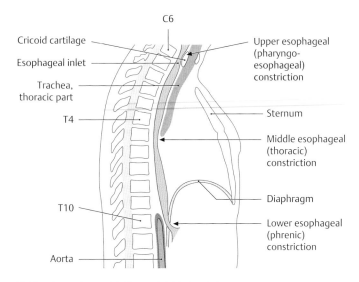

C6

Cricoid cartilage

Esophageal inlet

Trachea, thoracic part

T4

T10

Aorta

Upper esophageal (pharyngo-esophageal) constriction

Sternum

Middle esophageal (thoracic) constriction

Diaphragm

Lower esophageal (phrenic) constriction

B Esophageal constrictions, right lateral view.

Fig. 9.23 Esophagus in situ
Anterior view.

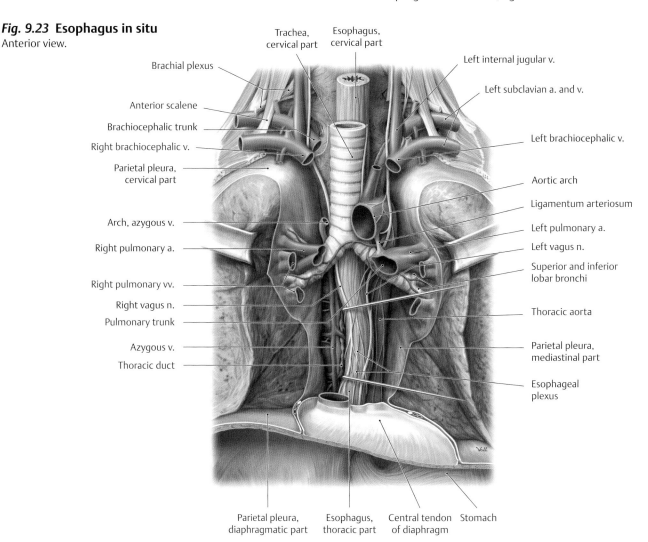

Trachea, cervical part

Esophagus, cervical part

Brachial plexus

Anterior scalene

Brachiocephalic trunk

Right brachiocephalic v.

Parietal pleura, cervical part

Arch, azygous v.

Right pulmonary a.

Right pulmonary vv.

Right vagus n.

Pulmonary trunk

Azygous v.

Thoracic duct

Left internal jugular v.

Left subclavian a. and v.

Left brachiocephalic v.

Aortic arch

Ligamentum arteriosum

Left pulmonary a.

Left vagus n.

Superior and inferior lobar bronchi

Thoracic aorta

Parietal pleura, mediastinal part

Esophageal plexus

Parietal pleura, diaphragmatic part

Esophagus, thoracic part

Central tendon of diaphragm

Stomach

Fig. 9.24 Structure of the esophagus

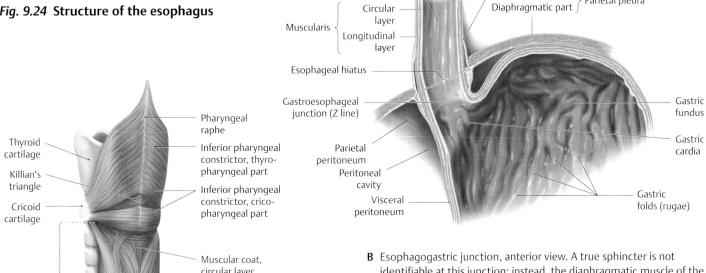

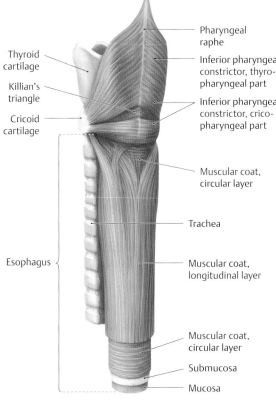

A Esophageal wall, oblique left posterior view. Pharynx (**p. 612**); trachea (**p. 120**).

B Esophagogastric junction, anterior view. A true sphincter is not identifiable at this junction; instead, the diaphragmatic muscle of the esophageal hiatus functions as a sphincter. It is often referred to as the "Z line" because of its zigzag form.

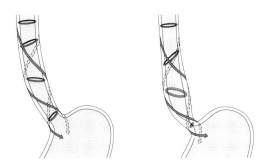

C Functional architecture of esophageal muscle.

Clinical box 9.6

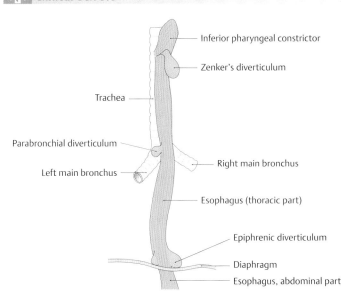

Esophageal diverticula

Diverticula (abnormal outpouchings or sacs) generally develop at weak spots in the esophageal wall. There are three main types of esophageal diverticula:

- Hypopharyngeal (pharyngo-esophageal) diverticula: Outpouchings occurring at the junction of the pharynx and the esophagus. These include Zenker's diverticula (70% of cases).

- "True" traction diverticula: Protrusion of all wall layers, not typically occurring at characteristic weak spots. However, they generally result from an inflammatory process (e.g., lymphangitis) and are thus common at sites where the esophagus closely approaches the bronchi and bronchial lymph nodes (thoracic or parabronchial diverticula).

- "False" pulsion diverticula: Herniations of the mucosa and submucosa through weak spots in the muscular coat due to a rise in esophageal pressure (e.g., during normal swallowing). These include parahiatal and epiphrenic diverticula occurring above the esophageal aperture of the diaphragm (10% of cases).

Neurovasculature of the Esophagus

Sympathetic innervation: Preganglionic fibers arise from the T2–T6 spinal cord segments. Postganglionic fibers arise from the sympathetic chain to join the esophageal plexus. Parasympathetic innervation: Preganglionic fibers arise from the dorsal vagal nucleus and travel in the vagus nerves to form the extensive esophageal plexus. *Note:* The postganglionic neurons are in the wall of the esophagus. Fibers to the cervical portion of the esophagus travel in the recurrent laryngeal nerves.

***Fig. 9.25* Autonomic innervation of the esophagus**

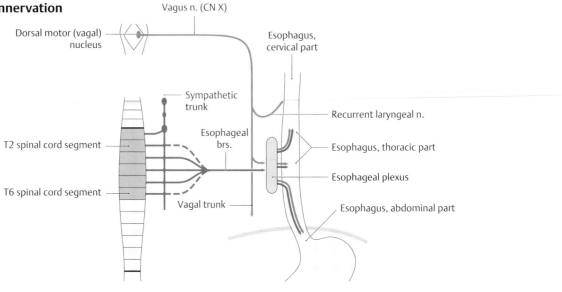

***Fig. 9.26* Esophageal plexus**

The left and right vagus nerves initially descend on the left and right sides of the esophagus. As they begin to contribute to the esophageal plexus, they shift to anterior and posterior positions, respectively. As the vagus nerves continue into the abdomen, they are named the anterior and posterior vagal trunks.

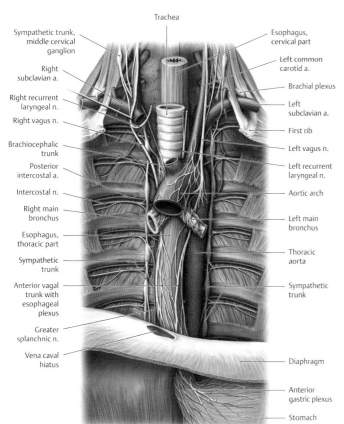

A Esophageal plexus in situ. Anterior view.

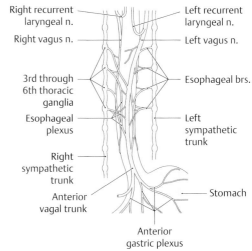

B Anterior view. Note the postganglionic sympathetic contribution to the esophageal plexus.

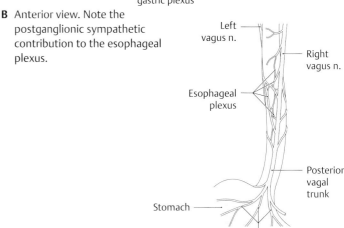

C Posterior view.

Fig. 9.27 **Esophageal arteries**
Anterior view.

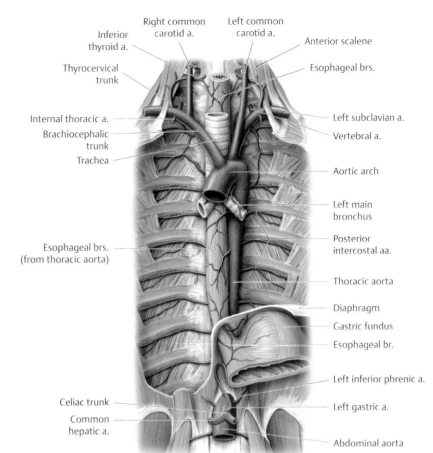

Fig. 9.28 **Esophageal veins**
Anterior view.

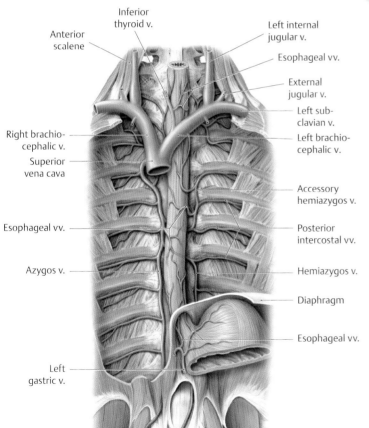

Table 9.6	Blood vessels of the esophagus	
Part	**Origin of esophageal arteries**	**Drainage of esophageal veins**
Cervical	Inferior thyroid a.	Inferior thyroid v.
	Rarely direct brs. from thyrocervical trunk or common carotid a.	Left brachiocephalic v.
Thoracic	Aorta (four or five esophageal aa.)	Upper left: Accessory hemiazygos v. or left brachiocephalic v.
		Lower left: Hemiazygos v.
		Right side: Azygos v.
Abdominal	Left gastric a.	Left gastric v.

Lymphatics of the Mediastinum

The superior phrenic lymph nodes drain lymph from the diaphragm, pericardium, lower esophagus, lung, and liver into the bronchomediastinal trunk. The inferior phrenic lymph nodes, found in the abdomen, collect lymph from the diaphragm and lower lobes of the lung and convey it to the lumbar trunk. *Note:* The pericardium may also drain superiorly to the brachiocephalic lymph nodes.

Fig. 9.29 Lymph nodes of the mediastinum and thoracic cavity
Left anterior oblique view.

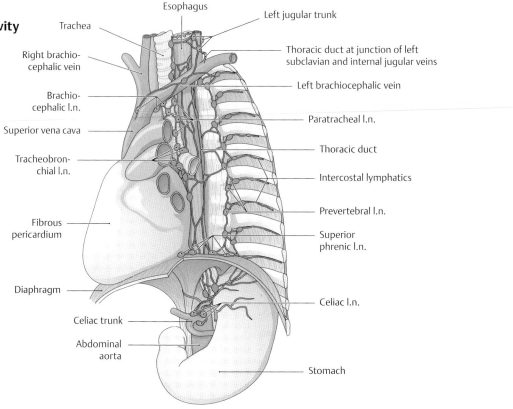

Fig. 9.30 Lymphatic drainage of the heart

A unique "crossed" drainage pattern exists in the heart: lymph from the left atrium and ventricle drains to the right venous junction, whereas lymph from the right atrium and ventricle drains to the left venous junction.

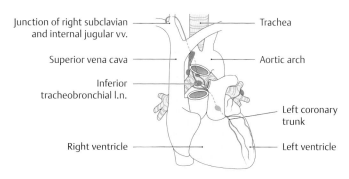

A Lymphatic drainage of the left chambers, anterior view.

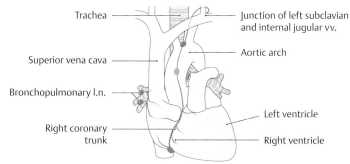

B Lymphatic drainage of the right chambers, anterior view.

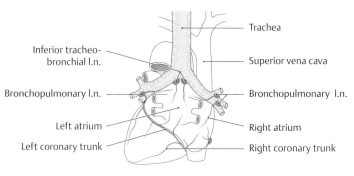

C Posterior view.

The paraesophageal nodes drain the esophagus. Lymphatic drainage of the cervical part of the esophagus is primarily cranial, to the deep cervical lymph nodes and then to the jugular trunk. The thoracic part of the esophagus drains to the bronchomediastinal trunks in two parts: the upper half drains cranially, and the lower half drains inferiorly via the superior phrenic lymph nodes. The bronchopulmonary and paratracheal nodes drain lymph from the lungs, bronchi, and trachea into the bronchomediastinal trunk (see **p. 128**).

Fig. 9.31 **Mediastinal lymph nodes**

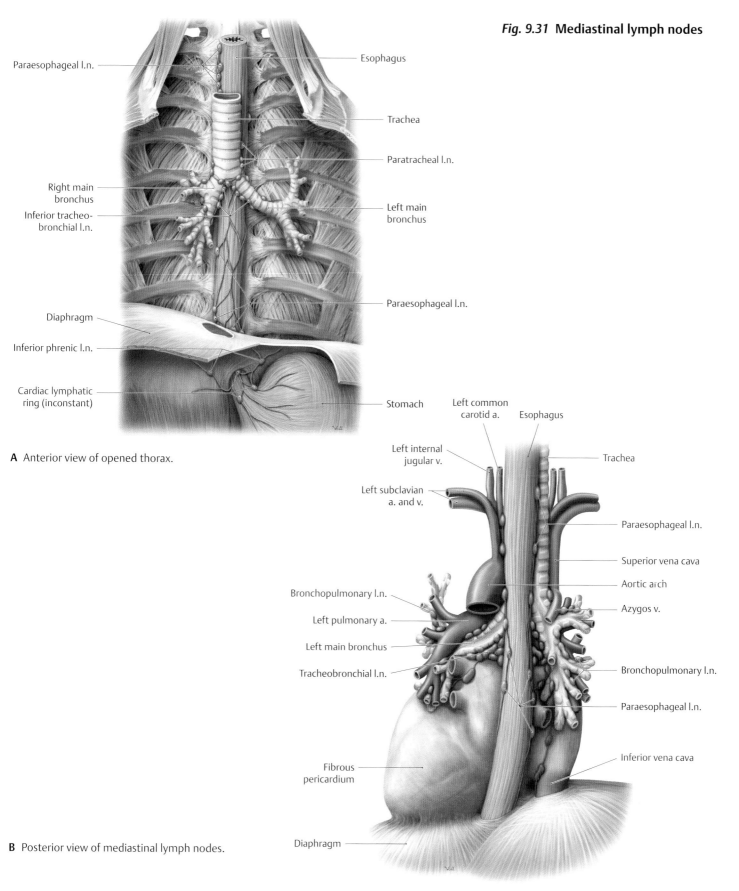

A Anterior view of opened thorax.

B Posterior view of mediastinal lymph nodes.

Pulmonary Cavities

The paired pulmonary cavities contain the left and right lungs. They are completely separated from each other by the mediastinum and are under negative atmospheric pressure (see respiratory mechanics, **pp. 122–123**). The left pulmonary cavity is slightly smaller than the right, especially anteriorly, due to the asymmetrical position of the heart in the mediastinum, with the greater mass on the left. This causes a shift of some of the boundaries of the parietal pleura and lung on the left side at the level of the heart, as reflected in the difference in thoracic landmarks found at the intersection of the anterior border of the pulmonary cavities with certain reference lines on the left and right.

Fig. 10.1 **Boundaries of the lungs and pulmonary cavities**
The upper red dot on each reference line is the inferior boundary of the lung and the lower blue dot is the inferior boundary of the pulmonary cavity.

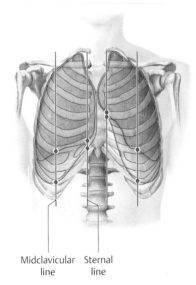

Midclavicular line   Sternal line

A Anterior view.

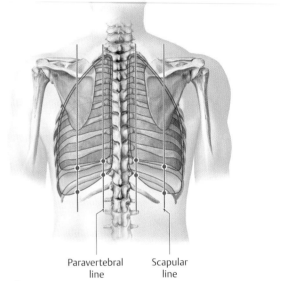

Paravertebral line   Scapular line

B Posterior view.

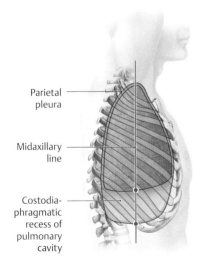

Parietal pleura

Midaxillary line

Costodiaphragmatic recess of pulmonary cavity

C Right lateral view.

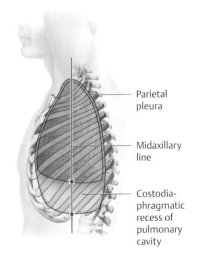

Parietal pleura

Midaxillary line

Costodiaphragmatic recess of pulmonary cavity

D Left lateral view.

Table 10.1	Pulmonary cavity boundaries and reference points			
Reference line	**Right lung**	**Right parietal pleura**	**Left lung**	**Left parietal pleura**
Sternal line (STL)	6th rib	7th rib	4th rib	4th rib
Midclavicular line (MCL)	6th rib	8th costal cartilage	6th rib	8th rib
Midaxillary line (MAL)	8th rib	10th rib	8th rib	10th rib
Scapular line (SL)	10th rib	11th rib	10th rib	11th rib
Paravertebral line (PV)	10th rib	T12 vertebra	10th rib	T12 vertebra

Fig. 10.2 Parietal pleura

The pulmonary cavity is bounded by two serous layers. The visceral pleura covering the lungs, and parietal pleura lining the inner surfaces of the thoracic cavity. The four divisions of the parietal pleura (costal, diaphragmatic, mediastinal, and cervical) are continuous.

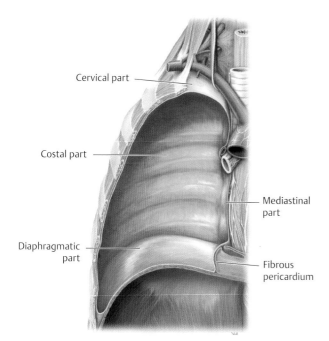

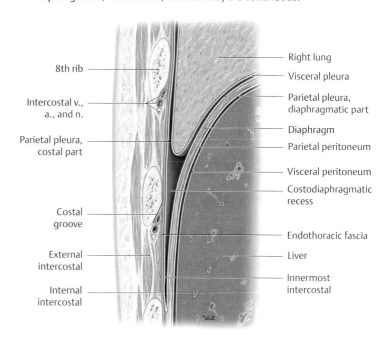

A Parts of the parietal pleura. *Opened:* Right pleural cavity, anterior view.

B Costodiaphragmatic recess, coronal section, anterior view. Reflection of the diaphragmatic pleura onto the inner thoracic wall (becoming the costal pleura) forms the costodiaphragmatic recess.

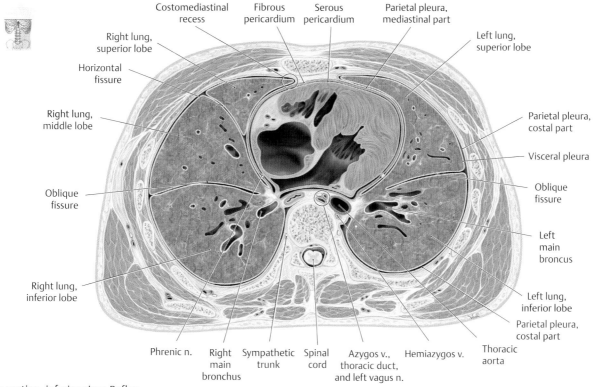

C Transverse section, inferior view. Reflection of the costal pleura onto the pericardium forms the costomediastinal recess.

113

Pleura: Subdivisions, Recesses & Innervation

Fig. 10.3 **Pleura and its divisions**

The anterior thoracic wall and costal portion of the parietal pleura have been removed to show the lungs in situ.

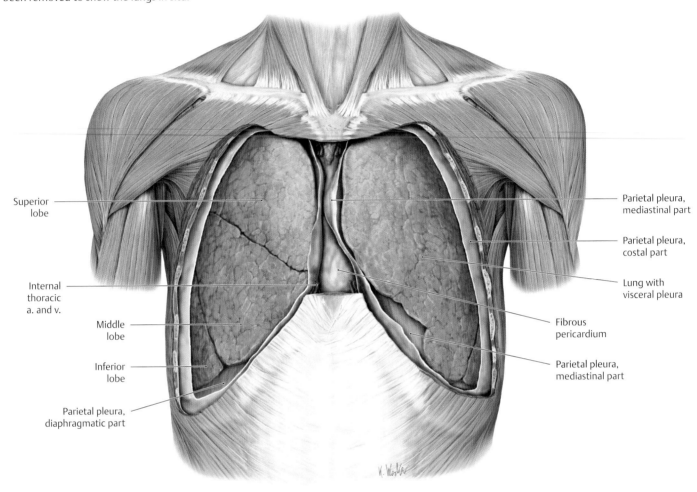

Superior lobe

Internal thoracic a. and v.

Middle lobe

Inferior lobe

Parietal pleura, diaphragmatic part

Parietal pleura, mediastinal part

Parietal pleura, costal part

Lung with visceral pleura

Fibrous pericardium

Parietal pleura, mediastinal part

✚ *Clinical box 10.1*

Percutaneous liver biopsy

Percutaneous liver biopsy is usually performed 2–3 cm superior to the inferior border of the liver at the right midaxillary line. The biopsy needle traverses the skin, thoracic wall, costal parietal pleura, costodiaphragmatic recess, diaphragmatic parietal pleura, diaphragm, then enters the liver in the abdominal cavity. The lower margin of the right lung rarely descends into the costodiaphragmatic recess during quiet inspiration and the costal and diaphragmatic parietal pleura are opposed by surface tension forces. Before inserting the biopsy needle, the physician will ask the patient to exhale and hold his or her breath. This increases the opposition of the costal and diaphragmatic pleura, more tightly closing the costodiaphrag-matic recess, and further decreasing the risk of pneumothorax, the introduc-tion of air in the interpleural space, when the biopsy needle is inserted. Pnemothorax, if severe, can produce lung collapse.

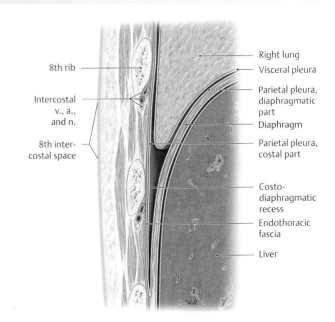

8th rib

Intercostal v., a., and n.

8th inter-costal space

Right lung

Visceral pleura

Parietal pleura, diaphragmatic part

Diaphragm

Parietal pleura, costal part

Costo-diaphragmatic recess

Endothoracic fascia

Liver

Fig. 10.4 **Costomediastinal and costodiaphragmatic recesses**

On the left side of the thorax, an examiner's fingertips are placed in the costomediastinal and costodiaphragmatic recesses. These recesses are formed by the acute reflection of the costal part of the parietal pleura onto the fibrous pericardium as mediastinal pleura (costomediastinal) or diaphragm as diaphragmatic pleura (costodiaphragmatic).

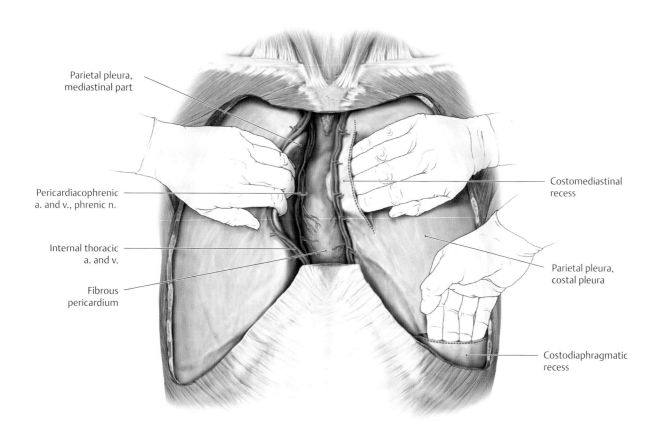

Parietal pleura, mediastinal part

Pericardiacophrenic a. and v., phrenic n.

Internal thoracic a. and v.

Fibrous pericardium

Costomediastinal recess

Parietal pleura, costal pleura

Costodiaphragmatic recess

Fig. 10.5 **Innervation of the pleura**

The costal and cervical portions and the periphery of the diaphragmatic portion of the parietal pleura are innervated by the intercostal nerves. The mediastinal and central portions of the diaphragmatic pleura are innervated by the phrenic nerves. The visceral pleura covering the lung itself receives its innervation from the autonomic nervous system.

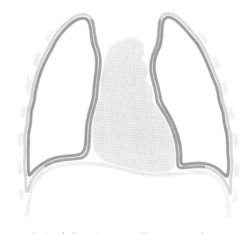

Parietal pleura innervated by intercostal nn.

Parietal pleura innervated by phrenic n.

Visceral pleura innervated by autonomic nn.

Lungs

Fig. 10.6 Lungs in situ

The left and right lungs occupy the full volume of the pleural cavity. Note that the left lung is slightly smaller than the right due to the asymmetrical position of the heart.

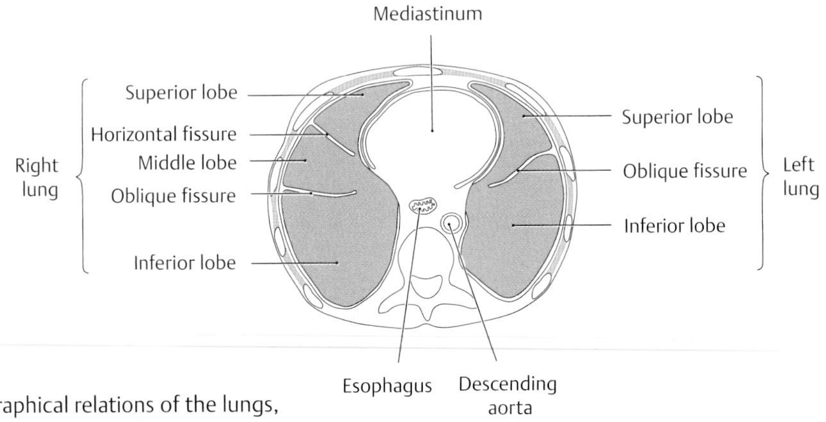

Mediastinum

Superior lobe

Horizontal fissure

Middle lobe

Oblique fissure

Right lung

Inferior lobe

Superior lobe

Oblique fissure

Inferior lobe

Left lung

Esophagus

Descending aorta

A Topographical relations of the lungs, transverse section, inferior view.

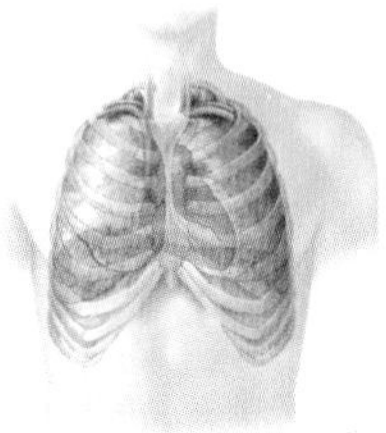

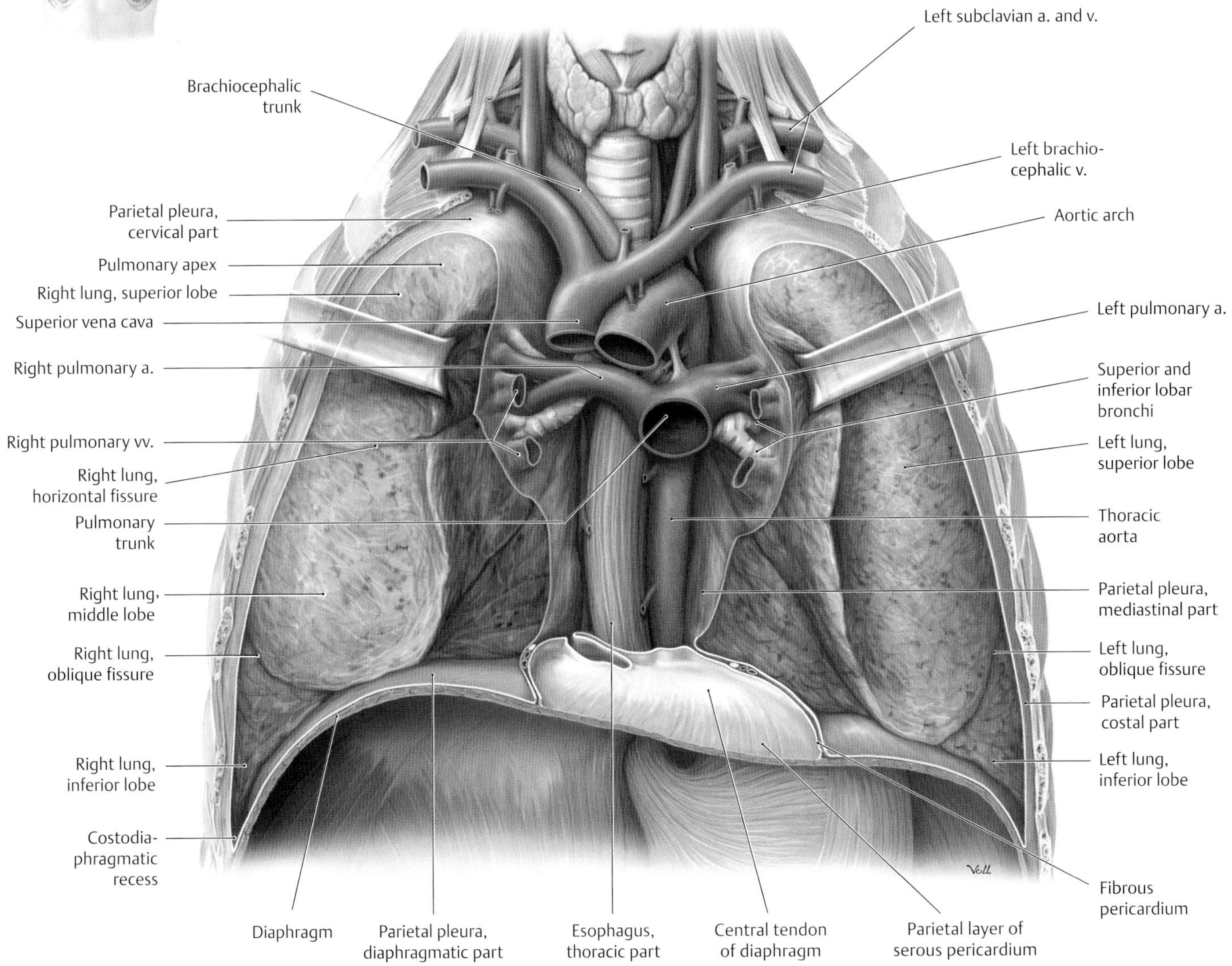

Left subclavian a. and v.

Brachiocephalic trunk

Left brachio-cephalic v.

Parietal pleura, cervical part

Aortic arch

Pulmonary apex

Right lung, superior lobe

Superior vena cava

Left pulmonary a.

Right pulmonary a.

Superior and inferior lobar bronchi

Right pulmonary vv.

Left lung, superior lobe

Right lung, horizontal fissure

Pulmonary trunk

Thoracic aorta

Right lung, middle lobe

Parietal pleura, mediastinal part

Left lung, oblique fissure

Right lung, oblique fissure

Parietal pleura, costal part

Right lung, inferior lobe

Left lung, inferior lobe

Costodia-phragmatic recess

Fibrous pericardium

Diaphragm

Parietal pleura, diaphragmatic part

Esophagus, thoracic part

Central tendon of diaphragm

Parietal layer of serous pericardium

B Anterior view with lungs retracted.

The oblique and horizontal fissures divide the right lung into three lobes: superior, middle, and inferior. The oblique fissure divides the left lung into two lobes: superior and inferior.

The apex of each lung extends into the root of the neck. The hilum is the location at which the bronchi and neurovascular structures connect to the lung.

Fig. 10.7 **Gross anatomy of the lungs**

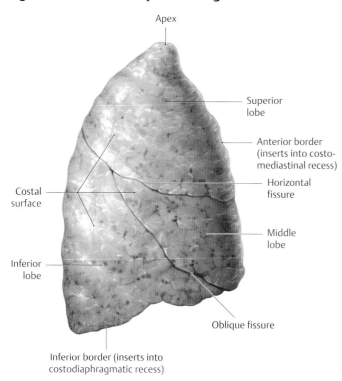

Apex

Superior lobe

Anterior border (inserts into costo-mediastinal recess)

Horizontal fissure

Middle lobe

Costal surface

Inferior lobe

Oblique fissure

Inferior border (inserts into costodiaphragmatic recess)

A Right lung, lateral view.

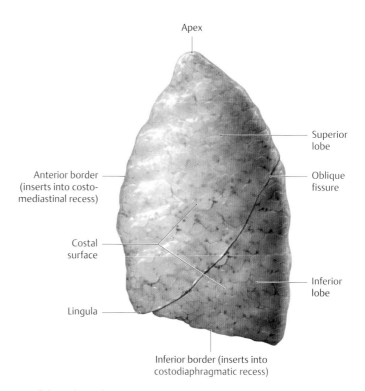

Apex

Superior lobe

Oblique fissure

Anterior border (inserts into costo-mediastinal recess)

Costal surface

Inferior lobe

Lingula

Inferior border (inserts into costodiaphragmatic recess)

B Left lung, lateral view.

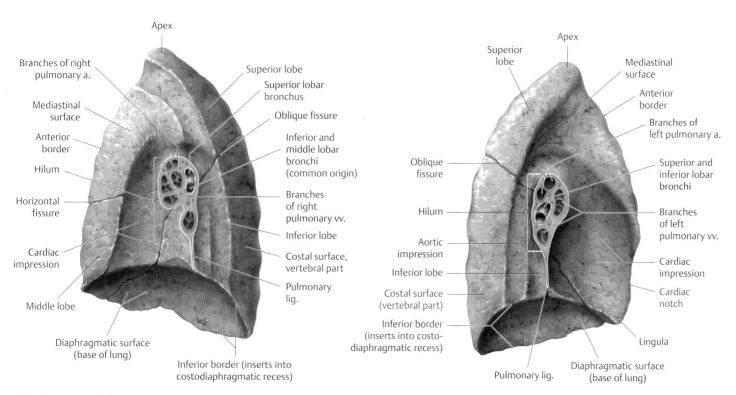

Apex

Branches of right pulmonary a.

Superior lobe

Superior lobar bronchus

Oblique fissure

Mediastinal surface

Inferior and middle lobar bronchi (common origin)

Anterior border

Hilum

Branches of right pulmonary vv.

Horizontal fissure

Inferior lobe

Costal surface, vertebral part

Cardiac impression

Pulmonary lig.

Middle lobe

Diaphragmatic surface (base of lung)

Inferior border (inserts into costodiaphragmatic recess)

C Right lung, medial view.

Apex

Superior lobe

Mediastinal surface

Anterior border

Branches of left pulmonary a.

Oblique fissure

Superior and inferior lobar bronchi

Hilum

Aortic impression

Branches of left pulmonary vv.

Inferior lobe

Cardiac impression

Costal surface (vertebral part)

Cardiac notch

Inferior border (inserts into costo-diaphragmatic recess)

Lingula

Pulmonary lig.

Diaphragmatic surface (base of lung)

D Left lung, medial view.

Bronchopulmonary Segments of the Lungs

 The lung lobes are subdivided into bronchopulmonary segments, the smallest resectable portion of a lung, each supplied by a tertiary (segmental) bronchus. *Note:* These subdivisions are not defined by surface boundaries but by origin.

Fig. 10.8 **Segmentation of the lung**
Anterior view. See **pp. 120–121** for details of the trachea and bronchial tree.

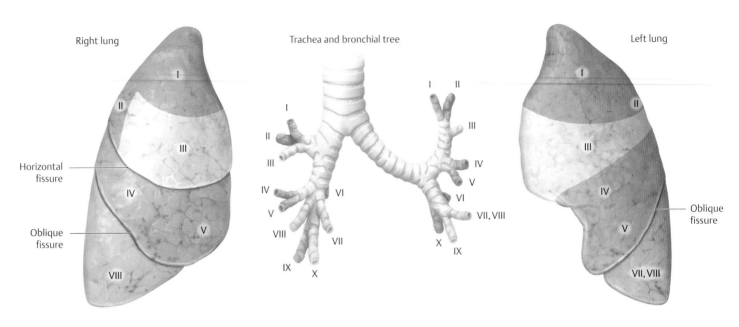

Right lung

Trachea and bronchial tree

Left lung

Horizontal fissure

Oblique fissure

Oblique fissure

Fig. 10.9 **Anteroposterior bronchogram**
Anterior view of right lung.

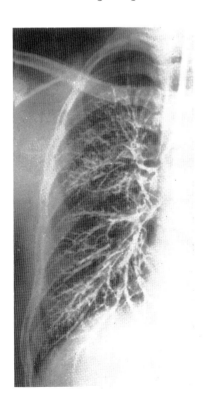

Table 10.2	Segmental architecture of the lungs

Each segment is supplied by a segmental bronchus of the same name (e.g., the apical segmental bronchus supplies the apical segment). See **pp. 120–121** for details of the trachea and bronchial tree.

	Right lung	Left lung	
Superior lobe			
I	Apical segment	Apicoposterior segment	I
II	Posterior segment		II
III	Anterior segment		III
Middle lobe		**Lingula**	
IV	Lateral segment	Superior lingular segment	IV
V	Medial segment	Inferior lingular segment	V
Inferior lobe			
VI	Superior segment		VI
VII	Medial basal segment		VII
VIII	Anterior basal segment		VIII
IX	Lateral basal segment		IX
X	Posterior basal segment		X

Fig. 10.10 Right lung: Bronchopulmonary segments

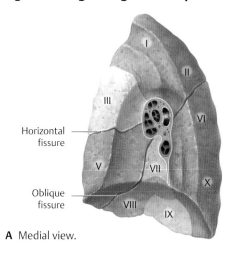

Horizontal fissure

Oblique fissure

A Medial view.

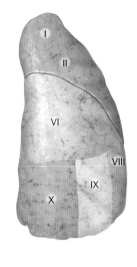

B Posterior view.

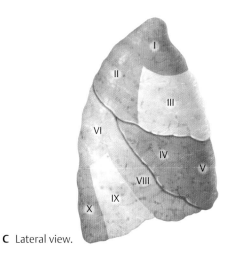

C Lateral view.

Fig. 10.11 Left lung: Bronchopulmonary segments

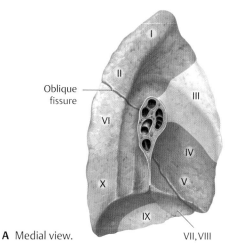

Oblique fissure

A Medial view.   VII, VIII

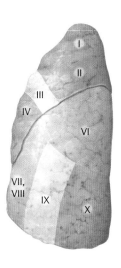

B Posterior view.

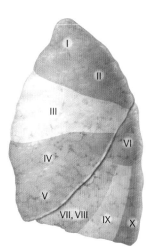

C Lateral view.

⚕ *Clinical box 10.2*

Lung resections

Lung cancer, emphysema, or tuberculosis may necessitate the surgical removal of damaged portions of the lung. Surgeons exploit the anatomical subdivision of the lungs into lobes and segments when excising damaged tissue.

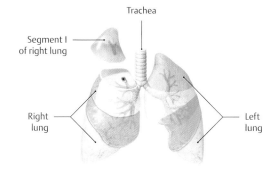

Trachea

Segment I of right lung

Right lung

Left lung

A Segmentectomy (wedge resection): Removal of one or more segments.

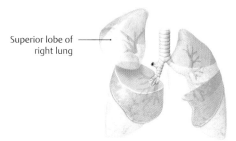

Superior lobe of right lung

B Lobectomy: Removal of lobe.

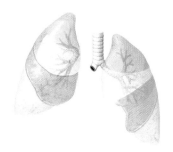

C Pneumonectomy: Removal of entire lung.

Trachea & Bronchial Tree

 At or near the level of the sternal angle, the lowest tracheal cartilage extends anteroposteriorly, forming the carina. The trachea bifurcates at the carina into the right and left main bronchi. Each bronchus gives off lobar branches to the corresponding lung.

Fig. 10.12 **Trachea**
See **p. 634** for the structures of the thyroid.

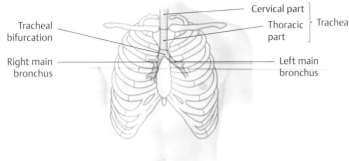

A Projection of trachea onto chest.

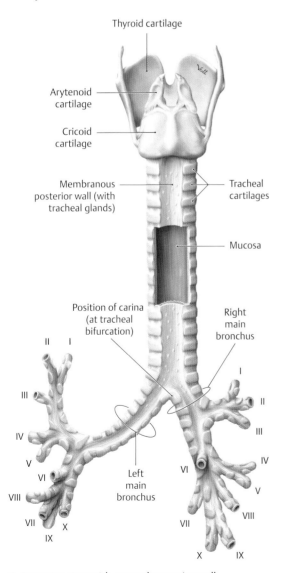

C Posterior view with opened posterior wall.

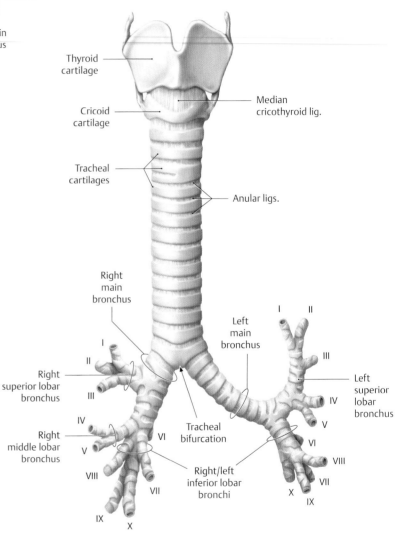

B Anterior view.

Foreign body aspiration
Toddlers are at particularly high risk of potentially fatal aspiration of foreign bodies. In general, foreign bodies are more likely to become lodged in the right main bronchus than the left: the left bronchus diverges more sharply at the tracheal bifurcation to pass more horizontally over the heart, whereas the right bronchus is relatively straight and more in line with the trachea.

The conducting portion of the bronchial tree extends from the tracheal bifurcation to the terminal bronchiole, inclusive. The respiratory portion consists of the respiratory bronchiole, alveolar ducts, alveolar sacs, and alveoli.

Fig. 10.13 Bronchial tree

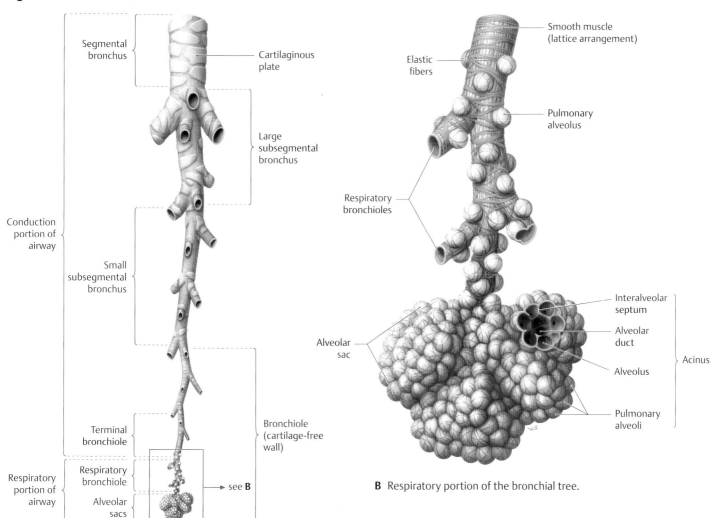

A Divisions of the bronchial tree.

B Respiratory portion of the bronchial tree.

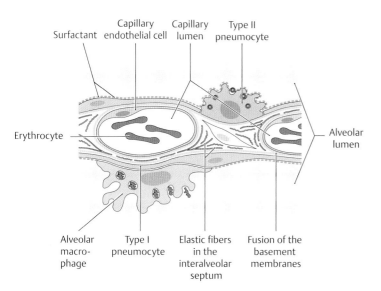

C Epithelial lining of the alveoli.

Respiratory Mechanics

The mechanics of respiration are based on a rhythmic increase and decrease in thoracic volume, with an associated expansion and contraction of the lungs. *Inspiration* (red): Contraction of the diaphragm leaflets lowers the diaphragm into the inspiratory position, increasing the volume of the pleural cavity along the vertical axis. Contraction of the thoracic muscles (external intercostals with the scalene, intercartilaginous, and posterior serratus muscles) elevates the ribs, expanding the pleural cavity along the sagittal and transverse axes (**Fig. 10.15A,B**). Surface tension in the pleural space causes the visceral and parietal pleura to adhere; thus, changes in thoracic volume alter the volume of the lungs.

This is particularly evident in the pleural recesses: at functional residual capacity (resting position between inspiration and expiration), the lung does not fully occupy the pleural cavity. As the pleural cavity expands, a negative intrapleural pressure is generated. The air pressure differential results in an influx of air (inspiration). *Expiration* (blue): During passive expiration, the muscles of the thoracic cage relax and the diaphragm returns to its expiratory position. Contraction of the lungs increases the pulmonary pressure and expels air from the lungs. For forcible expiration, the internal intercostal muscles (with the transverse thoracic and subcostal mucosa) can actively lower the rib cage more rapidly and to a greater extent than through passive elastic recoil.

Fig. 10.14 **Respiratory changes in thoracic volume**
Inspiratory position (red); expiratory position (blue).

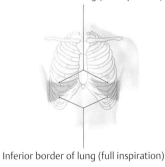

Fig. 10.15 **Inspiration: Pleural cavity expansion**

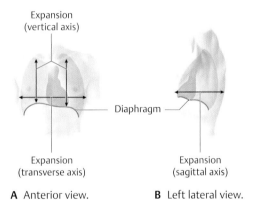

A Anterior view.   **B** Left lateral view.   **C** Anterolateral view.

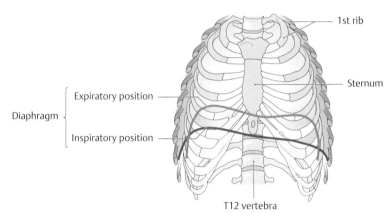

Fig. 10.17 **Respiratory changes in lung volume**

Fig. 10.16 **Expiration: Pleural cavity contraction**

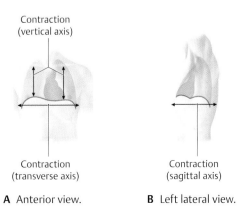

A Anterior view.   **B** Left lateral view.   **C** Anterolateral view.

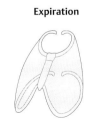

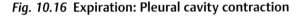

Fig. 10.18 Inspiration: Lung expansion

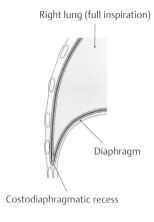

Right lung (full inspiration)

Diaphragm

Costodiaphragmatic recess

Fig. 10.19 Expiration: Lung contraction

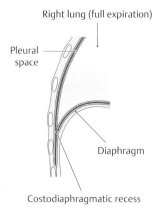

Right lung (full expiration)

Pleural space

Diaphragm

Costodiaphragmatic recess

Fig. 10.20 Movements of the lung and bronchial tree

As the volume of the lung changes with the thoracic cavity, the entire bronchial tree moves within the lung. These structural movements are more pronounced in portions of the bronchial tree distant from the pulmonary hilum.

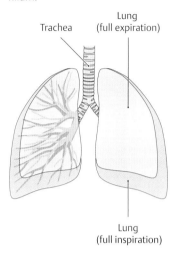

Trachea

Lung (full expiration)

Lung (full inspiration)

✳ Clinical box 10.5

Pneumothorax

The pleural space is normally sealed from the outside environment. Injury to the parietal pleura, visceral pleura, or lung allows air to enter the pleural cavity (pneumothorax). The lung collapses due to its inherent elasticity, and the patient's ability to breathe is compromised. The uninjured lung continues to function under normal pressure variations, resulting in "mediastinal flutter": the mediastinum shifts toward the normal side during inspiration and returns to the midline during expiration. Tension (valve) pneumothorax occurs when traumatically detached and displaced tissue covers the defect in the thoracic wall from the inside. This mobile flap allows air to enter, but not escape, the pleural cavity, causing a pressure buildup. The mediastinum shifts to the normal side, which may cause kinking of the great vessels and prevent the return of venous blood to the heart. Without treatment, tension pneumothorax is invariably fatal.

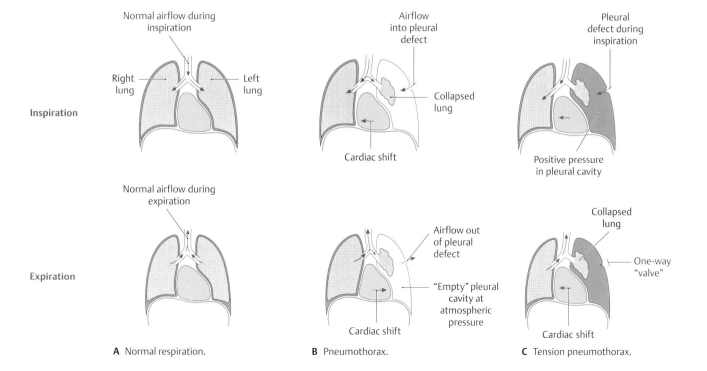

A Normal respiration.   **B** Pneumothorax.   **C** Tension pneumothorax.

Pulmonary Arteries & Veins

 The pulmonary trunk arises from the right ventricle and divides into a left and right pulmonary artery for each lung. The paired pulmonary veins open into the left atrium on each side. The pulmonary arteries accompany and follow the branching of the bronchial tree, whereas the pulmonary veins do not, being located at the margins of the pulmonary lobules.

Fig. 10.21 **Pulmonary arteries and veins**
Anterior view.

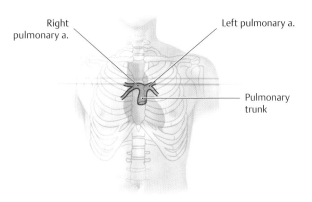

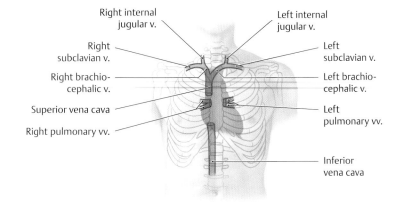

A Projection of pulmonary arteries on chest wall.

B Projection of pulmonary veins on chest wall.

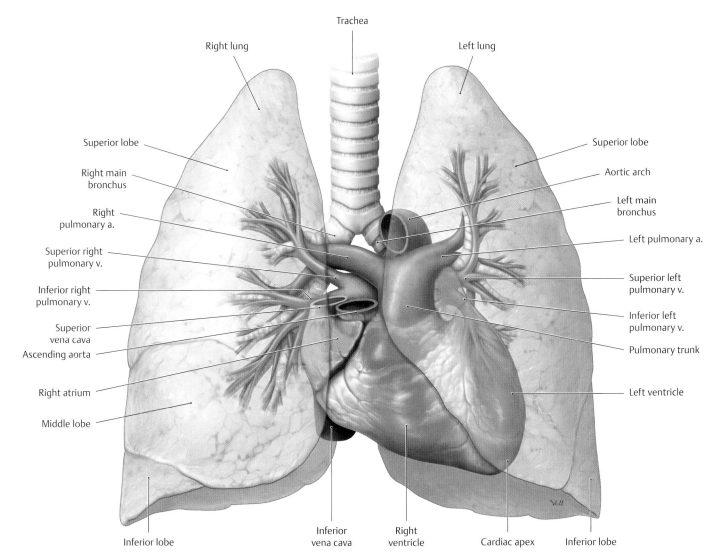

C Distribution of the pulmonary arteries and veins, anterior view.

Fig. 10.22 Pulmonary arteries

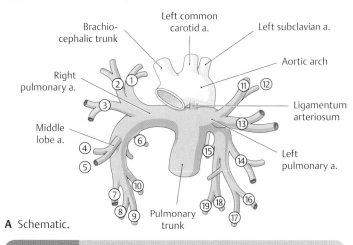

A Schematic.

Table 10.3	**Pulmonary arteries and their branches**	
Right pulmonary artery		**Left pulmonary artery**

	Superior lobe arteries	
①	Apical segmental a.	⑪
②	Posterior segmental a.	⑫
③	Anterior segmental a.	⑬
	Middle lobe arteries	
④	Lateral segmental a.	Lingular a.	⑭
⑤	Medial segmental a.	
	Inferior lobe arteries	
⑥	Superior segmental a.	⑮
⑦	Anterior basal segmental a.	⑯
⑧	Lateral basal segmental a.	⑰
⑨	Posterior basal segmental a.	⑱
⑩	Medial basal segmental a.	⑲

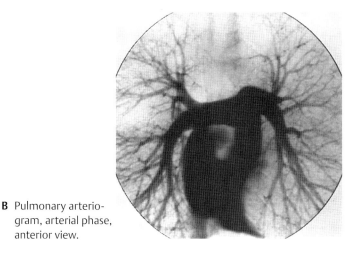

B Pulmonary arterio-
gram, arterial phase,
anterior view.

Fig. 10.23 Pulmonary veins

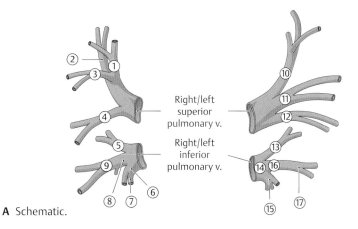

A Schematic.

Table 10.4	**Pulmonary veins and their tributaries**	
Right pulmonary vein		**Left pulmonary vein**

	Superior pulmonary veins		
①	Apical v.	Apicoposterior v.	⑩
②	Posterior v.		
③	Anterior v.	Anterior v.	⑪
④	Middle lobe v.	Lingular v.	⑫
	Inferior pulmonary veins		
⑤	Superior v.		⑬
⑥	Common basal v.		⑭
⑦	Inferior basal v.		⑮
⑧	Superior basal v.		⑯
⑨	Anterior basal v.		⑰

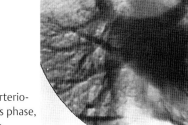

B Pulmonary arterio-
gram, venous phase,
anterior view.

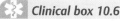 **Clinical box 10.6**

Pulmonary embolism

Potentially life-threatening pulmonary embolism occurs when blood
clots migrate through the venous system and become lodged in one of
the arteries supplying the lungs. Symptoms include dyspnea (difficulty
breathing) and tachycardia (increased heart rate). Most pulmonary emboli
originate from stagnant blood in the veins of the lower limb and pelvis
(venous thromboemboli). Causes include immobilization, disordered blood
coagulation, and trauma. *Note*: A thromboembolus is a thrombus (blood clot)
that has migrated (embolized).

Neurovasculature of the Tracheobronchial Tree

Fig. 10.24 Pulmonary vasculature

The pulmonary system is responsible for gaseous exchange within the lung. Pulmonary arteries (shown in blue) carry *deoxygenated* blood and follow the bronchial tree. The pulmonary vein and its tributaries (red) is the only vein in the body carrying *oxygenated* blood, which it receives from the alveolar capillaries at the periphery of the lobule.

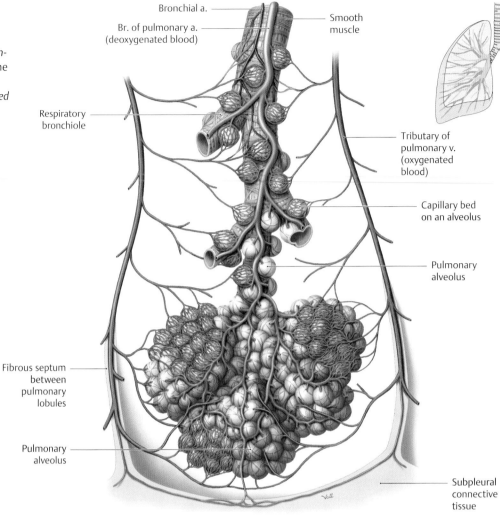

Fig. 10.25 Arteries of the tracheobronchial tree

The bronchial tree receives its nutrients via the bronchial arteries, found in the adventitia of the airways. Typically, there are one to three bronchial arteries arising directly from the aorta. Origin from a posterior intercostal artery may also occur.

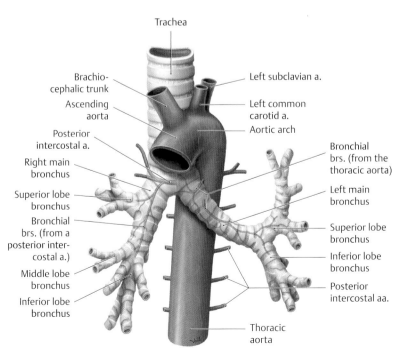

Fig. 10.26 **Veins of the tracheobronchial tree**

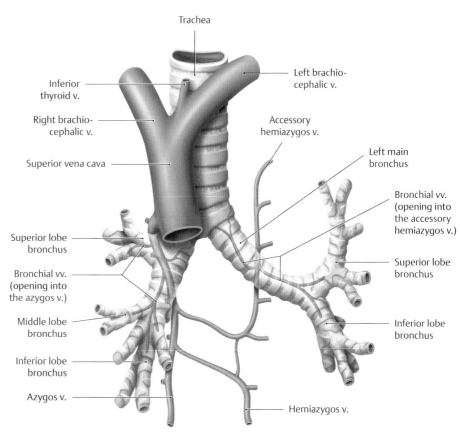

Fig. 10.27 **Autonomic innervation of the tracheobronchial tree**
Sympathetic innervation (red); parasympathetic innervation (blue).

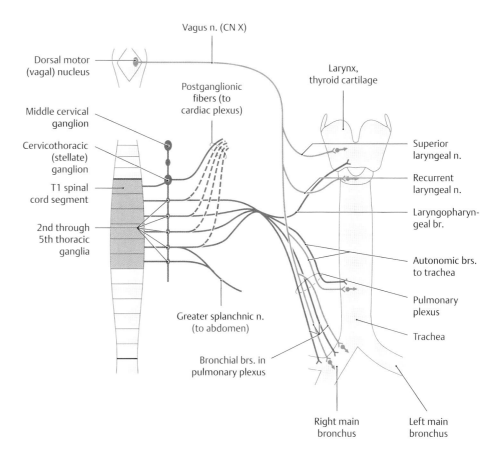

Lymphatics of the Pleural Cavity

 The lungs and bronchi are drained by two lymphatic drainage systems. The peribronchial network follows the bronchial tree, draining lymph from the bronchi and most of the lungs. The subpleural network collects lymph from the peripheral lung and visceral pleura.

Fig. 10.28 **Lymphatic drainage of the pleural cavity**

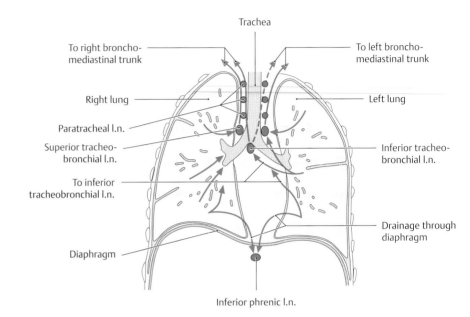

A Peribronchial network, coronal section, anterior view. (Intra)pulmonary nodes along the bronchial tree drain lymph from the lungs into the bronchopulmonary (hilar) nodes. Lymph then passes sequentially through the inferior and superior tracheobronchial nodes, paratracheal nodes, bronchomediastinal trunk, and finally to the right lymphatic or thoracic duct.
Note: Significant amounts of lymph from the left lower lobe drain to the right superior tracheobronchial nodes.

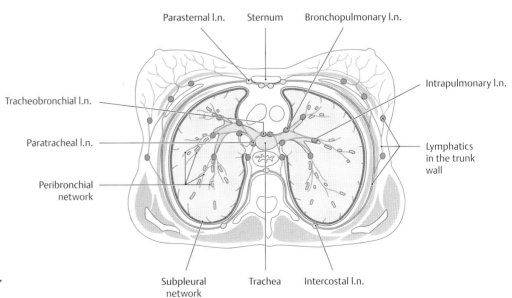

B Subpleural network, transverse section, superior view.

Fig. 10.29 **Lymph nodes of the pleural cavity**
Anterior view of pulmonary nodes.

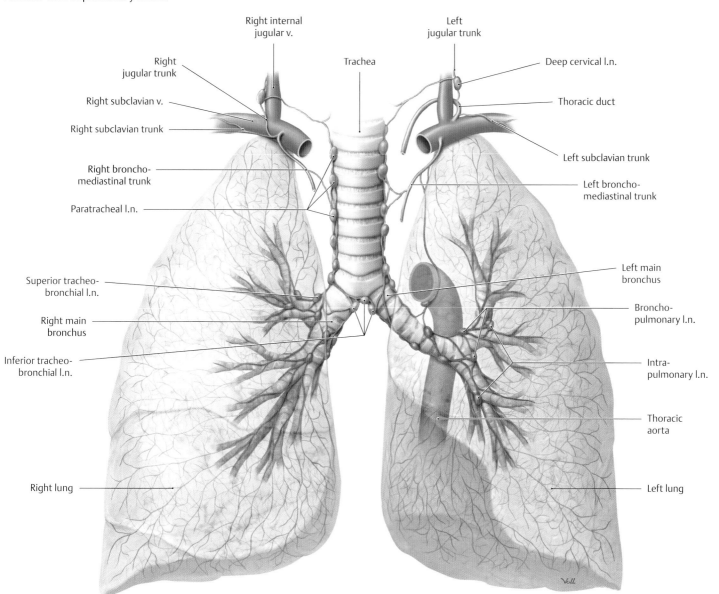

Right internal jugular v.

Right jugular trunk

Right subclavian v.

Right subclavian trunk

Right broncho-mediastinal trunk

Paratracheal l.n.

Superior tracheo-bronchial l.n.

Right main bronchus

Inferior tracheo-bronchial l.n.

Right lung

Trachea

Left jugular trunk

Deep cervical l.n.

Thoracic duct

Left subclavian trunk

Left broncho-mediastinal trunk

Left main bronchus

Broncho-pulmonary l.n.

Intra-pulmonary l.n.

Thoracic aorta

Left lung

Sectional Anatomy of the Thorax

Fig. 11.1 Transverse section through the thoracic inlet region of the thorax
Inferior view.

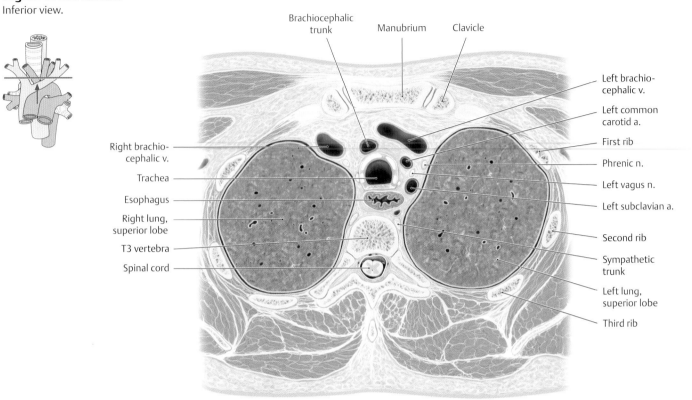

Brachiocephalic trunk — Manubrium — Clavicle

Left brachio-cephalic v.

Left common carotid a.

First rib

Phrenic n.

Left vagus n.

Left subclavian a.

Second rib

Sympathetic trunk

Left lung, superior lobe

Third rib

Right brachio-cephalic v.

Trachea

Esophagus

Right lung, superior lobe

T3 vertebra

Spinal cord

Fig. 11.2 Transverse section through the mid region of the thorax
Inferior view.

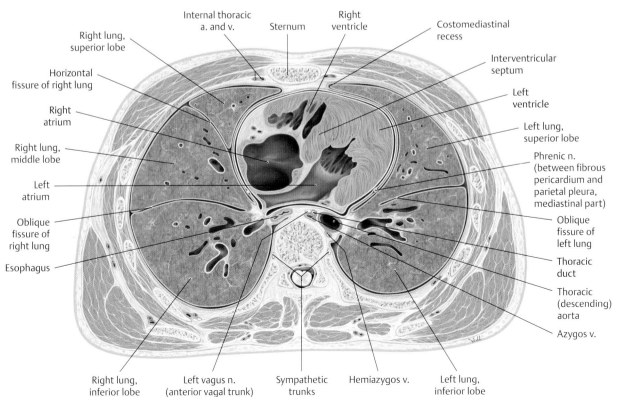

Right lung, superior lobe

Horizontal fissure of right lung

Right atrium

Right lung, middle lobe

Left atrium

Oblique fissure of right lung

Esophagus

Internal thoracic a. and v. — Sternum — Right ventricle

Costomediastinal recess

Interventricular septum

Left ventricle

Left lung, superior lobe

Phrenic n. (between fibrous pericardium and parietal pleura, mediastinal part)

Oblique fissure of left lung

Thoracic duct

Thoracic (descending) aorta

Azygos v.

Right lung, inferior lobe — Left vagus n. (anterior vagal trunk) — Sympathetic trunks — Hemiazygos v. — Left lung, inferior lobe

Fig. 11.3 Coronal section through the heart
Anterior view.

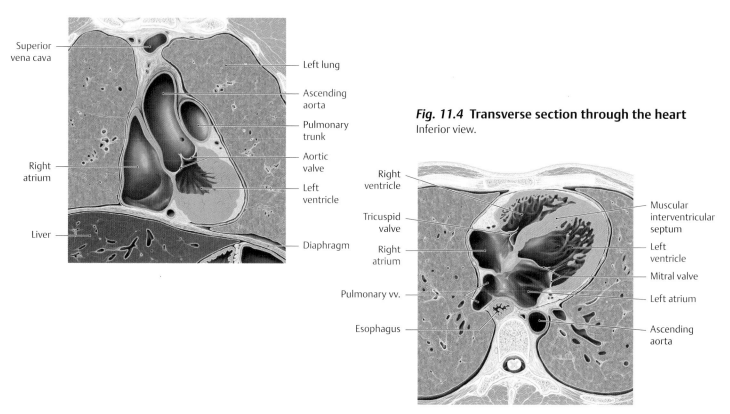

Superior vena cava

Right atrium

Liver

Left lung

Ascending aorta

Pulmonary trunk

Aortic valve

Left ventricle

Diaphragm

Fig. 11.4 Transverse section through the heart
Inferior view.

Right ventricle

Tricuspid valve

Right atrium

Pulmonary vv.

Esophagus

Muscular interventricular septum

Left ventricle

Mitral valve

Left atrium

Ascending aorta

Fig. 11.5 Pleural recesses
Transverse section, superior view.

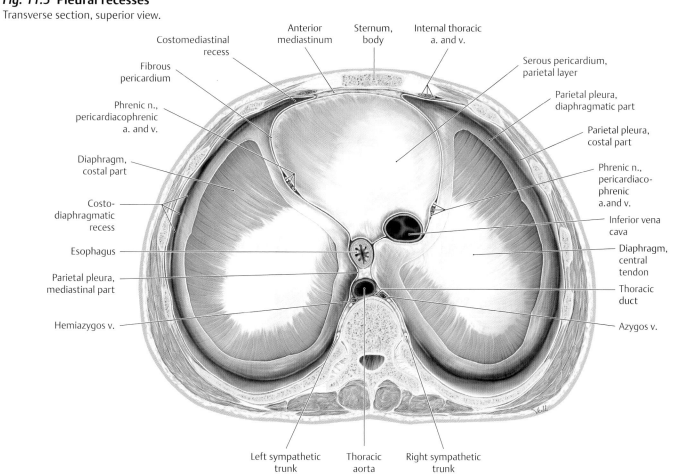

Costomediastinal recess

Fibrous pericardium

Phrenic n., pericardiacophrenic a. and v.

Diaphragm, costal part

Costo-diaphragmatic recess

Esophagus

Parietal pleura, mediastinal part

Hemiazygos v.

Anterior mediastinum

Sternum, body

Internal thoracic a. and v.

Serous pericardium, parietal layer

Parietal pleura, diaphragmatic part

Parietal pleura, costal part

Phrenic n., pericardiaco-phrenic a. and v.

Inferior vena cava

Diaphragm, central tendon

Thoracic duct

Azygos v.

Left sympathetic trunk

Thoracic aorta

Right sympathetic trunk

131

Radiographic Anatomy of the Thorax (I)

Fig. 11.6 Radiographic appearance of the heart

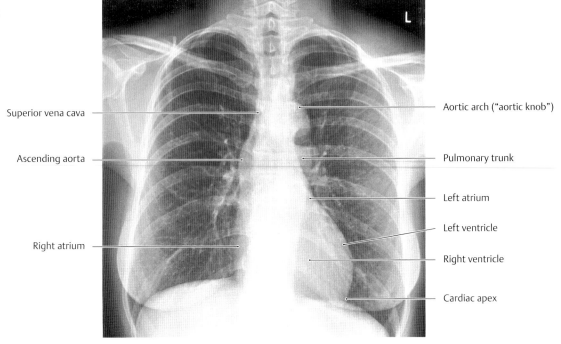

Superior vena cava

Ascending aorta

Right atrium

Aortic arch ("aortic knob")

Pulmonary trunk

Left atrium

Left ventricle

Right ventricle

Cardiac apex

A Anteroposterior chest radiograph. Anterior view.

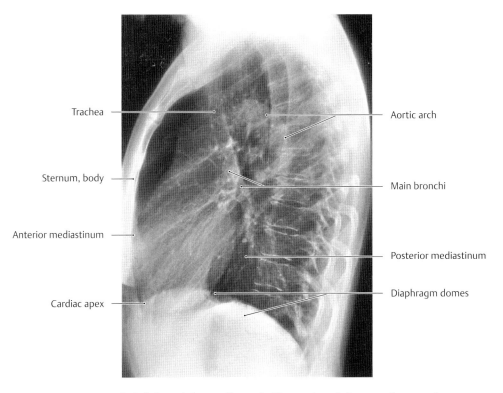

Trachea

Sternum, body

Anterior mediastinum

Cardiac apex

Aortic arch

Main bronchi

Posterior mediastinum

Diaphragm domes

B Left lateral chest radiograph. The aortic arch forms a sling over the main left bronchus. Note the narrowness of the anterior mediastinum relative to the posterior mediastinum.

Fig. 11.7 Left bronchogram
Anteroposterior view.

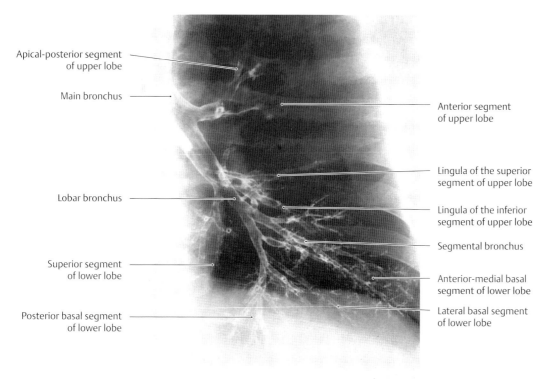

Apical-posterior segment of upper lobe

Main bronchus

Lobar bronchus

Superior segment of lower lobe

Posterior basal segment of lower lobe

Anterior segment of upper lobe

Lingula of the superior segment of upper lobe

Lingula of the inferior segment of upper lobe

Segmental bronchus

Anterior-medial basal segment of lower lobe

Lateral basal segment of lower lobe

Fig. 11.8 MRI of the thorax
Coronal view.

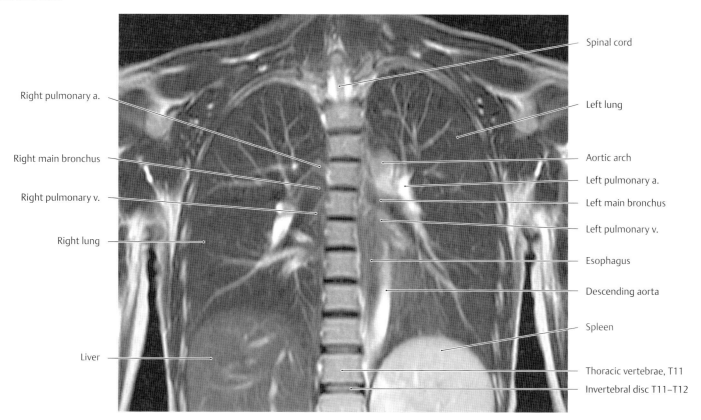

Right pulmonary a.

Right main bronchus

Right pulmonary v.

Right lung

Liver

Spinal cord

Left lung

Aortic arch

Left pulmonary a.

Left main bronchus

Left pulmonary v.

Esophagus

Descending aorta

Spleen

Thoracic vertebrae, T11

Invertebral disc T11–T12

Radiographic Anatomy of the Thorax (II)

Fig. 11.9 Selective coronary angiography of the left coronary artery in a right anterior oblique position

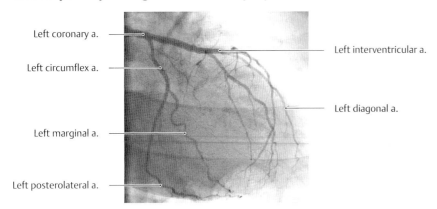

Left coronary a.

Left circumflex a.

Left marginal a.

Left posterolateral a.

Left interventricular a.

Left diagonal a.

Fig. 11.10 Selective coronary angiography of the right coronary artery in a left anterior oblique projection

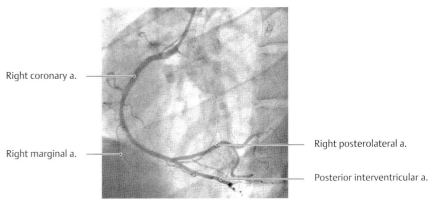

Right coronary a.

Right marginal a.

Right posterolateral a.

Posterior interventricular a.

Fig. 11.11 CT of the heart
CT angiography.

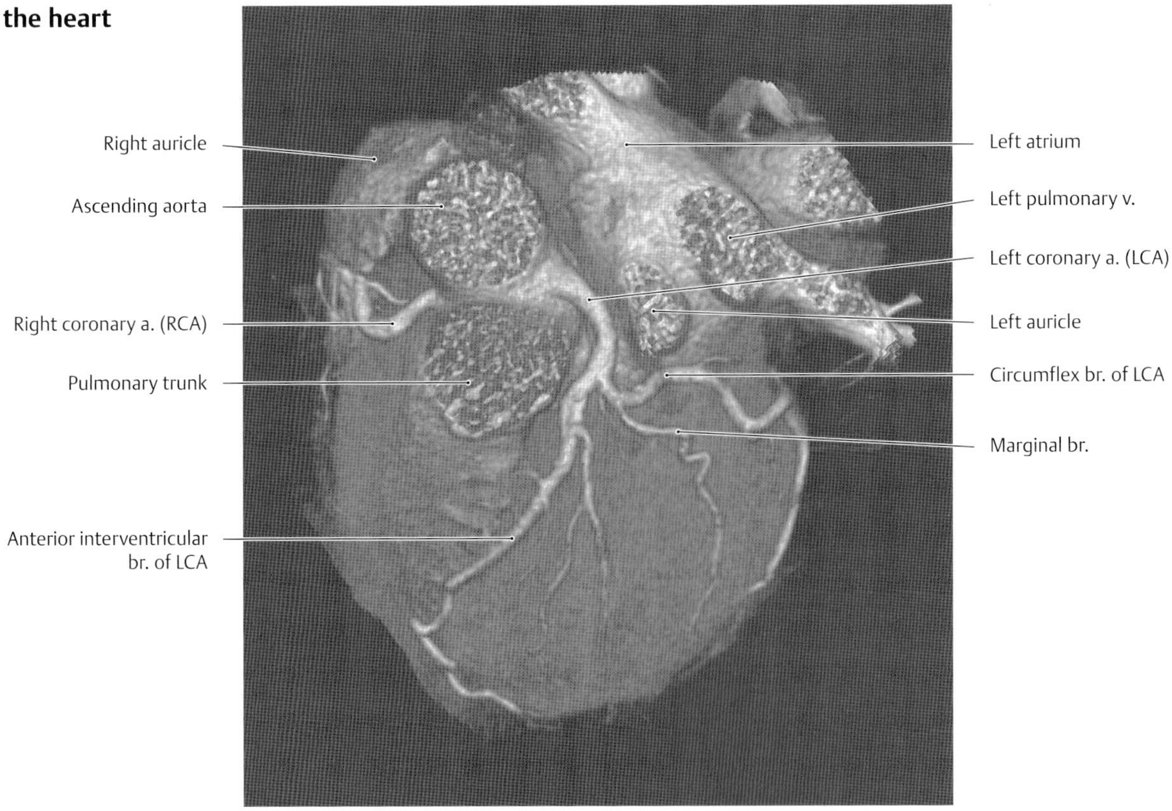

Right auricle

Ascending aorta

Right coronary a. (RCA)

Pulmonary trunk

Anterior interventricular br. of LCA

Left atrium

Left pulmonary v.

Left coronary a. (LCA)

Left auricle

Circumflex br. of LCA

Marginal br.

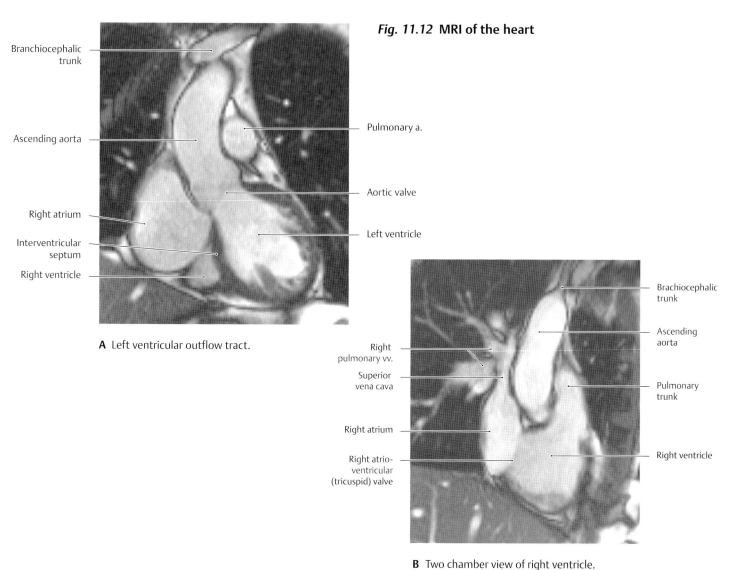

Fig. 11.12 MRI of the heart

Branchiocephalic trunk

Ascending aorta

Right atrium

Interventricular septum

Right ventricle

Pulmonary a.

Aortic valve

Left ventricle

A Left ventricular outflow tract.

Right pulmonary vv.

Superior vena cava

Right atrium

Right atrio-ventricular (tricuspid) valve

Branchiocephalic trunk

Ascending aorta

Pulmonary trunk

Right ventricle

B Two chamber view of right ventricle.

Fig. 11.13 Aortic arch angiogram
Left lateral view.

Right thyrocervical trunk
Right common carotid a.
Right vertebral a.
Right subclavian a.

Brachiocephalic trunk

Aortic arch

Ascending aorta

Left thyrocervical trunk

Left vertebral a.

Left subclavian a.

Left common carotid a.

Descending aorta

Radiographic Anatomy of the Thorax (III)

Fig. 11.14 CT of the thorax

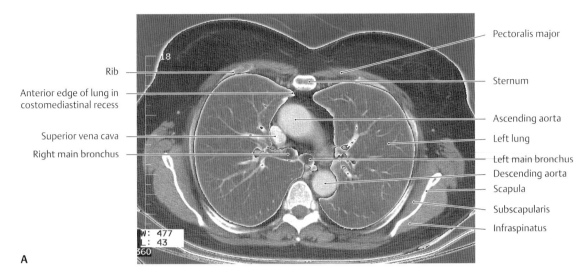

Rib
Anterior edge of lung in costomediastinal recess
Superior vena cava
Right main bronchus

Pectoralis major
Sternum
Ascending aorta
Left lung
Left main bronchus
Descending aorta
Scapula
Subscapularis
Infraspinatus

W: 477
L: 43

A

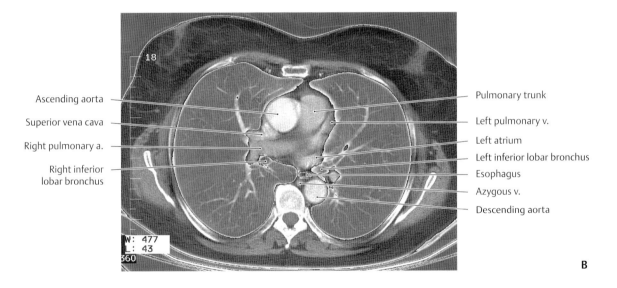

Ascending aorta
Superior vena cava
Right pulmonary a.
Right inferior lobar bronchus

Pulmonary trunk
Left pulmonary v.
Left atrium
Left inferior lobar bronchus
Esophagus
Azygous v.
Descending aorta

W: 477
L: 43

B

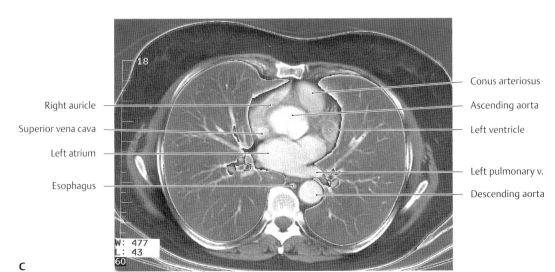

Right auricle
Superior vena cava
Left atrium
Esophagus

Conus arteriosus
Ascending aorta
Left ventricle
Left pulmonary v.
Descending aorta

W: 477
L: 43

C

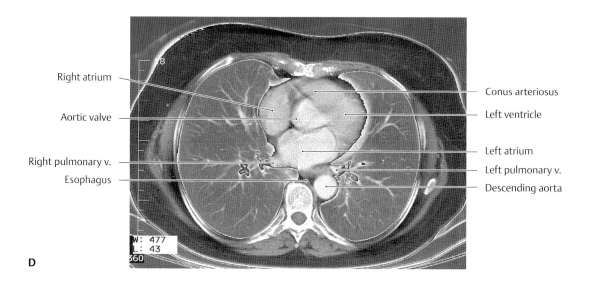

Right atrium —
Aortic valve —
Right pulmonary v. —
Esophagus —

— Conus arteriosus
— Left ventricle
— Left atrium
— Left pulmonary v.
— Descending aorta

W: 477
L: 43
360

D

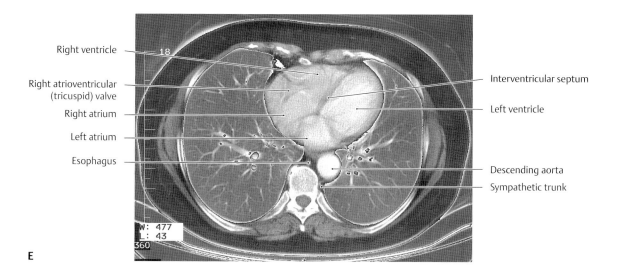

Right ventricle —
Right atrioventricular (tricuspid) valve —
Right atrium —
Left atrium —
Esophagus —

— Interventricular septum
— Left ventricle
— Descending aorta
— Sympathetic trunk

W: 477
L: 43
360

E

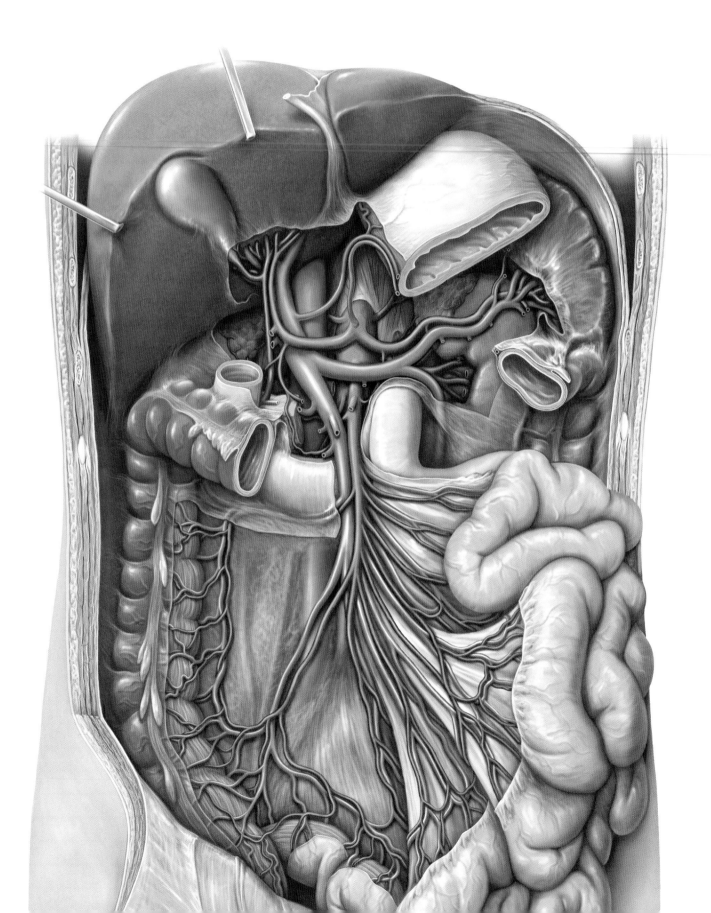

Abdomen

Surface Anatomy

Fig. 12.1 Palpable structures of the abdomen and pelvis

Anterior view. See **pp. 2–3** for structures of the back.

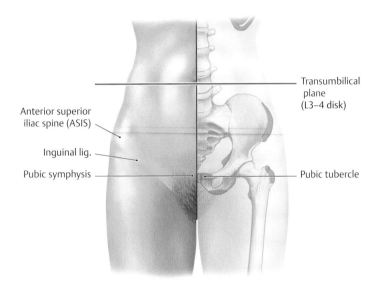

A Bony prominences.

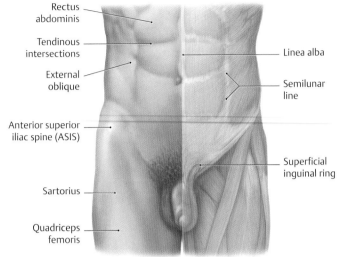

B Musculature.

Fig. 12.2 Quadrants and layers of the abdominopelvic cavity

Anterior view. The location of the organs of the abdomen and pelvis can be described by quadrant and layer.

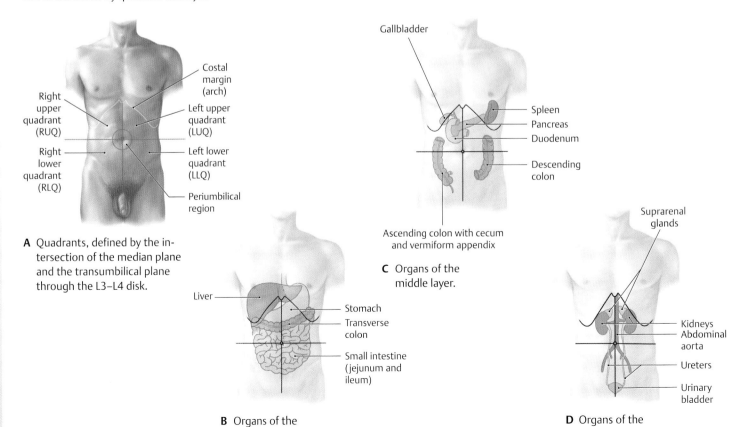

A Quadrants, defined by the intersection of the median plane and the transumbilical plane through the L3–L4 disk.

B Organs of the anterior layer.

C Organs of the middle layer.

D Organs of the posterior layer.

Table 12.1	Transverse planes through the abdomen
① Transpyloric plane	Transverse plane midway between the superior borders of the pubic symphysis and the manubrium
② Subcostal plane	Plane at the lowest level of the costal margin (the inferior margin of the tenth costal cartilage)
③ Supracrestal plane	Plane passing through the summits of the iliac crests
④ Transtubercular plane	Plane at the level of the iliac tubercles (the iliac tubercle lies ~5 cm posterolateral to the anterior superior iliac spine)
⑤ Interspinous plane	Plane at the level of the anterior superior iliac spines

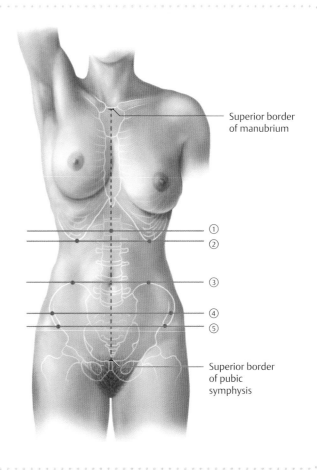

Superior border of manubrium

Superior border of pubic symphysis

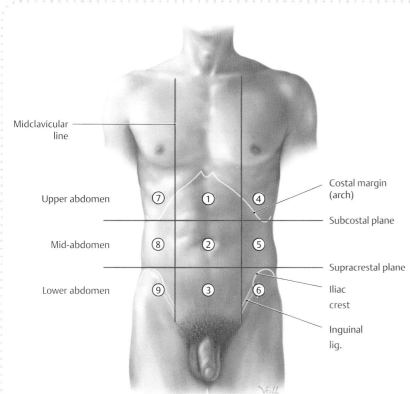

Midclavicular line

Upper abdomen

Mid-abdomen

Lower abdomen

Costal margin (arch)

Subcostal plane

Supracrestal plane

Iliac crest

Inguinal lig.

Table 12.2	Regions of the abdomen
① Epigastric region	
② Umbilical region	
③ Pubic region	
④ Left hypochondriac region	
⑤ Left lateral (lumbar) region	
⑥ Left inguinal region	
⑦ Right hypochondriac region	
⑧ Right lateral (lumbar) region	
⑨ Right inguinal region	

Bony Framework for the Abdominal Wall

Fig. 13.1 Bony framework of the abdomen
Anterior view. These bones are the site of attachment for the muscles and ligaments of the anterolateral abdominal wall and form a bony cage that protects certain abdominal organs.

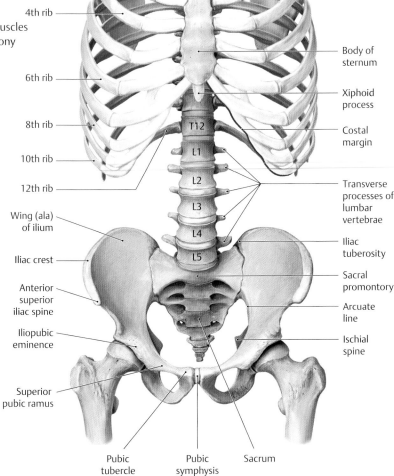

Fig. 13.2 Ligaments of the pelvis

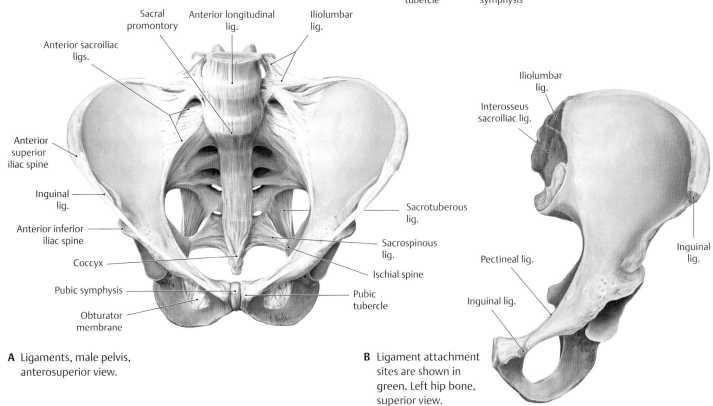

A Ligaments, male pelvis, anterosuperior view.

B Ligament attachment sites are shown in green. Left hip bone, superior view.

Fig. 13.3 **Abdominal wall muscle attachment sites**

Left hip bone. Muscle origins are in red, insertions in blue.

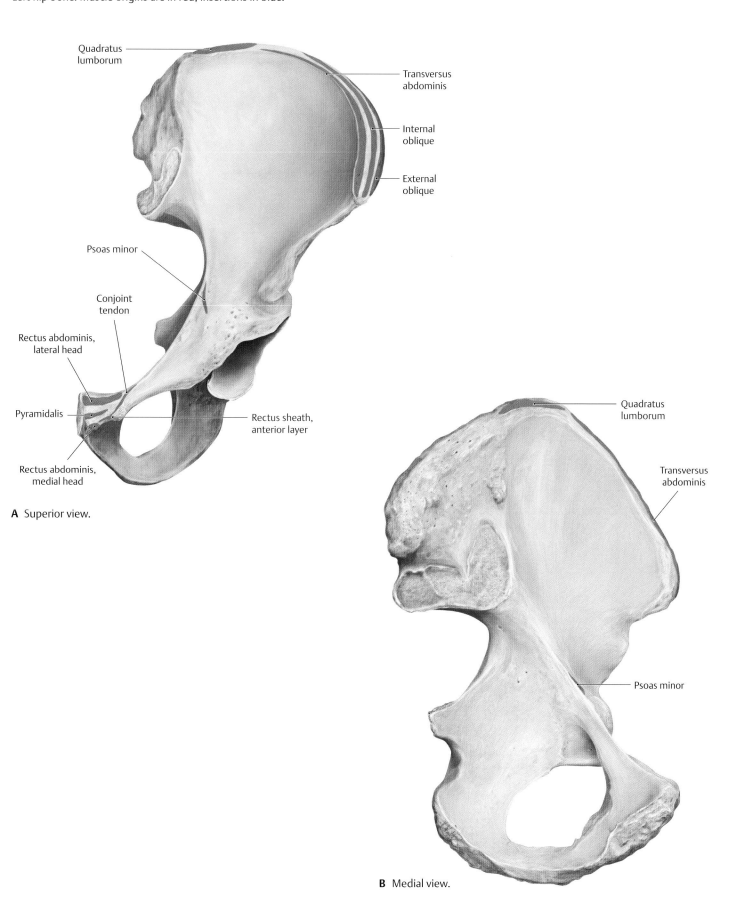

Quadratus lumborum

Transversus abdominis

Internal oblique

External oblique

Psoas minor

Conjoint tendon

Rectus abdominis, lateral head

Pyramidalis

Rectus abdominis, medial head

Rectus sheath, anterior layer

A Superior view.

Quadratus lumborum

Transversus abdominis

Psoas minor

B Medial view.

Muscles of the Anterolateral Abdominal Wall

 The oblique muscles of the anterolateral abdominal wall consist of the external and internal obliques and the transversus abdominis. The posterior or deep abdominal wall muscles (notably the psoas major) are functionally hip muscles (see **p. 148**).

Fig. 13.4 **Muscles of the abdominal wall**
Right side, anterior view.

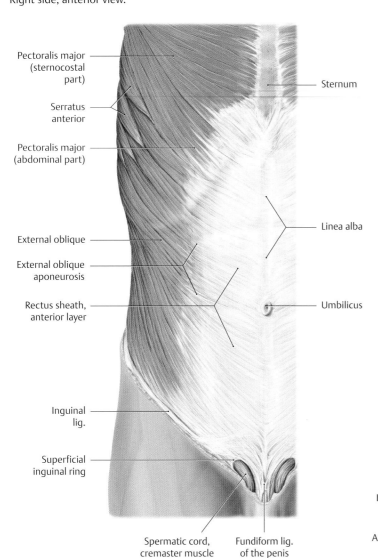

Pectoralis major
(sternocostal
part)

Serratus
anterior

Pectoralis major
(abdominal part)

External oblique

External oblique
aponeurosis

Rectus sheath,
anterior layer

Inguinal
lig.

Superficial
inguinal ring

Spermatic cord,
cremaster muscle

Fundiform lig.
of the penis

Sternum

Linea alba

Umbilicus

A Superficial abdominal wall muscles.

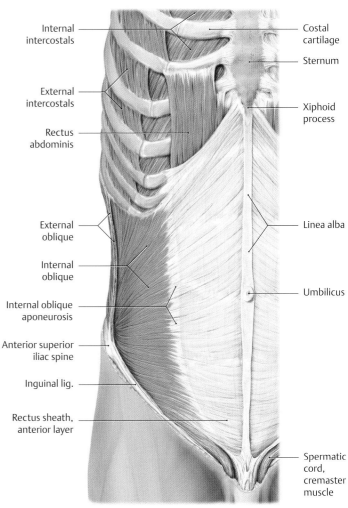

Internal
intercostals

External
intercostals

Rectus
abdominis

External
oblique

Internal
oblique

Internal oblique
aponeurosis

Anterior superior
iliac spine

Inguinal lig.

Rectus sheath,
anterior layer

Costal
cartilage

Sternum

Xiphoid
process

Linea alba

Umbilicus

Spermatic
cord,
cremaster
muscle

B *Removed:* External oblique, pectoralis major, and serratus anterior.

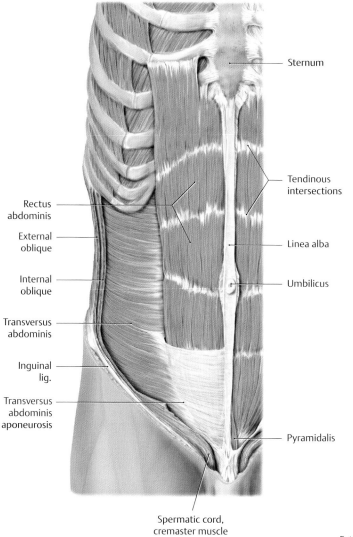

Sternum

Tendinous
intersections

Rectus
abdominis

External
oblique

Linea alba

Internal
oblique

Umbilicus

Transversus
abdominis

Inguinal
lig.

Transversus
abdominis
aponeurosis

Pyramidalis

Spermatic cord,
cremaster muscle

C *Removed:* Internal oblique.

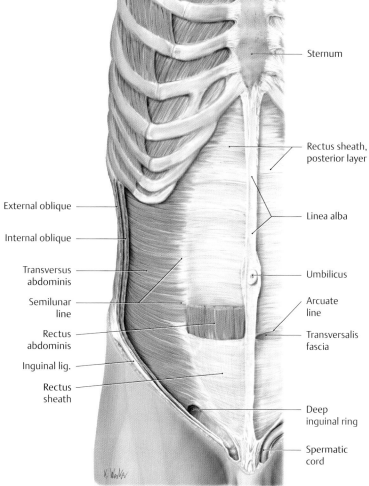

Sternum

External oblique

Rectus sheath,
posterior layer

Internal oblique

Linea alba

Transversus
abdominis

Umbilicus

Semilunar
line

Arcuate
line

Rectus
abdominis

Transversalis
fascia

Inguinal lig.

Rectus
sheath

Deep
inguinal ring

Spermatic
cord

D *Removed:* Rectus abdominis.

145

Muscles of the Posterior Abdominal Wall & Diaphragm

Fig. 13.5 **Muscles of the posterior abdominal wall**

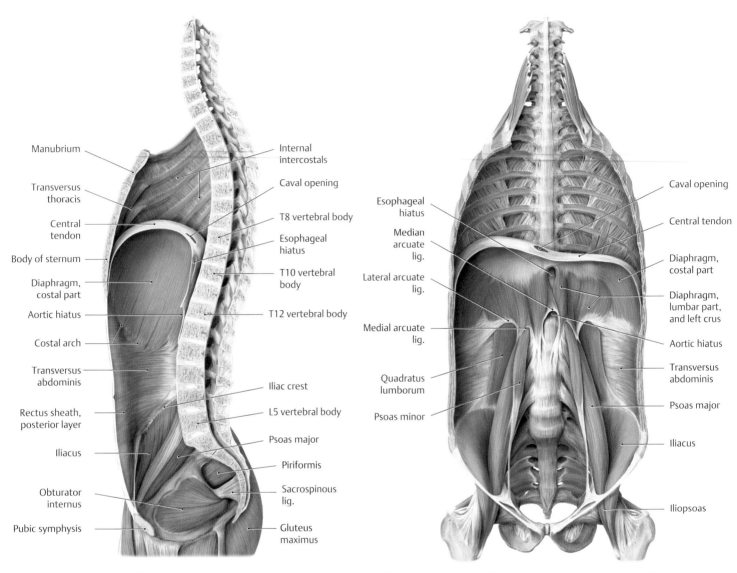

A Midsagittal section with diagraphm in intermediate position.

B Coronal section with diaphragm in intermediate position.

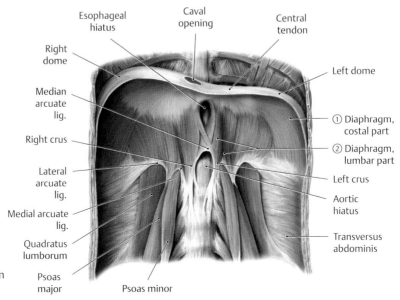

C Coronal section with diaphragm in intermediate position.

Fig. 13.6 Diaphragm in situ

The diaphragm, which separates the thorax from the abdomen, has two asymmetric domes and three apertures (for the aorta, vena cava, and esophagus).

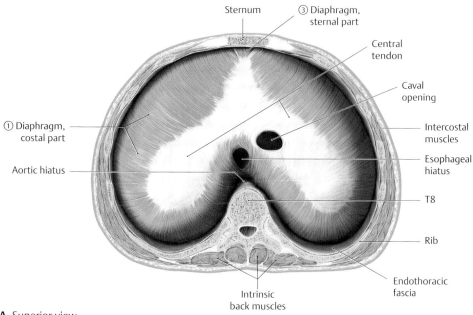

A Superior view.

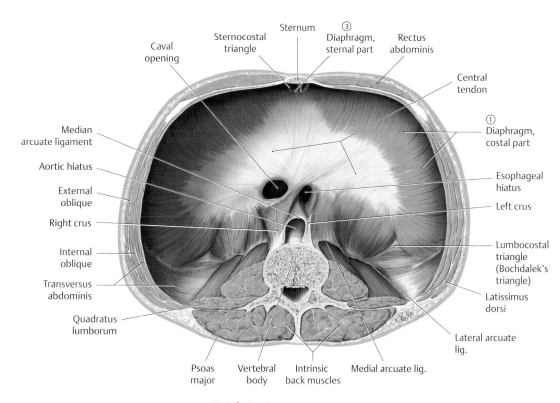

B Inferior view.

Table 13.1	Diaphragm				
Muscle		Origin	Insertion	Innervation	Action
Diaphragm	① Costal part	7th to 12th ribs (inner surface; lower margin of costal arch)	Central tendon	Phrenic n. (C3–C5, cervical plexus)	Principal muscle of respiration (diaphragmatic and thoracic breathing); aids in compressing abdominal viscera (abdominal press)
	② Lumbar part	Medial part: L1–L3 vertebral bodies, intervertebral disks, and anterior longitudinal lig. as right and left crura			
		Lateral parts: lateral and medial arcuate ligs.			
	③ Sternal part	Xiphoid process (posterior surface)			

Abdominal Wall Muscle Facts

Fig. 13.7 Anterior abdominal wall muscles
Anterior view.

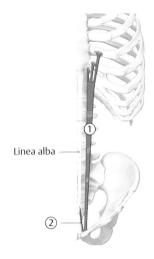

Linea alba

Fig. 13.8 Anterolateral abdominal wall muscles
Anterior view.

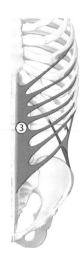

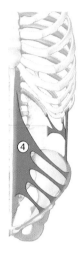

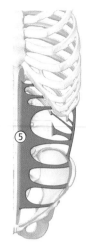

A External oblique.

B Internal oblique.

C Transversus abdominis.

Fig. 13.9 Posterior abdominal wall muscles
Anterior view. The psoas major and iliacus are together known as the iliopsoas.

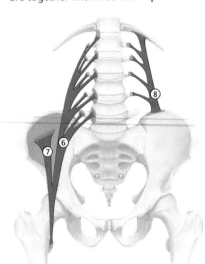

Table 13.2	Abdominal wall muscles			
Muscle	**Origin**	**Insertion**	**Innervation**	**Action**
Anterior abdominal wall muscles				
① Rectus abdominis	*Lateral head:* Crest of pubis to pubic tubercle *Medial head:* Anterior region of pubic symphysis	Cartilages of 5th to 7th ribs, xiphoid process of sternum	Intercostal nn. (T5–T11) , subcostal n. (T12)	Flexes trunk, compresses abdomen, stabilizes pelvis
② Pyramidalis	Pubis (anterior to rectus abdominis)	Linea alba (runs within the rectus sheath)	Subcostal n. (T12)	Tenses linea alba
Anterolateral abdominal wall muscles				
③ External oblique	5th to 12th ribs (outer surface)	Linea alba, pubic tubercle, anterior iliac crest	Intercostal nn. (T7–T11) , subcostal n. (T12)	*Unilateral:* Bends trunk to same side, rotates trunk to opposite side
④ Internal oblique	Thoracolumbar fascia (deep layer), iliac crest (intermediate line), anterior superior iliac spine, iliopsoas fascia	10th to 12th ribs (lower borders), linea alba (anterior and posterior layers)	Intercostal nn. (T7–T11) , subcostal n. (T12) iliohypogastric n., ilioinguinal n.	*Bilateral:* Flexes trunk, compresses abdomen, stabilizes pelvis
⑤ Transversus abdominis	7th to 12th costal cartilages (inner surfaces), thoracolumbar fascia (deep layer), iliac crest, anterior superior iliac spine (inner lip), iliopsoas fascia	Linea alba, pubic crest		*Unilateral:* Rotates trunk to same side *Bilateral:* Compresses abdomen
Posterior abdominal wall muscles				
Psoas minor* (see **Fig. 31.17**)	T12, L1 vertebrae and intervertebral disk (lateral surfaces)	Pectineal line, iliopubic ramus, iliac fascia; lowermost fibers may reach inguinal lig.		Weak flexor of the trunk
⑥ Psoas major — Superficial layer	T12–L4 vertebral bodies and associated intervertebral disks (lateral surfaces)	Femur (lesser trochanter), joint insertion as iliopsoas muscle	L1–L2 (L3) spinal nn.	Hip joint: Flexion and external rotation Lumbar spine (with femur fixed): *Unilateral:* Contraction bends trunk laterally *Bilateral:* Contraction raises trunk from supine position
⑥ Psoas major — Deep layer	L1–L5 (costal processes)			
⑦ Iliacus	Iliac fossa		Femoral n. (L2–L4)	
⑧ Quadratus lumborum	Iliac crest and iliolumbar lig. (not shown)	12th rib, L1–L4 vertebrae (costal processes)	Subcostal n. (T12), L1–L4 spinal nn.	*Unilateral:* Bends trunk to same side *Bilateral:* Bearing down and expiration, stabilizes 12th rib

* Approximately 50% of the population has this muscle. For the diaphragm see **pp. 64–65.**

Fig. 13.10 Anterior, anterolateral, and posterior abdominal wall muscles
Anterior view.

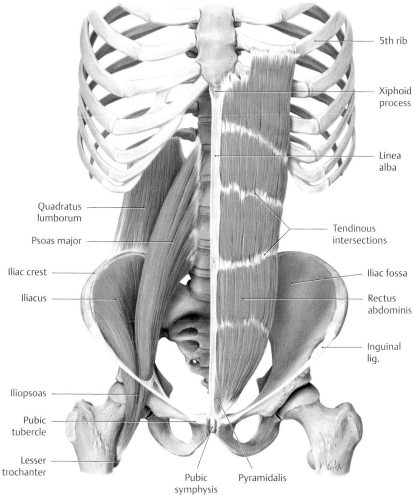

A Anterior and posterior muscles.

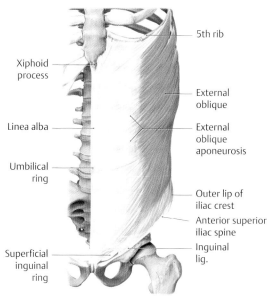

B External oblique.

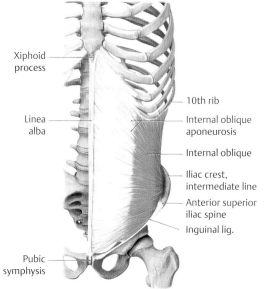

C Internal oblique.

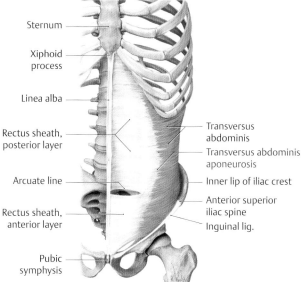

D Transversus abdominis.

Inguinal Region & Canal

The inguinal region is the junction of the anterior abdominal wall and the anterior thigh. The inguinal canal is an important site for the passage of structures into and out of the abdominal cavity (e.g., components of the spermatic cord).

***Fig. 13.11* Inguinal region**
Right side, anterior view.

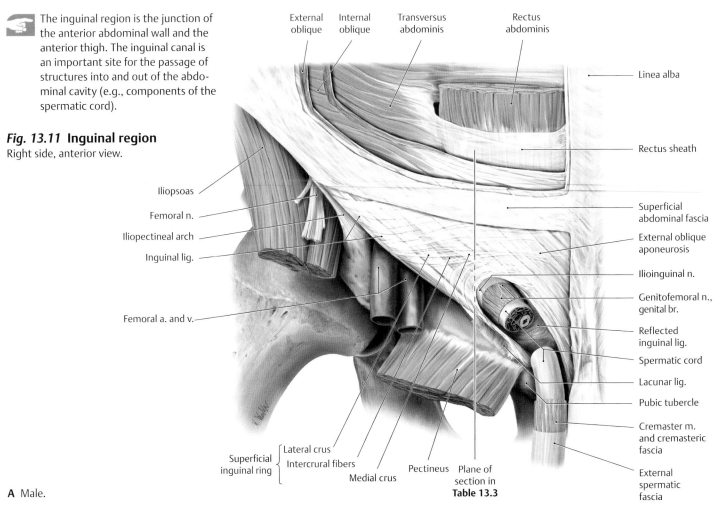

External oblique
Internal oblique
Transversus abdominis
Rectus abdominis
Linea alba
Rectus sheath
Superficial abdominal fascia
External oblique aponeurosis
Ilioinguinal n.
Genitofemoral n., genital br.
Reflected inguinal lig.
Spermatic cord
Lacunar lig.
Pubic tubercle
Cremaster m. and cremasteric fascia
External spermatic fascia

Iliopsoas
Femoral n.
Iliopectineal arch
Inguinal lig.
Femoral a. and v.
Superficial inguinal ring {
Lateral crus
Intercrural fibers
Medial crus
Pectineus
Plane of section in
Table 13.3

A Male.

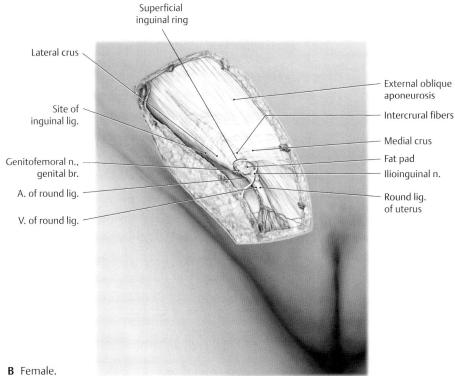

Superficial inguinal ring
Lateral crus
Site of inguinal lig.
Genitofemoral n., genital br.
A. of round lig.
V. of round lig.
External oblique aponeurosis
Intercrural fibers
Medial crus
Fat pad
Ilioinguinal n.
Round lig. of uterus

B Female.

Table 13.3	Structures of the inguinal canal		
Structures			**Formed by**
Wall	Anterior wall	①	External oblique aponeurosis
	Roof	②	Internal oblique muscle
		③	Transversus abdominis
	Posterior wall	④	Transversalis fascia
		⑤	Parietal peritoneum
	Floor	⑥	Inguinal lig. (densely interwoven fibers of the lower external oblique aponeurosis and adjacent fascia lata of thigh)
Openings	Superficial inguinal ring		Opening in external oblique aponeurosis; bounded by medial and lateral crus, intercrural fibers, and reflected inguinal lig.
	Deep inguinal ring		Outpouching of the transversalis fascia lateral to the lateral umbilical fold (inferior epigastric vessels)

Sagittal section through plane in **Fig. 13.11A.**

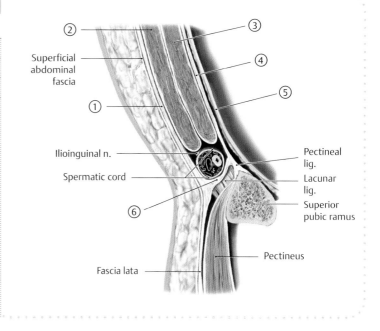

Fig. 13.12 **Dissection of the inguinal region**
Right side, anterior view.

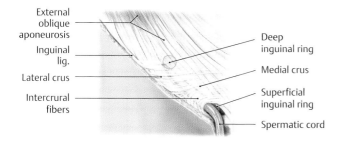

A Superficial layer.

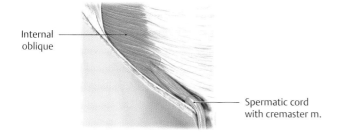

B *Removed:* External oblique aponeurosis.

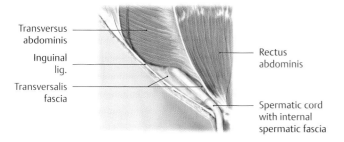

C *Removed:* Internal oblique.

Fig. 13.13 **Opening of the inguinal canal**
Right side, anterior view.

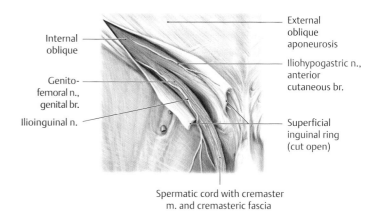

A *Divided:* External oblique aponeurosis.

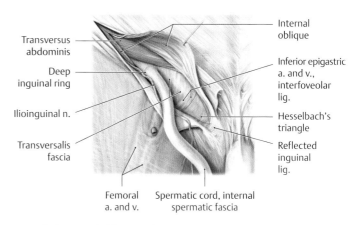

B *Divided:* Internal oblique and cremaster.

Spermatic Cord, Scrotum & Testis

The coverings of the scrotum, testis, and spermatic cord are continuations of muscular and fascial layers of the anterior abdominal wall, as are those of the inguinal canal.

Fig. 13.14 Scrotum and spermatic cord
Anterior view. *Removed:* Skin over the scrotum and spermatic cord.

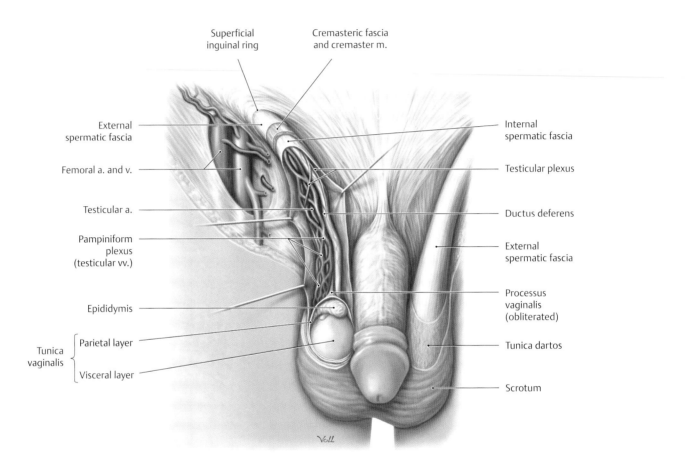

Superficial inguinal ring — Cremasteric fascia and cremaster m.

External spermatic fascia — Internal spermatic fascia

Femoral a. and v. — Testicular plexus

Testicular a. — Ductus deferens

Pampiniform plexus (testicular vv.) — External spermatic fascia

Epididymis — Processus vaginalis (obliterated)

Tunica vaginalis { Parietal layer — Tunica dartos

Visceral layer } — Scrotum

Fig. 13.15 Spermatic cord: Contents
Cross section.

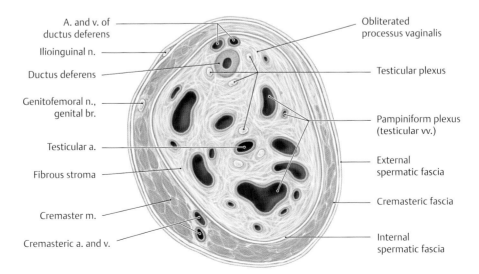

A. and v. of ductus deferens — Obliterated processus vaginalis

Ilioinguinal n. —

Ductus deferens — Testicular plexus

Genitofemoral n., genital br. — Pampiniform plexus (testicular vv.)

Testicular a. — External spermatic fascia

Fibrous stroma — Cremasteric fascia

Cremaster m. — Internal spermatic fascia

Cremasteric a. and v. —

Fig. 13.16 Testis and epididymis

Left lateral view.

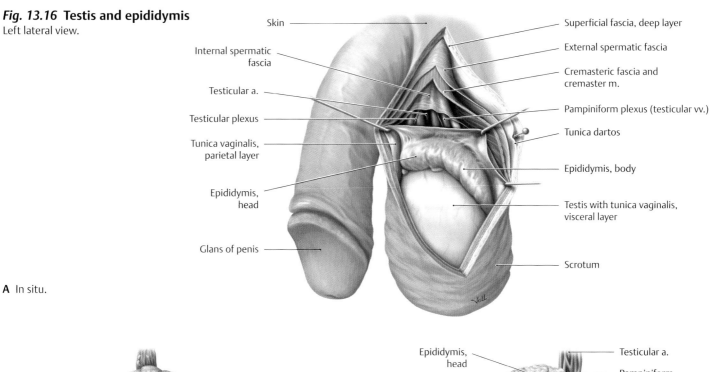

Skin — Superficial fascia, deep layer

Internal spermatic fascia — External spermatic fascia

Testicular a. — Cremasteric fascia and cremaster m.

Testicular plexus — Pampiniform plexus (testicular vv.)

Tunica vaginalis, parietal layer — Tunica dartos

Epididymis, head — Epididymis, body

Glans of penis — Testis with tunica vaginalis, visceral layer

Scrotum

A In situ.

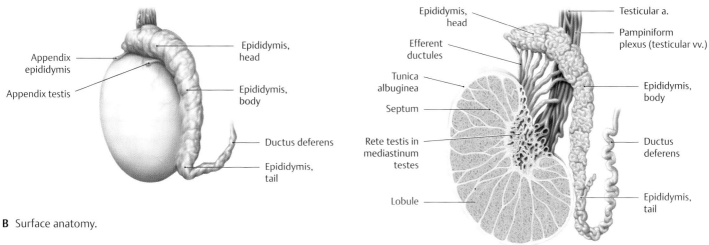

Appendix epididymis — Epididymis, head

Appendix testis — Epididymis, body

Ductus deferens

Epididymis, tail

B Surface anatomy.

Epididymis, head — Testicular a.

Efferent ductules — Pampiniform plexus (testicular vv.)

Tunica albuginea — Epididymis, body

Septum

Rete testis in mediastinum testes — Ductus deferens

Lobule — Epididymis, tail

C Sagittal section.

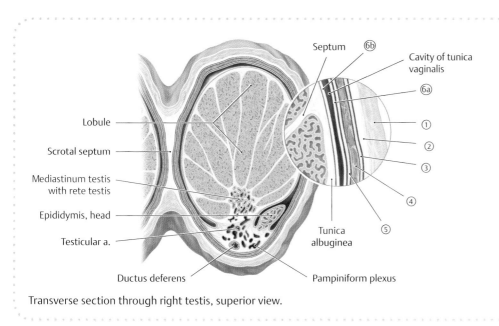

Septum ⑥b

Cavity of tunica vaginalis

⑥a

Lobule

Scrotal septum ②

Mediastinum testis with rete testis ③

Epididymis, head

Testicular a. ⑤

④

Ductus deferens — Tunica albuginea

Pampiniform plexus

Transverse section through right testis, superior view.

Table 13.4	Coverings of the testis	
Covering layer		**Derived from**
①	Scrotal skin	Abdominal skin
②	Tunica dartos	Dartos fascia and m.
③	External spermatic fascia	External oblique fascia
④	Cremaster m. and/or cremasteric fascia	Internal oblique
⑤	Internal spermatic fascia	Transversalis fascia
⑥a	Tunica vaginalis, parietal layer	Peritoneum
⑥b	Tunica vaginalis, visceral layer	

* The transversus abdominis has no contribution to the spermatic cord or covering of the testis.

153

Anterior Abdominal Wall & Inguinal Hernias

The rectus sheath is created by fusion of the aponeuroses of the transversus abdominis and abdominal oblique muscles. The inferior edge of the posterior layer of the rectus sheath is called the arcuate line.

***Fig. 13.17* Anterior abdominal wall and rectus sheath**

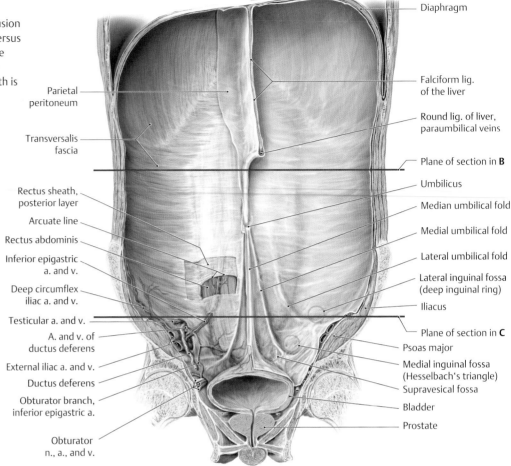

A Coronal section, male, posterior (internal) view of anterior abdominal wall. The three fossae of the anterior abdominal wall (circled) are sites of potential herniation through the wall.

Labels (left): Parietal peritoneum; Transversalis fascia; Rectus sheath, posterior layer; Arcuate line; Rectus abdominis; Inferior epigastric a. and v.; Deep circumflex iliac a. and v.; Testicular a. and v.; A. and v. of ductus deferens; External iliac a. and v.; Ductus deferens; Obturator branch, inferior epigastric a.; Obturator n., a., and v.

Labels (right): Diaphragm; Falciform lig. of the liver; Round lig. of liver, paraumbilical veins; Plane of section in **B**; Umbilicus; Median umbilical fold; Medial umbilical fold; Lateral umbilical fold; Lateral inguinal fossa (deep inguinal ring); Iliacus; Plane of section in **C**; Psoas major; Medial inguinal fossa (Hesselbach's triangle); Supravesical fossa; Bladder; Prostate

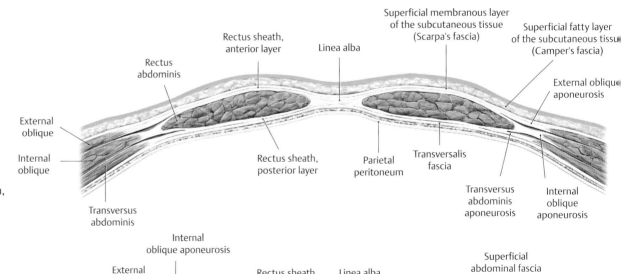

B Transverse section, superior to the arcuate line.

Labels: Rectus abdominis; External oblique; Internal oblique; Transversus abdominis; Rectus sheath, anterior layer; Linea alba; Superficial membranous layer of the subcutaneous tissue (Scarpa's fascia); Superficial fatty layer of the subcutaneous tissue (Camper's fascia); External oblique aponeurosis; Internal oblique aponeurosis; Transversus abdominis aponeurosis; Transversalis fascia; Parietal peritoneum; Rectus sheath, posterior layer

C Transverse section, inferior to the arcuate line.

Labels: External oblique aponeurosis; Internal oblique aponeurosis; Transversus abdominis aponeurosis; Rectus sheath; Linea alba; Transversalis fascia; Parietal peritoneum; Superficial abdominal fascia

Fig. 13.18 **Inferior anterior abdominal wall: Structure and fossae**

Coronal section, posterior (internal) view of left inferior portion of the anterior abdominal wall.

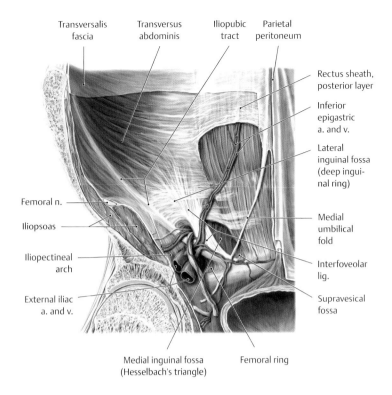

![] **Clinical box 13.1**

Inguinal and femoral hernias

Indirect inguinal hernias occur in younger males and may be congenital or acquired; direct inguinal hernias generally occur in older males and are always acquired. Femoral hernias are acquired and more common in females.

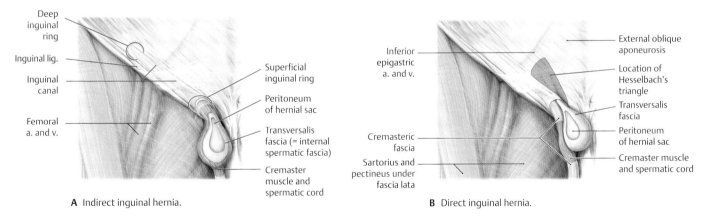

A Indirect inguinal hernia.

B Direct inguinal hernia.

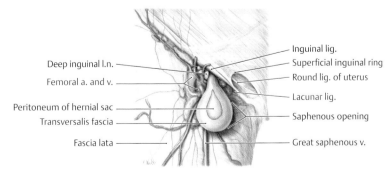

C Femoral hernia.

Divisions of the Abdominopelvic Cavity

 Organs in the abdominopelvic cavity are classified by the presence of surrounding peritoneum (the serous membrane lining the cavity) and a mesentery (a double layer of peritoneum that connects the organ to the abdominal wall) (see **Table 14.1**).

Fig. 14.1 **Peritoneal cavity**

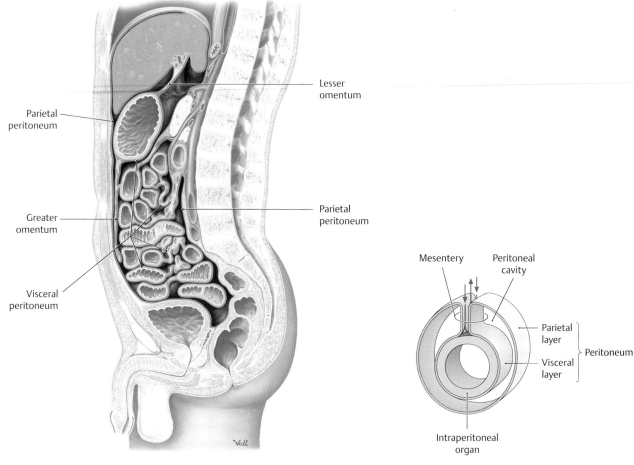

A Midsagittal section through the male abdominopelvic cavity, viewed from the left. The peritoneum is shown in red.

B An intraperitoneal organ, showing the mesentery and surrounding peritoneum. Arrows indicate location of blood vessels in the mesentery.

Table 14.1	Organs of the abdominopelvic cavity classified by their relationship to the peritoneum		
Location	**Organs**		
Intraperitoneal organs: These organs have a mesentery and are completely covered by the peritoneum.			
Abdominal peritoneal	• Stomach • Small intestine (jejunum, ileum, some of the superior part of the duodenum) • Spleen • Liver	• Gallbladder • Cecum with vermiform appendix (portions of variable size may be retroperitoneal) • Large intestine (transverse and sigmoid colons)	
Pelvic peritoneal	• Uterus (fundus and body)	• Ovaries	• Uterine tubes
Extraperitoneal organs: These organs either have no mesentery or lost it during development.			
Retroperitoneal	Primarily	• Kidneys and ureters	• Suprarenal glands	• Uterine cervix
	Secondarily	• Duodenum (descending, horizontal, and ascending) • Pancreas	• Ascending and descending colon and cecum • Rectum (upper 2/3)	
Infraperitoneal/subperitoneal		• Urinary bladder • Distal ureters • Prostate	• Seminal vesicle • Uterine cervix	• Vagina • Rectum (lower 1/3)

Fig. 14.2 **Peritoneal relationships of the abdominopelvic organs**

Midsagittal section through the male abdomino-pelvic cavity, viewed from the left.

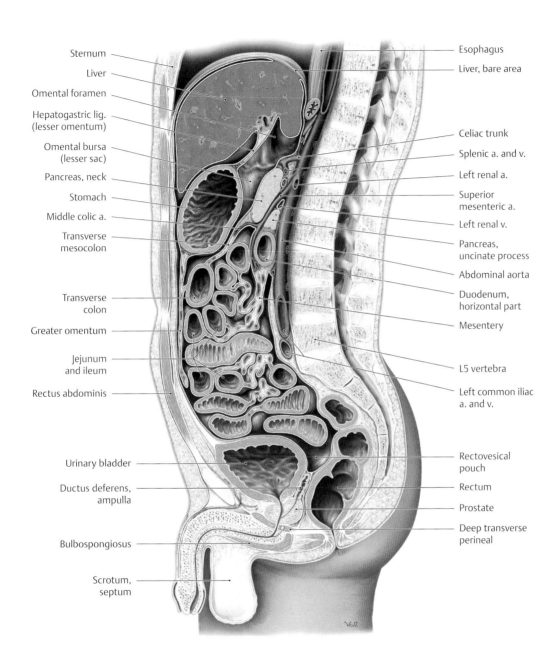

Sternum
Liver
Omental foramen
Hepatogastric lig. (lesser omentum)
Omental bursa (lesser sac)
Pancreas, neck
Stomach
Middle colic a.
Transverse mesocolon
Transverse colon
Greater omentum
Jejunum and ileum
Rectus abdominis
Urinary bladder
Ductus deferens, ampulla
Bulbospongiosus
Scrotum, septum

Esophagus
Liver, bare area
Celiac trunk
Splenic a. and v.
Left renal a.
Superior mesenteric a.
Left renal v.
Pancreas, uncinate process
Abdominal aorta
Duodenum, horizontal part
Mesentery
L5 vertebra
Left common iliac a. and v.
Rectovesical pouch
Rectum
Prostate
Deep transverse perineal

 Clinical box 14.1

Acute abdominal pain

Acute abdominal pain ("acute abdomen") may be so severe that the abdominal wall becomes extremely sensitive to touch ("guarding") and the intestines stop functioning. Causes include organ inflammation such as appendicitis, perforation due to a gastric ulcer (see **p. 165**), or organ blockage by a stone, tumor, etc. In women, gynecological processes or ectopic pregnancies may produce severe abdominal pain.

Peritoneal Cavity & Greater Sac

The peritoneal cavity is divided into the large greater sac and small omental bursa (lesser sac). The greater omentum is an apron-like fold of peritoneum suspended from the greater curvature of the stomach and covering the anterior surface of the transverse colon. The attachment of the transverse mesocolon on the anterior surface of the descending part of the duodenum and the pancreas divides the peritoneal cavity into a supracolic compartment (liver, gallbladder, and stomach) and an infracolic compartment (intestines).

Fig. 14.3 **Dissection of the peritoneal cavity**
Anterior view.

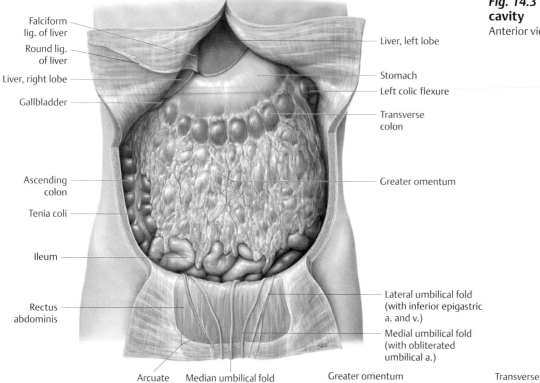

Falciform lig. of liver
Round lig. of liver
Liver, right lobe
Gallbladder
Ascending colon
Tenia coli
Ileum
Rectus abdominis
Arcuate line
Median umbilical fold (with obliterated urachus)
Liver, left lobe
Stomach
Left colic flexure
Transverse colon
Greater omentum
Lateral umbilical fold (with inferior epigastric a. and v.)
Medial umbilical fold (with obliterated umbilical a.)

A Greater sac. *Retracted:* Abdominal wall.

Greater omentum (reflected superiorly)
Transverse colon
Transverse mesocolon with middle colic a. and v.
Parietal peritoneum
Jejunum (covered by visceral peritoneum)
Ascending colon
Tenia coli
Ileum
Rectus abdominis
Arcuate line
Median umbilical fold (with obliterated urachus)
Lateral umbilical fold (with inferior epigastric a. and v.)
Medial umbilical fold (with obliterated umbilical a.)

B Infracolic compartment, the portion of the peritoneal cavity below the attachment of the transverse mesocolon. *Reflected:* Greater omentum and transverse colon.

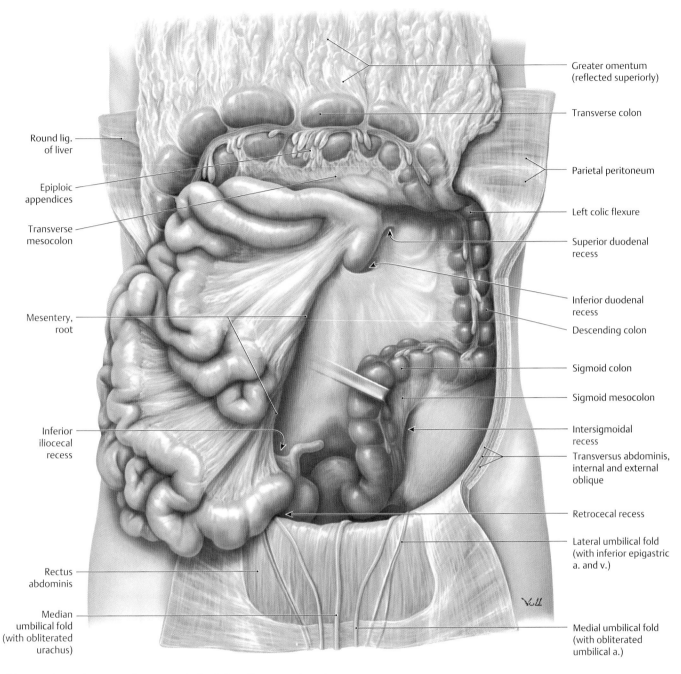

Round lig. of liver

Epiploic appendices

Transverse mesocolon

Mesentery, root

Inferior iliocecal recess

Rectus abdominis

Median umbilical fold (with obliterated urachus)

Greater omentum (reflected superiorly)

Transverse colon

Parietal peritoneum

Left colic flexure

Superior duodenal recess

Inferior duodenal recess

Descending colon

Sigmoid colon

Sigmoid mesocolon

Intersigmoidal recess

Transversus abdominis, internal and external oblique

Retrocecal recess

Lateral umbilical fold (with inferior epigastric a. and v.)

Medial umbilical fold (with obliterated umbilical a.)

C Mesenteries and mesenteric recesses in the infracolic compartment. *Reflected:* Greater omentum, transverse colon, small intestines, and sigmoid colon.

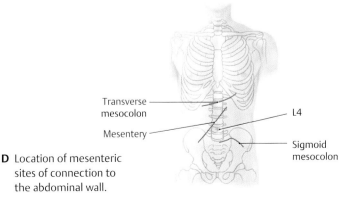

Transverse mesocolon

Mesentery

L4

Sigmoid mesocolon

D Location of mesenteric sites of connection to the abdominal wall.

159

Omental Bursa, or Lesser Sac

 The omental bursa, or lesser sac, is the portion of the peritoneal cavity behind the stomach and the lesser omentum (a double-layered peritoneal structure connecting the lesser curvature of the stomach and the proximal part of the duodenum to the liver).

The omental bursa communicates with the greater sac via the omental (epiploic) foramen, located posterior to the free edge of the lesser omentum.

Fig. 14.4 Omental bursa (lesser sac)

Anterior view. The omental bursa (lesser sac) is the portion of the peritoneal cavity located behind the lesser omentum and stomach.

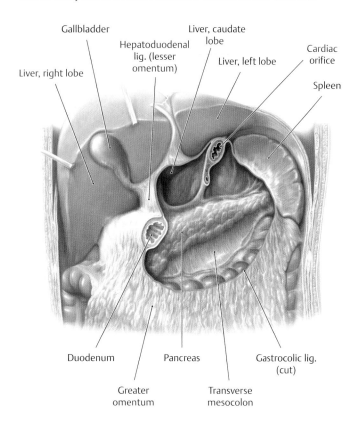

A Boundaries of the omental bursa (lesser sac).

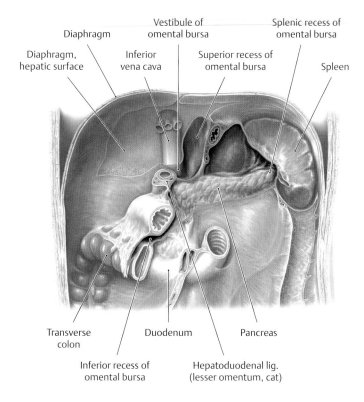

B Posterior wall of the omental bursa (lesser sac).

Fig. 14.5 Location of the omental bursa

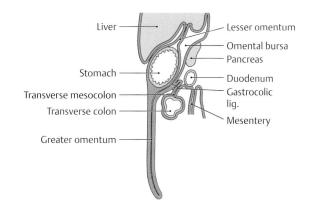

A Sagittal section.

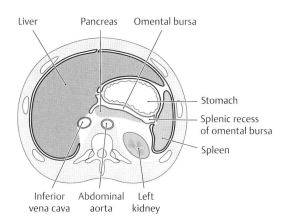

B Transverse section, inferior view.

Fig. 14.6 Omental bursa in situ

Anterior view. *Divided:* Gastrocolic ligament. *Retracted:* Liver.
Reflected: Stomach.

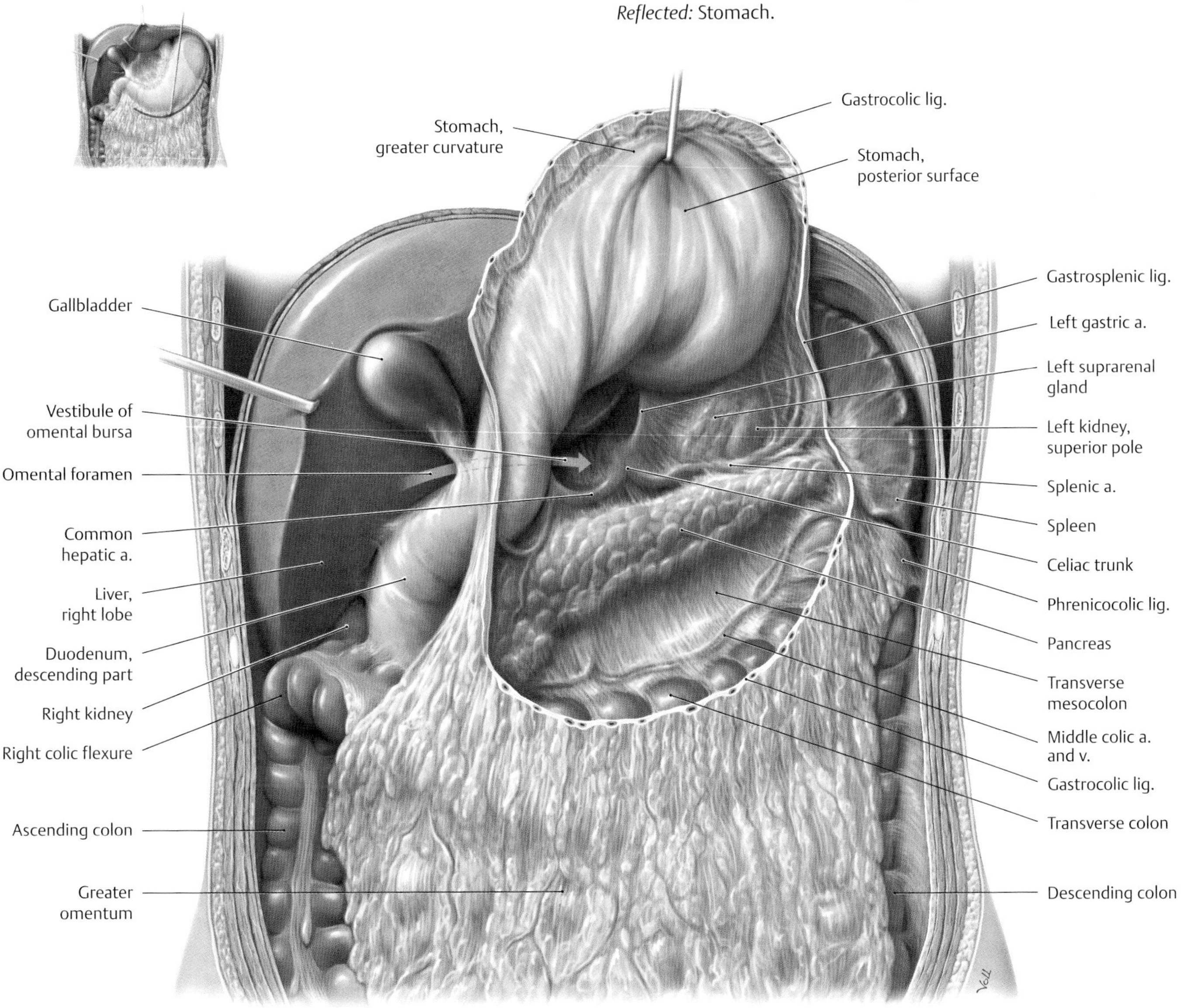

Table 14.2	Boundaries of the omental bursa	
Direction	**Boundary**	**Recess**
Anterior	Lesser omentum, gastrocolic lig.	—
Inferior	Transverse mesocolon	Inferior recess
Superior	Liver (with caudate lobe)	Superior recess
Posterior	Pancreas, aorta (abdominal part), celiac trunk, splenic a. and v., gastrosplenic fold, left suprarenal gland, left kidney (superior pole)	—
Right	Liver, duodenal bulb	—
Left	Spleen, gastrosplenic lig.	Splenic recess

Table 14.3	Boundaries of the omental foramen

The communication between the greater sac and lesser sac (omental bursa) is the omental (epiploic) foramen (see arrow in **Fig. 14.6**).

Direction	**Boundary**
Anterior	Hepatoduodenal lig. with the portal v., proper hepatic a., and bile duct
Inferior	Duodenum (superior part)
Posterior	Inferior vena cava, diaphragm (right crus)
Superior	Liver (caudate lobe)

Mesenteries & Posterior Wall

Fig. 14.7 **Mesenteries and organs of the peritoneal cavity**

Anterior view. *Removed:* Stomach, jejunum, and ileum. *Reflected:* Liver.

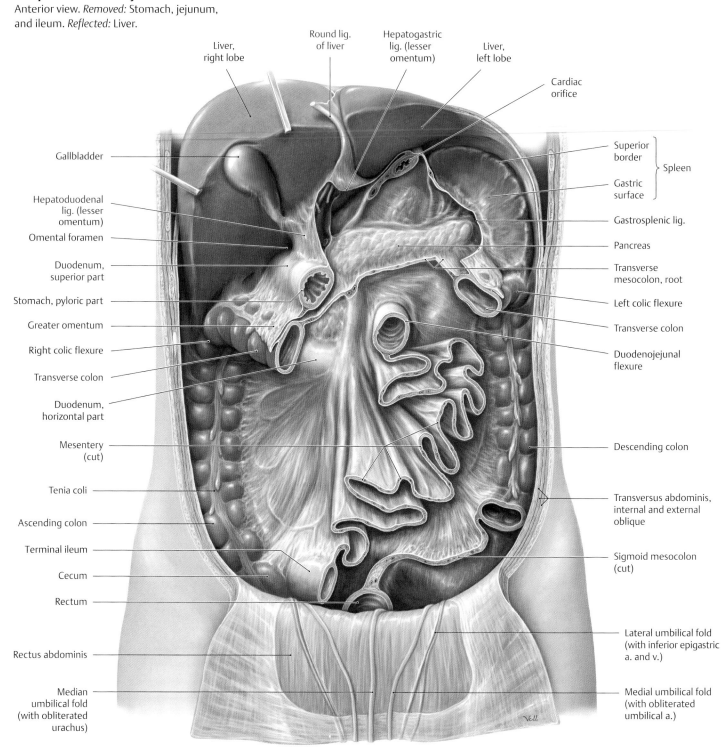

Liver, right lobe

Round lig. of liver

Hepatogastric lig. (lesser omentum)

Liver, left lobe

Cardiac orifice

Gallbladder

Hepatoduodenal lig. (lesser omentum)

Omental foramen

Duodenum, superior part

Stomach, pyloric part

Greater omentum

Right colic flexure

Transverse colon

Duodenum, horizontal part

Mesentery (cut)

Tenia coli

Ascending colon

Terminal ileum

Cecum

Rectum

Rectus abdominis

Median umbilical fold (with obliterated urachus)

Superior border

Gastric surface

Spleen

Gastrosplenic lig.

Pancreas

Transverse mesocolon, root

Left colic flexure

Transverse colon

Duodenojejunal flexure

Descending colon

Transversus abdominis, internal and external oblique

Sigmoid mesocolon (cut)

Lateral umbilical fold (with inferior epigastric a. and v.)

Medial umbilical fold (with obliterated umbilical a.)

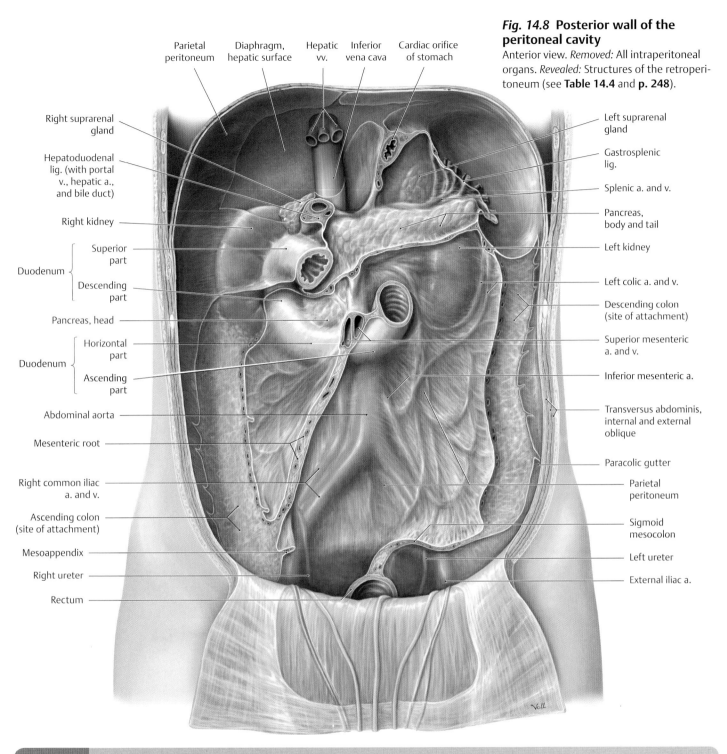

Fig. 14.8 Posterior wall of the peritoneal cavity

Anterior view. *Removed:* All intraperitoneal organs. *Revealed:* Structures of the retroperitoneum (see **Table 14.4** and **p. 248**).

Parietal peritoneum

Diaphragm, hepatic surface

Hepatic vv.

Inferior vena cava

Cardiac orifice of stomach

Right suprarenal gland

Hepatoduodenal lig. (with portal v., hepatic a., and bile duct)

Right kidney

Duodenum — Superior part

Duodenum — Descending part

Pancreas, head

Duodenum — Horizontal part

Duodenum — Ascending part

Abdominal aorta

Mesenteric root

Right common iliac a. and v.

Ascending colon (site of attachment)

Mesoappendix

Right ureter

Rectum

Left suprarenal gland

Gastrosplenic lig.

Splenic a. and v.

Pancreas, body and tail

Left kidney

Left colic a. and v.

Descending colon (site of attachment)

Superior mesenteric a. and v.

Inferior mesenteric a.

Transversus abdominis, internal and external oblique

Paracolic gutter

Parietal peritoneum

Sigmoid mesocolon

Left ureter

External iliac a.

Table 14.4   Structures of the retroperitoneum

See **pp. 194, 202, 215** for neurovascular structures of the retroperitoneum.

Classification	Organs	Vessels	Nerves

Primarily retroperitoneal (no mesentery; retroperitoneal when formed)	• Kidneys
	• Suprarenal glands
	• Ureters
		• Aorta (abdominal part)
		• Inferior vena cava and tributaries
		• Ascending lumbar vv.
		• Portal v. and tributaries
		• Lumbar, sacral, and iliac l.n.
		• Lumbar trunks and cisterna chyli
			• Lumbar plexus brs.
			  ○ Iliohypogastric n.
			  ○ Ilioinguinal n.
			  ○ Genitofemoral n.
			  ○ Lateral femoral cutaneous n.
			  ○ Femoral n.
			  ○ Obturator n.
			• Sympathetic trunk
			• Autonomic ganglia and plexuses

Secondarily retroperitoneal (mesentery lost during development)	• Pancreas • Duodenum (descending and horizontal parts; some of ascending part) • Ascending and descending colon • Cecum (portions; variable) • Rectum (upper 2/3)		

Stomach

Fig. 15.1 Stomach: Location

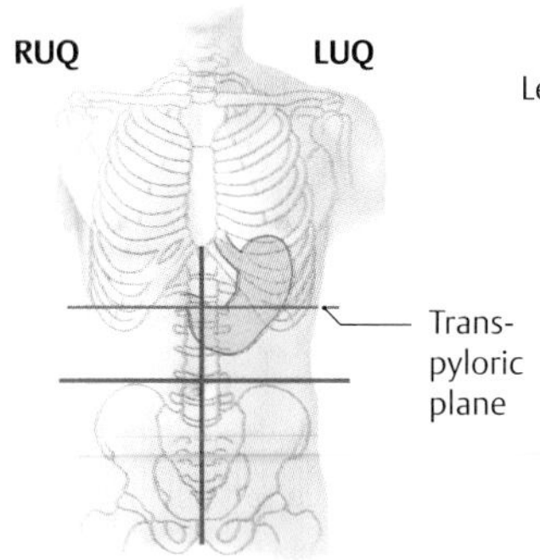

A Anterior view.

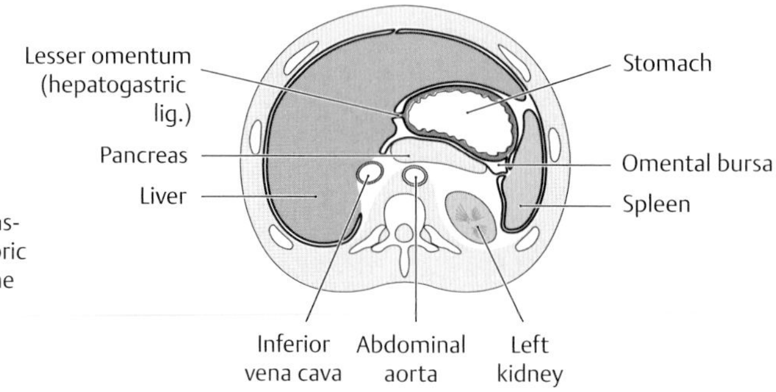

B Transverse section, inferior view.

Fig. 15.2 Relations of the stomach

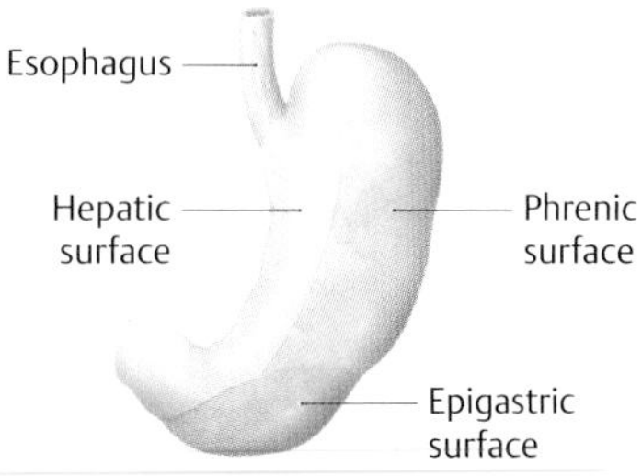

A Anterior view.

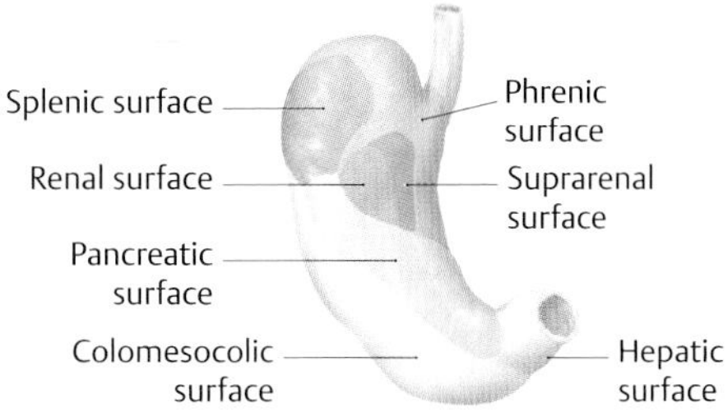

B Posterior view.

Fig. 15.3 Stomach
Anterior view.

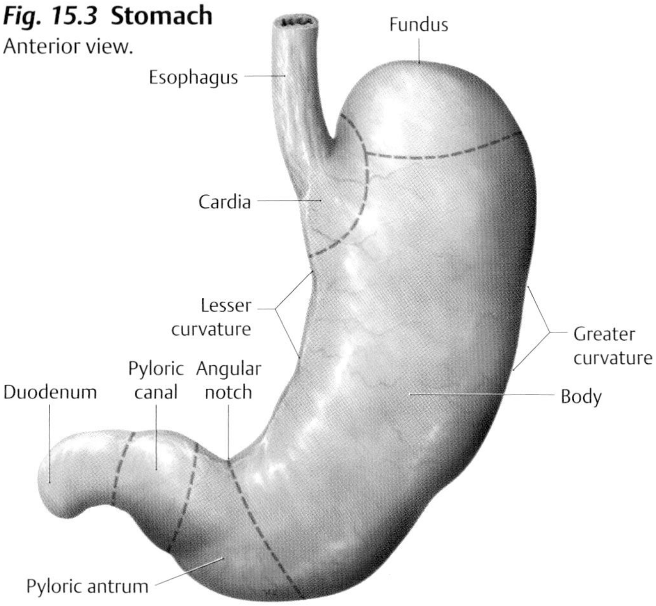

A Anterior wall.

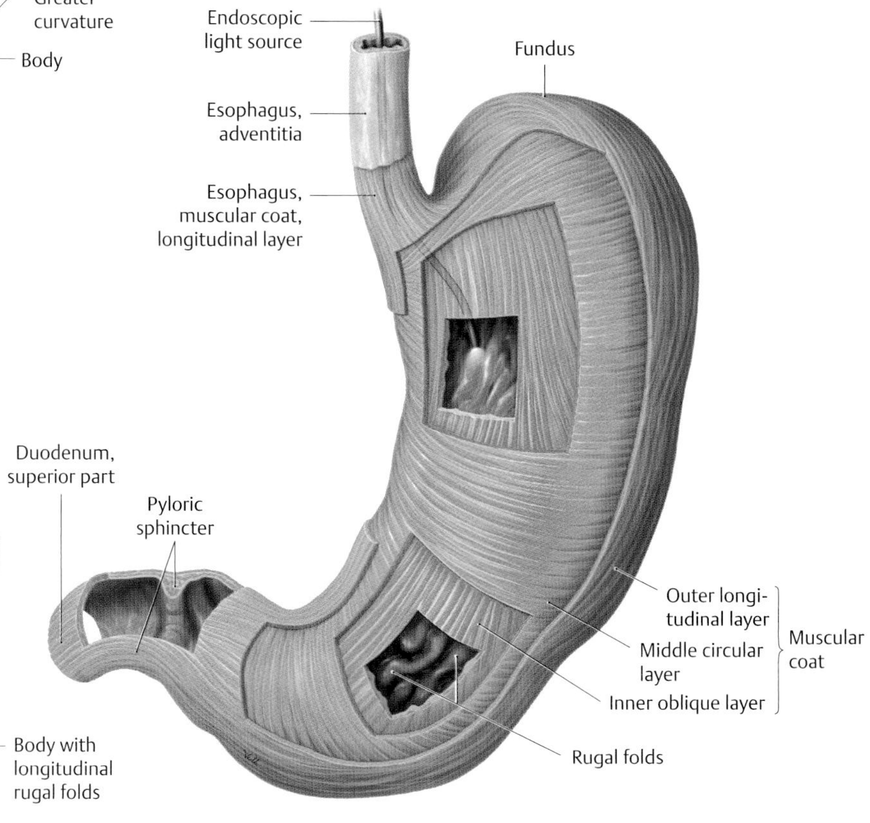

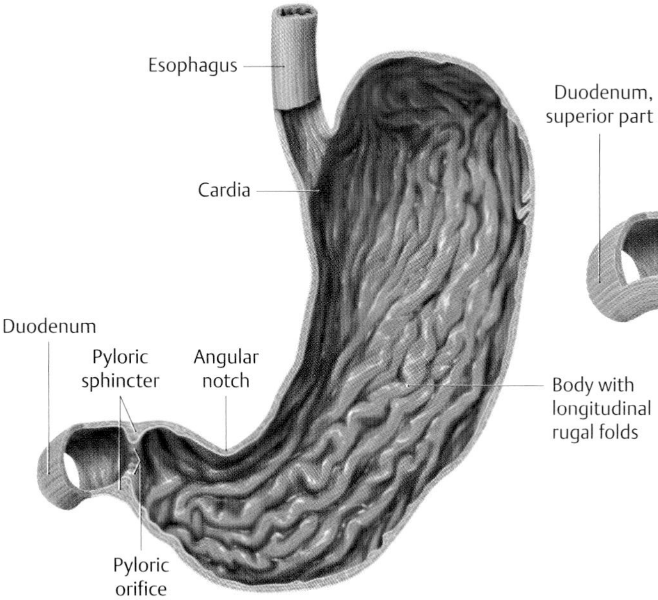

C Interior. *Removed:* Anterior wall.

B Muscular layers. *Removed:* Serosa and subserosa. *Windowed:* Muscular coat.

The stomach resides primarily in the left upper quadrant. It is intraperitoneal, its mesenteries being the lesser and greater omenta.

Fig. 15.4 **Stomach in situ**
Anterior view of the opened upper abdomen. Arrow indicates the omental foramen.

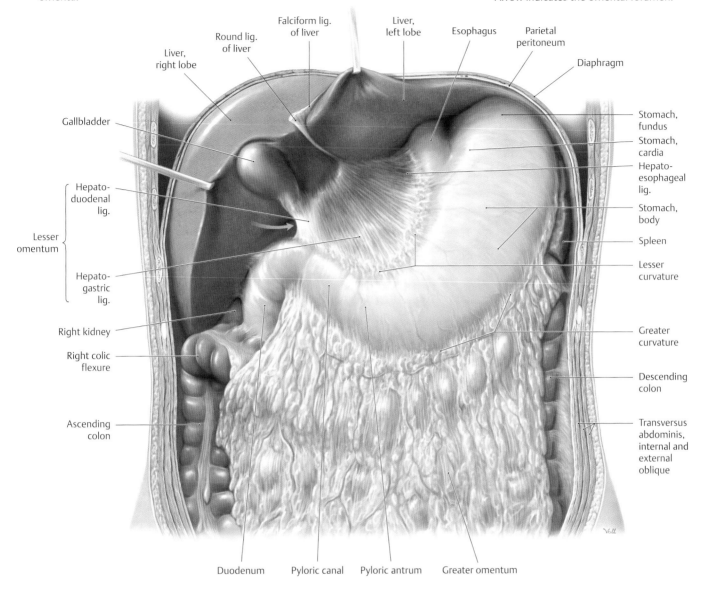

Falciform lig. of liver

Round lig. of liver

Liver, right lobe

Liver, left lobe

Esophagus

Parietal peritoneum

Diaphragm

Gallbladder

Stomach, fundus

Stomach, cardia

Hepato-esophageal lig.

Hepato-duodenal lig.

Lesser omentum

Hepato-gastric lig.

Stomach, body

Spleen

Lesser curvature

Right kidney

Right colic flexure

Greater curvature

Descending colon

Ascending colon

Transversus abdominis, internal and external oblique

Duodenum   Pyloric canal   Pyloric antrum   Greater omentum

 Clinical box 15.1

Gastritis and gastric ulcers

Gastritis and gastric ulcers, the two most common diseases of the stomach, are associated with increased acid production and are caused by alcohol, drugs such as aspirin, and the bacterium *Helicobacter pylori*. Symptoms include lessened appetite, pain, and even bleeding, which manifests as black stool or dark brown material, often described as resembling "coffee grounds," in vomit. Gastritis is limited to the inner surface of the stomach, whereas gastric ulcers extend into the stomach wall. The gastric ulcer in **C** is covered with fibrin and shows hematin spots.

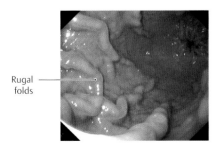

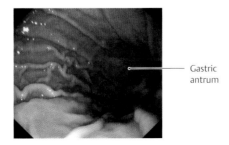

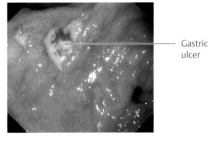

Rugal folds

Gastric antrum

Gastric ulcer

A Body of normal stomach.

B Normal pyloric antrum.

C Gastric ulcer.

Duodenum

 The small intestine consists of the duodenum, jejunum, and ileum (see **p. 168**). The duodenum is primarily retroperitoneal and is divided into four parts: superior, descending, horizontal, and ascending.

Fig. 15.5 **Duodenum: Location**
Anterior view.

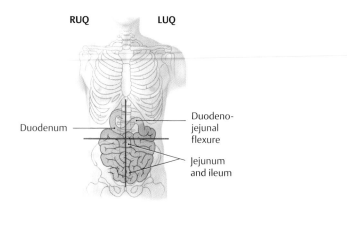

RUQ   LUQ

Duodenum

Duodeno-jejunal flexure

Jejunum and ileum

Fig. 15.6 **Parts of the duodenum**
Anterior view.

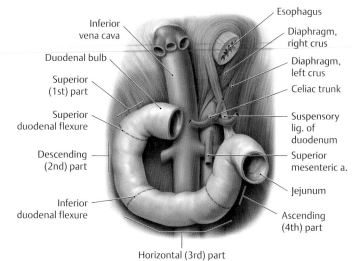

Inferior vena cava

Esophagus

Diaphragm, right crus

Duodenal bulb

Superior (1st) part

Diaphragm, left crus

Celiac trunk

Superior duodenal flexure

Suspensory lig. of duodenum

Descending (2nd) part

Superior mesenteric a.

Inferior duodenal flexure

Jejunum

Ascending (4th) part

Horizontal (3rd) part

Fig. 15.7 **Duodenum**
Anterior view with the anterior wall opened.

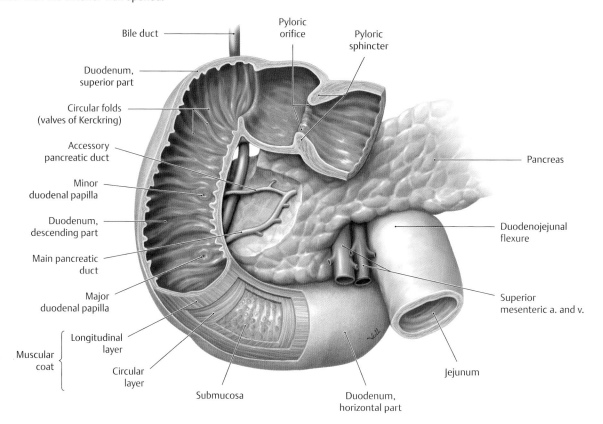

Bile duct

Pyloric orifice

Pyloric sphincter

Duodenum, superior part

Circular folds (valves of Kerckring)

Accessory pancreatic duct

Pancreas

Minor duodenal papilla

Duodenum, descending part

Duodenojejunal flexure

Main pancreatic duct

Major duodenal papilla

Superior mesenteric a. and v.

Longitudinal layer

Muscular coat

Circular layer

Jejunum

Submucosa

Duodenum, horizontal part

Fig. 15.8 Duodenum in situ

Anterior view. *Removed:* Stomach, liver, small intestine, and large portions of the transverse colon. *Thinned:* Retroperitoneal fat and connective tissue.

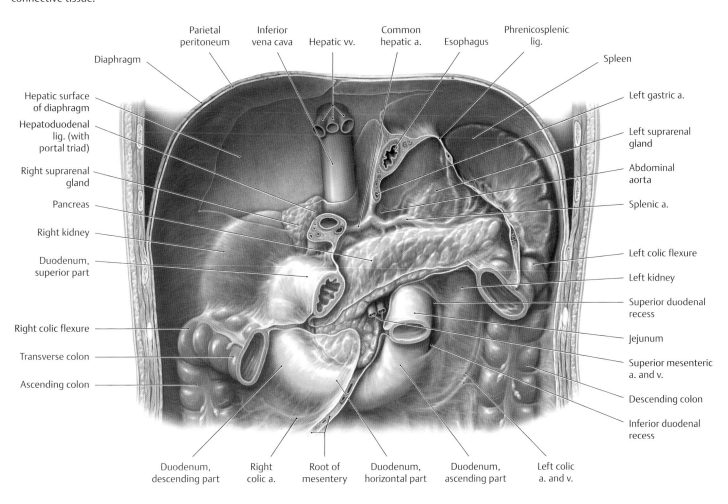

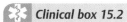

Clinical box 15.2

Endoscopy of the papillary region

Two important ducts end in the descending portion of the duodenum: the common bile duct and the pancreatic duct (see **Fig. 15.7**). These ducts may be examined by X-ray through endoscopic retrograde

cholangiopancreatography (ERCP), in which dye is injected endoscopically into the duodenal papilla. Duodenal diverticula (generally harmless outpouchings) may complicate the procedure.

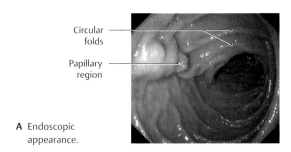

A Endoscopic appearance.

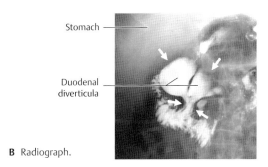

B Radiograph.

Jejunum & Ileum

Fig. 15.9 Jejunum and ileum: Location

Anterior view. The intraperitoneal jejunum and ileum are enclosed by the mesentery proper.

Fig. 15.10 Wall structure of the jejunum and ileum

Macroscopic views of the longitudinally opened small intestine.

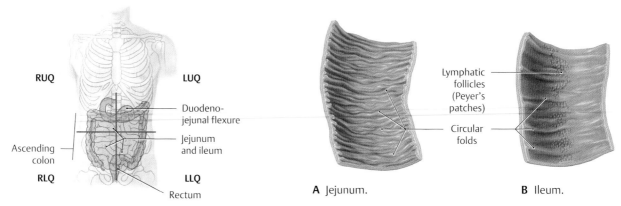

RUQ

LUQ

Duodeno-jejunal flexure

Jejunum and ileum

Ascending colon

RLQ

LLQ

Rectum

Lymphatic follicles (Peyer's patches)

Circular folds

A Jejunum.

B Ileum.

Fig. 15.11 Jejunum and ileum in situ

Anterior view. *Reflected:* Transverse colon.

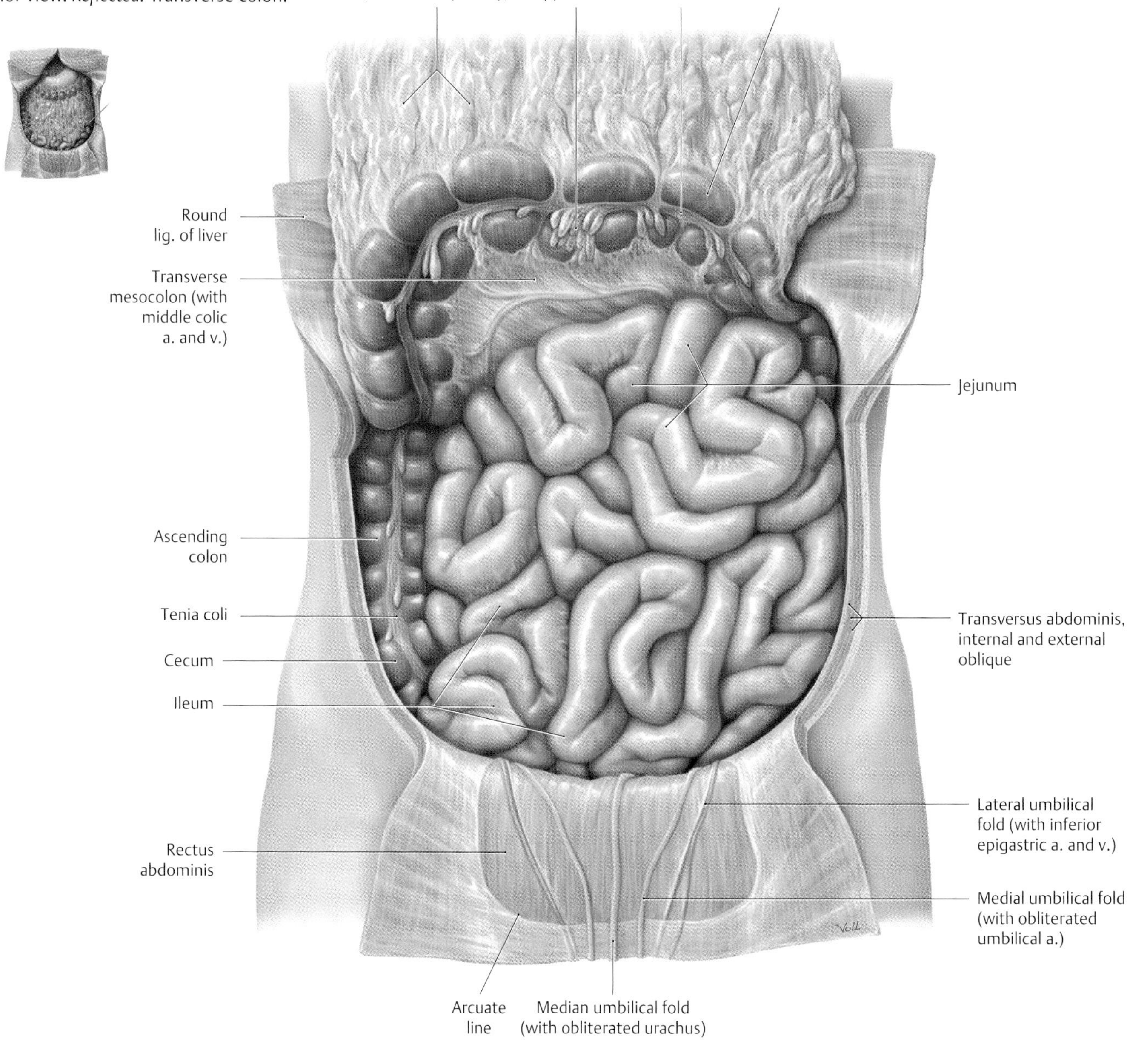

Greater omentum (reflected superiorly)

Epiploic appendices

Tenia coli

Transverse colon

Round lig. of liver

Transverse mesocolon (with middle colic a. and v.)

Ascending colon

Tenia coli

Cecum

Ileum

Rectus abdominis

Jejunum

Transversus abdominis, internal and external oblique

Lateral umbilical fold (with inferior epigastric a. and v.)

Medial umbilical fold (with obliterated umbilical a.)

Arcuate line

Median umbilical fold (with obliterated urachus)

Crohn's disease

Crohn's disease, a chronic inflammation of the digestive tract, occurs most often in the terminal ileum (30% of cases). Patients are generally young and suffer from abdominal pain, nausea, elevated body temperature, and diarrhea. Initially, these symptoms can be confused with appendicitis.

Complications of the chronic inflammation in Crohn's disease often lead to fistula formation (in this case, an abnormal passage between two gastrointestinal regions) (**B**).

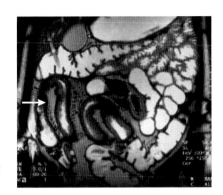

A MRI showing thickened wall of terminal ileum.

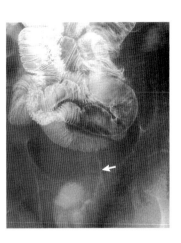

B Double-contrast radiograph, showing ileorectal fistula (arrow).

Fig. 15.12 **Mesentery of the small intestine**

Anterior view. *Removed:* Stomach, jejunum, and ileum. *Reflected:* Liver.

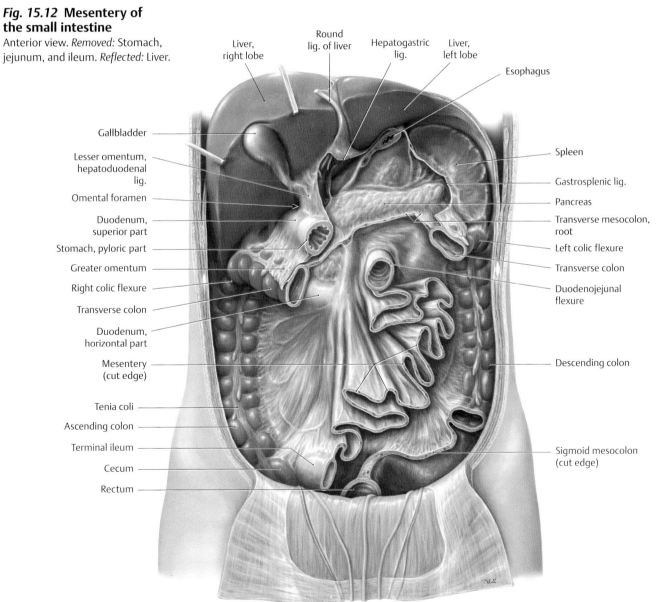

Cecum, Appendix & Colon

 The ascending and descending colon are normally secondarily retroperitoneal, but sometimes they are suspended by a short mesentery from the posterior abdominal wall. *Note:* In the clinical setting, the left colic flexure is often referred to as the splenic flexure and the right colic flexure, as the hepatic flexure.

Fig. 15.13 **Large intestine: Location**
Anterior view.

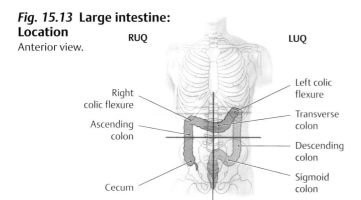

Fig. 15.14 **Ileocecal orifice**
Anterior view of longitudinal coronal section.

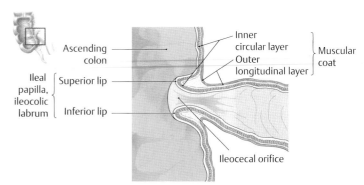

Fig. 15.15 **Large intestine**
Anterior view.

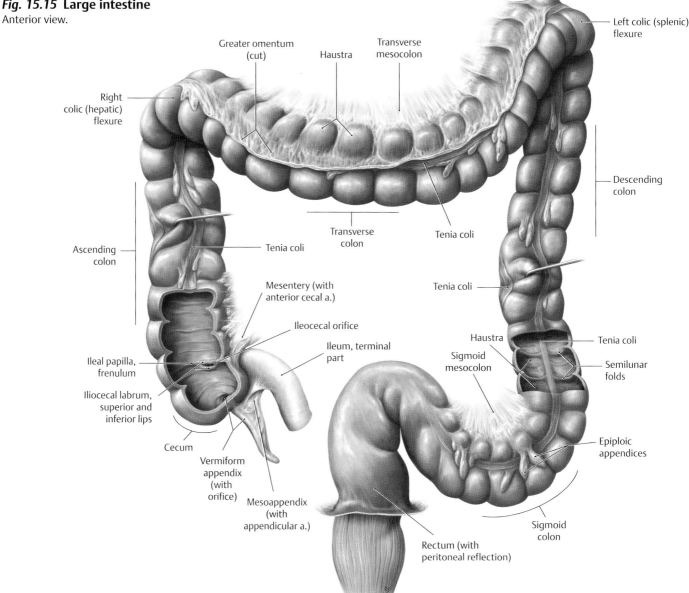

Fig. 15.16 Large intestine in situ
Anterior view. *Reflected:* Transverse colon and greater omentum. *Removed:* Intraperitoneal small intestine.

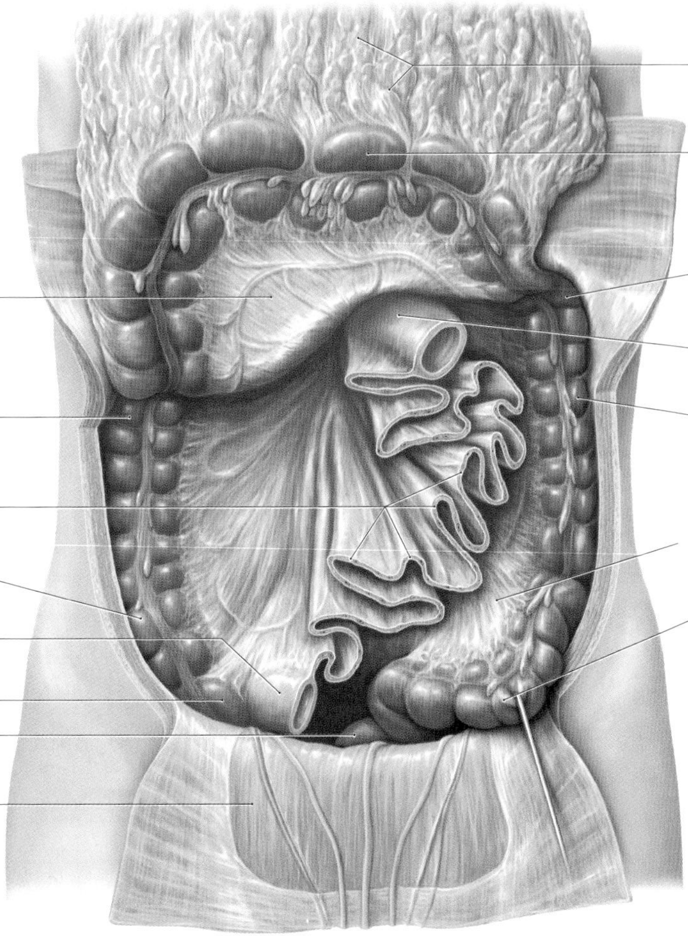

Greater omentum
Transverse colon
Left colic (splenic) flexure
Duodenojejunal flexure
Descending colon
Sigmoid mesocolon
Sigmoid colon
Transverse mesocolon
Right colic (hepatic) flexure
Mesentery (cut)
Ascending colon
Terminal ileum
Cecum
Rectum
Rectus abdominis

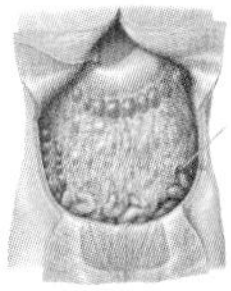

Clinical box 15.4

Colitis

Ulcerative colitis is a chronic inflammation of the large intestine, often starting in the rectum. Typical symptoms include diarrhea (sometimes with blood), pain, weight loss, and inflammation of other organs. Patients are also at higher risk for colorectal carcinomas.

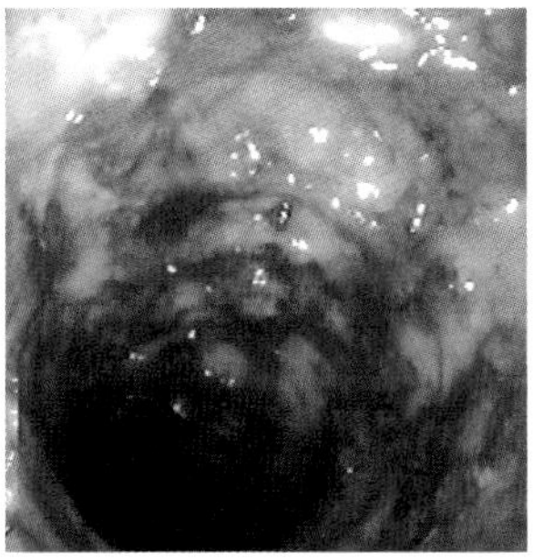

A Colonoscopy of ulcerative colitis.

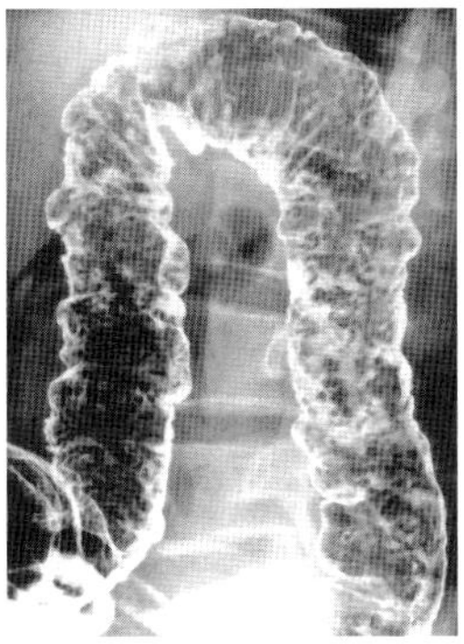

B Early-phase colitis. Double-contrast radiograph, anterior view.

Clinical box 15.5

Colon carcinoma

Malignant tumors of the colon and rectum are among the most frequent solid tumors. More than 90% occur in patients over the age of 50. In early stages, the tumor may be asymptomatic; later symptoms include loss of appetite, changes in bowel movements, and weight loss. Blood in the stools is particularly incriminating, necessitating a thorough examination. Hemorrhoids are not a sufficient explanation for blood in stools unless all other tests (including a colonoscopy) are negative.

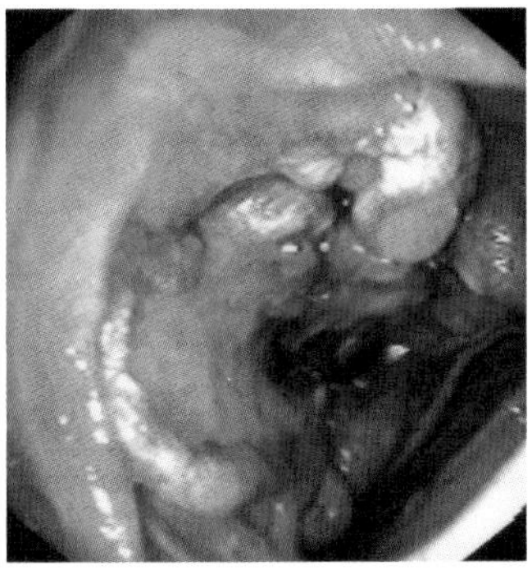

Colonoscopy of colon carcinoma. The tumor partially blocks the lumen of the colon.

Liver: Overview

Fig. 15.17 Liver: Location

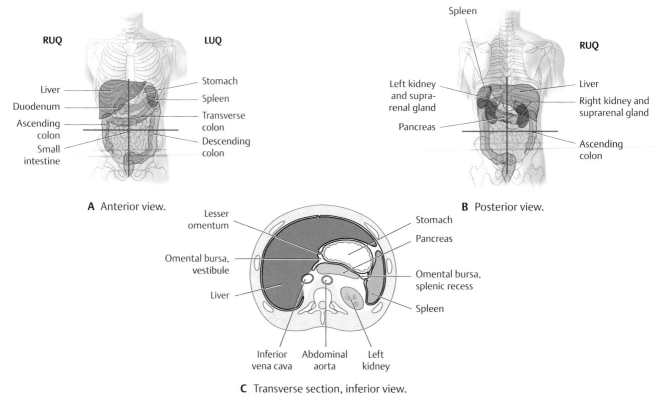

A Anterior view.

RUQ · LUQ

Liver — Stomach
Duodenum — Spleen
Ascending colon — Transverse colon
Small intestine — Descending colon

Spleen

B Posterior view.

RUQ

Left kidney and supra-renal gland — Liver
Pancreas — Right kidney and suprarenal gland
Ascending colon

C Transverse section, inferior view.

Lesser omentum — Stomach
Omental bursa, vestibule — Pancreas
Liver — Omental bursa, splenic recess
Spleen
Inferior vena cava · Abdominal aorta · Left kidney

Fig. 15.18 Liver in situ

Anterior view. The liver is intraperitoneal except for its "bare area" (see **Fig. 15.23**); its mesenteries include the falciform, coronary, and triangular ligaments (see **Fig. 15.22A**).

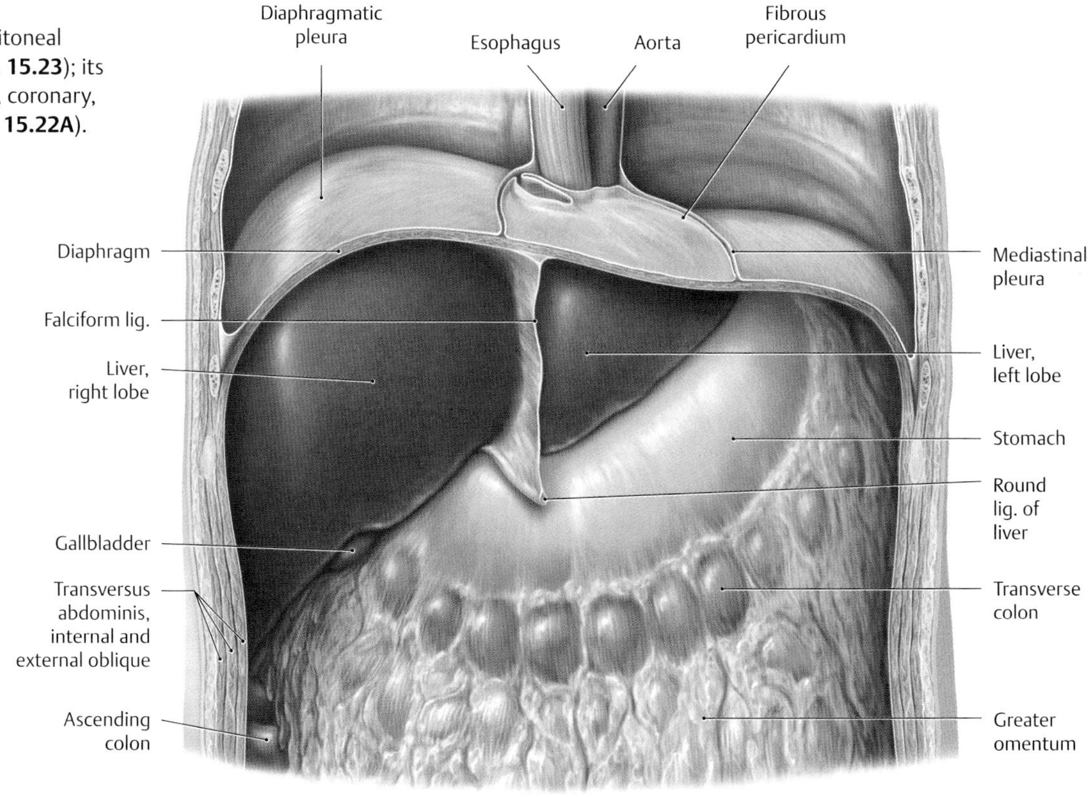

Diaphragmatic pleura · Esophagus · Aorta · Fibrous pericardium

Diaphragm
Falciform lig.
Liver, right lobe
Mediastinal pleura
Liver, left lobe
Stomach
Round lig. of liver
Gallbladder
Transversus abdominis, internal and external oblique
Transverse colon
Ascending colon
Greater omentum

Fig. 15.19 Liver in situ: Inferior surface

The liver is retracted to show the gallbladder on its inferior surface.

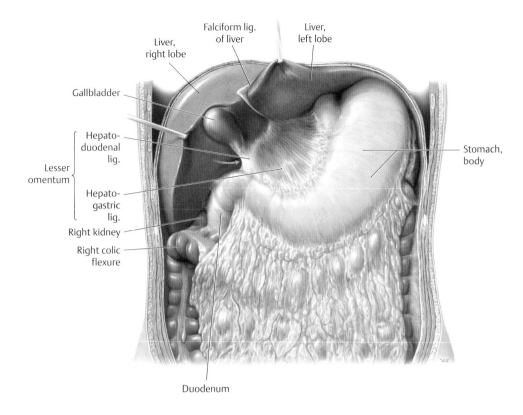

Falciform lig. of liver

Liver, left lobe

Liver, right lobe

Gallbladder

Hepato-duodenal lig.

Lesser omentum

Hepato-gastric lig.

Right kidney

Right colic flexure

Stomach, body

Duodenum

Fig. 15.20 Relations of the liver

Visceral surface, inferior view.

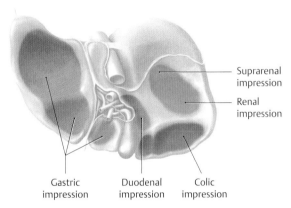

Suprarenal impression

Renal impression

Gastric impression

Duodenal impression

Colic impression

Fig. 15.21 Attachment of liver to diaphragm

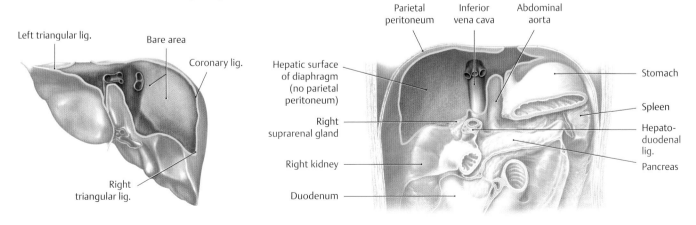

Left triangular lig.

Bare area

Coronary lig.

Right triangular lig.

A Diaphragmatic surface of the liver, posterior view.

Parietal peritoneum

Inferior vena cava

Abdominal aorta

Hepatic surface of diaphragm (no parietal peritoneum)

Right suprarenal gland

Right kidney

Duodenum

Stomach

Spleen

Hepato-duodenal lig.

Pancreas

B Hepatic surface of the diaphragm, anterior view.

Liver: Lobes & Segments

Fig. 15.22 **Surfaces of the liver**

The liver is divided into four lobes by its ligaments: right, left, caudate, and quadrate. The falciform ligament, a double layer of parietal peritoneum that reflects off the anterior abdominal wall and extends to the liver, spreading out over its surface as visceral peritoneum, divides the liver into right and left anatomical lobes. The round ligament of the liver is found in the free edge of the falciform ligament and is the obliterated umbilical vein, which once extended from the umbilicus to the liver.

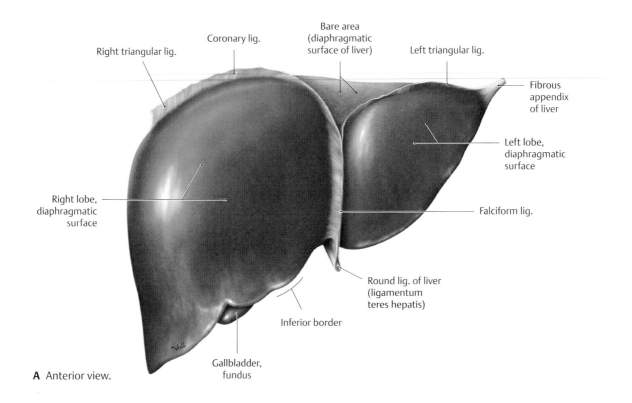

Right triangular lig. Coronary lig. Bare area (diaphragmatic surface of liver) Left triangular lig.

Fibrous appendix of liver

Left lobe, diaphragmatic surface

Right lobe, diaphragmatic surface

Falciform lig.

Round lig. of liver (ligamentum teres hepatis)

Inferior border

Gallbladder, fundus

A Anterior view.

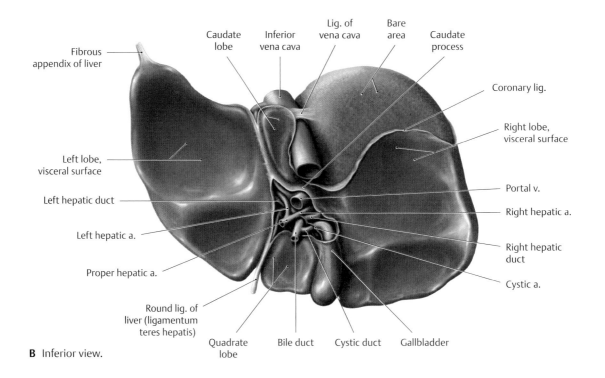

Fibrous appendix of liver

Caudate lobe Inferior vena cava Lig. of vena cava Bare area Caudate process

Coronary lig.

Right lobe, visceral surface

Left lobe, visceral surface

Left hepatic duct

Portal v.

Right hepatic a.

Left hepatic a.

Right hepatic duct

Proper hepatic a.

Cystic a.

Round lig. of liver (ligamentum teres hepatis)

Quadrate lobe Bile duct Cystic duct Gallbladder

B Inferior view.

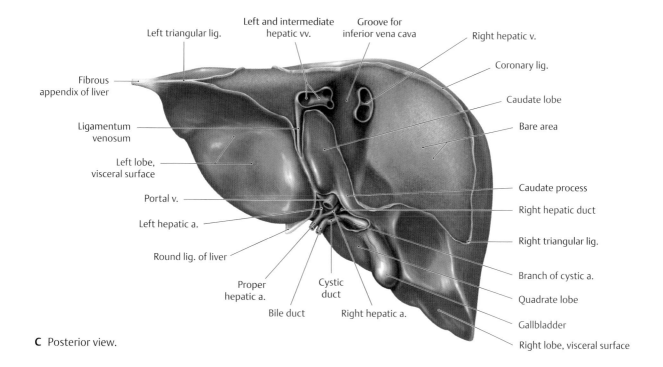

C Posterior view.

Fig. 15.23 Segmentation of the liver

The liver is divided into functional divisions, which are further divided into segments (see **Table 15.1**). Each segment is served by tertiary branches of the hepatic artery, the portal vein, and the common hepatic duct, which together make up the portal triad.

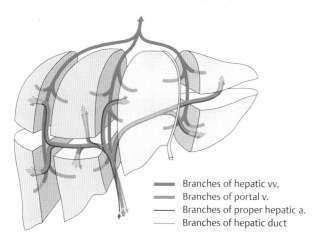

— Branches of hepatic vv.
— Branches of portal v.
— Branches of proper hepatic a.
— Branches of hepatic duct

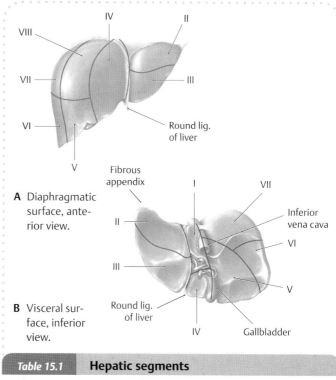

A Diaphragmatic surface, anterior view.

B Visceral surface, inferior view.

Table 15.1	Hepatic segments		
Part	**Division**	**Segment**	
Left part	Posterior part	I	Caudate lobe
	Left lateral division	II	Left posterolateral
		III	Left anterolateral
	Left medial division	IV	Left medial
Right part	Right medial division	V	Right anteromedial
		VI	Right anterolateral
	Right lateral division	VII	Right posterolateral
		VIII	Right posteromedial

Gallbladder & Bile Ducts

Fig. 15.24 **Gallbladder: Location**

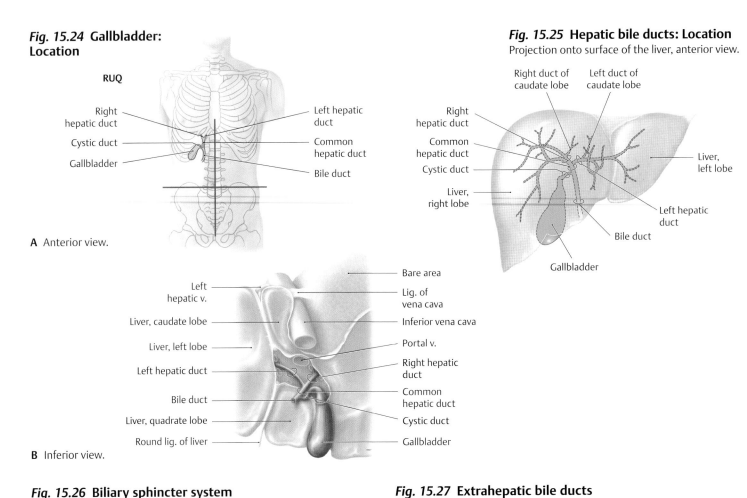

RUQ

Right hepatic duct

Cystic duct

Gallbladder

Left hepatic duct

Common hepatic duct

Bile duct

A Anterior view.

Left hepatic v.

Liver, caudate lobe

Liver, left lobe

Left hepatic duct

Bile duct

Liver, quadrate lobe

Round lig. of liver

Bare area

Lig. of vena cava

Inferior vena cava

Portal v.

Right hepatic duct

Common hepatic duct

Cystic duct

Gallbladder

B Inferior view.

Fig. 15.25 **Hepatic bile ducts: Location**

Projection onto surface of the liver, anterior view.

Right duct of caudate lobe

Left duct of caudate lobe

Right hepatic duct

Common hepatic duct

Cystic duct

Liver, right lobe

Liver, left lobe

Left hepatic duct

Bile duct

Gallbladder

Fig. 15.26 **Biliary sphincter system**

Duodenum wall

Hepato-pancreatic ampulla

Sphincter of bile duct

Sphincter of pancreatic duct

Sphincter of hepatopancreatic ampulla

A Sphincters of the pancreatic and bile ducts.

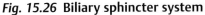

Duodenum, muscular coat

Longitudinal layer

Circular layer

Bile duct

Longitudinal slips of duodenal muscle on bile duct

Sphincter of hepato-pancreatic ampulla

Pancreatic duct

B Sphincter system in the duodenal wall.

Fig. 15.27 **Extrahepatic bile ducts**

Anterior view. *Opened:* Gallbladder and duodenum.

Right hepatic duct

Cystic duct

Neck

Infundibulum

Gall-bladder

Body

Fundus

Left hepatic duct

Common hepatic duct

Duodenum, superior part

Bile duct

Accessory pancreatic duct

Pancreatic duct

Minor duodenal papilla

Major duodenal papilla

Duodenum, descending part

Duodenum, horizontal part

Fig. 15.28 Biliary tract in situ

Anterior view. *Removed:* Stomach, small intestine, transverse colon, and large portions of the liver. The gallbladder is intraperitoneal, covered by visceral peritoneum where it is not attached to the liver.

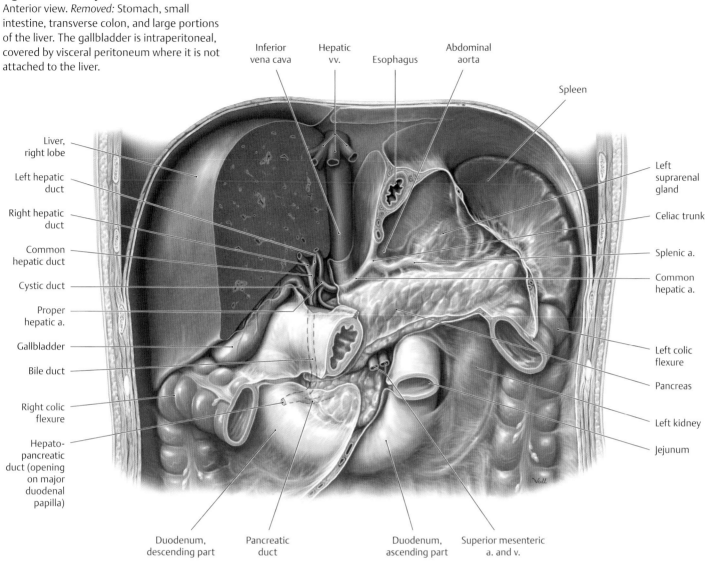

Liver, right lobe

Left hepatic duct

Right hepatic duct

Common hepatic duct

Cystic duct

Proper hepatic a.

Gallbladder

Bile duct

Right colic flexure

Hepato-pancreatic duct (opening on major duodenal papilla)

Inferior vena cava

Hepatic vv.

Esophagus

Abdominal aorta

Spleen

Left suprarenal gland

Celiac trunk

Splenic a.

Common hepatic a.

Left colic flexure

Pancreas

Left kidney

Jejunum

Duodenum, descending part

Pancreatic duct

Duodenum, ascending part

Superior mesenteric a. and v.

✚ Clinical box 15.6

Obstruction of the bile duct

As bile is stored and concentrated in the gallbladder, certain substances, such as cholesterol, may crystallize, resulting in the formation of gallstones. Migration of gallstones into the bile duct causes severe pain (colic). Gallstones may also block the pancreatic duct in the papillary regions, causing highly acute or even life-threatening pancreatitis.

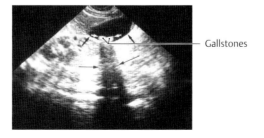

Gallstones

Ultrasound appearance of two gallstones. Black arrows mark the echo-free area behind the stones.

Pancreas & Spleen

Fig. 15.29 Pancreas and spleen: Location

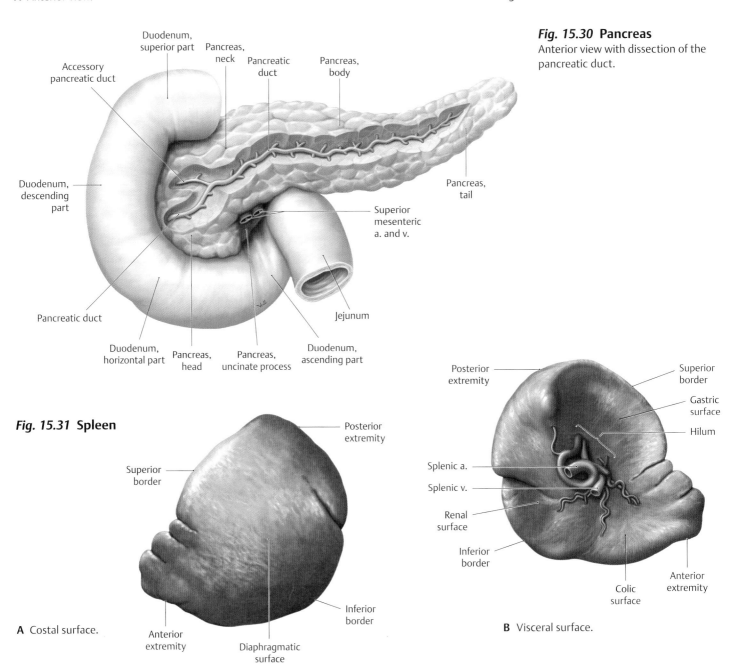

A Anterior view.

RUQ   LUQ

Pancreas   Spleen

B Left lateral view.

10th rib

C Transverse section through L1 vertebra, inferior view.

Lesser omentum (hepatogastric lig.)

Pancreas

Liver

Stomach

Gastrosplenic lig.

Omental bursa, splenic recess

Splenorenal lig.

Spleen

Inferior vena cava   Abdominal aorta   Left kidney

Fig. 15.30 Pancreas
Anterior view with dissection of the pancreatic duct.

Duodenum, superior part

Pancreas, neck

Pancreatic duct

Pancreas, body

Accessory pancreatic duct

Duodenum, descending part

Pancreatic duct

Pancreas, tail

Superior mesenteric a. and v.

Jejunum

Duodenum, horizontal part

Pancreas, head

Pancreas, uncinate process

Duodenum, ascending part

Fig. 15.31 Spleen

Superior border

Posterior extremity

A Costal surface.

Anterior extremity

Diaphragmatic surface

Inferior border

Posterior extremity

Splenic a.

Splenic v.

Renal surface

Inferior border

Superior border

Gastric surface

Hilum

Colic surface

Anterior extremity

B Visceral surface.

Fig. 15.32 Pancreas and spleen in situ

Anterior view. *Removed:* Liver, stomach, small intestine, and large intestine. The pancreas is retroperitoneal, whereas the spleen is intraperitoneal.

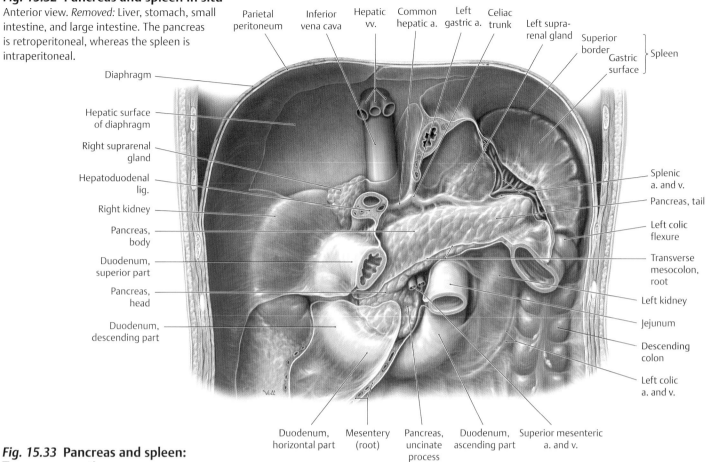

Fig. 15.33 Pancreas and spleen: Transverse section

Superior view. Section through L1 vertebra.

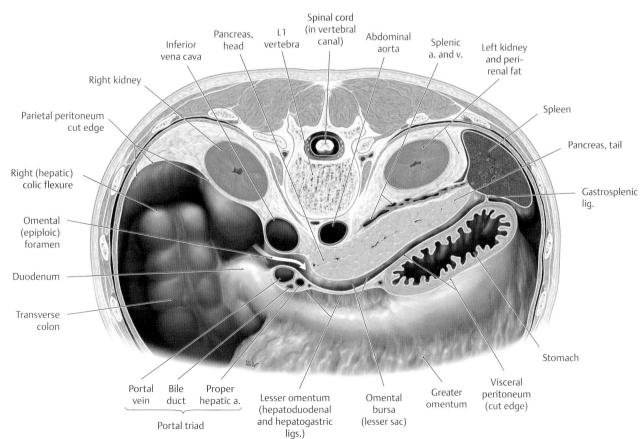

Kidneys & Suprarenal Glands (I)

Fig. 15.34 Kidneys and suprarenal glands: Location

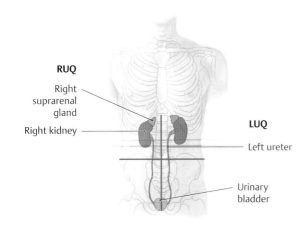

RUQ

Right suprarenal gland

Right kidney

LUQ

Left ureter

Urinary bladder

A Anterior view.

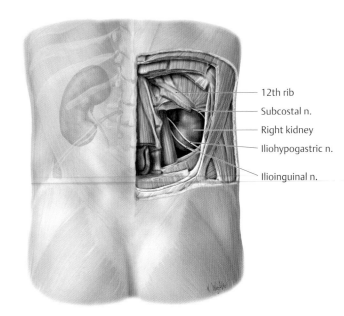

12th rib

Subcostal n.

Right kidney

Iliohypogastric n.

Ilioinguinal n.

Fig. 15.35 Relations of the kidneys: areas of organ contact.
Anterior view.

B Posterior view. Right side windowed.

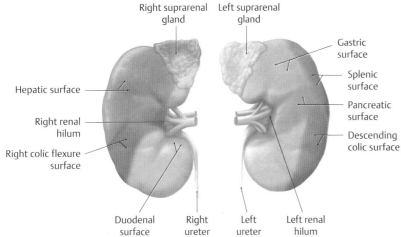

Right suprarenal gland

Left suprarenal gland

Gastric surface

Splenic surface

Pancreatic surface

Descending colic surface

Hepatic surface

Right renal hilum

Right colic flexure surface

Duodenal surface

Right ureter

Left ureter

Left renal hilum

Fig. 15.36 Right kidney in the renal bed
Sagittal section through the right renal bed.

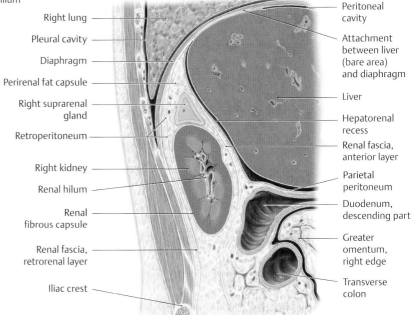

Right lung

Pleural cavity

Diaphragm

Perirenal fat capsule

Right suprarenal gland

Retroperitoneum

Right kidney

Renal hilum

Renal fibrous capsule

Renal fascia, retrorenal layer

Iliac crest

Peritoneal cavity

Attachment between liver (bare area) and diaphragm

Liver

Hepatorenal recess

Renal fascia, anterior layer

Parietal peritoneum

Duodenum, descending part

Greater omentum, right edge

Transverse colon

Fig. 15.37 **Kidneys and suprarenal glands in the retroperitoneum**

Anterior view. Both the kidneys and suprarenal glands are retroperitoneal.

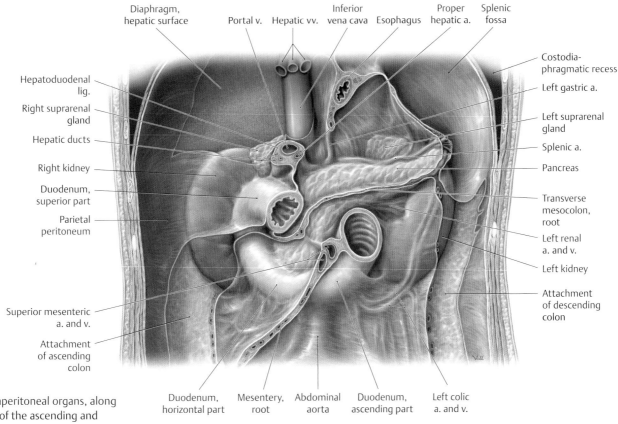

Diaphragm, hepatic surface — Portal v. — Hepatic vv. — Inferior vena cava — Esophagus — Proper hepatic a. — Splenic fossa — Costodiaphragmatic recess — Left gastric a. — Left suprarenal gland — Splenic a. — Pancreas — Transverse mesocolon, root — Left renal a. and v. — Left kidney — Attachment of descending colon

Hepatoduodenal lig. — Right suprarenal gland — Hepatic ducts — Right kidney — Duodenum, superior part — Parietal peritoneum — Superior mesenteric a. and v. — Attachment of ascending colon

Duodenum, horizontal part — Mesentery, root — Abdominal aorta — Duodenum, ascending part — Left colic a. and v.

A *Removed:* Intraperitoneal organs, along with portions of the ascending and descending colon.

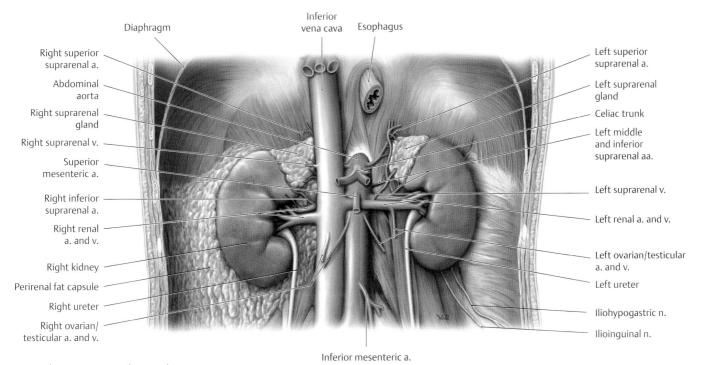

Diaphragm — Inferior vena cava — Esophagus

Right superior suprarenal a. — Abdominal aorta — Right suprarenal gland — Right suprarenal v. — Superior mesenteric a. — Right inferior suprarenal a. — Right renal a. and v. — Right kidney — Perirenal fat capsule — Right ureter — Right ovarian/testicular a. and v.

Left superior suprarenal a. — Left suprarenal gland — Celiac trunk — Left middle and inferior suprarenal aa. — Left suprarenal v. — Left renal a. and v. — Left ovarian/testicular a. and v. — Left ureter — Iliohypogastric n. — Ilioinguinal n.

Inferior mesenteric a.

B *Removed:* Peritoneum, spleen and gastrointestinal organs, along with fat capsule (left side) *Retracted:* Esophagus

Kidneys & Suprarenal Glands (II)

Fig. 15.38 **Kidney: Structure**
Right kidney with suprarenal gland.

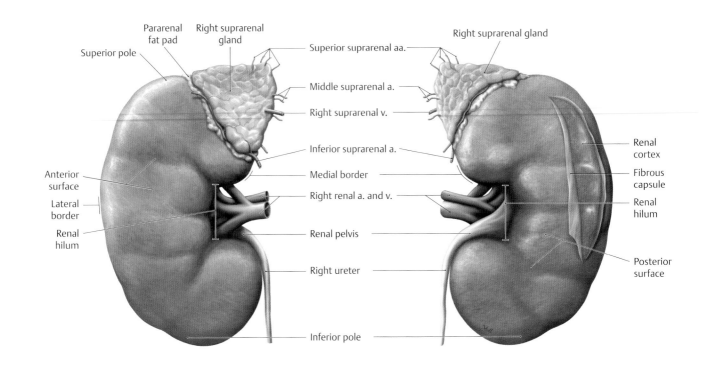

A Anterior view.

B Posterior view.

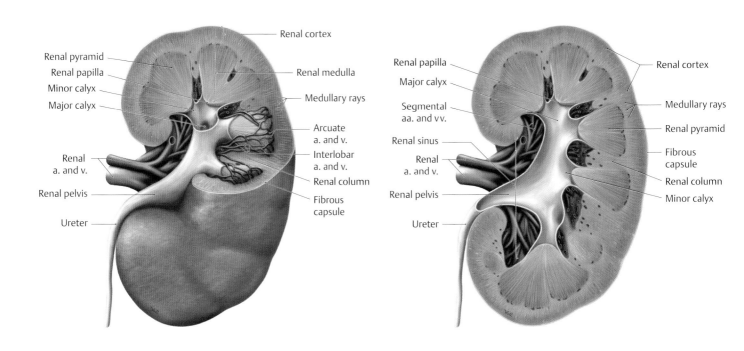

C Posterior view with upper half partially removed.

D Posterior view, midsagittal section.

Fig. 15.39 **Right kidney and suprarenal gland**

Anterior view. *Removed:* Perirenal fat capsule.
Retracted: Inferior vena cava.

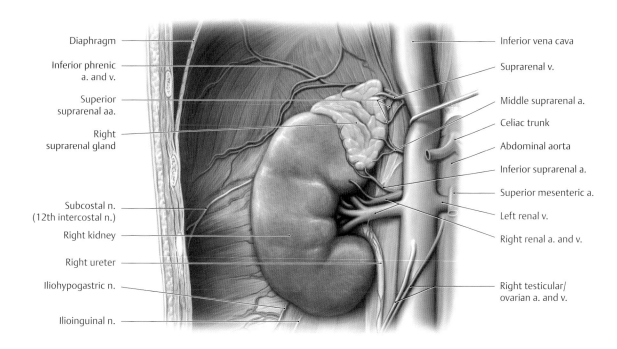

Diaphragm

Inferior phrenic
a. and v.

Superior
suprarenal aa.

Right
suprarenal gland

Subcostal n.
(12th intercostal n.)

Right kidney

Right ureter

Iliohypogastric n.

Ilioinguinal n.

Inferior vena cava

Suprarenal v.

Middle suprarenal a.

Celiac trunk

Abdominal aorta

Inferior suprarenal a.

Superior mesenteric a.

Left renal v.

Right renal a. and v.

Right testicular/
ovarian a. and v.

Fig. 15.40 **Left kidney and suprarenal gland**

Anterior view. *Removed:* Perirenal fat capsule.
Retracted: Pancreas.

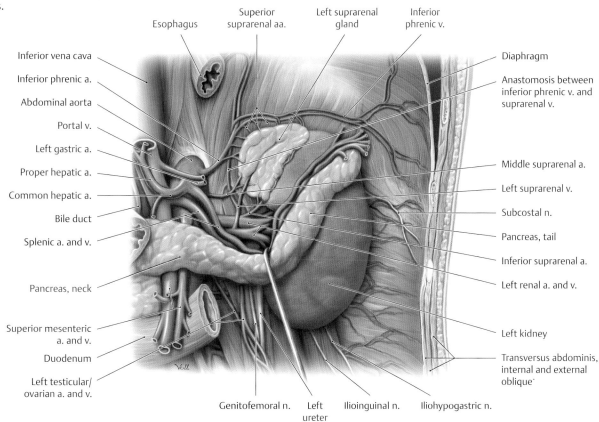

Esophagus

Superior
suprarenal aa.

Left suprarenal
gland

Inferior
phrenic v.

Inferior vena cava

Inferior phrenic a.

Abdominal aorta

Portal v.

Left gastric a.

Proper hepatic a.

Common hepatic a.

Bile duct

Splenic a. and v.

Pancreas, neck

Superior mesenteric
a. and v.

Duodenum

Left testicular/
ovarian a. and v.

Genitofemoral n.

Left
ureter

Ilioinguinal n.

Iliohypogastric n.

Diaphragm

Anastomosis between
inferior phrenic v. and
suprarenal v.

Middle suprarenal a.

Left suprarenal v.

Subcostal n.

Pancreas, tail

Inferior suprarenal a.

Left renal a. and v.

Left kidney

Transversus abdominis,
internal and external
oblique

183

Arteries of the Abdomen

Fig. 16.1 Abdominal aorta and major branches

Anterior view. The abdominal aorta enters the abdomen at the T12 level through the aortic hiatus of the diaphragm (see **p. 66**). Before bifurcating at L4 into its terminal branches, the common iliac arteries, the abdominal aorta gives off the renal arteries (see **p. 183**) and three major trunks that supply the organs of the gastrointestinal system:

Celiac trunk: Supplies the structures of the foregut, the anterior portion of the alimentary canal. The foregut consists of the esophagus (abdominal 1.25 cm), stomach, duodenum (proximal half), liver, gallbladder, and pancreas (superior portion).

Superior mesenteric artery: Supplies the structures of the midgut: the duodenum (distal half), jejunum and ileum, cecum and appendix, ascending colon, right colic flexure, and the proximal one half of the transverse colon.

Inferior mesenteric artery: Supplies the structures of the hindgut: the transverse colon (distal half), left colic flexure, descending and sigmoid colons, rectum, and anal canal (upper part).

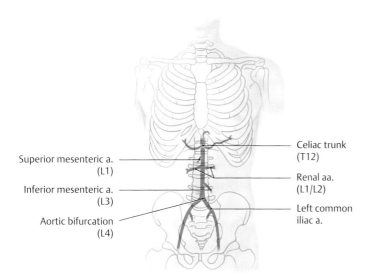

Fig. 16.2 Arteries of the abdominal wall

The superior and inferior epigastric arteries form a potential anastomosis, or bypass for blood, from the subclavian and femoral arteries. This effectively allows blood to potentially bypass the abdominal aorta.

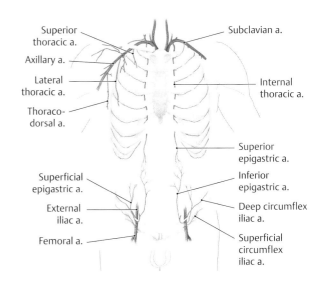

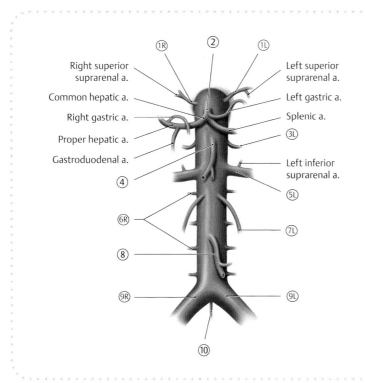

| Table 16.1 | Branches of the abdominal aorta |

The abdominal aorta gives rise to three major unpaired trunks (bold) and the unpaired median sacral artery, as well as six paired branches.

Branch from abdominal aorta			Branches	
①R	①L	Inferior phrenic aa. (paired)	Superior suprarenal aa.	
②		**Celiac trunk**	Left gastric a.	
			Splenic a.	
			Common hepatic a.	Proper hepatic a.
				Right gastric a.
				Gastroduodenal a.
③R	③L	Middle suprarenal aa. (paired)		
④		**Superior mesenteric a.**		
⑤R	⑤L	Renal aa. (paired)	Inferior suprarenal aa.	
⑥R	⑥L	Lumbar aa. (1st through 4th, paired)		
⑦R	⑦L	Testicular/ovarian aa. (paired)		
⑧		**Inferior mesenteric a.**		
⑨R	⑨L	Common iliac aa. (paired)	External iliac a.	
			Internal iliac a.	
⑩		Median sacral a.		

Fig. 16.3 Celiac trunk

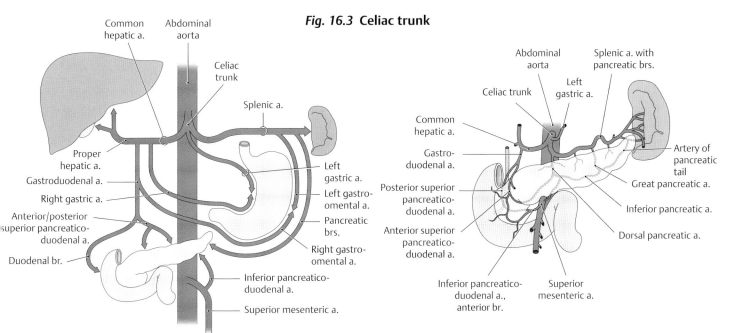

A Celiac trunk distribution.

B Arterial supply to the pancreas

Fig. 16.4 Superior mesenteric artery

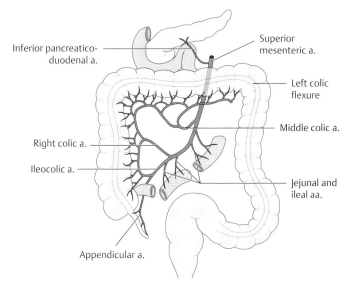

Fig. 16.5 Inferior mesenteric artery

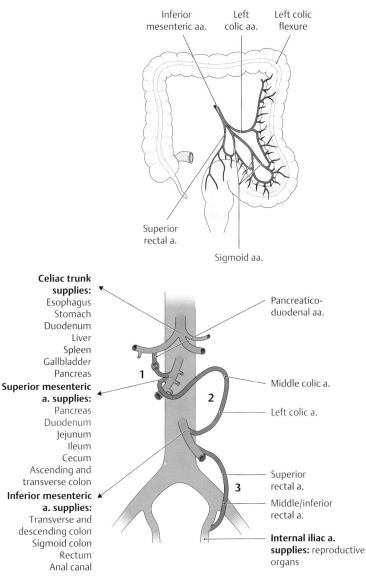

Fig. 16.6 Abdominal arterial anastomoses

Three major anastomoses provide overlap in the arterial supply to abdominal areas to ensure adequate blood flow.
1–Between the celiac trunk and the superior mesenteric artery via the pancreaticoduodenal arteries.
2–Between the superior and inferior mesenteric arteries via the middle and left colic arteries.
3–Between the inferior mesenteric and the internal iliac arteries via the superior and middle or inferior rectal arteries.

Abdominal Aorta & Renal Arteries

Fig. 16.7 **Abdominal aorta**

Anterior view of the female abdomen. *Removed:* All organs except the left kidney and suprarenal gland. The abdominal aorta is the distal continuation of the thoracic aorta (see **p. 80**). It enters the abdomen at the T12 level and bifurcates into the common iliac arteries at L4.

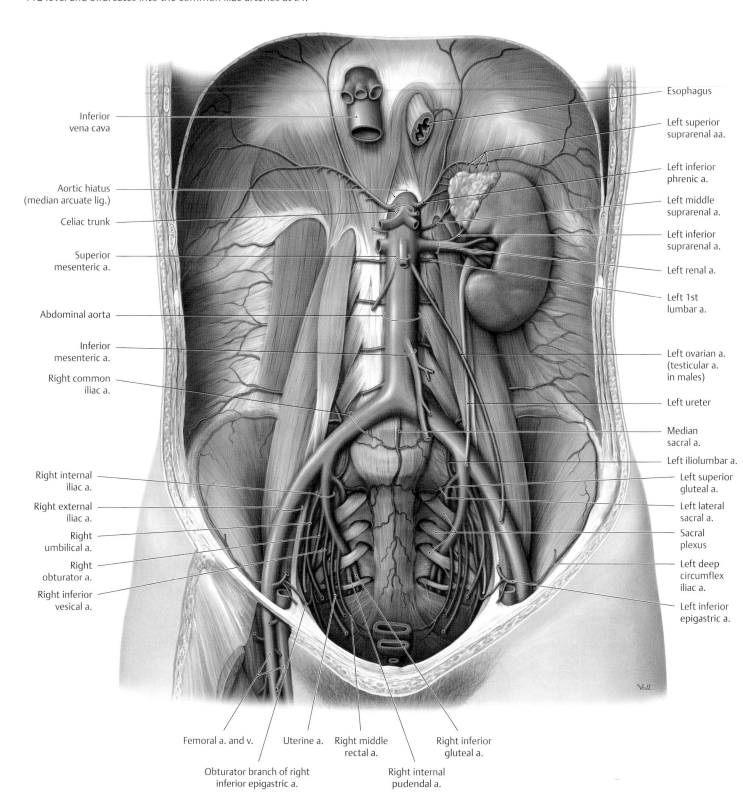

Inferior vena cava

Aortic hiatus (median arcuate lig.)

Celiac trunk

Superior mesenteric a.

Abdominal aorta

Inferior mesenteric a.

Right common iliac a.

Right internal iliac a.

Right external iliac a.

Right umbilical a.

Right obturator a.

Right inferior vesical a.

Esophagus

Left superior suprarenal aa.

Left inferior phrenic a.

Left middle suprarenal a.

Left inferior suprarenal a.

Left renal a.

Left 1st lumbar a.

Left ovarian a. (testicular a. in males)

Left ureter

Median sacral a.

Left iliolumbar a.

Left superior gluteal a.

Left lateral sacral a.

Sacral plexus

Left deep circumflex iliac a.

Left inferior epigastric a.

Femoral a. and v.

Obturator branch of right inferior epigastric a.

Uterine a.

Right middle rectal a.

Right internal pudendal a.

Right inferior gluteal a.

Fig. 16.8 Renal arteries

Left kidney, anterior view. The renal arteries arise at approximately the level of L2. Each renal artery divides into an anterior and a posterior branch. The anterior branch further divides into four segmental arteries (circled).

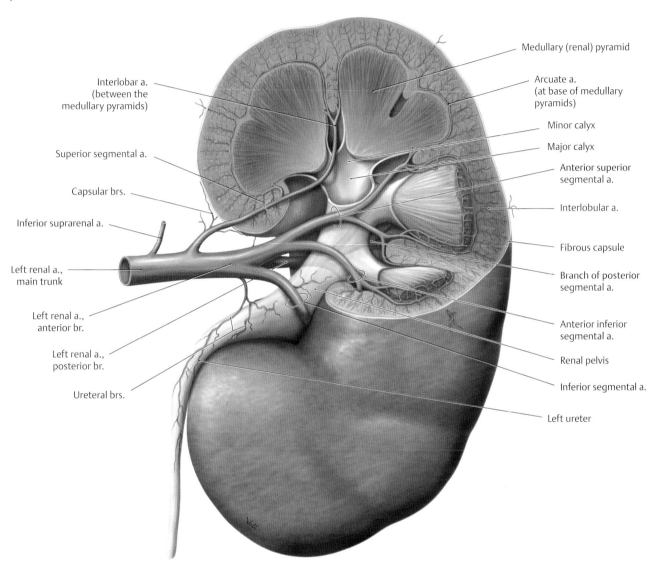

- Medullary (renal) pyramid
- Arcuate a. (at base of medullary pyramids)
- Minor calyx
- Major calyx
- Anterior superior segmental a.
- Interlobular a.
- Fibrous capsule
- Branch of posterior segmental a.
- Anterior inferior segmental a.
- Renal pelvis
- Inferior segmental a.
- Left ureter

- Interlobar a. (between the medullary pyramids)
- Superior segmental a.
- Capsular brs.
- Inferior suprarenal a.
- Left renal a., main trunk
- Left renal a., anterior br.
- Left renal a., posterior br.
- Ureteral brs.

Clinical box 16.1

Renal hypertension

The kidney is an important blood pressure sensor and regulator. Stenosis (narrowing) of the renal artery reduces blood flow through the kidney and stimulates increased production of renin, an enzyme that cleaves angiotensinogen to form angiotensin I. Subsequent cleavage yields angiotensin II, which induces vasoconstriction and an increase in blood pressure. Renal hypertension must be excluded (or confirmed) when diagnosing high blood pressure.

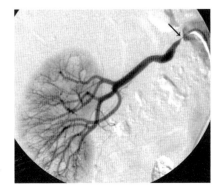

Stenosis of the right renal artery (*arrow*), visible via arteriography.

Celiac Trunk

The distribution of the celiac trunk is shown on **p. 185**.

***Fig. 16.9* Celiac trunk: Stomach, liver, and gallbladder**
Anterior view. *Opened:* Lesser omentum. *Incised:* Greater omentum. The
celiac trunk arises from the abdominal aorta at about the level of T12/L1.

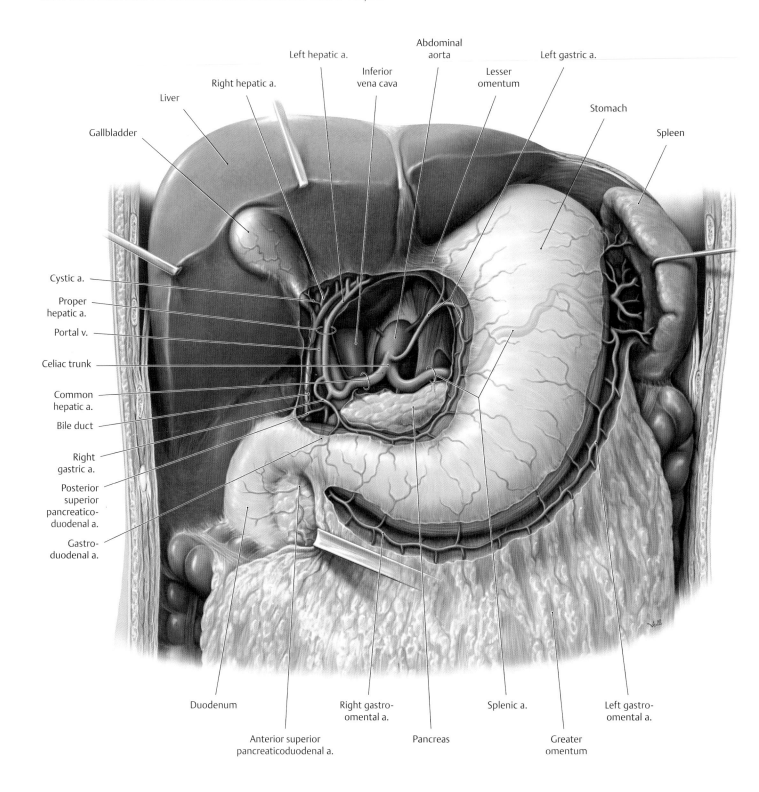

Labels (clockwise / as positioned):

- Left hepatic a.
- Abdominal aorta
- Left gastric a.
- Right hepatic a.
- Inferior vena cava
- Lesser omentum
- Liver
- Stomach
- Gallbladder
- Spleen
- Cystic a.
- Proper hepatic a.
- Portal v.
- Celiac trunk
- Common hepatic a.
- Bile duct
- Right gastric a.
- Posterior superior pancreatico- duodenal a.
- Gastro- duodenal a.
- Duodenum
- Anterior superior pancreaticoduodenal a.
- Right gastro- omental a.
- Pancreas
- Splenic a.
- Greater omentum
- Left gastro- omental a.

Abdomen

188

Fig. 16.10 Celiac trunk: Pancreas, duodenum, and spleen

Anterior view. *Removed:* Stomach (body) and lesser omentum.

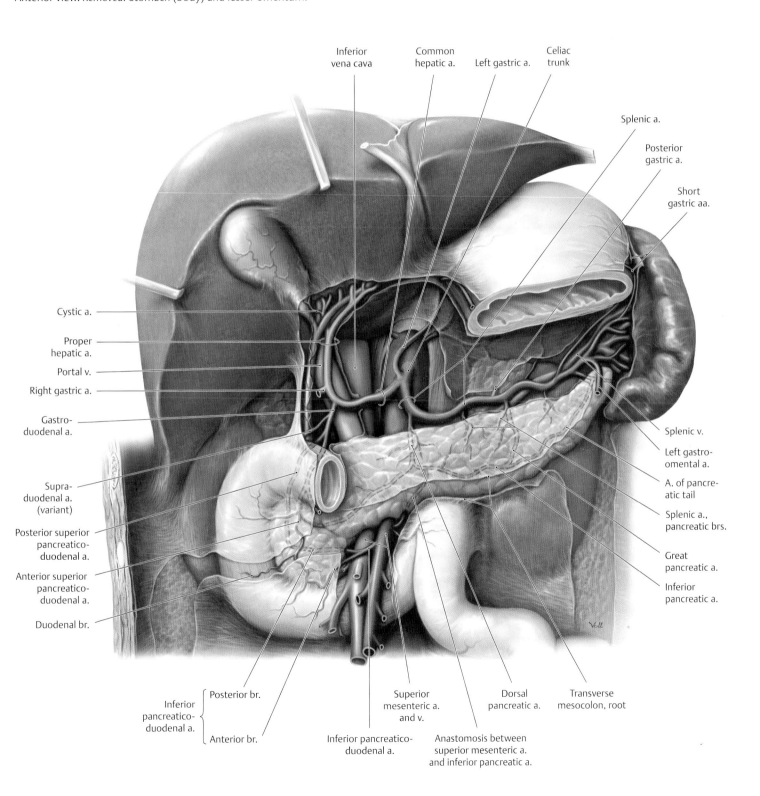

Inferior vena cava

Common hepatic a.

Left gastric a.

Celiac trunk

Splenic a.

Posterior gastric a.

Short gastric aa.

Cystic a.

Proper hepatic a.

Portal v.

Right gastric a.

Gastro-duodenal a.

Supra-duodenal a. (variant)

Posterior superior pancreatico-duodenal a.

Anterior superior pancreatico-duodenal a.

Duodenal br.

Splenic v.

Left gastro-omental a.

A. of pancre-atic tail

Splenic a., pancreatic brs.

Great pancreatic a.

Inferior pancreatic a.

Inferior pancreatico-duodenal a. { Posterior br.

Anterior br.

Superior mesenteric a. and v.

Inferior pancreatico-duodenal a.

Dorsal pancreatic a.

Anastomosis between superior mesenteric a. and inferior pancreatic a.

Transverse mesocolon, root

Superior & Inferior Mesenteric Arteries

Fig. 16.11 **Superior mesenteric artery**

Anterior view. *Partially removed:* Stomach, duodenum, and peritoneum. *Reflected:* Liver and gallbladder. *Note:* The middle colic artery
has been truncated (see **Fig. 16.12**). The superior and inferior mesenteric arteries arise from the aorta opposite L1 and L3, respectively.

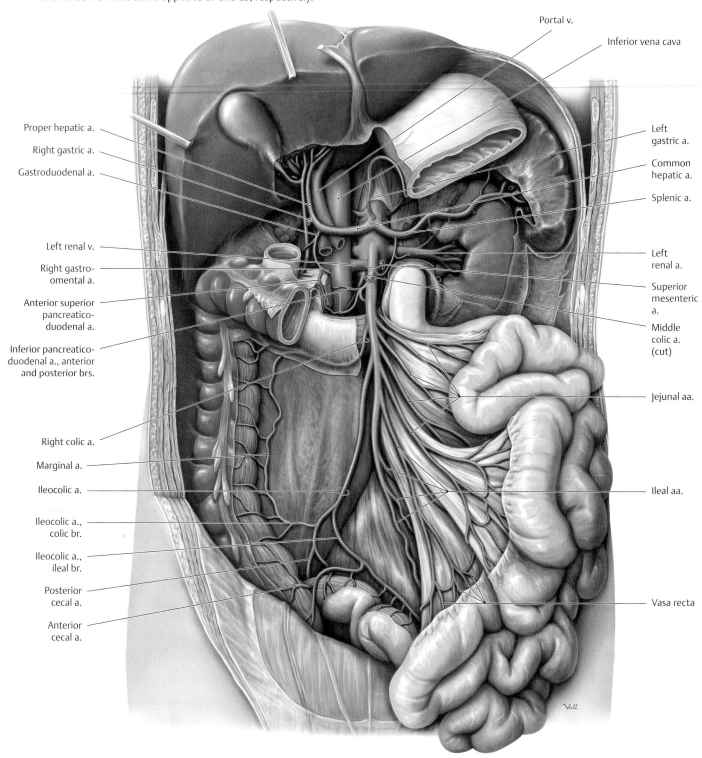

Portal v.

Inferior vena cava

Proper hepatic a.

Right gastric a.

Gastroduodenal a.

Left
gastric a.

Common
hepatic a.

Splenic a.

Left renal v.

Right gastro-
omental a.

Anterior superior
pancreatico-
duodenal a.

Inferior pancreatico-
duodenal a., anterior
and posterior brs.

Left
renal a.

Superior
mesenteric
a.

Middle
colic a.
(cut)

Right colic a.

Jejunal aa.

Marginal a.

Ileocolic a.

Ileal aa.

Ileocolic a.,
colic br.

Ileocolic a.,
ileal br.

Posterior
cecal a.

Anterior
cecal a.

Vasa recta

***Fig. 16.12* Inferior mesenteric artery**
Anterior view. *Removed:* Jejunum and ileum. *Reflected:* Transverse colon.

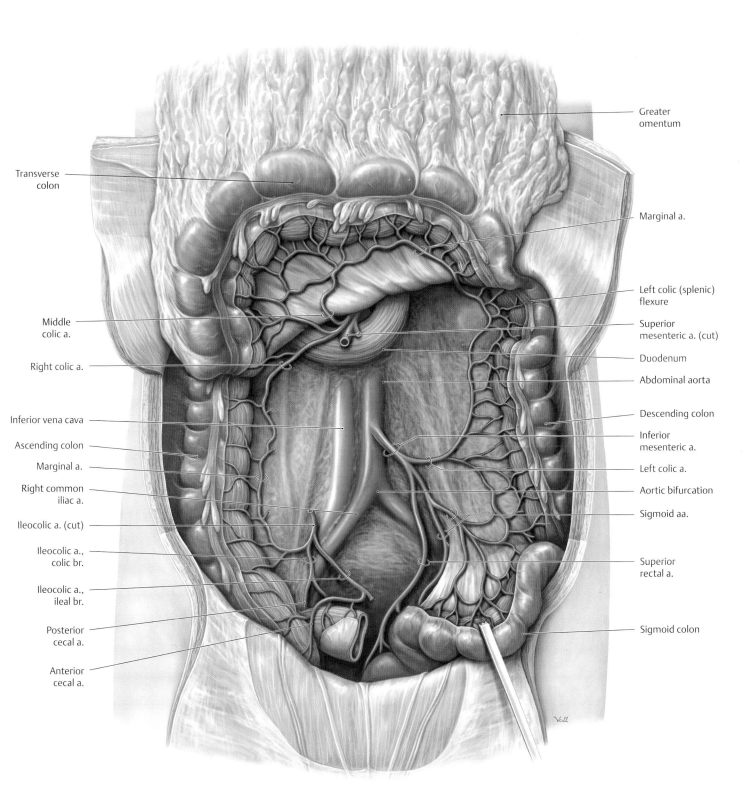

Transverse colon

Greater omentum

Marginal a.

Left colic (splenic) flexure

Middle colic a.

Superior mesenteric a. (cut)

Right colic a.

Duodenum

Abdominal aorta

Inferior vena cava

Descending colon

Ascending colon

Inferior mesenteric a.

Marginal a.

Left colic a.

Right common iliac a.

Aortic bifurcation

Ileocolic a. (cut)

Sigmoid aa.

Ileocolic a., colic br.

Superior rectal a.

Ileocolic a., ileal br.

Posterior cecal a.

Anterior cecal a.

Sigmoid colon

Veins of the Abdomen

Fig. 16.13 Inferior vena cava: Location

Anterior view.

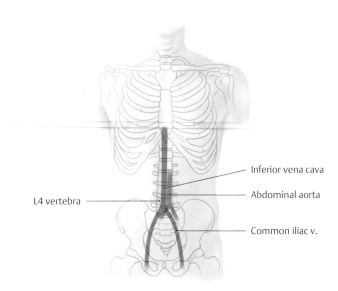

Fig. 16.14 Tributaries of the renal veins

Anterior view.

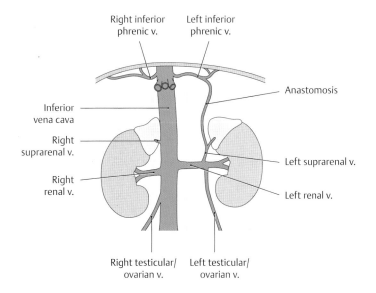

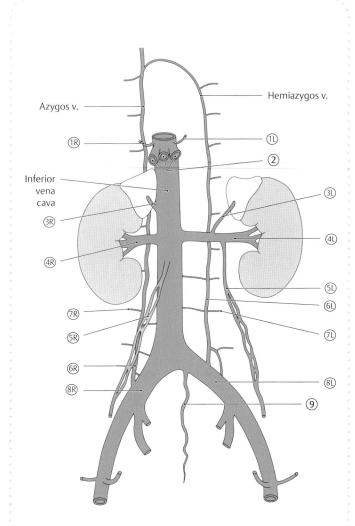

Table 16.2		Tributaries of the inferior vena cava
①R	①L	Inferior phrenic vv. (paired)
	②	Hepatic vv. (3)
③R	③L	Suprarenal vv. (the right vein is a direct tributary)
④R	④L	Renal vv. (paired)
⑤R	⑤L	Testicular/ovarian vv. (the right vein is a direct tributary)
⑥R	⑥L	Ascending lumbar vv. (paired), not direct tributaries
⑦R	⑦L	Lumbar vv.
⑧R	⑧L	Common iliac vv. (paired)
	⑨	Median sacral v.

Fig. 16.15 **Portal vein**

The portal vein (see **p. 196**) drains venous blood from the abdominopelvic organs supplied by the celiac trunk and superior and inferior mesenteric arteries.

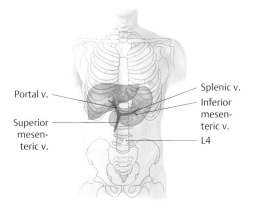

A Location, anterior view.

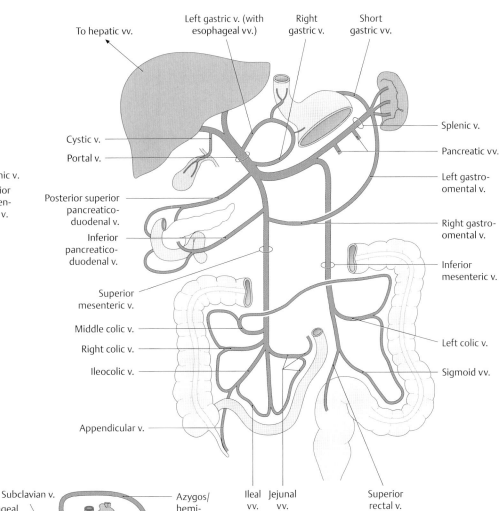

B Portal vein distribution.

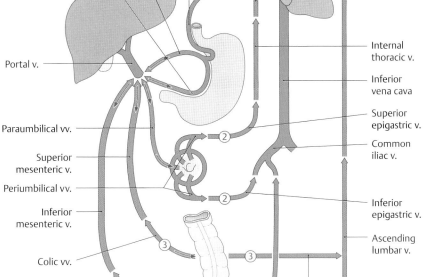

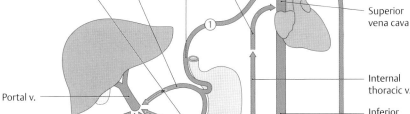

Clinical box 16.2

Cancer metastases

Tumors in the region drained by the superior rectal vein may spread through the portal venous system to the capillary bed of the liver (hepatic metastasis). Tumors drained by the middle or inferior rectal veins may metastasize to the capillary bed of the lung (pulmonary metastasis) via the inferior vena cava and right heart.

C Collateral pathways between the portal and systemic systems. When the portal system is compromised, the portal vein can divert blood away from the liver back to its supplying veins, which return this nutrient-rich blood to the heart via the venae cavae. The red arrows indicate the flow reversal in the (1) esophageal veins, (2) paraumbilical veins, (3) the colic veins, and (4) the middle and inferior rectal veins.

Inferior Vena Cava & Renal Veins

Fig. 16.16 Inferior vena cava
Anterior view of the female abdomen. *Removed:* All organs except the left kidney and suprarenal gland.

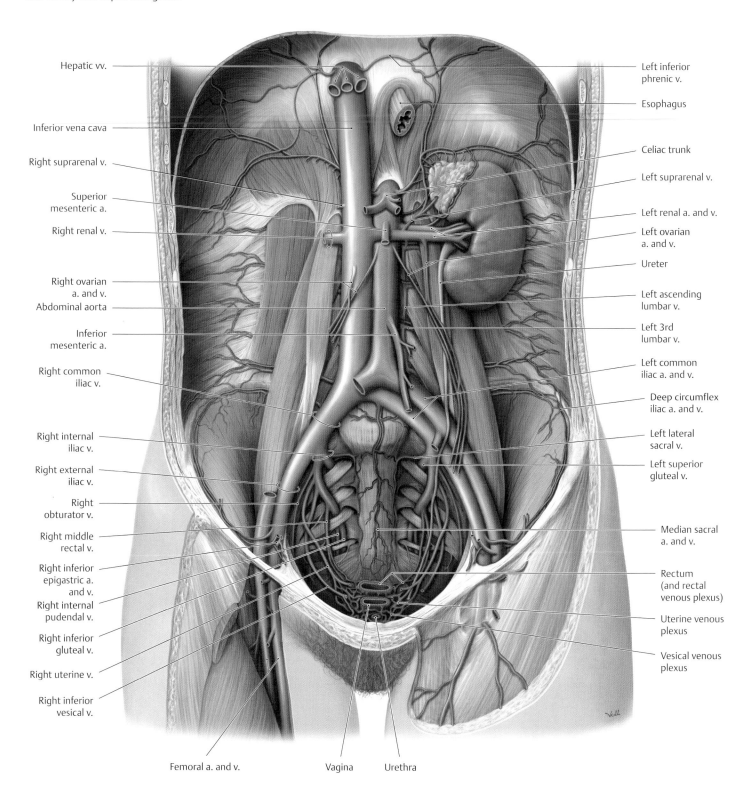

Hepatic vv.

Inferior vena cava

Right suprarenal v.

Superior mesenteric a.

Right renal v.

Right ovarian a. and v.

Abdominal aorta

Inferior mesenteric a.

Right common iliac v.

Right internal iliac v.

Right external iliac v.

Right obturator v.

Right middle rectal v.

Right inferior epigastric a. and v.

Right internal pudendal v.

Right inferior gluteal v.

Right uterine v.

Right inferior vesical v.

Left inferior phrenic v.

Esophagus

Celiac trunk

Left suprarenal v.

Left renal a. and v.

Left ovarian a. and v.

Ureter

Left ascending lumbar v.

Left 3rd lumbar v.

Left common iliac a. and v.

Deep circumflex iliac a. and v.

Left lateral sacral v.

Left superior gluteal v.

Median sacral a. and v.

Rectum (and rectal venous plexus)

Uterine venous plexus

Vesical venous plexus

Femoral a. and v.

Vagina

Urethra

Fig. 16.17 **Renal veins**

Anterior view. See **p. 187** for the renal arteries in isolation.
Removed: All organs except kidneys and suprarenal glands.

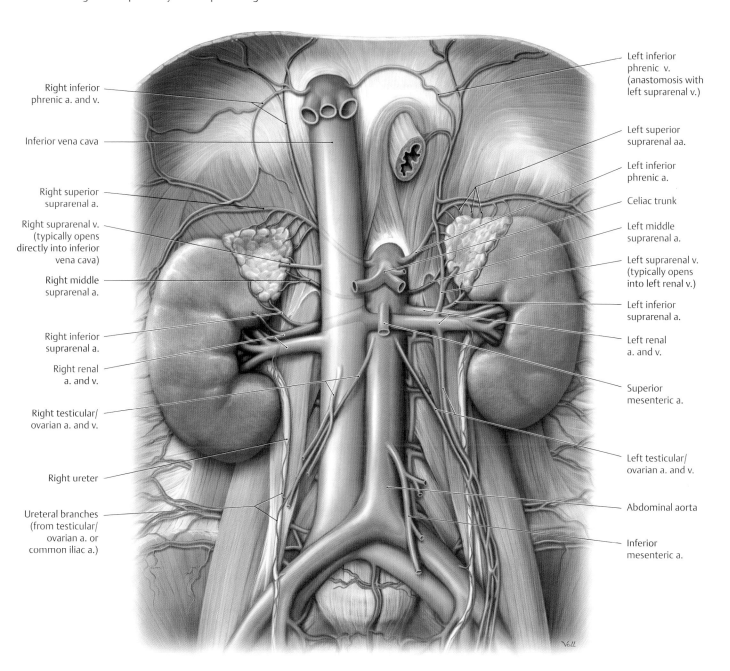

Right inferior
phrenic a. and v.

Inferior vena cava

Right superior
suprarenal a.

Right suprarenal v.
(typically opens
directly into inferior
vena cava)

Right middle
suprarenal a.

Right inferior
suprarenal a.

Right renal
a. and v.

Right testicular/
ovarian a. and v.

Right ureter

Ureteral branches
(from testicular/
ovarian a. or
common iliac a.)

Left inferior
phrenic v.
(anastomosis with
left suprarenal v.)

Left superior
suprarenal aa.

Left inferior
phrenic a.

Celiac trunk

Left middle
suprarenal a.

Left suprarenal v.
(typically opens
into left renal v.)

Left inferior
suprarenal a.

Left renal
a. and v.

Superior
mesenteric a.

Left testicular/
ovarian a. and v.

Abdominal aorta

Inferior
mesenteric a.

Portal Vein

 The portal vein is typically formed by the union of the superior mesenteric and the splenic veins posterior to the neck of the pancreas. The distribution of the portal vein is shown on **p. 193.**

Fig. 16.18 **Portal vein: Stomach and duodenum**
Anterior view. *Removed:* Liver, lesser omentum, and peritoneum.
Opened: Greater omentum.

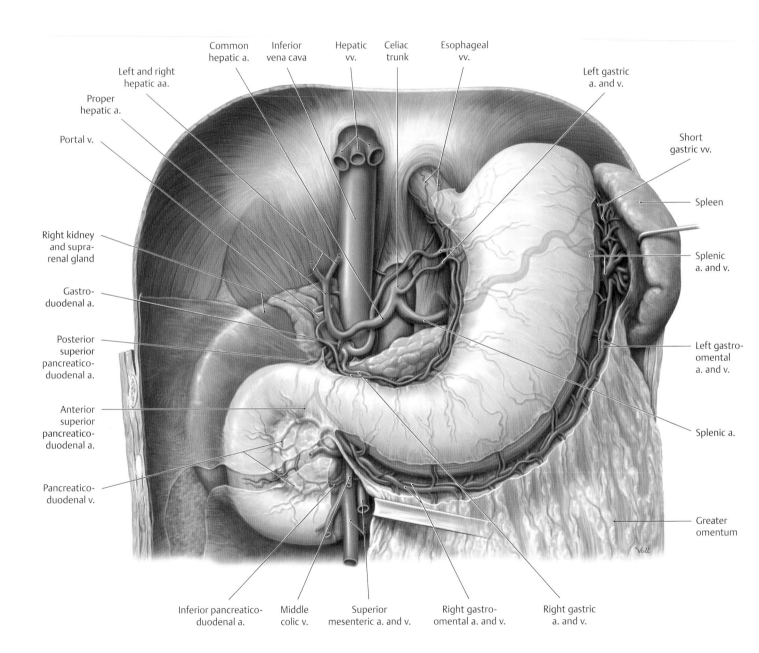

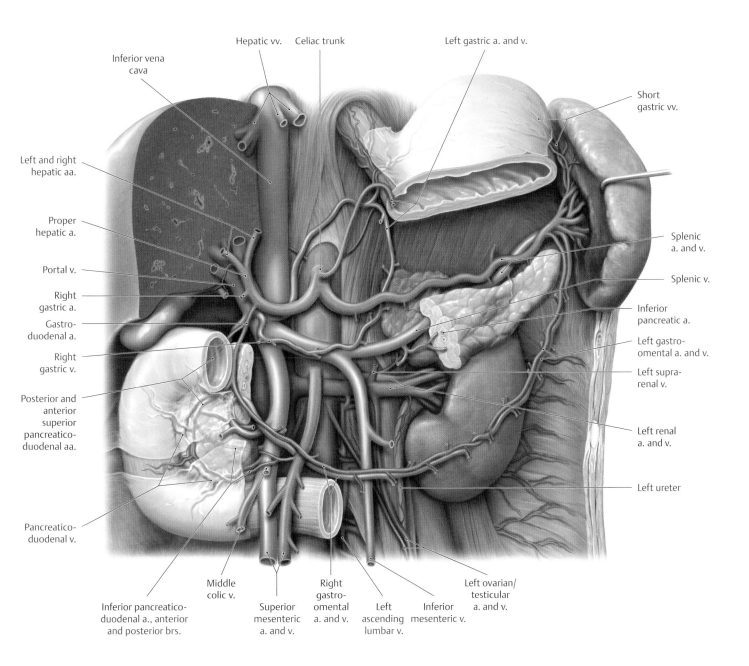

Fig. 16.19 **Portal vein: Pancreas and spleen**

Anterior view. *Partially removed:* Liver, stomach, pancreas, and peritoneum.

Hepatic vv. Celiac trunk

Left gastric a. and v.

Inferior vena cava

Short gastric vv.

Left and right hepatic aa.

Proper hepatic a.

Splenic a. and v.

Portal v.

Splenic v.

Right gastric a.

Inferior pancreatic a.

Gastro-duodenal a.

Left gastro-omental a. and v.

Right gastric v.

Left supra-renal v.

Posterior and anterior superior pancreatico-duodenal aa.

Left renal a. and v.

Left ureter

Pancreatico-duodenal v.

Inferior pancreatico-duodenal a., anterior and posterior brs.

Middle colic v.

Superior mesenteric a. and v.

Right gastro-omental a. and v.

Left ascending lumbar v.

Inferior mesenteric v.

Left ovarian/testicular a. and v.

Superior & Inferior Mesenteric Veins

***Fig. 16.20* Superior mesenteric vein**
Anterior view. *Partially removed*: Stomach, duodenum, and peritoneum.
Removed: Pancreas, greater omentum, and transverse colon.
Reflected: Liver and gallbladder. *Displaced*: Small intestine.

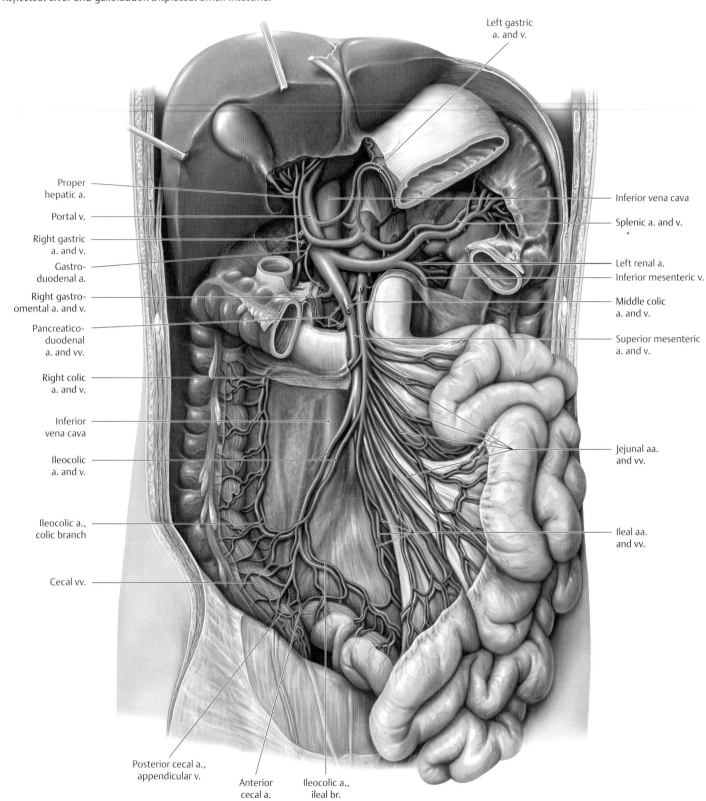

Left gastric
a. and v.

Proper
hepatic a.

Portal v.

Right gastric
a. and v.

Gastro-
duodenal a.

Right gastro-
omental a. and v.

Pancreatico-
duodenal
a. and vv.

Right colic
a. and v.

Inferior
vena cava

Ileocolic
a. and v.

Ileocolic a.,
colic branch

Cecal vv.

Posterior cecal a.,
appendicular v.

Anterior
cecal a.

Ileocolic a.,
ileal br.

Inferior vena cava

Splenic a. and v.

Left renal a.

Inferior mesenteric v.

Middle colic
a. and v.

Superior mesenteric
a. and v.

Jejunal aa.
and vv.

Ileal aa.
and vv.

Fig. 16.21 Inferior mesenteric vein

Anterior view. *Partially removed*: Stomach, duodenum, and peritoneum. *Removed*: Pancreas, greater omentum, transverse colon, and small intestine. *Reflected*: Liver and gallbladder.

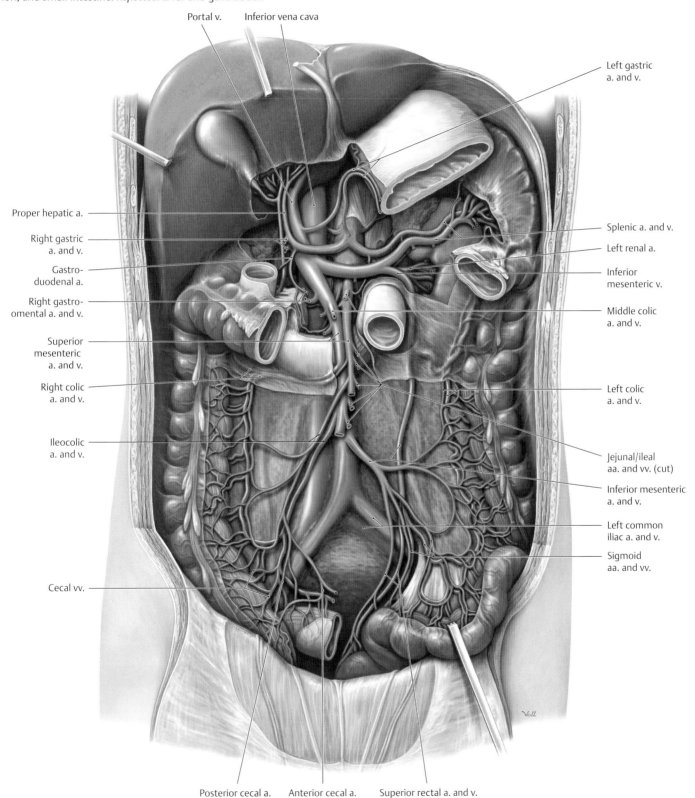

Portal v. Inferior vena cava

Left gastric a. and v.

Proper hepatic a.

Right gastric a. and v.

Gastro-duodenal a.

Right gastro-omental a. and v.

Superior mesenteric a. and v.

Right colic a. and v.

Ileocolic a. and v.

Cecal vv.

Splenic a. and v.

Left renal a.

Inferior mesenteric v.

Middle colic a. and v.

Left colic a. and v.

Jejunal/ileal aa. and vv. (cut)

Inferior mesenteric a. and v.

Left common iliac a. and v.

Sigmoid aa. and vv.

Posterior cecal a. Anterior cecal a. Superior rectal a. and v.

Lymphatics of the Abdominal Organs

Fig. 16.22 **Lymphatic drainage of the internal organs**

See **Table 16.3** for numbering. Lymph drainage from the abdomen, pelvis, and lower limb ultimately passes through the lumbar lymph nodes (clinically, the aortic nodes). The lumbar lymph nodes consist of the right lateral aortic (caval) and left lateral aortic nodes, the preaortic nodes, and the retroaortic nodes.

Efferent lymph vessels from the lateral aortic lymph nodes and the retroaortic nodes form the lumbar trunks and those from the preaortic nodes form the intestinal trunks, respectively. The lumbar and intestinal trunks terminate in the cisterna chyli.

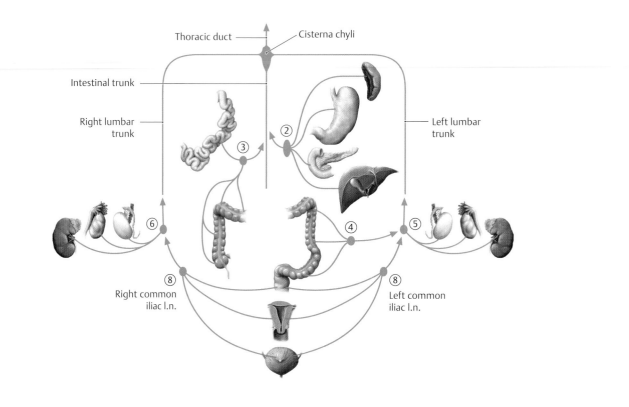

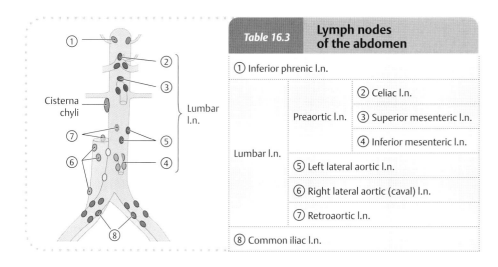

Table 16.3	Lymph nodes of the abdomen		
① Inferior phrenic l.n.			
Lumbar l.n.	Preaortic l.n.	② Celiac l.n.	
		③ Superior mesenteric l.n.	
		④ Inferior mesenteric l.n.	
	⑤ Left lateral aortic l.n.		
	⑥ Right lateral aortic (caval) l.n.		
	⑦ Retroaortic l.n.		
⑧ Common iliac l.n.			

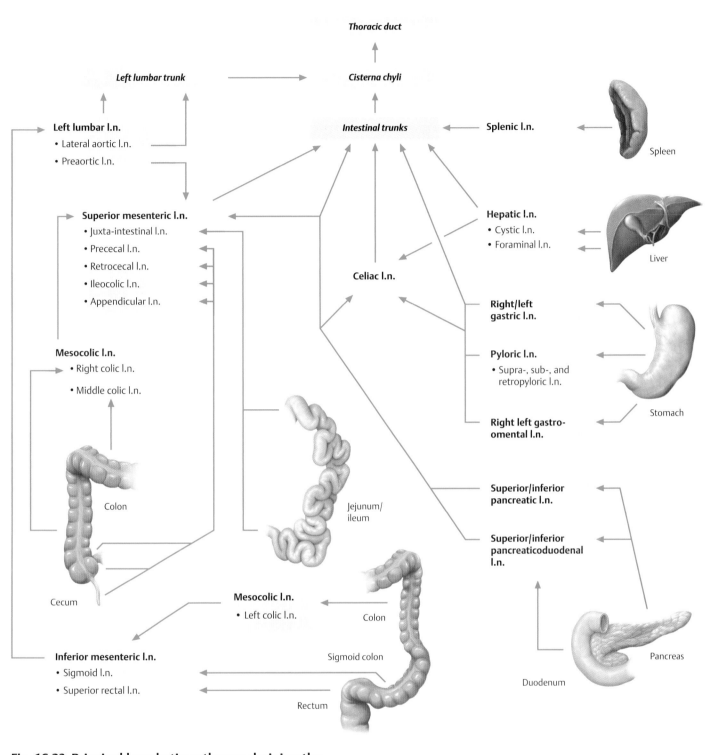

Fig. 16.23 Principal lymphatic pathways draining the digestive organs and spleen

Lymph from the spleen and most digestive organs drains directly from regional lymph nodes or through intervening collecting nodes to the intestinal trunks, except for the descending and sigmoid colon and the upper part of the rectum, which are drained by the left lumbar trunk.

The three large collecting nodes are:

• *Celiac lymph nodes* collect lymph from the stomach, duodenum, pancreas, spleen, and liver. Topographically and at dissection they are often indistinguishable from the regional lymph nodes of the nearby upper abdominal organs.

• *Superior mesenteric lymph nodes* collect lymph from the jejunum, ileum, ascending and transverse colon.

• *Inferior mesenteric lymph nodes* collect lymph from the descending and sigmoid colon and rectum.

These nodes drain principally through the intestinal trunks to the cisterna chyli, but there is an accessory drainage route by way of the left lumbar lymph nodes. Lymph from the pelvis also drains up into the inferior mesenteric and lateral aortic lymph nodes. A complete drainage pathway for lymph from the pelvis can be found on **p. 271.**

Lymph Nodes of the Posterior Abdominal Wall

Lymph nodes in the abdomen and pelvis may be classified as either parietal or visceral. The majority of the parietal lymph nodes are located on the posterior abdominal wall.

Fig. 16.24 **Parietal lymph nodes in the abdomen and pelvis**
Anterior view. *Removed:* All visceral structures except vessels.

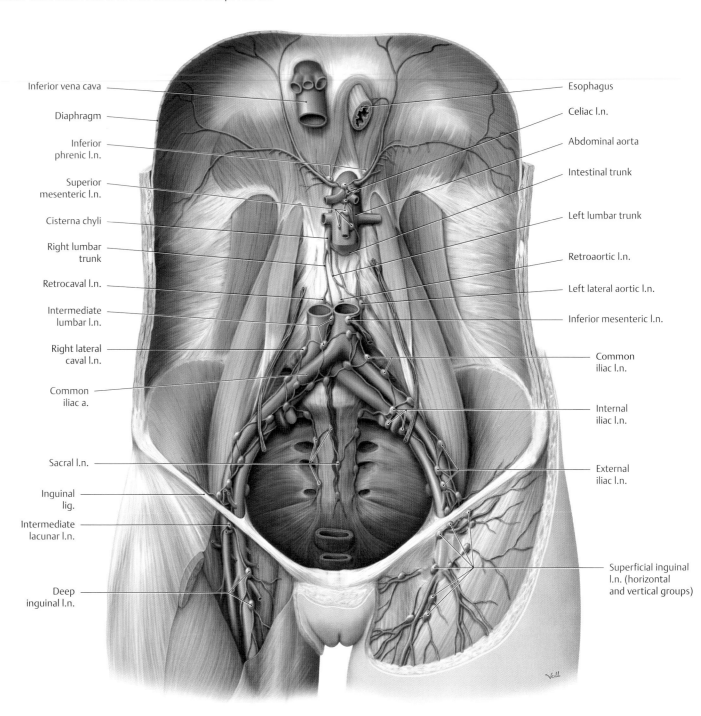

Inferior vena cava

Diaphragm

Inferior phrenic l.n.

Superior mesenteric l.n.

Cisterna chyli

Right lumbar trunk

Retrocaval l.n.

Intermediate lumbar l.n.

Right lateral caval l.n.

Common iliac a.

Sacral l.n.

Inguinal lig.

Intermediate lacunar l.n.

Deep inguinal l.n.

Esophagus

Celiac l.n.

Abdominal aorta

Intestinal trunk

Left lumbar trunk

Retroaortic l.n.

Left lateral aortic l.n.

Inferior mesenteric l.n.

Common iliac l.n.

Internal iliac l.n.

External iliac l.n.

Superficial inguinal l.n. (horizontal and vertical groups)

Fig. 16.25 Lymph nodes of the kidneys, ureters, and suprarenal glands

Anterior view.

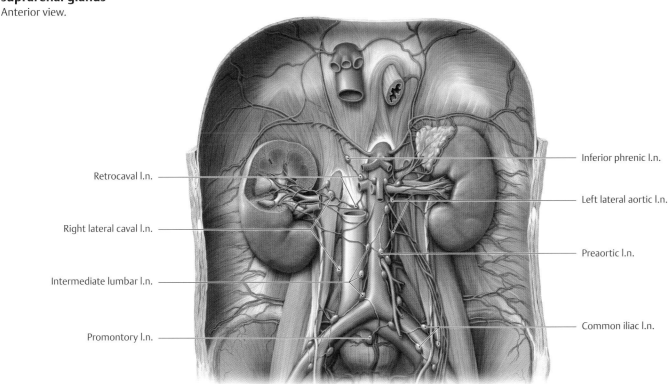

Retrocaval l.n.

Right lateral caval l.n.

Intermediate lumbar l.n.

Promontory l.n.

Inferior phrenic l.n.

Left lateral aortic l.n.

Preaortic l.n.

Common iliac l.n.

Fig. 16.26 Lymphatic drainage of the kidneys and gonads (with pelvic organs)

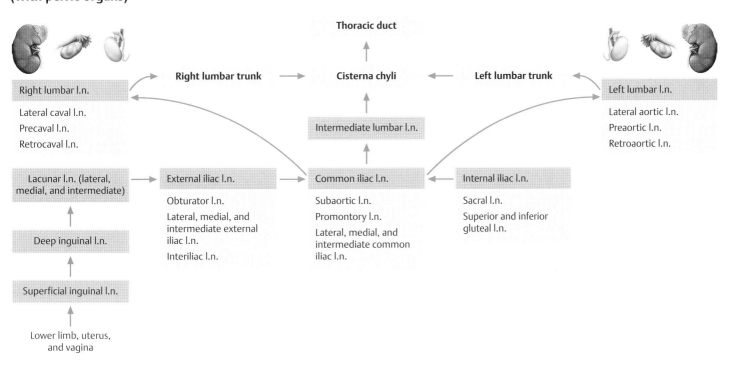

Thoracic duct

Right lumbar trunk → Cisterna chyli ← Left lumbar trunk

Right lumbar l.n.

Lateral caval l.n.
Precaval l.n.
Retrocaval l.n.

Left lumbar l.n.

Lateral aortic l.n.
Preaortic l.n.
Retroaortic l.n.

Intermediate lumbar l.n.

Lacunar l.n. (lateral, medial, and intermediate)

External iliac l.n.

Obturator l.n.
Lateral, medial, and intermediate external iliac l.n.
Interiliac l.n.

Common iliac l.n.

Subaortic l.n.
Promontory l.n.
Lateral, medial, and intermediate common iliac l.n.

Internal iliac l.n.

Sacral l.n.
Superior and inferior gluteal l.n.

Deep inguinal l.n.

Superficial inguinal l.n.

Lower limb, uterus, and vagina

Lymph Nodes of the Supracolic Organs

***Fig. 16.27* Lymph nodes of the stomach and liver**

Anterior view. *Removed:* Lesser omentum. *Opened:* Greater omentum. Arrows show direction of lymphatic drainage.

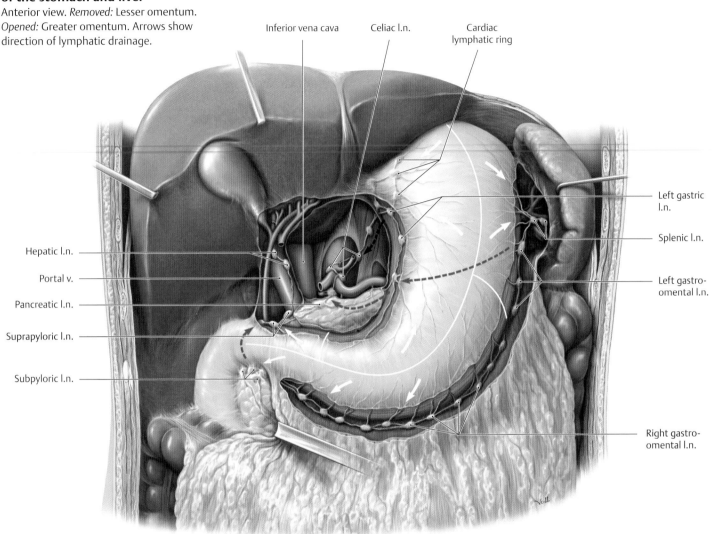

Inferior vena cava — Celiac l.n. — Cardiac lymphatic ring

Hepatic l.n.
Portal v.
Pancreatic l.n.
Suprapyloric l.n.
Subpyloric l.n.

Left gastric l.n.
Splenic l.n.
Left gastro-omental l.n.
Right gastro-omental l.n.

***Fig. 16.28* Lymphatic drainage of the liver and biliary tract**

Anterior view. In the region of the liver, the major lymph-producing organ, the important pathways are:

- *Liver and intrahepatic bile ducts:* Most lymph drains inferiorly through the hepatic nodes to the celiac nodes and then to the intestinal trunk and cisterna chyli, but it may take a more direct route bypassing the celiac nodes. A small amount drains cranially through the inferior phrenic nodes to the lumbar trunk. It also can drain through the diaphragm to the superior phrenic nodes and on to the bronchomediastinal trunk.
- *Gallbladder:* Lymph drains initially to the cystic node, then follows one of the pathways described above.
- *Common bile duct:* Lymph drains through the pyloric nodes (supra-, sub-, and retropyloric) and the foraminal node to the celiac nodes, then to the intestinal trunk.

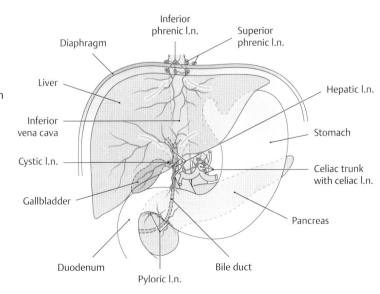

Inferior phrenic l.n.
Diaphragm — Superior phrenic l.n.
Liver
Inferior vena cava
Cystic l.n.
Gallbladder
Duodenum
Pyloric l.n.
Hepatic l.n.
Stomach
Celiac trunk with celiac l.n.
Pancreas
Bile duct

Fig. 16.29 Lymph nodes of the spleen, pancreas, and duodenum

Anterior view. *Removed:* Stomach and colon.

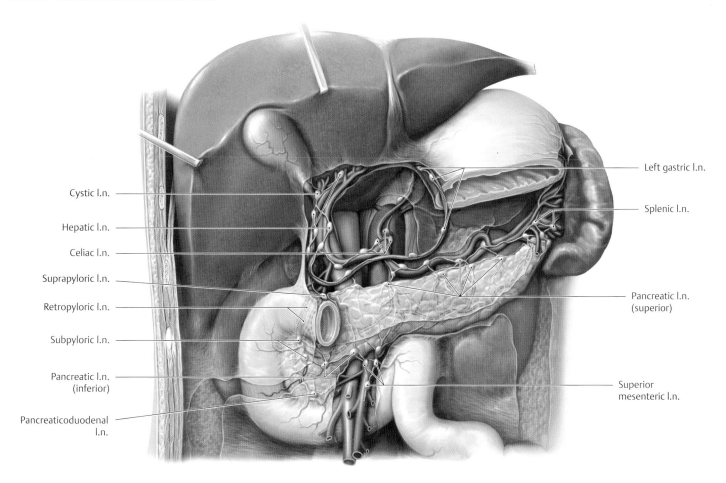

Cystic l.n.

Hepatic l.n.

Celiac l.n.

Suprapyloric l.n.

Retropyloric l.n.

Subpyloric l.n.

Pancreatic l.n. (inferior)

Pancreaticoduodenal l.n.

Left gastric l.n.

Splenic l.n.

Pancreatic l.n. (superior)

Superior mesenteric l.n.

Fig. 16.30 Lymphatic drainage of the stomach, liver, spleen, pancreas, and duodenum

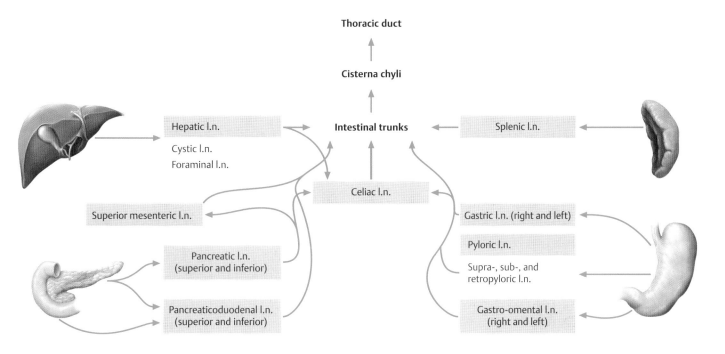

Thoracic duct

Cisterna chyli

Hepatic l.n.
Cystic l.n.
Foraminal l.n.

Intestinal trunks

Splenic l.n.

Celiac l.n.

Superior mesenteric l.n.

Gastric l.n. (right and left)

Pyloric l.n.

Supra-, sub-, and retropyloric l.n.

Pancreatic l.n. (superior and inferior)

Pancreaticoduodenal l.n. (superior and inferior)

Gastro-omental l.n. (right and left)

Lymph Nodes of the Infracolic Organs

Fig. 16.31 Lymph nodes of the jejunum and ileum
Anterior view. *Removed:* Stomach, liver, pancreas, and colon.

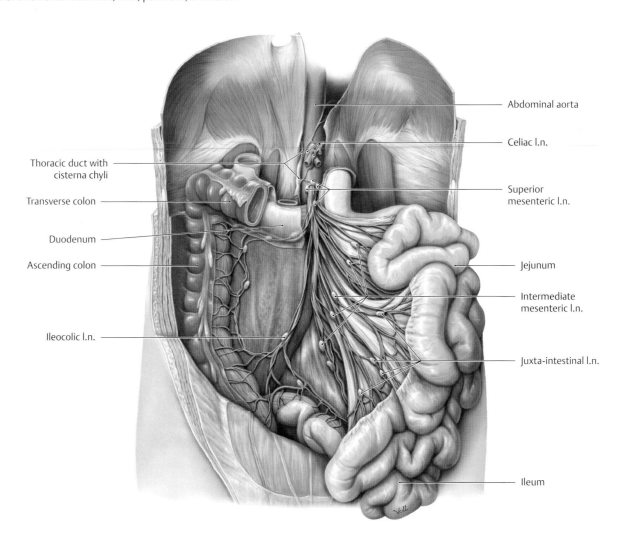

Fig. 16.32 Lymphatic drainage of the intestines

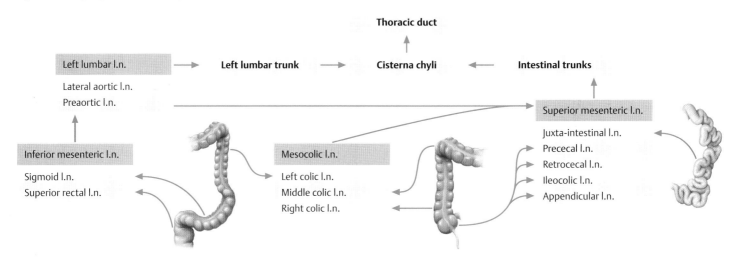

***Fig. 16.33* Lymph nodes of the large intestine**
Anterior view. *Reflected:* Transverse colon and greater omentum.

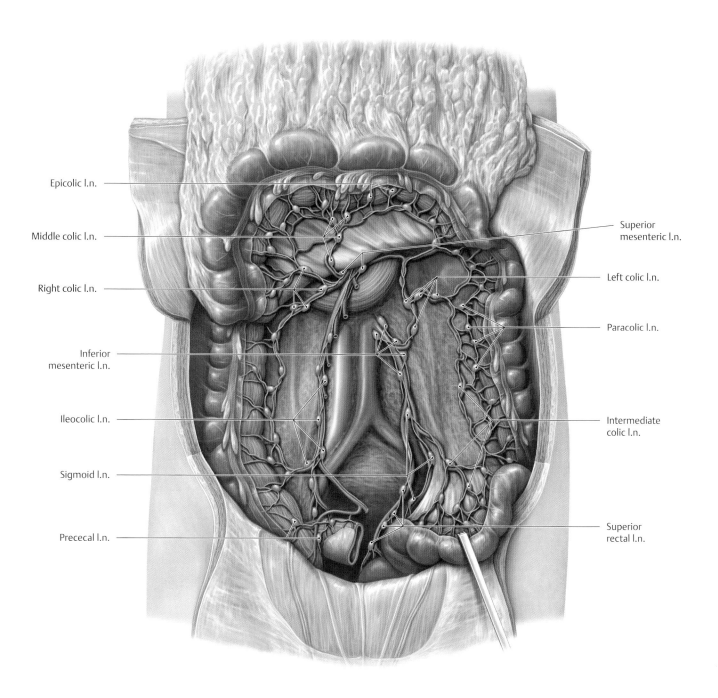

Epicolic l.n.

Middle colic l.n.

Right colic l.n.

Inferior
mesenteric l.n.

Ileocolic l.n.

Sigmoid l.n.

Prececal l.n.

Superior
mesenteric l.n.

Left colic l.n.

Paracolic l.n.

Intermediate
colic l.n.

Superior
rectal l.n.

Nerves of the Abdominal Wall

Fig. 16.34 **Somatic nerves of the abdomen and pelvis**
Anterior view.

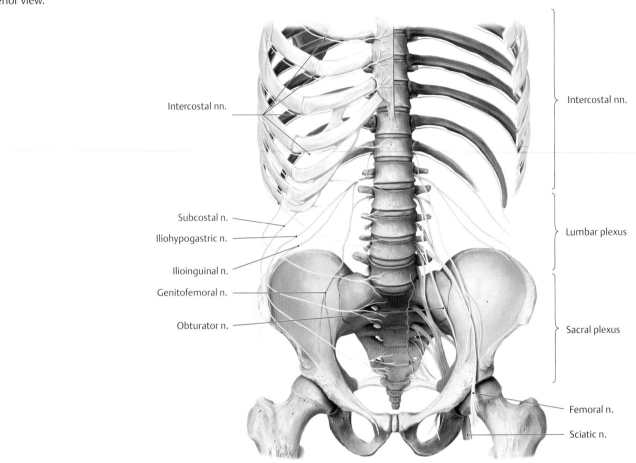

Intercostal nn.

Intercostal nn.

Subcostal n.

Iliohypogastric n.

Ilioinguinal n.

Genitofemoral n.

Obturator n.

Lumbar plexus

Sacral plexus

Femoral n.

Sciatic n.

Fig. 16.35 **Cutaneous innervation of the anterior trunk**
Anterior view.

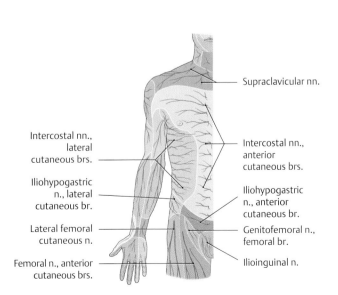

Supraclavicular nn.

Intercostal nn., lateral cutaneous brs.

Iliohypogastric n., lateral cutaneous br.

Lateral femoral cutaneous n.

Femoral n., anterior cutaneous brs.

Intercostal nn., anterior cutaneous brs.

Iliohypogastric n., anterior cutaneous br.

Genitofemoral n., femoral br.

Ilioinguinal n.

Fig. 16.36 **Dermatomes of the anterior trunk**
Anterior view.

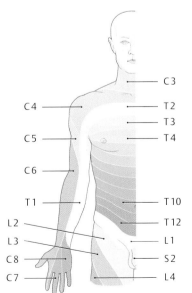

C 3

C 4

C 5

C 6

T 1

L 2

L 3

C 8

C 7

T 2

T 3

T 4

T 10

T 12

L 1

S 2

L 4

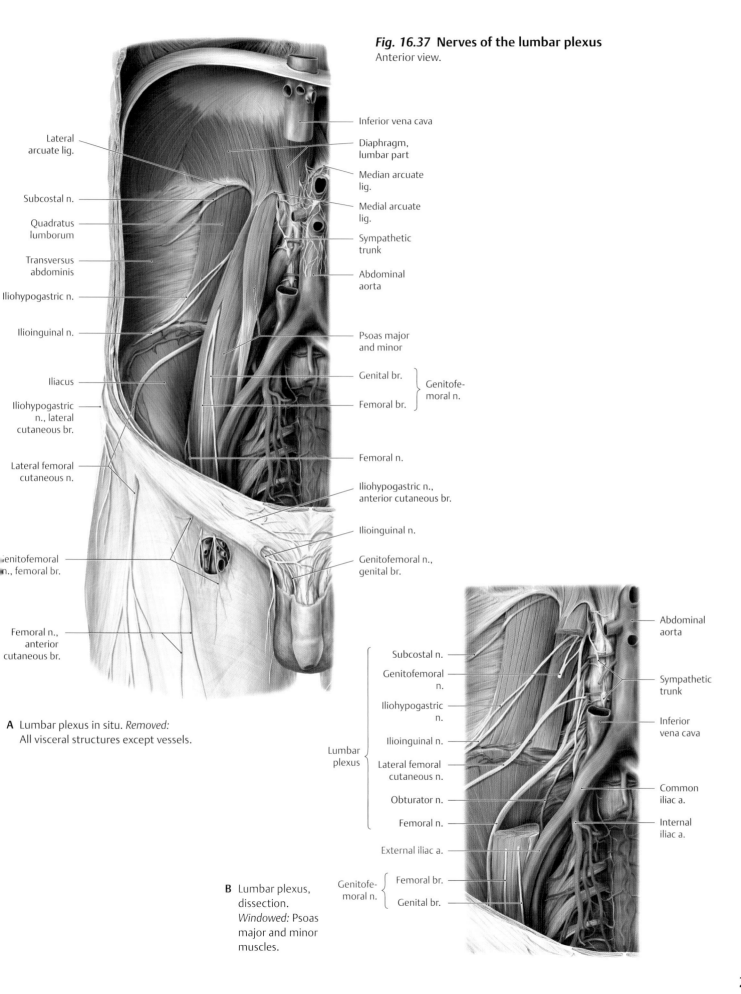

Fig. 16.37 **Nerves of the lumbar plexus**
Anterior view.

Inferior vena cava

Diaphragm, lumbar part

Median arcuate lig.

Medial arcuate lig.

Sympathetic trunk

Abdominal aorta

Lateral arcuate lig.

Subcostal n.

Quadratus lumborum

Transversus abdominis

Iliohypogastric n.

Ilioinguinal n.

Iliacus

Iliohypogastric n., lateral cutaneous br.

Lateral femoral cutaneous n.

Genitofemoral n., femoral br.

Femoral n., anterior cutaneous br.

Psoas major and minor

Genital br. ⎱ Genitofe-
Femoral br. ⎰ moral n.

Femoral n.

Iliohypogastric n., anterior cutaneous br.

Ilioinguinal n.

Genitofemoral n., genital br.

A Lumbar plexus in situ. *Removed:* All visceral structures except vessels.

Abdominal aorta

Sympathetic trunk

Inferior vena cava

Common iliac a.

Internal iliac a.

Subcostal n.

Genitofemoral n.

Iliohypogastric n.

Ilioinguinal n.

Lateral femoral cutaneous n.

Obturator n.

Femoral n.

Lumbar plexus

External iliac a.

Genitofe-moral n. ⎱ Femoral br.
⎰ Genital br.

B Lumbar plexus, dissection. *Windowed:* Psoas major and minor muscles.

Autonomic Innervation: Overview

Fig. 16.38 Sympathetic and parasympathetic nervous systems in the abdomen and pelvis

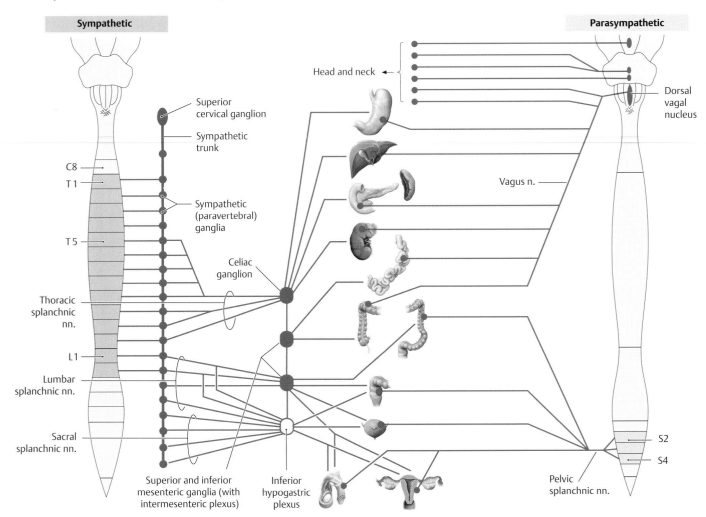

Table 16.4	Effects of the autonomic nervous system in the abdomen and pelvis		
Organ (organ system)		**Sympathetic effect**	**Parasympathetic effect**
Gastrointestinal tract	Longitudinal and circular muscle fibers	↓ motility	↑ motility
	Sphincter muscles	Contraction	Relaxation
	Glands	↓ secretions	↑ secretions
Splenic capsule		Contraction	
Liver		↑ glycogenolysis/gluconeogenesis	No effect
Pancreas	Endocrine pancreas	↓ insulin secretion	
	Exocrine pancreas	↓ secretion	↑ secretion
Urinary bladder	Detrusor vesicae	Relaxation	Contraction
	Functional bladder sphincter	Contraction	Inhibits contraction
Seminal vesicle and ductus deferens		Contraction (ejaculation)	
Uterus		Contraction or relaxation, depending on hormonal status	No effect
Arteries		Vasoconstriction	Vasodilation of the arteries of the penis and clitoris (erection)
Suprarenal glands (medulla)		Release of adrenalin	No effect
Urinary tract	Kidney	Vasoconstriction (↓ urine formation)	Vasodilation

Fig. 16.39 **Autonomic innervation of the intraperitoneal organs**

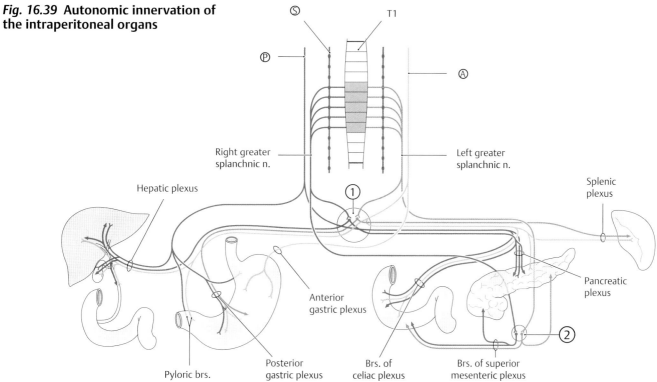

Ⓢ	Sympathetic trunk
Ⓟ	Posterior vagal trunk (from right vagus n.)
Ⓐ	Anterior vagal trunk (from left vagus n.)
①	Celiac ganglia
②	Superior mesenteric ganglion
③	Inferior mesenteric ganglion
④	Greater splanchnic n. (T5–T9)
⑤	Lesser splanchnic n. (T10–T11)
⑥	Least splanchnic n. (T12)
⑦	Lumbar splanchnic nn. (L1–L2)
⑧	Lumbar splanchnic nn. (from 3rd to 5th lumbar ganglia)
⑨	Sacral splanchnic nn. (from 1st to 3rd sacral ganglia)
⑩	Pelvic splanchnic nn. (S2–S4)

A Innervation of the foregut. As the left and right vagus nerves descend along the esophagus, they become the anterior and posterior vagal trunks, respectively. Each trunk produces a celiac, pyloric, and hepatic branch, and a gastric plexus.

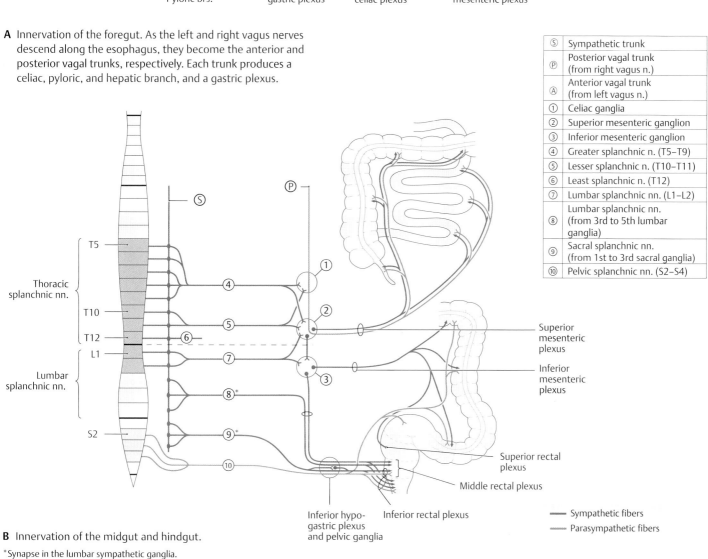

B Innervation of the midgut and hindgut.

*Synapse in the lumbar sympathetic ganglia.

— Sympathetic fibers
— Parasympathetic fibers

Autonomic Plexuses

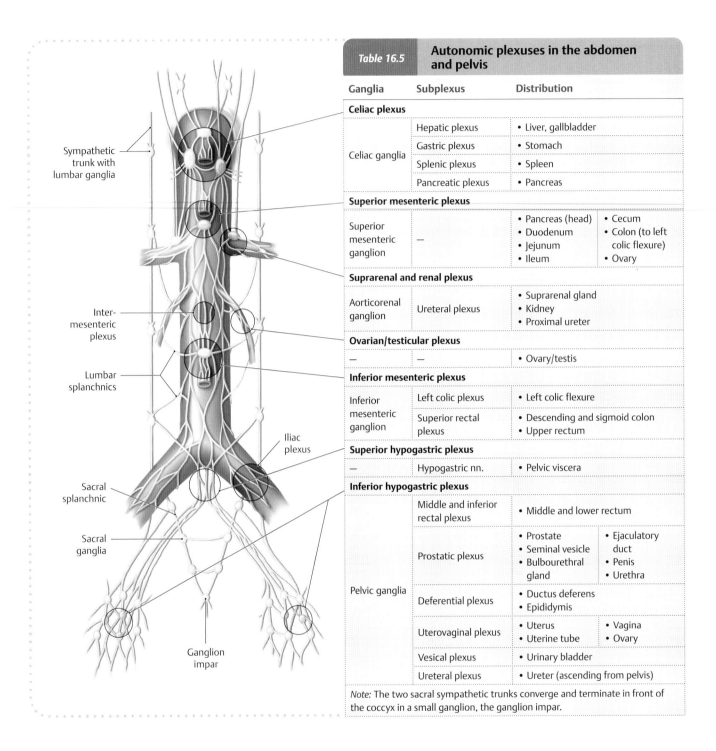

Sympathetic trunk with lumbar ganglia

Inter-mesenteric plexus

Lumbar splanchnics

Iliac plexus

Sacral splanchnic

Sacral ganglia

Ganglion impar

Table 16.5	Autonomic plexuses in the abdomen and pelvis	
Ganglia	**Subplexus**	**Distribution**
Celiac plexus		
Celiac ganglia	Hepatic plexus	• Liver, gallbladder
	Gastric plexus	• Stomach
	Splenic plexus	• Spleen
	Pancreatic plexus	• Pancreas
Superior mesenteric plexus		
Superior mesenteric ganglion	—	• Pancreas (head) • Cecum • Duodenum • Colon (to left colic flexure) • Jejunum • Ileum • Ovary
Suprarenal and renal plexus		
Aorticorenal ganglion	Ureteral plexus	• Suprarenal gland • Kidney • Proximal ureter
Ovarian/testicular plexus		
—	—	• Ovary/testis
Inferior mesenteric plexus		
Inferior mesenteric ganglion	Left colic plexus	• Left colic flexure
	Superior rectal plexus	• Descending and sigmoid colon • Upper rectum
Superior hypogastric plexus		
—	Hypogastric nn.	• Pelvic viscera
Inferior hypogastric plexus		
Pelvic ganglia	Middle and inferior rectal plexus	• Middle and lower rectum
	Prostatic plexus	• Prostate • Ejaculatory duct • Seminal vesicle • Penis • Bulbourethral gland • Urethra
	Deferential plexus	• Ductus deferens • Epididymis
	Uterovaginal plexus	• Uterus • Vagina • Uterine tube • Ovary
	Vesical plexus	• Urinary bladder
	Ureteral plexus	• Ureter (ascending from pelvis)

Note: The two sacral sympathetic trunks converge and terminate in front of the coccyx in a small ganglion, the ganglion impar.

Fig. 16.40 Autonomic plexuses in the abdomen and pelvis

Anterior view of the male abdomen and pelvis. *Removed:* Peritoneum, majority of the stomach, and all other abdominal organs except kidneys and suprarenal glands.

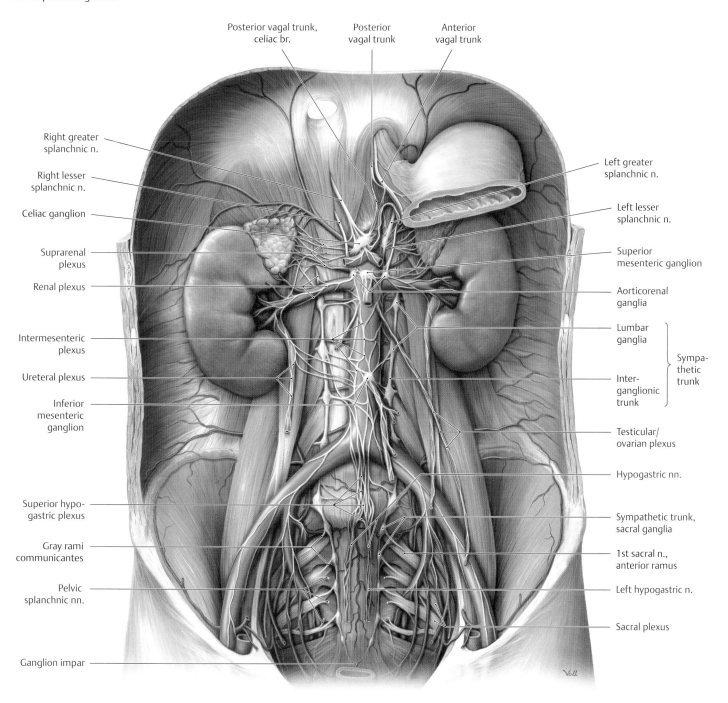

Posterior vagal trunk, celiac br.

Posterior vagal trunk

Anterior vagal trunk

Right greater splanchnic n.

Right lesser splanchnic n.

Celiac ganglion

Suprarenal plexus

Renal plexus

Intermesenteric plexus

Ureteral plexus

Inferior mesenteric ganglion

Superior hypo-gastric plexus

Gray rami communicantes

Pelvic splanchnic nn.

Ganglion impar

Left greater splanchnic n.

Left lesser splanchnic n.

Superior mesenteric ganglion

Aorticorenal ganglia

Lumbar ganglia

Inter-ganglionic trunk

Sympa-thetic trunk

Testicular/ovarian plexus

Hypogastric nn.

Sympathetic trunk, sacral ganglia

1st sacral n., anterior ramus

Left hypogastric n.

Sacral plexus

Innervation of the Abdominal Organs

Fig. 16.41 Innervation of the anterior abdominal organs
Anterior view. *Removed:* Lesser omentum, ascending colon, and parts of the transverse colon. *Opened:* Omental bursa. The anterior and posterior vagal trunks each produce a celiac, hepatic, and pyloric branch, and a gastric plexus. See **p. 210** for schematic.

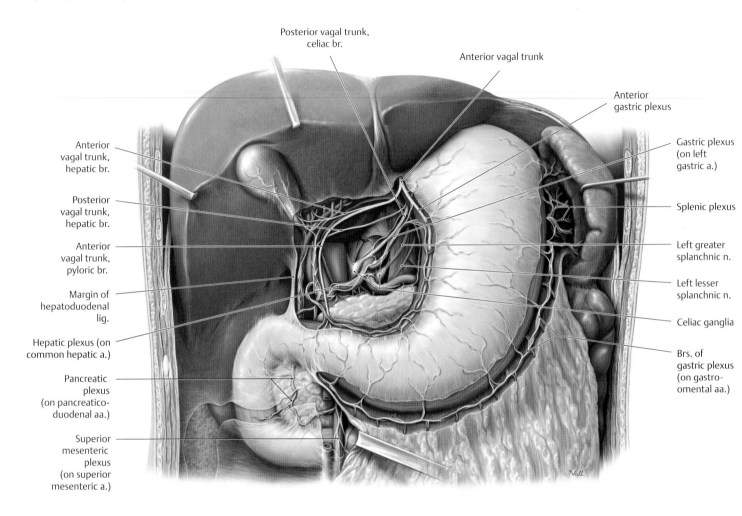

Fig. 16.42 Innervation of the urinary organs

Anterior view of the male abdomen and pelvis. *Removed:* Peritoneum, majority of stomach, and abdominal organs except kidneys, suprarenal glands, and bladder. See **p. 276** for schematic.

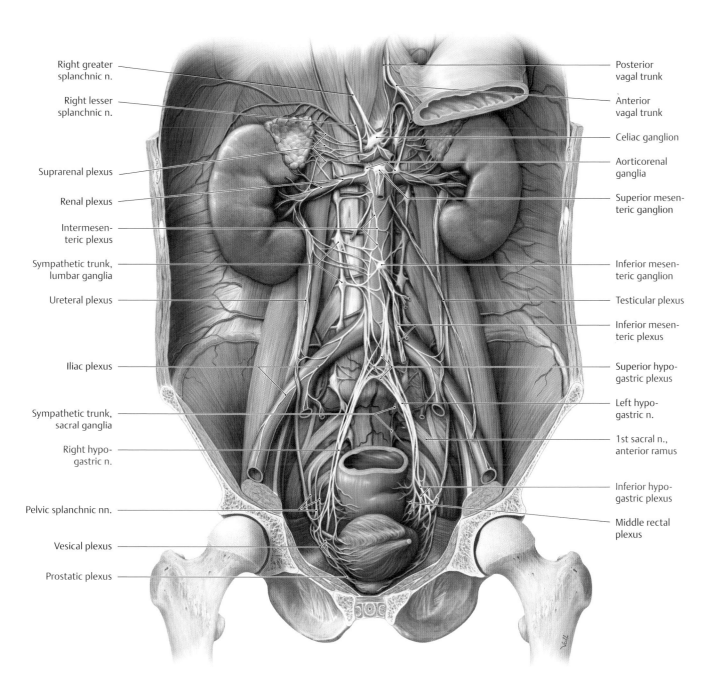

Right greater splanchnic n.

Right lesser splanchnic n.

Suprarenal plexus

Renal plexus

Intermesenteric plexus

Sympathetic trunk, lumbar ganglia

Ureteral plexus

Iliac plexus

Sympathetic trunk, sacral ganglia

Right hypogastric n.

Pelvic splanchnic nn.

Vesical plexus

Prostatic plexus

Posterior vagal trunk

Anterior vagal trunk

Celiac ganglion

Aorticorenal ganglia

Superior mesenteric ganglion

Inferior mesenteric ganglion

Testicular plexus

Inferior mesenteric plexus

Superior hypogastric plexus

Left hypogastric n.

1st sacral n., anterior ramus

Inferior hypogastric plexus

Middle rectal plexus

Innervation of the Intestines

Fig. 16.43 Innervation of the small intestine
Anterior view. *Partially removed:* Stomach, pancreas,
and transverse colon (distal part). See **p. 210** for schematic.

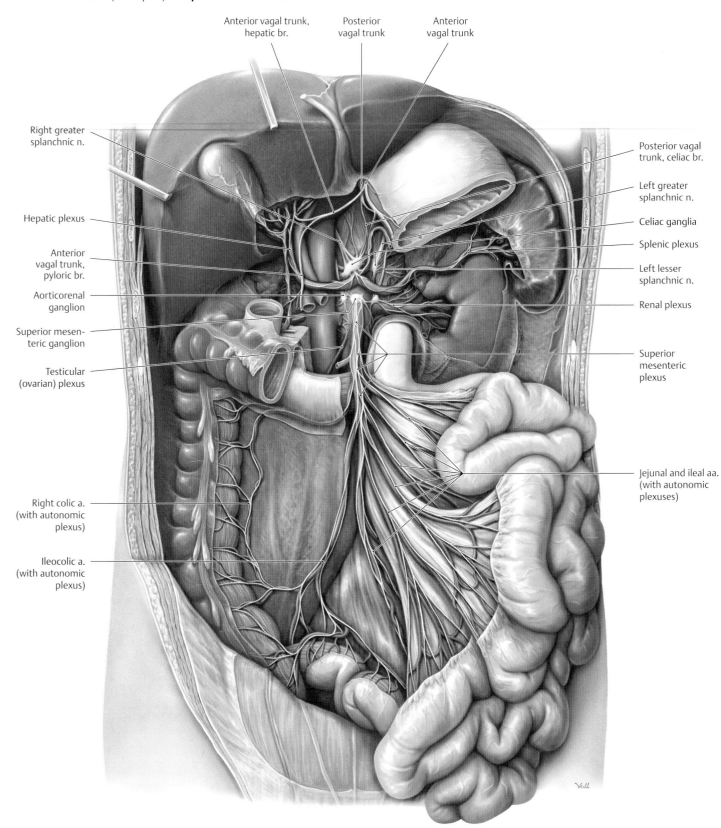

Anterior vagal trunk,
hepatic br.

Posterior
vagal trunk

Anterior
vagal trunk

Right greater
splanchnic n.

Hepatic plexus

Anterior
vagal trunk,
pyloric br.

Aorticorenal
ganglion

Superior mesen-
teric ganglion

Testicular
(ovarian) plexus

Right colic a.
(with autonomic
plexus)

Ileocolic a.
(with autonomic
plexus)

Posterior vagal
trunk, celiac br.

Left greater
splanchnic n.

Celiac ganglia

Splenic plexus

Left lesser
splanchnic n.

Renal plexus

Superior
mesenteric
plexus

Jejunal and ileal aa.
(with autonomic
plexuses)

Fig. 16.44 Innervation of the large intestine

Anterior view. *Removed:* Small intestine.
Reflected: Transverse and sigmoid colons. See **p. 210** for schematic.

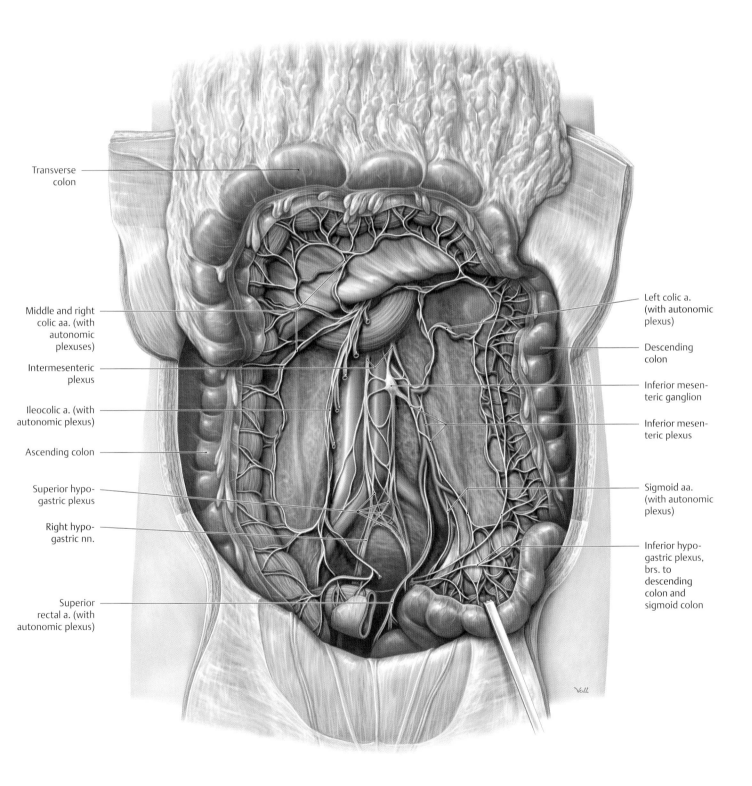

Transverse colon

Middle and right colic aa. (with autonomic plexuses)

Intermesenteric plexus

Ileocolic a. (with autonomic plexus)

Ascending colon

Superior hypogastric plexus

Right hypogastric nn.

Superior rectal a. (with autonomic plexus)

Left colic a. (with autonomic plexus)

Descending colon

Inferior mesenteric ganglion

Inferior mesenteric plexus

Sigmoid aa. (with autonomic plexus)

Inferior hypogastric plexus, brs. to descending colon and sigmoid colon

Sectional Anatomy of the Abdomen

Fig. 17.1 **Transverse sections of the abdomen**
Inferior view.

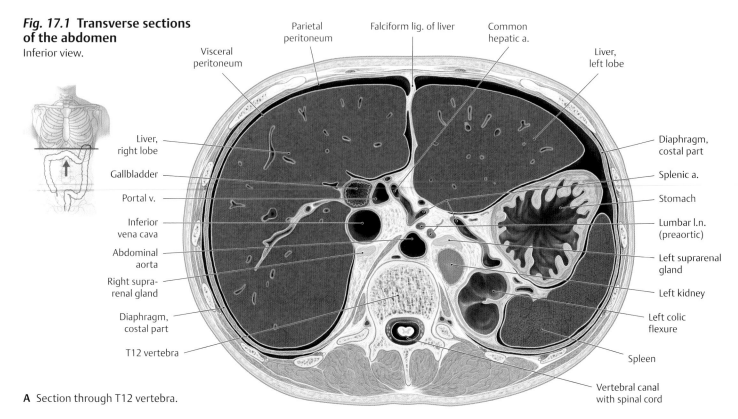

A Section through T12 vertebra.

Labels (top figure):
Parietal peritoneum — Falciform lig. of liver — Common hepatic a. — Liver, left lobe — Visceral peritoneum — Liver, right lobe — Gallbladder — Portal v. — Inferior vena cava — Abdominal aorta — Right supra-renal gland — Diaphragm, costal part — T12 vertebra — Diaphragm, costal part — Splenic a. — Stomach — Lumbar l.n. (preaortic) — Left suprarenal gland — Left kidney — Left colic flexure — Spleen — Vertebral canal with spinal cord

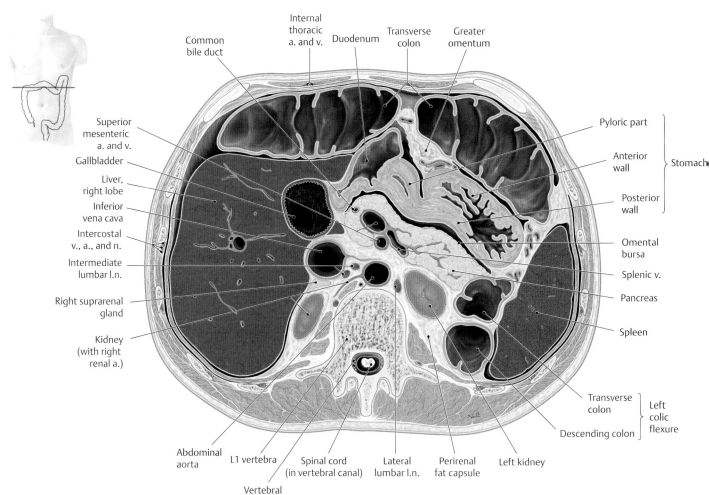

B Section through L1 vertebra.

Labels (bottom figure):
Common bile duct — Internal thoracic a. and v. — Duodenum — Transverse colon — Greater omentum — Superior mesenteric a. and v. — Gallbladder — Liver, right lobe — Inferior vena cava — Intercostal v., a., and n. — Intermediate lumbar l.n. — Right suprarenal gland — Kidney (with right renal a.) — Abdominal aorta — L1 vertebra — Spinal cord (in vertebral canal) — Vertebral venous plexus — Lateral lumbar l.n. — Perirenal fat capsule — Left kidney — Pyloric part — Anterior wall — Stomach — Posterior wall — Omental bursa — Splenic v. — Pancreas — Spleen — Transverse colon — Descending colon — Left colic flexure

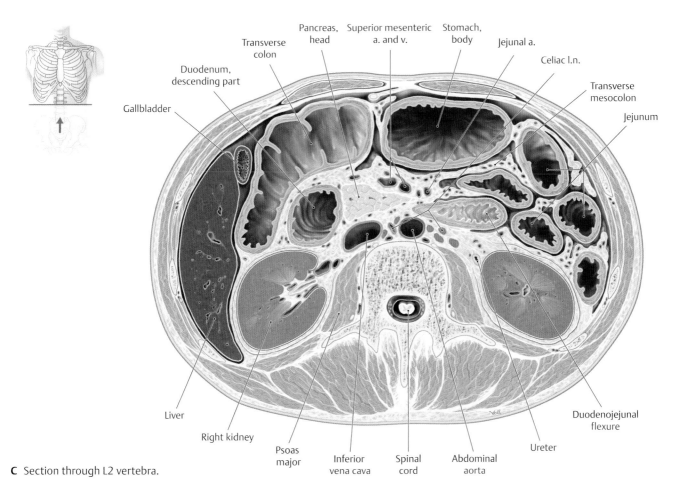

C Section through L2 vertebra.

Radiographic Anatomy of the Abdomen (I)

Fig. 17.2 **CT of the abdomen**
Inferior view.

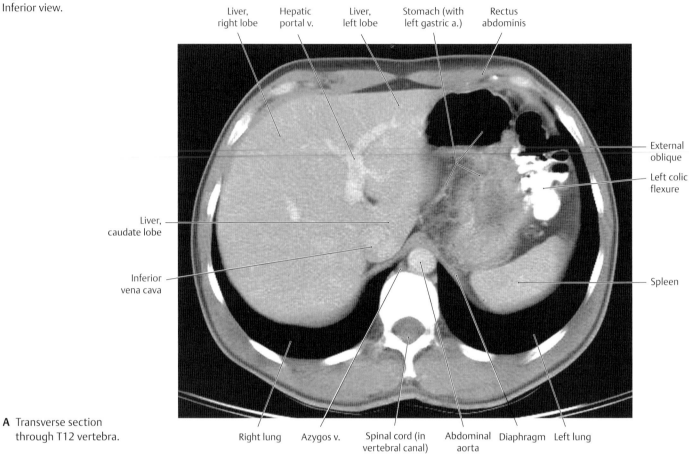

A Transverse section through T12 vertebra.

Labels (clockwise): Liver, right lobe — Hepatic portal v. — Liver, left lobe — Stomach (with left gastric a.) — Rectus abdominis — External oblique — Left colic flexure — Spleen — Left lung — Diaphragm — Abdominal aorta — Spinal cord (in vertebral canal) — Azygos v. — Right lung — Inferior vena cava — Liver, caudate lobe

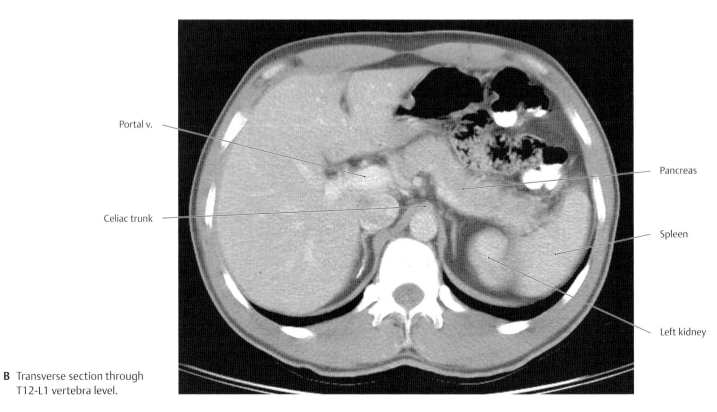

B Transverse section through T12–L1 vertebra level.

Labels: Portal v. — Celiac trunk — Pancreas — Spleen — Left kidney

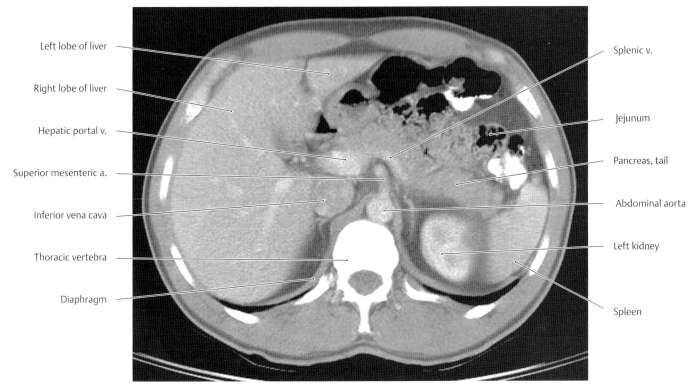

Left lobe of liver

Right lobe of liver

Hepatic portal v.

Superior mesenteric a.

Inferior vena cava

Thoracic vertebra

Diaphragm

Splenic v.

Jejunum

Pancreas, tail

Abdominal aorta

Left kidney

Spleen

C Transverse view through
L1 vertebra.

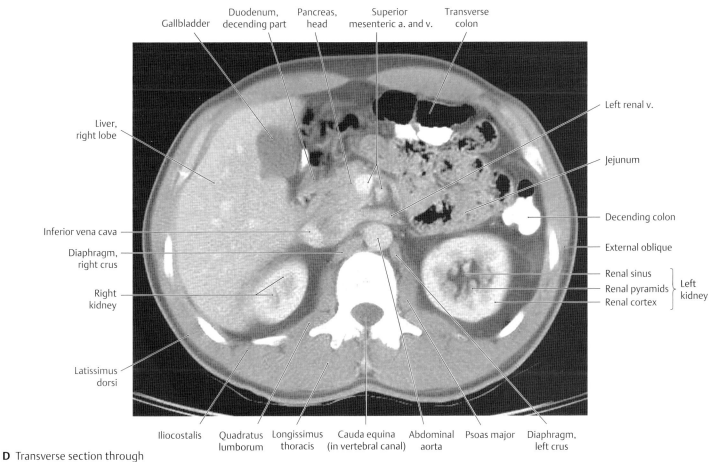

Gallbladder

Duodenum,
decending part

Pancreas,
head

Superior
mesenteric a. and v.

Transverse
colon

Liver,
right lobe

Inferior vena cava

Diaphragm,
right crus

Right
kidney

Latissimus
dorsi

Left renal v.

Jejunum

Decending colon

External oblique

Renal sinus
Renal pyramids } Left
Renal cortex } kidney

Iliocostalis

Quadratus
lumborum

Longissimus
thoracis

Cauda equina
(in vertebral canal)

Abdominal
aorta

Psoas major

Diaphragm,
left crus

D Transverse section through
L1-L2 vertebral level.

221

Radiographic Anatomy of the Abdomen (II)

Fig. 17.3 **CT of the abdomen**
Inferior view.

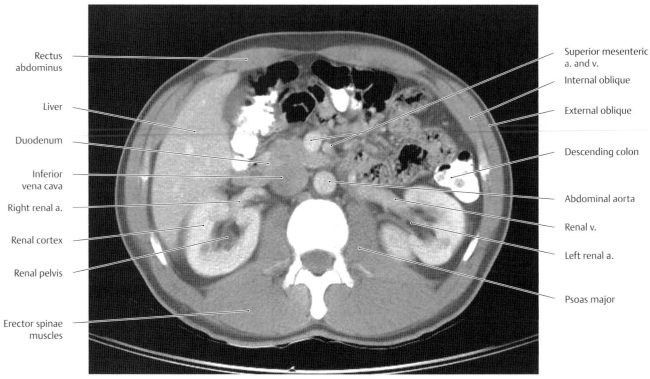

Rectus abdominus — Liver — Duodenum — Inferior vena cava — Right renal a. — Renal cortex — Renal pelvis — Erector spinae muscles

Superior mesenteric a. and v. — Internal oblique — External oblique — Descending colon — Abdominal aorta — Renal v. — Left renal a. — Psoas major

A Transverse section through L2-L3 vertebral level.

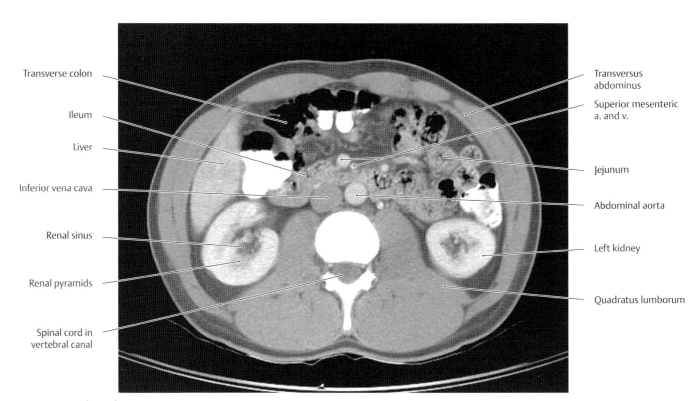

Transverse colon — Ileum — Liver — Inferior vena cava — Renal sinus — Renal pyramids — Spinal cord in vertebral canal

Transversus abdominus — Superior mesenteric a. and v. — Jejunum — Abdominal aorta — Left kidney — Quadratus lumborum

B Transverse section through L3-L4 vertebral level.

Fig. 17.4 Radiograph of double contrast barium enema of the small intestine
Anterior view.

Circular folds   Jejunum

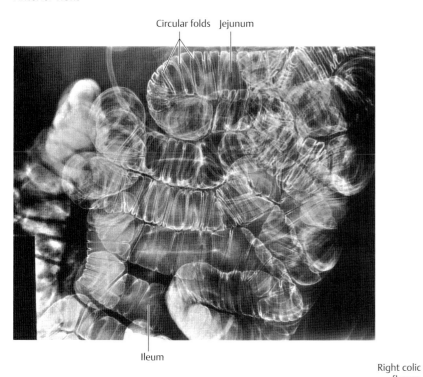

Ileum

Fig. 17.5 Radiograph of double contrast barium enema of the large intestine
Anterior view.

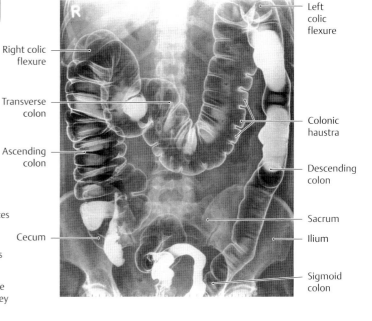

Right colic flexure

Transverse colon

Ascending colon

Cecum

Left colic flexure

Colonic haustra

Descending colon

Sacrum

Ilium

Sigmoid colon

Fig. 17.6 Radiograph of intravenous pylegram
Anterior view.

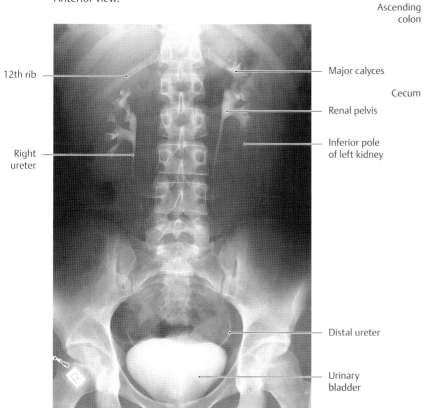

12th rib

Right ureter

Major calyces

Renal pelvis

Inferior pole of left kidney

Distal ureter

Urinary bladder

223

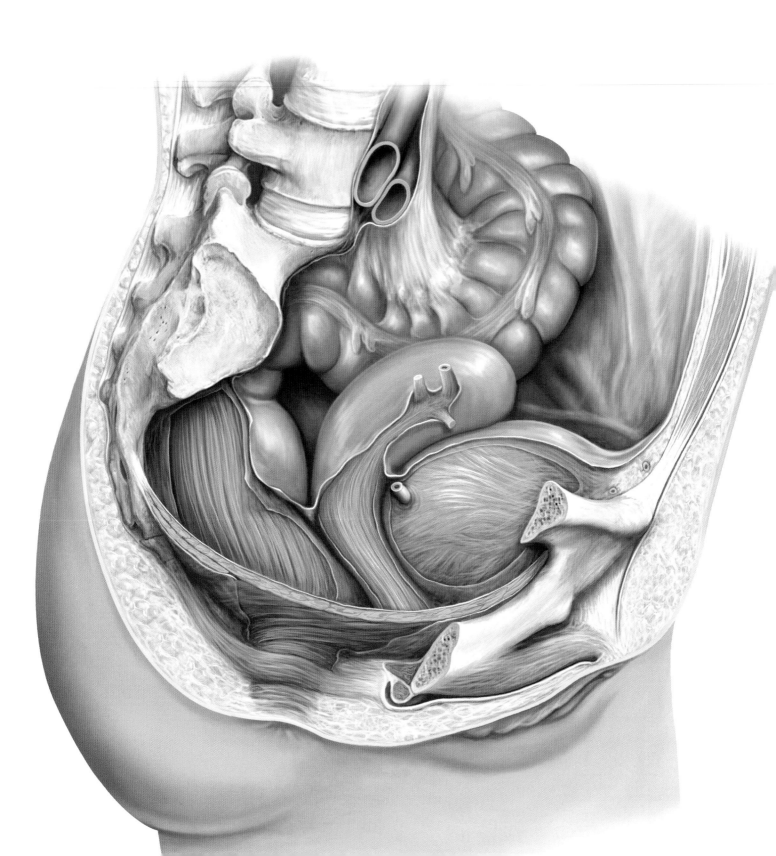

Pelvis & Perineum

Surface Anatomy

Fig. 18.1 **Palpable structures of the pelvis**

Anterior view. The structures are common to both male and female. See **pp. 2–3** for structures of the back.

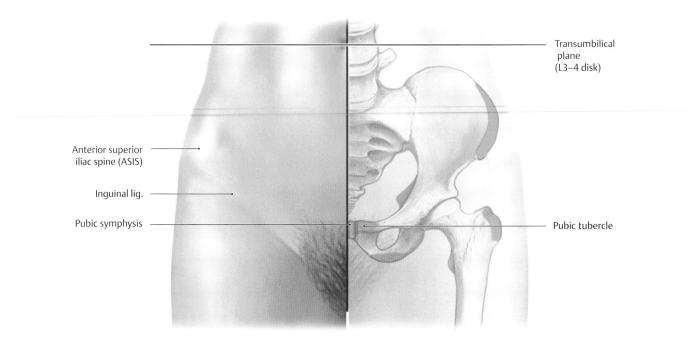

A Bony prominences, female pelvis.

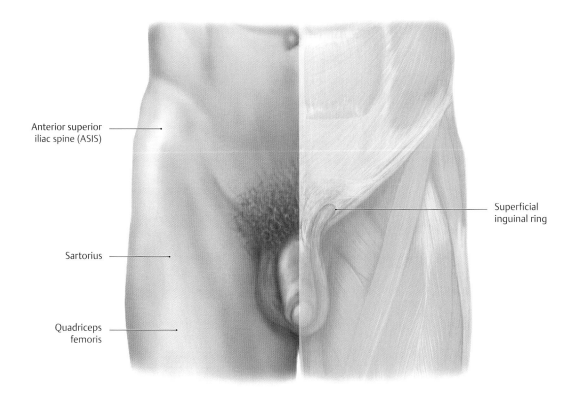

B Musculature, male pelvis.

The *perineum* is the inferiormost portion of the trunk, between the thighs and buttocks, extending from the pubis to the coccyx and superiorly to the inferior fascia of the pelvic diaphragm, including all of the structures of the anal and urogenital triangles

(**Fig. 18.2A**). The bilateral boundaries of the perineum are the pubic symphysis, ischiopubic ramus, ischial tuberosity, sacrotuberous ligament, and coccyx.

Fig. 18.2 Regions of the female perineum
Lithotomy position.

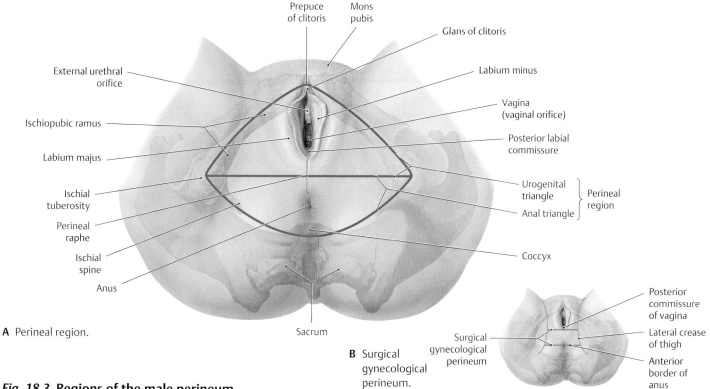

A Perineal region.

B Surgical gynecological perineum.

Fig. 18.3 Regions of the male perineum
Lithotomy position.

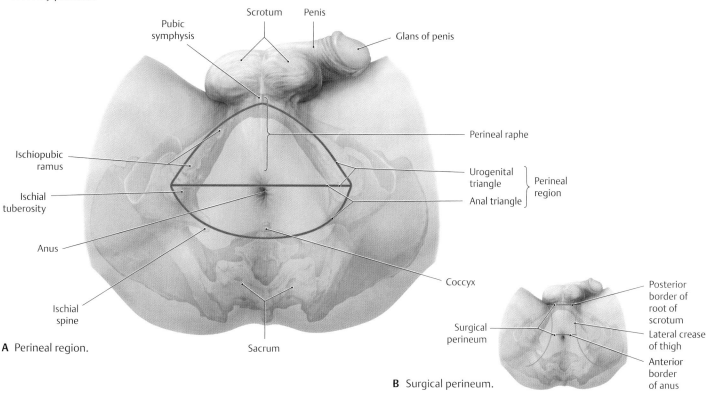

A Perineal region.

B Surgical perineum.

Pelvic Girdle

 The pelvis is the region of the body inferior to the abdomen and surrounded by the pelvic girdle, which is the two hip bones and the sacrum that connect the vertebral column to the femur. The two hip bones are connected to each other at the cartilaginous pubic symphysis and to the sacrum via the sacroiliac joints, creating the pelvic brim (red, **Fig. 19.1**). The stability of the pelvic girdle is necessary for the transfer of trunk loads to the lower limb, which occurs in normal gait.

Fig. 19.1 Pelvic girdle
Anterosuperior view. The pelvic girdle consists of the two hip bones and the sacrum.

Fig. 19.2 Hip bone
Right hip bone (male).

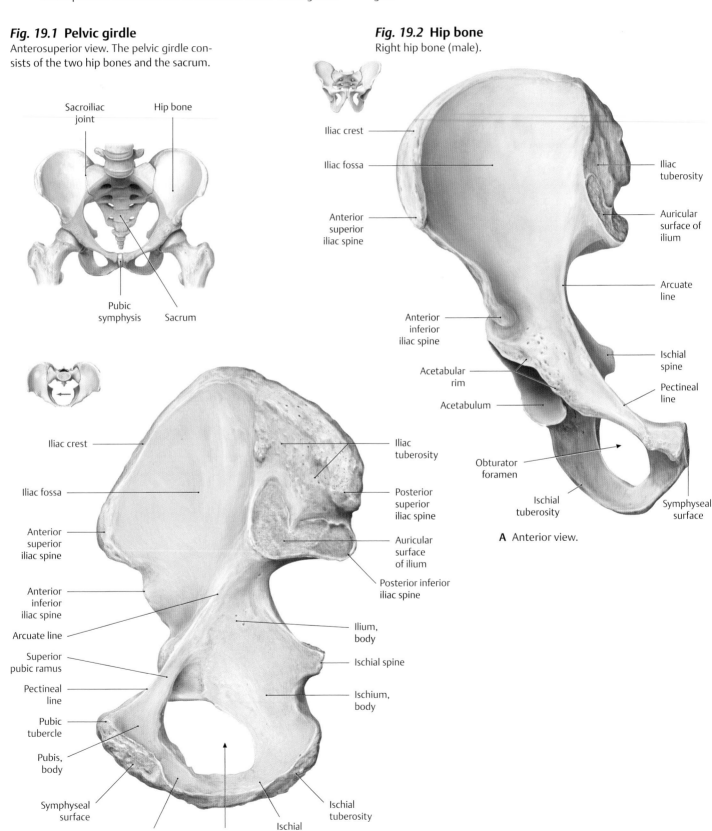

A Anterior view.

B Medial view.

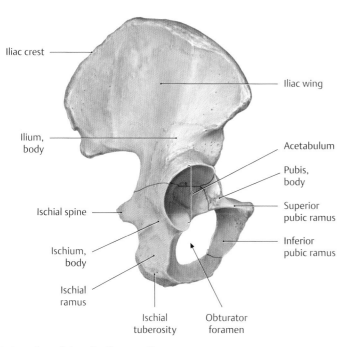

Iliac crest

Iliac wing

Ilium, body

Acetabulum

Pubis, body

Ischial spine

Superior pubic ramus

Inferior pubic ramus

Ischium, body

Ischial ramus

Ischial tuberosity

Obturator foramen

A Junction of the triradiate cartilage.

Fig. 19.3 Triradiate cartilage of the hip bone

Right hip bone, lateral view. The hip bone consists of the ilium, ischium, and pubis.

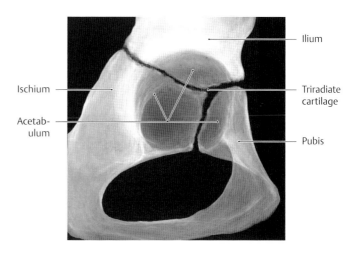

Ilium

Ischium

Triradiate cartilage

Acetabulum

Pubis

B Radiograph of a child's acetabulum.

Fig. 19.4 Hip bone: Lateral view

Right hip bone (male).

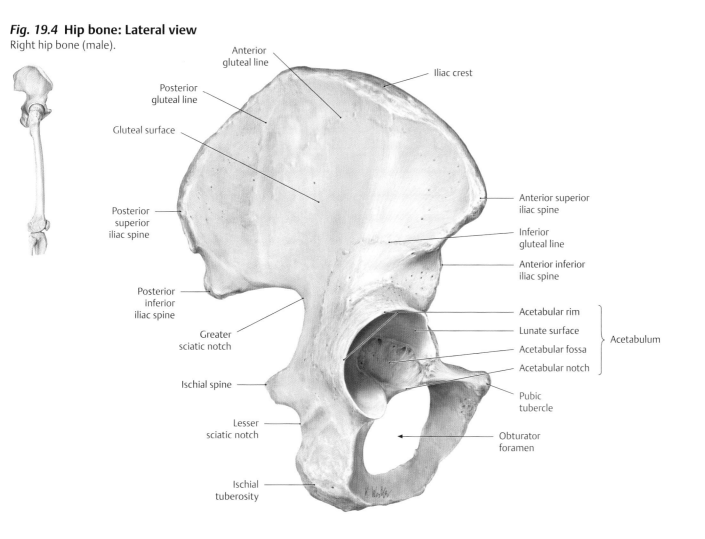

Anterior gluteal line

Posterior gluteal line

Gluteal surface

Posterior superior iliac spine

Posterior inferior iliac spine

Greater sciatic notch

Ischial spine

Lesser sciatic notch

Ischial tuberosity

Iliac crest

Anterior superior iliac spine

Inferior gluteal line

Anterior inferior iliac spine

Acetabular rim

Lunate surface

Acetabular fossa

Acetabular notch

Acetabulum

Pubic tubercle

Obturator foramen

Female & Male Pelvis

Fig. 19.5 Female pelvis

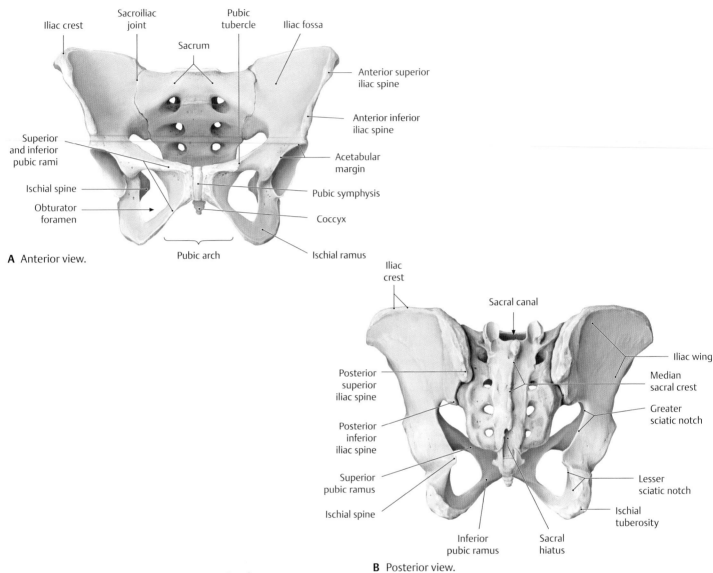

A Anterior view.

Iliac crest — Sacroiliac joint — Sacrum — Pubic tubercle — Iliac fossa — Anterior superior iliac spine — Anterior inferior iliac spine — Acetabular margin — Pubic symphysis — Coccyx — Ischial ramus — Pubic arch — Obturator foramen — Ischial spine — Superior and inferior pubic rami

B Posterior view.

Iliac crest — Sacral canal — Iliac wing — Median sacral crest — Greater sciatic notch — Lesser sciatic notch — Ischial tuberosity — Sacral hiatus — Inferior pubic ramus — Ischial spine — Superior pubic ramus — Posterior inferior iliac spine — Posterior superior iliac spine

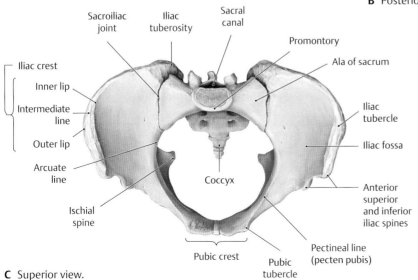

C Superior view.

Sacroiliac joint — Iliac tuberosity — Sacral canal — Promontory — Ala of sacrum — Iliac tubercle — Iliac fossa — Anterior superior and inferior iliac spines — Pectineal line (pecten pubis) — Pubic tubercle — Pubic crest — Ischial spine — Arcuate line — Coccyx — Outer lip — Intermediate line — Inner lip — Iliac crest

✳ Clinical box 19.1

Childbirth

A non-optimal relation between the maternal pelvis and the fetal head may lead to complications during childbirth, potentially necessitating a caesarean section. Maternal causes include earlier pelvic trauma and innate malformations. Fetal causes include hydrocephalus (disturbed circulation of cerebrospinal fluid, leading to brain dilation and cranial expansion).

Fig. 19.6 **Male pelvis**

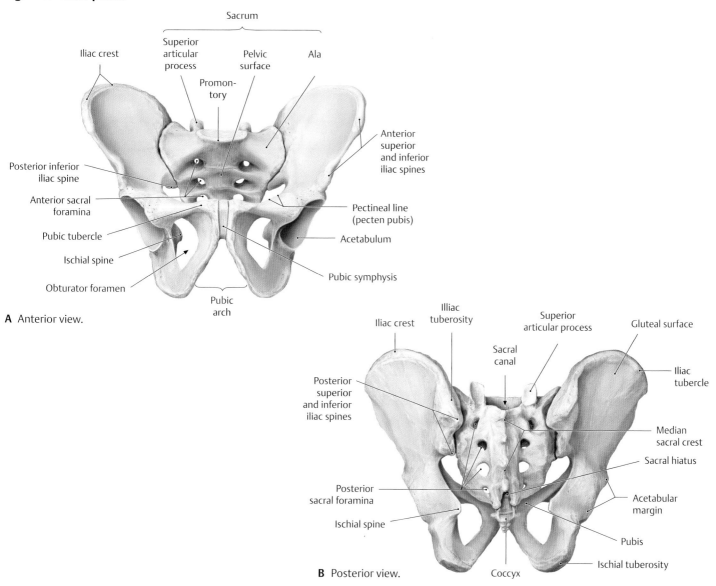

A Anterior view.

B Posterior view.

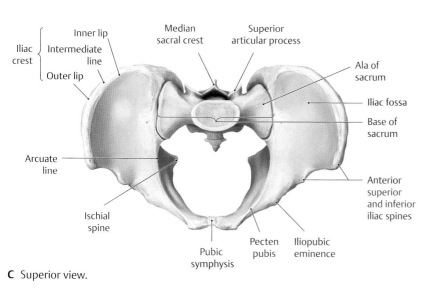

C Superior view.

Female & Male Pelvic Measurements

 The *pelvic inlet*, the superior aperture of the pelvis, is the boundary between the abdominal and pelvic cavities. It is defined by the plane that passes through its edge, the *pelvic brim*, which is the prominence of the sacrum, the arcuate and pectineal lines, and the upper margin of the pubic symphysis. Occasionally, the terms *pelvic inlet* and *pelvic brim* are used interchangeably. The *pelvic outlet* is the plane of the inferior aperture, passing through the pubic arch, the ischial tuberosities, the inferior margin of the sacrotuberous ligament, and the tip of the coccyx.

Table 19.1	Gender-specific features of the pelvis	
Structure	♀	♂
False pelvis	Wide and shallow	Narrow and deep
Pelvic inlet	Transversely oval	Heart-shaped
Pelvic outlet	Roomy and round	Narrow and oblong
Ischial tuberosities	Everted	Inverted
Pelvic cavity	Roomy and shallow	Narrow and deep
Sacrum	Short, wide, and flat	Long, narrow, and convex
Subpubic angle	90–100 degrees	70 degrees

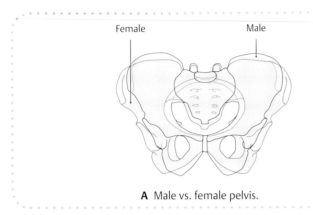

A Male vs. female pelvis.

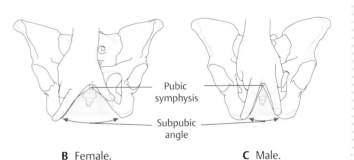

B Female.　　　　**C** Male.

Fig. 19.7 True and false pelvis

The pelvis is the region of the body inferior to the abdomen, surrounded by the pelvic girdle. The *false pelvis* is immediately inferior to the abdominal cavity, between the iliac alae, and superior to the pelvic inlet. The *true pelvis* is the bony-walled space between the pelvic inlet and the pelvic outlet. It is bounded inferiorly by the pelvic diaphragm, also called the pelvic floor.

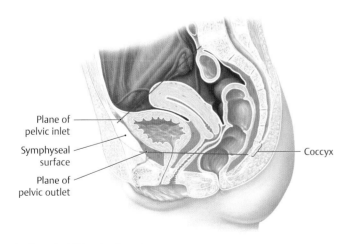

A Female. Midsagittal section, viewed from left side.

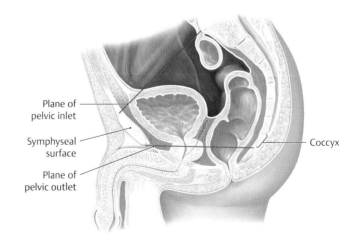

B Male. Midsagittal section, viewed from left side.

Fig. 19.8 Narrowest diameter of female pelvic canal

The true conjugate, the distance between the promontory and the most posterosuperior point of the pubic symphysis, is the narrowest AP (anteroposterior) diameter of the pelvic (birth) canal. This diameter is difficult to measure due to the viscera, so the diagonal conjugate, the distance between the promontory and the inferior border of the pubic symphysis, is used to estimate it. The linea terminalis is part of the border defining the pelvic inlet.

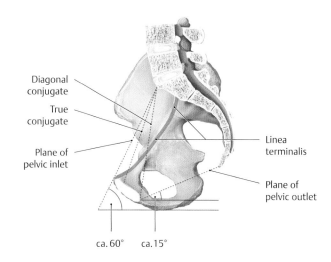

Fig. 19.9 Pelvic inlet and outlet

The measurements shown are applicable to both male and female. The transverse and oblique diameters of the female pelvic inlet are obstetrically important, as they are the measure of the diameter of the pelvic (birth) canal. The interspinous distance is the narrowest diameter of the pelvic outlet.

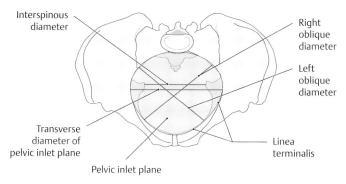

A Female pelvis, superior view. Pelvic inlet outlined in red.

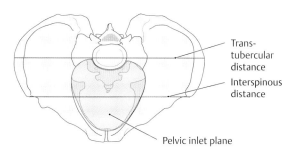

B Male pelvis, superior view. Pelvic inlet outlined in red.

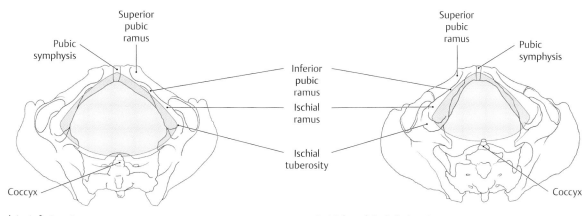

C Female pelvis, inferior view. Pelvic outlet outlined in red.

D Male pelvis, inferior view. Pelvic outlet outlined in red.

Pelvic Ligaments

Fig. 19.10 Ligaments of the pelvis
Male pelvis.

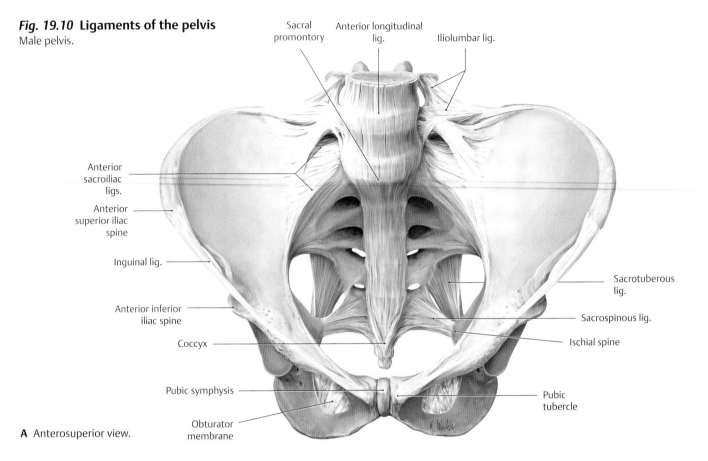

Sacral promontory

Anterior longitudinal lig.

Iliolumbar lig.

Anterior sacroiliac ligs.

Anterior superior iliac spine

Inguinal lig.

Anterior inferior iliac spine

Coccyx

Pubic symphysis

Obturator membrane

Sacrotuberous lig.

Sacrospinous lig.

Ischial spine

Pubic tubercle

A Anterosuperior view.

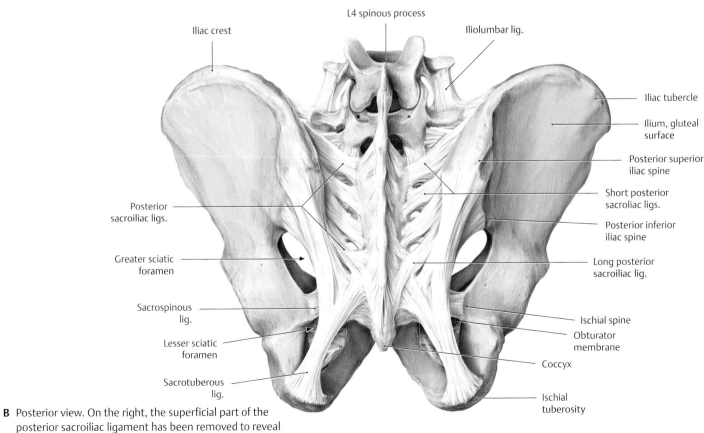

L4 spinous process

Iliac crest

Iliolumbar lig.

Iliac tubercle

Ilium, gluteal surface

Posterior superior iliac spine

Short posterior sacroiliac ligs.

Posterior inferior iliac spine

Long posterior sacroiliac lig.

Posterior sacroiliac ligs.

Greater sciatic foramen

Sacrospinous lig.

Lesser sciatic foramen

Sacrotuberous lig.

Ischial spine

Obturator membrane

Coccyx

Ischial tuberosity

B Posterior view. On the right, the superficial part of the posterior sacroiliac ligament has been removed to reveal long and short posterior sacroiliac ligaments which blend with the deeper interosseous sacroiliac ligament.

Fig. 19.11 Ligaments of the sacroiliac joint
Male pelvis.

Fig. 19.12 Pelvic ligament attachment sites on hip bone
Left hip bone, medial view. Ligament attachments are shown in green.

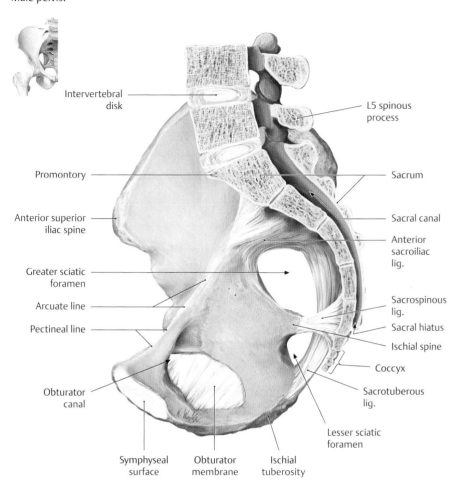

Intervertebral disk
L5 spinous process
Promontory
Sacrum
Anterior superior iliac spine
Sacral canal
Anterior sacroiliac lig.
Greater sciatic foramen
Arcuate line
Sacrospinous lig.
Pectineal line
Sacral hiatus
Ischial spine
Coccyx
Sacrotuberous lig.
Obturator canal
Lesser sciatic foramen
Symphyseal surface
Obturator membrane
Ischial tuberosity

A Right half of pelvis, medial view.

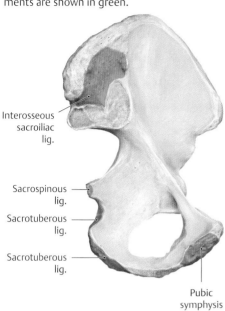

Interosseous sacroiliac lig.
Sacrospinous lig.
Sacrotuberous lig.
Sacrotuberous lig.
Pubic symphysis

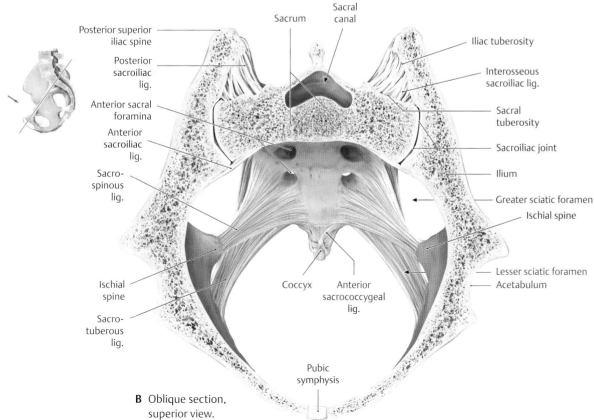

Posterior superior iliac spine
Sacrum
Sacral canal
Iliac tuberosity
Posterior sacroiliac lig.
Interosseous sacroiliac lig.
Anterior sacral foramina
Sacral tuberosity
Anterior sacroiliac lig.
Sacroiliac joint
Sacro-spinous lig.
Ilium
Greater sciatic foramen
Ischial spine
Ischial spine
Lesser sciatic foramen
Coccyx
Anterior sacrococcygeal lig.
Acetabulum
Sacro-tuberous lig.
Pubic symphysis

B Oblique section, superior view.

Muscles of the Pelvic Floor & Perineum

Fig. 19.13 Muscles of the pelvic floor

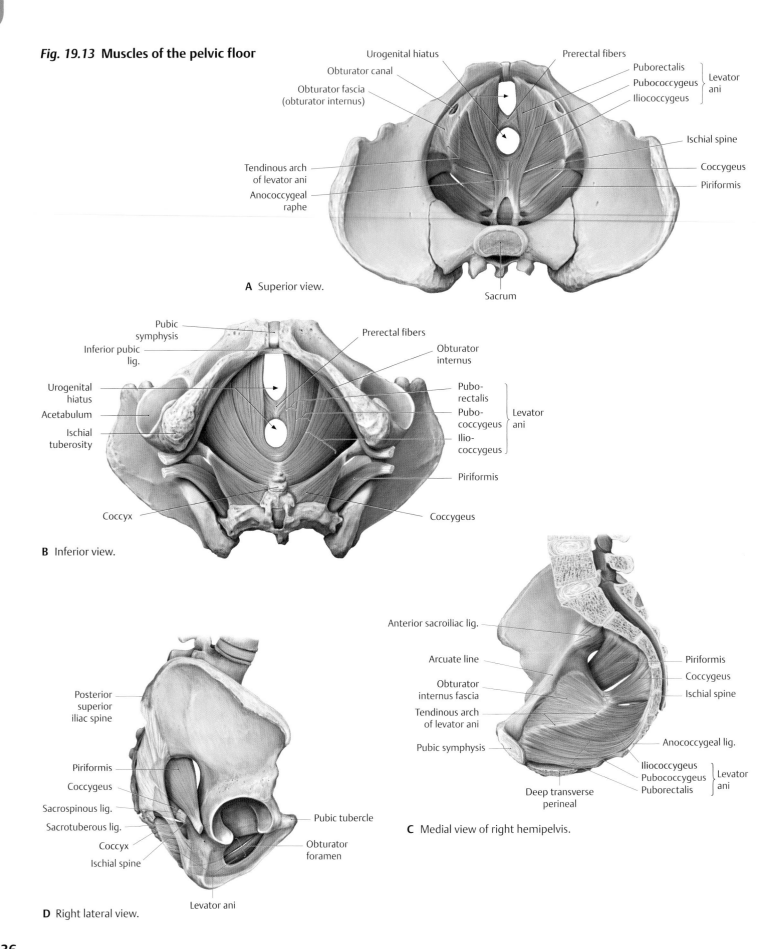

A Superior view.

- Urogenital hiatus
- Obturator canal
- Obturator fascia (obturator internus)
- Tendinous arch of levator ani
- Anococcygeal raphe
- Prerectal fibers
- Puborectalis
- Pubococcygeus
- Iliococcygeus
- Levator ani
- Ischial spine
- Coccygeus
- Piriformis
- Sacrum

B Inferior view.

- Pubic symphysis
- Inferior pubic lig.
- Urogenital hiatus
- Acetabulum
- Ischial tuberosity
- Coccyx
- Prerectal fibers
- Obturator internus
- Pubo-rectalis
- Pubo-coccygeus
- Ilio-coccygeus
- Levator ani
- Piriformis
- Coccygeus

D Right lateral view.

- Posterior superior iliac spine
- Piriformis
- Coccygeus
- Sacrospinous lig.
- Sacrotuberous lig.
- Coccyx
- Ischial spine
- Levator ani
- Pubic tubercle
- Obturator foramen

C Medial view of right hemipelvis.

- Anterior sacroiliac lig.
- Arcuate line
- Obturator internus fascia
- Tendinous arch of levator ani
- Pubic symphysis
- Piriformis
- Coccygeus
- Ischial spine
- Anococcygeal lig.
- Iliococcygeus
- Pubococcygeus
- Puborectalis
- Levator ani
- Deep transverse perineal

Fig. 19.14 Muscles and fascia of the pelvic floor and perineum, in situ

Lithotomy position. Removed on left side: Superficial perineal (Colle's) fascia, inferior fascia of the pelvic diaphragm, and obturator fascia.
Note: The green arrows are pointing forward to the anterior recess of the ischioanal fossa.

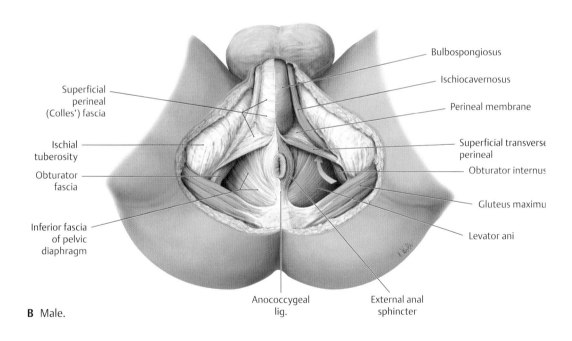

Superficial perineal (Colles') fascia
Perineal body
Ischial tuberosity
Obturator fascia
Inferior fascia of pelvic diaphragm
Anococcygeal lig.
Coccyx
Anal cleft

Bulbospongiosus
Ischiocavernosus
Perineal membrane
Superficial transverse perineal
Obturator internus
Gluteus maximus
Levator ani
External anal sphincter

A Female.

Superficial perineal (Colles') fascia
Ischial tuberosity
Obturator fascia
Inferior fascia of pelvic diaphragm
Anococcygeal lig.

Bulbospongiosus
Ischiocavernosus
Perineal membrane
Superficial transverse perineal
Obturator internus
Gluteus maximus
Levator ani
External anal sphincter

B Male.

Fig. 19.15 Gender-related differences in structure of the levator ani

Posterior view. Note the connective tissue gaps between muscular parts of the levator ani in the female.

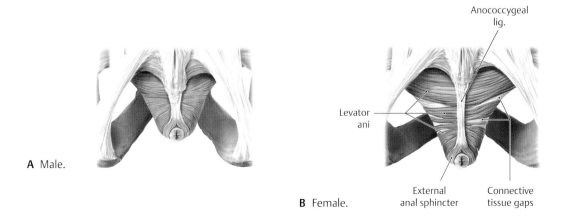

A Male.

Levator ani

Anococcygeal lig.

External anal sphincter
Connective tissue gaps

B Female.

237

Pelvic Floor & Perineal Muscle Facts

Fig. 19.16 Muscles of the pelvic floor
Superior view.

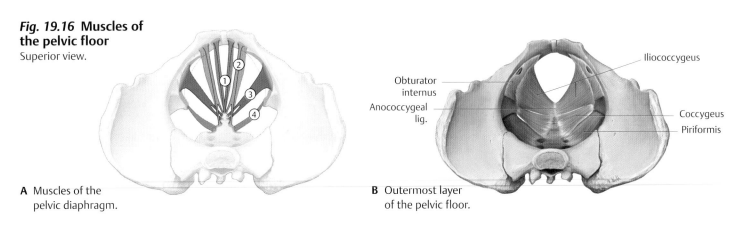

A Muscles of the pelvic diaphragm.

B Outermost layer of the pelvic floor.

Table 19.2		Muscles of the pelvic floor			
Muscle		**Origin**	**Insertion**	**Innervation**	**Action**
Muscles of the pelvic diaphragm					
Levator ani	① Puborectalis	Superior pubic ramus (both sides of pubic symphysis)	Anococcygeal lig.	Nerve to levator ani (S4), inferior rectal n.	Pelvic diaphragm: Supports pelvic viscera
	② Pubococcygeus	Pubis (lateral to origin of puborectalis)	Anococcygeal lig., coccyx		
	③ Iliococcygeus	Internal obturator fascia of levator ani (tendinous arch)			
④ Coccygeus		Lateral surface of coccyx and S5 segment	Ischial spine	Direct branches from sacral plexus (S4–S5)	Supports pelvic viscera, flexes coccyx
Muscles of the pelvic wall (parietal muscles)					
Piriformis*		Sacrum (pelvic surface)	Femur (apex of greater trochanter)	Direct branches from sacral plexus (S1–S2)	Hip joint: External rotation, stabilization, and abduction of flexed hip
Obturator internus*		Obturator membrane and bony boundaries (inner surface)	Femur (greater trochanter, medial surface)	Direct branches from sacral plexus (L5–S1)	Hip joint: External rotation and abduction of flexed hip

*The piriformis and obturator internus are considered muscles of the hip (see **p. 420**).
The female and male external genitalia are shown on **pp. 278, 280.**

Fig. 19.17 Muscles of the perineum
Inferior view.

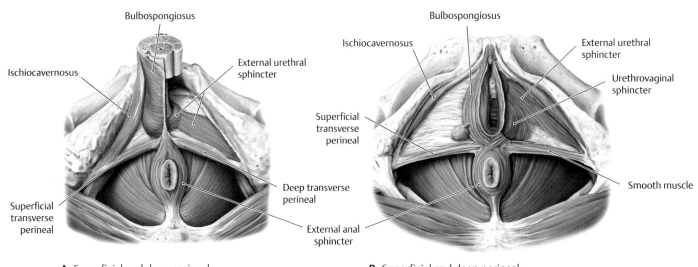

A Superficial and deep perineal muscles in the male.

B Superficial and deep perineal muscles in the female.

Table 19.3	Muscles of the perineum			
Muscle	**Origin**	**Insertion**	**Innervation**	**Action**
① Ischiocavernosus	Ischial ramus	Crus of clitoris or penis	Pudendal n. (S2–S4)	Maintains erection by squeezing blood into corpus cavernosum of clitoris or penis
② Bulbospongiosus	Runs anteriorly from perineal body to clitoris (females) or penile raphe (males)			Females: Compresses greater vestibular gland Males: Assists in erection
③ Superficial transverse perineal	Ischial ramus	Perineal body		Helps hold perineal body in median plane, holds the pelvic organs in place, and supports visceral canals through the muscles of the perineum
④ Deep transverse perineal*	Inferior pubic ramus, ischial ramus	Perineal body and external anal sphincter		
⑤ External urethral sphincter	Encircles urethra (division of deep transverse perineal muscle), in males ascends anteriorly to neck of the bladder; in females, some fibers surround the vagina as the urethrovaginal sphincter			Closes urethra
⑥ External anal sphincter	Encircles anus (runs posteriorly from perineal body to anococcygeal lig.)			Closes anus

* Typically, this muscle is not developed in females and is replaced by smooth muscle tissue. When developed, it provides dynamic support to the pelvic organs.

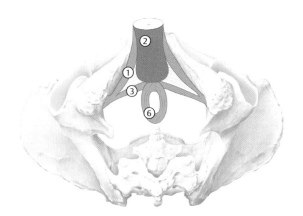

C Muscles of the superficial pouch in the male.

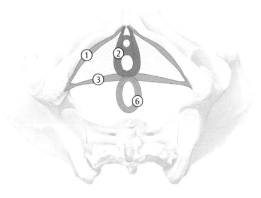

D Muscles of the superficial pouch in the female.

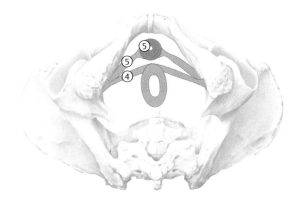

E Muscles of the deep pouch in the male.

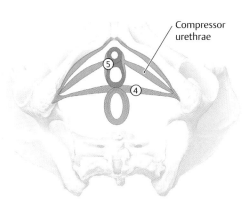

Compressor urethrae

F Muscles of the deep pouch in the female.

Contents of the Pelvis

***Fig. 20.1* Male pelvis**
Parasagittal section, viewed from the right side.

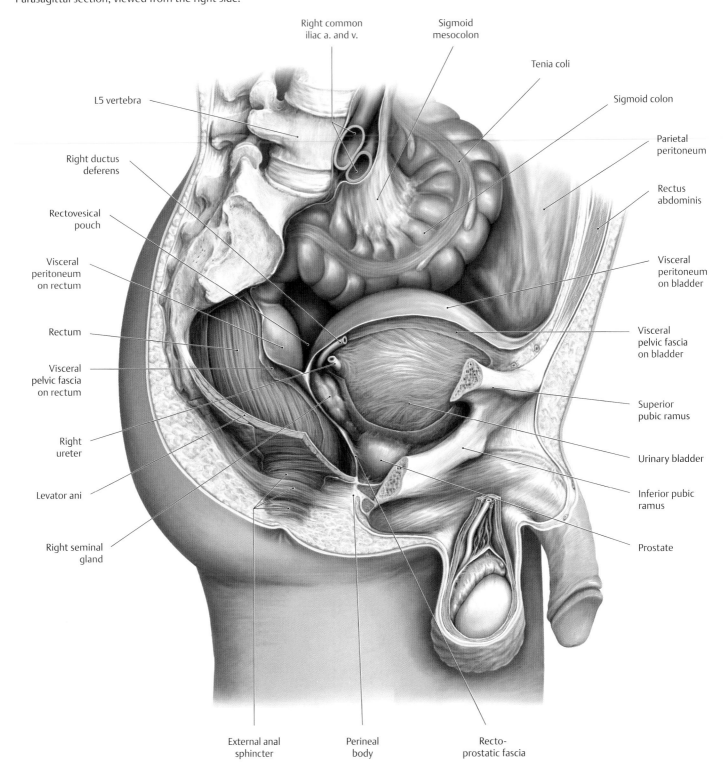

Right common
iliac a. and v.

Sigmoid
mesocolon

Tenia coli

Sigmoid colon

L5 vertebra

Parietal
peritoneum

Right ductus
deferens

Rectus
abdominis

Rectovesical
pouch

Visceral
peritoneum
on rectum

Visceral
peritoneum
on bladder

Rectum

Visceral
pelvic fascia
on bladder

Visceral
pelvic fascia
on rectum

Superior
pubic ramus

Right
ureter

Urinary bladder

Levator ani

Inferior pubic
ramus

Right seminal
gland

Prostate

External anal
sphincter

Perineal
body

Recto-
prostatic fascia

Fig. 20.2 **Female pelvis**

Parasagittal section, viewed from the right side.

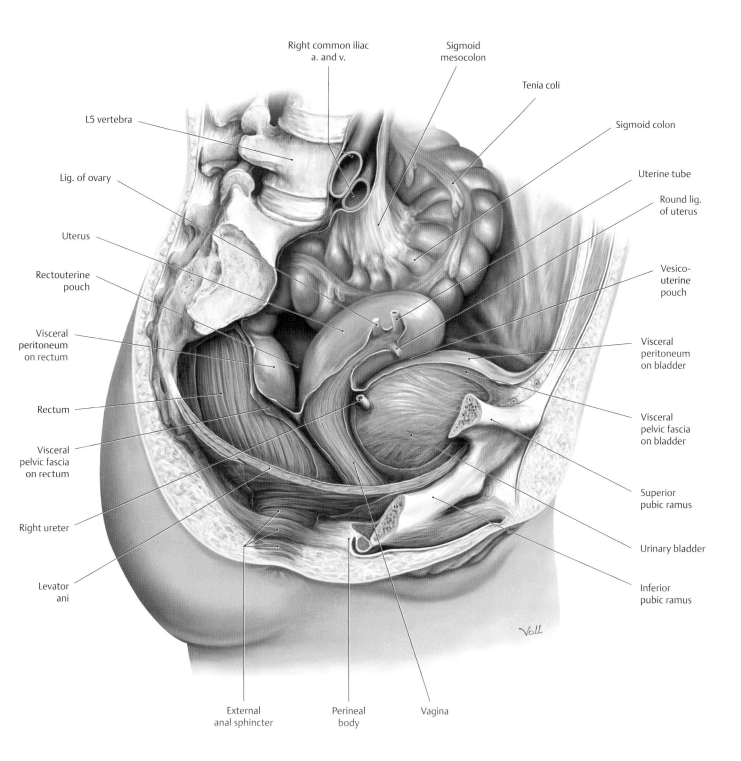

Right common iliac a. and v.

Sigmoid mesocolon

Tenia coli

Sigmoid colon

L5 vertebra

Uterine tube

Round lig. of uterus

Lig. of ovary

Uterus

Vesico-uterine pouch

Rectouterine pouch

Visceral peritoneum on rectum

Visceral peritoneum on bladder

Rectum

Visceral pelvic fascia on bladder

Visceral pelvic fascia on rectum

Right ureter

Superior pubic ramus

Levator ani

Urinary bladder

Inferior pubic ramus

External anal sphincter

Perineal body

Vagina

Voll

Peritoneal Relationships

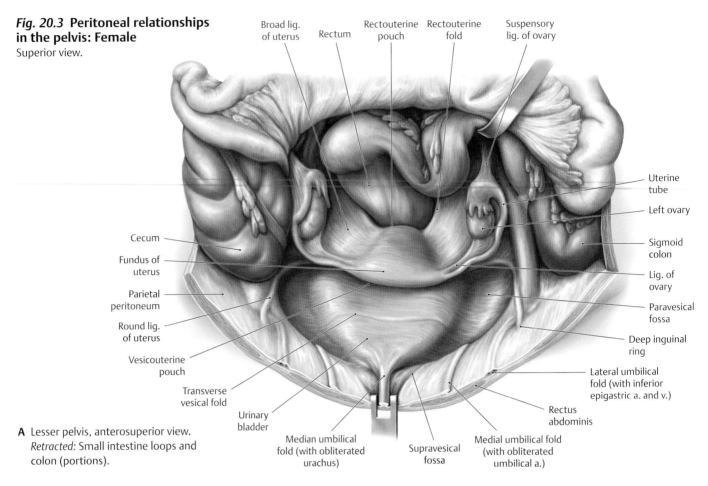

Fig. 20.3 **Peritoneal relationships in the pelvis: Female**
Superior view.

Labels: Broad lig. of uterus · Rectum · Rectouterine pouch · Rectouterine fold · Suspensory lig. of ovary · Uterine tube · Left ovary · Sigmoid colon · Lig. of ovary · Paravesical fossa · Deep inguinal ring · Lateral umbilical fold (with inferior epigastric a. and v.) · Rectus abdominis · Medial umbilical fold (with obliterated umbilical a.) · Supravesical fossa · Median umbilical fold (with obliterated urachus) · Urinary bladder · Transverse vesical fold · Vesicouterine pouch · Round lig. of uterus · Parietal peritoneum · Fundus of uterus · Cecum

A Lesser pelvis, anterosuperior view.
Retracted: Small intestine loops and colon (portions).

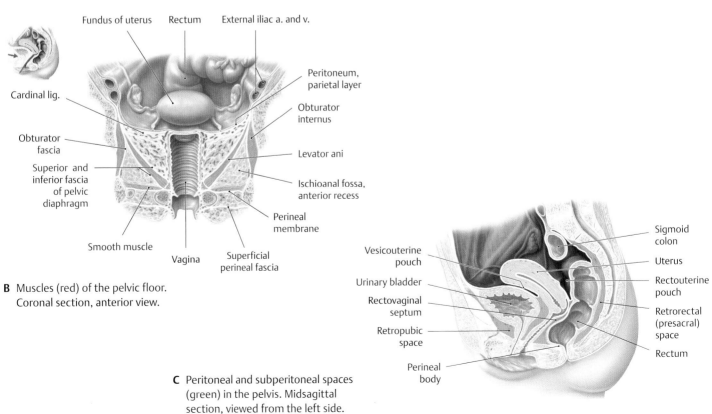

Labels (B): Fundus of uterus · Rectum · External iliac a. and v. · Peritoneum, parietal layer · Obturator internus · Levator ani · Ischioanal fossa, anterior recess · Perineal membrane · Superficial perineal fascia · Vagina · Smooth muscle · Superior and inferior fascia of pelvic diaphragm · Obturator fascia · Cardinal lig.

B Muscles (red) of the pelvic floor. Coronal section, anterior view.

Labels (C): Vesicouterine pouch · Urinary bladder · Rectovaginal septum · Retropubic space · Perineal body · Sigmoid colon · Uterus · Rectouterine pouch · Retrorectal (presacral) space · Rectum

C Peritoneal and subperitoneal spaces (green) in the pelvis. Midsagittal section, viewed from the left side.

242

Fig. 20.4 Peritoneal relationships in the pelvis: Male
Superior view.

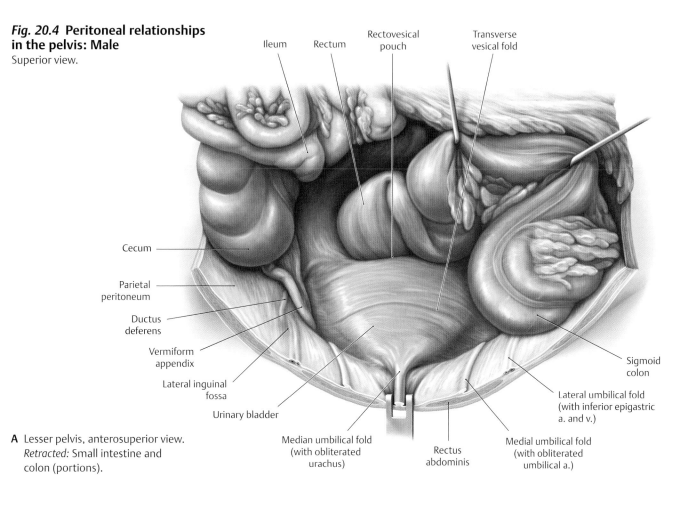

A Lesser pelvis, anterosuperior view.
Retracted: Small intestine and colon (portions).

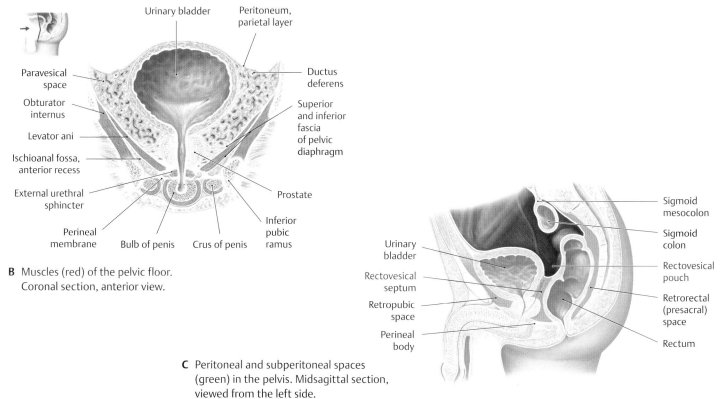

B Muscles (red) of the pelvic floor. Coronal section, anterior view.

C Peritoneal and subperitoneal spaces (green) in the pelvis. Midsagittal section, viewed from the left side.

Pelvis & Perineum

Pelvis & Perineum

The *pelvis* is the region of the body inferior to the abdomen, surrounded by the pelvic girdle. The *false*, or greater, *pelvis* is immediately inferior to the abdominal cavity, between the iliac alae, and superior to the pelvic inlet. The *true*, or lesser, *pelvis* is found between the pelvic inlet and the pelvic outlet and extends inferiorly to the pelvic diaphragm (levator ani and coccygeus), a muscular sling attached to the boundaries of the pelvic outlet. The *perineum* is the inferior most portion of the trunk, between the thighs and buttocks, extending from the pubis to the coccyx and superiorly to the pelvic diaphragm. The *superficial perineal* pouch lies between the membranous layer of the subcutaneous tissue (Colle's fascia) and the perineal membrane. The *deep perineal* pouch lies between the perineal membrane and the inferior fascia of the pelvic diaphragm.

Table 20.1 Divisions of the pelvis and perineum

The levels of the pelvis are determined by bony landmarks (iliac alae and pelvic inlet/brim). The contents of the perineum are separated from the true pelvis by the pelvic diaphragm and two fascial layers.

Iliac crest		
Pelvis	**False pelvis**	• Ileum (coils)
		• Cecum and appendix
		• Sigmoid colon
		• Common and external iliac aa. and vv.
		• Lumbar plexus (brs.)
	Pelvic inlet	
	True pelvis	• Distal ureters
		• Urinary bladder
		• Rectum
		♀: Vagina, uterus, uterine tubes, and ovaries
		♂: Ductus deferens, seminal gland, and prostate
		• Internal iliac a. and v. and brs.
		• Sacral plexus
		• Inferior hypogastric plexus
Pelvic diaphragm (levator ani & coccygeus)		
Perineum	**Deep pouch**	• Sphincter urethrae and deep transverse perineal mm.
		• Urethra (membranous)
		• Vagina
		• Rectum
		• Bulbourethral gland
		• Ischioanal fossa
		• Internal pudendal a. and v., pudendal n. and brs.
	Perineal membrane	
	Superficial pouch	• Ischiocavernosus, bulbospongiosus, and superficial transverse perineal mm.
		• Urethra (penile)
		• Clitoris and penis
		• Internal pudendal a. and v., pudendal n. and branches
	Superficial perineal (Colles') fascia	
	Subcutaneous perineal space	• Fat
Skin		

Fig. 20.5 Pelvis and urogenital triangle

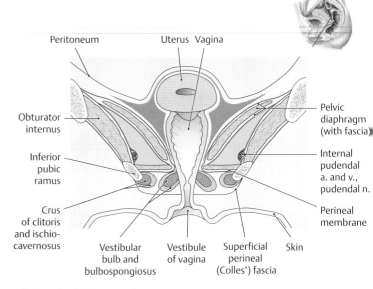

Peritoneum — Uterus — Vagina — Obturator internus — Inferior pubic ramus — Crus of clitoris and ischiocavernosus — Vestibular bulb and bulbospongiosus — Vestibule of vagina — Superficial perineal (Colles') fascia — Skin — Perineal membrane — Internal pudendal a. and v., pudendal n. — Pelvic diaphragm (with fascia)

A Female. Oblique section.

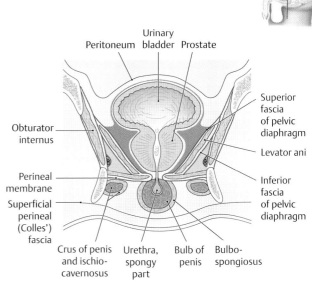

Peritoneum — Urinary bladder — Prostate — Obturator internus — Perineal membrane — Superficial perineal (Colles') fascia — Crus of penis and ischiocavernosus — Urethra, spongy part — Bulb of penis — Bulbospongiosus — Superior fascia of pelvic diaphragm — Levator ani — Inferior fascia of pelvic diaphragm

B Male. Coronal section.

☐ Peritoneal cavity ▨ Subperitoneal space ☐ Ischioanal fossa — — Visceral pelvic fascia — Parietal pelvic fascia

Fig. 20.6 Pelvis: Oblique section

Anterior view.

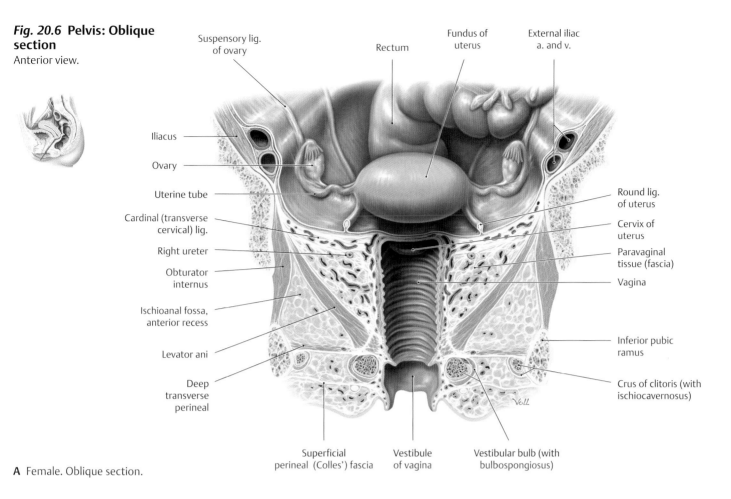

Suspensory lig. of ovary — **Rectum** — **Fundus of uterus** — **External iliac a. and v.**

Iliacus

Ovary

Uterine tube

Cardinal (transverse cervical) lig.

Right ureter

Obturator internus

Ischioanal fossa, anterior recess

Levator ani

Deep transverse perineal

Round lig. of uterus

Cervix of uterus

Paravaginal tissue (fascia)

Vagina

Inferior pubic ramus

Crus of clitoris (with ischiocavernosus)

Superficial perineal (Colles') fascia — Vestibule of vagina — Vestibular bulb (with bulbospongiosus)

A Female. Oblique section.

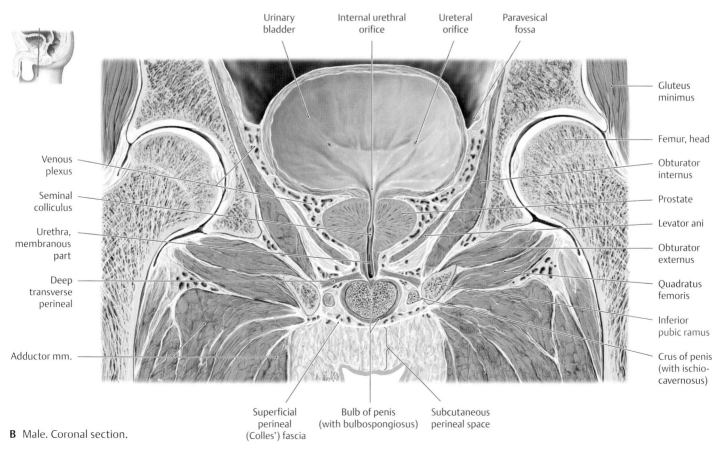

Urinary bladder — Internal urethral orifice — Ureteral orifice — Paravesical fossa

Venous plexus

Seminal colliculus

Urethra, membranous part

Deep transverse perineal

Adductor mm.

Gluteus minimus

Femur, head

Obturator internus

Prostate

Levator ani

Obturator externus

Quadratus femoris

Inferior pubic ramus

Crus of penis (with ischiocavernosus)

Superficial perineal (Colles') fascia — Bulb of penis (with bulbospongiosus) — Subcutaneous perineal space

B Male. Coronal section.

Rectum & Anal Canal

Fig. 21.1 **Rectum: Location**

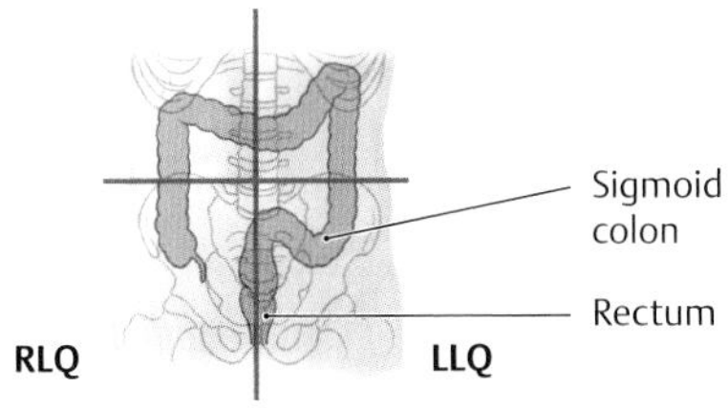

Sigmoid colon

Rectum

RLQ   **LLQ**

A Anterior view.

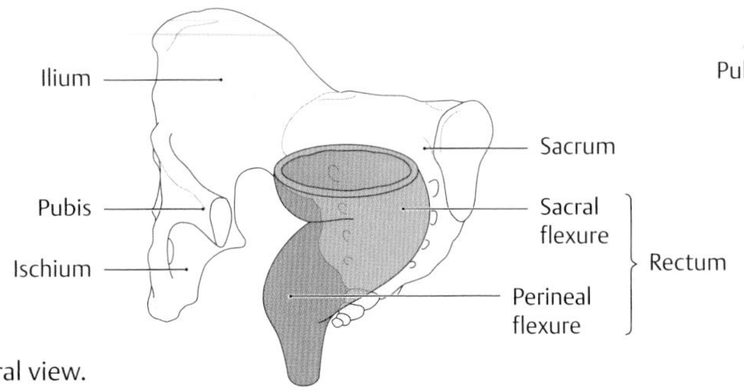

Ilium

Pubis

Ischium

Sacrum

Sacral flexure

Rectum

Perineal flexure

B Left anterolateral view.

Fig. 21.2 **Closure of the rectum**
Left lateral view. The puborectalis acts as a muscular sling that kinks the anorectal junction. It functions in the maintenance of fecal continence.

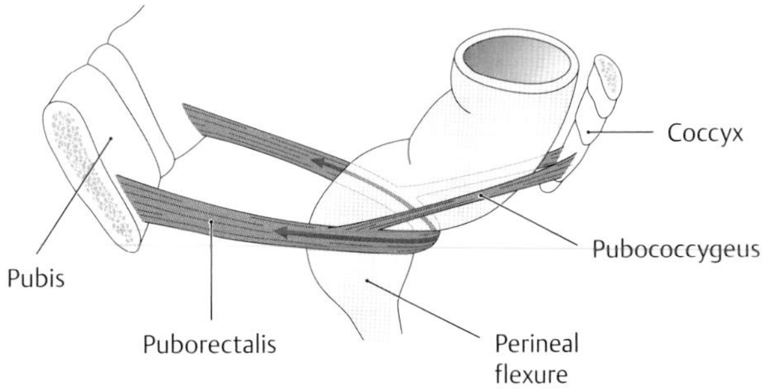

Pubis

Puborectalis

Coccyx

Pubococcygeus

Perineal flexure

Fig. 21.3 **Rectum in situ**
Coronal section, anterior view of the female pelvis. The upper third of the rectum is covered with visceral peritoneum on its anterior and lateral sides. The middle third is covered only anteriorly and the lower third is inferior to the parietal peritoneum.

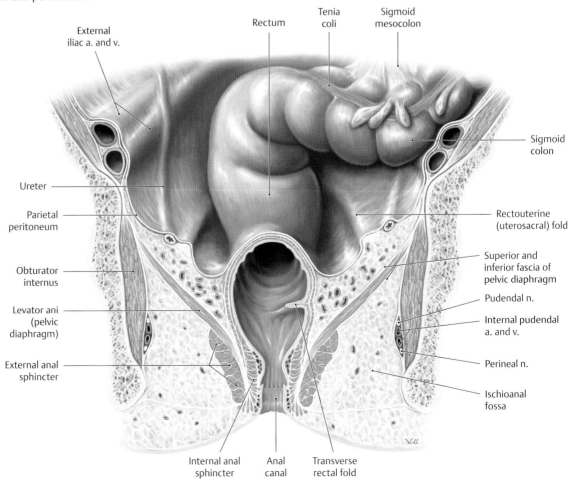

External iliac a. and v.

Rectum

Tenia coli

Sigmoid mesocolon

Ureter

Parietal peritoneum

Obturator internus

Levator ani (pelvic diaphragm)

External anal sphincter

Sigmoid colon

Rectouterine (uterosacral) fold

Superior and inferior fascia of pelvic diaphragm

Pudendal n.

Internal pudendal a. and v.

Perineal n.

Ischioanal fossa

Internal anal sphincter

Anal canal

Transverse rectal fold

Fig. 21.4 Rectum and anal canal

Coronal section, anterior view with the anterior wall removed.

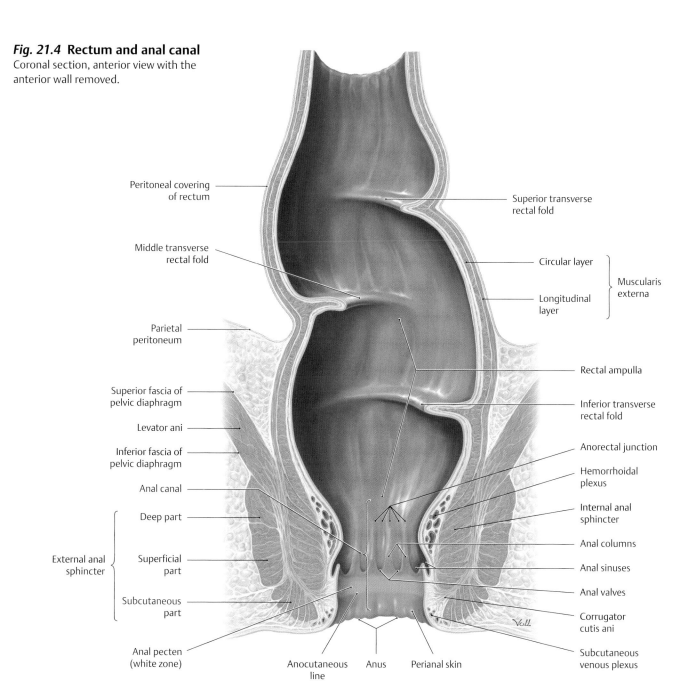

Peritoneal covering of rectum

Middle transverse rectal fold

Parietal peritoneum

Superior fascia of pelvic diaphragm

Levator ani

Inferior fascia of pelvic diaphragm

Anal canal

External anal sphincter
- Deep part
- Superficial part
- Subcutaneous part

Anal pecten (white zone)

Anocutaneous line

Anus

Perianal skin

Superior transverse rectal fold

Circular layer

Longitudinal layer

} Muscularis externa

Rectal ampulla

Inferior transverse rectal fold

Anorectal junction

Hemorrhoidal plexus

Internal anal sphincter

Anal columns

Anal sinuses

Anal valves

Corrugator cutis ani

Subcutaneous venous plexus

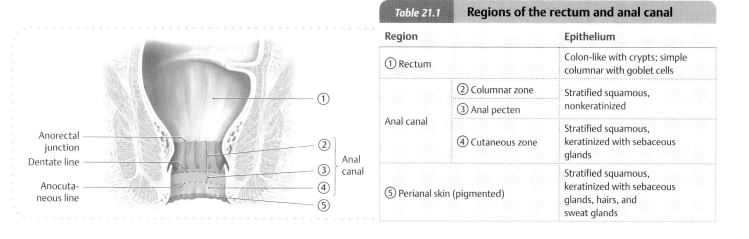

Anorectal junction

Dentate line

Anocutaneous line

① ② ③ ④ ⑤ — Anal canal

Table 21.1	Regions of the rectum and anal canal	
Region		**Epithelium**
① Rectum		Colon-like with crypts; simple columnar with goblet cells
Anal canal	② Columnar zone	Stratified squamous, nonkeratinized
	③ Anal pecten	
	④ Cutaneous zone	Stratified squamous, keratinized with sebaceous glands
⑤ Perianal skin (pigmented)		Stratified squamous, keratinized with sebaceous glands, hairs, and sweat glands

Ureters

 The ureters cross the common iliac artery at its bifurcation into the external and internal iliac arteries.

Fig. 21.5 **Ureters in situ**

Anterior view, male abdomen. *Removed:* Non-urinary organs and rectal stump. The ureters are retroperitoneal.

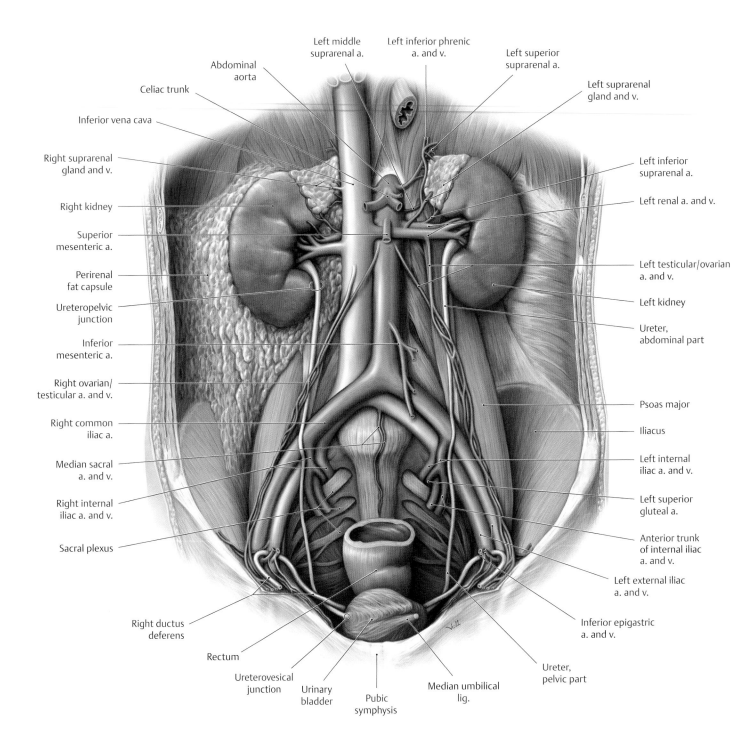

Fig. 21.6 Ureter in the male pelvis

Superior view.

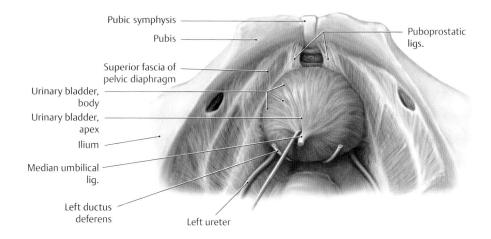

Pubic symphysis

Pubis

Puboprostatic ligs.

Superior fascia of pelvic diaphragm

Urinary bladder, body

Urinary bladder, apex

Ilium

Median umbilical lig.

Left ductus deferens

Left ureter

Fig. 21.7 Ureter in the female pelvis

Pelvis viewed from above. *Removed from left side:* Peritoneum and broad ligament of uterus. The pelvic ureters pass under the uterine artery approximately 2 cm lateral to the cervix.

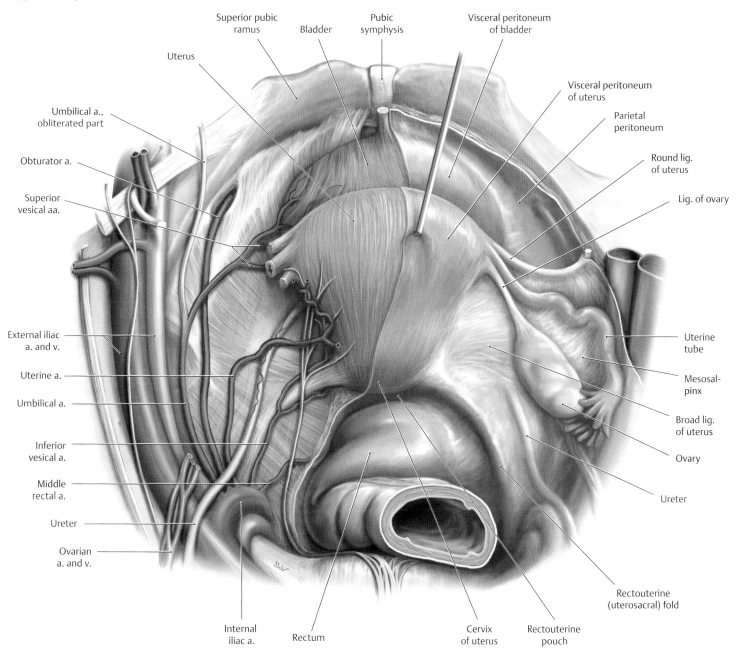

Superior pubic ramus

Uterus

Bladder

Pubic symphysis

Visceral peritoneum of bladder

Umbilical a., obliterated part

Obturator a.

Superior vesical aa.

External iliac a. and v.

Uterine a.

Umbilical a.

Inferior vesical a.

Middle rectal a.

Ureter

Ovarian a. and v.

Internal iliac a.

Rectum

Cervix of uterus

Rectouterine pouch

Visceral peritoneum of uterus

Parietal peritoneum

Round lig. of uterus

Lig. of ovary

Uterine tube

Mesosalpinx

Broad lig. of uterus

Ovary

Ureter

Rectouterine (uterosacral) fold

Urinary Bladder & Urethra

Fig. 21.8 Female urinary bladder and urethra

Suspensory lig. of ovary
(with ovarian a. and v.)

Right uterine tube

Right external iliac a. and v.

Rectus abdominis

Fundus of uterus

Round lig. of uterus

Left common iliac a. and v.

L5 vertebra

Right ureter

Right ovary and lig. of ovary

Body of uterus

Urinary bladder

Pubic symphysis

Vagina

Clitoris

Urethra

Rectum

Cervix of uterus

Posterior vaginal fornix

Anterior vaginal fornix

Levator ani

External anal sphincter

Perineal membrane

A Midsagittal section of pelvis, viewed from the left side. Right hemipelvis.

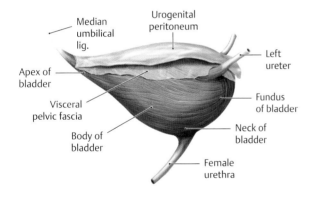

Median umbilical lig.

Urogenital peritoneum

Left ureter

Apex of bladder

Visceral pelvic fascia

Body of bladder

Fundus of bladder

Neck of bladder

Female urethra

B Bladder and urethra, left lateral view.

Fig. 21.9 Urethral sphincter mechanism in the female
Anterolateral view.

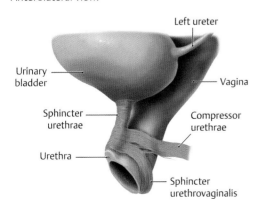

Left ureter

Urinary bladder

Sphincter urethrae

Urethra

Vagina

Compressor urethrae

Sphincter urethrovaginalis

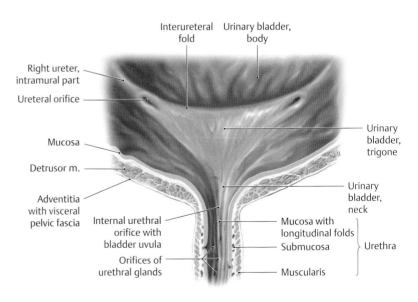

Interureteral fold

Urinary bladder, body

Right ureter, intramural part

Ureteral orifice

Mucosa

Detrusor m.

Adventitia with visceral pelvic fascia

Internal urethral orifice with bladder uvula

Orifices of urethral glands

Urinary bladder, trigone

Urinary bladder, neck

Mucosa with longitudinal folds

Submucosa

Muscularis

Urethra

C Trigone and urethra, coronal section, anterior view.

Fig. 21.10 Male urinary bladder and urethra

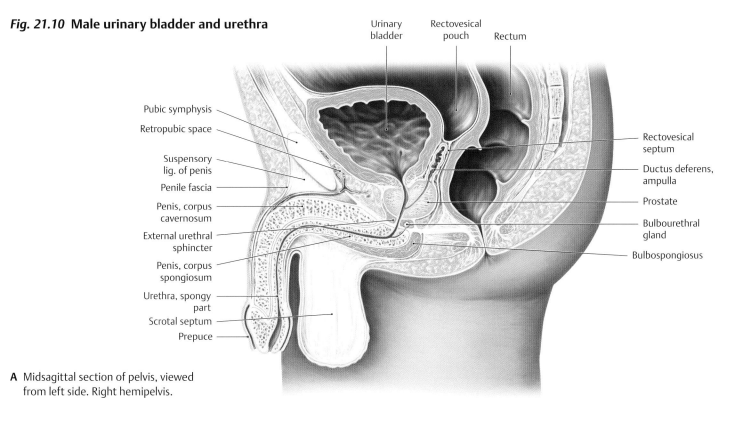

Pubic symphysis

Retropubic space

Suspensory lig. of penis

Penile fascia

Penis, corpus cavernosum

External urethral sphincter

Penis, corpus spongiosum

Urethra, spongy part

Scrotal septum

Prepuce

Urinary bladder

Rectovesical pouch

Rectum

Rectovesical septum

Ductus deferens, ampulla

Prostate

Bulbourethral gland

Bulbospongiosus

A Midsagittal section of pelvis, viewed from left side. Right hemipelvis.

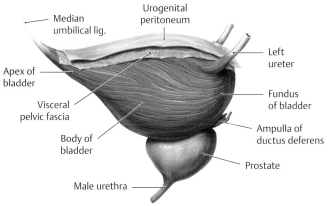

Median umbilical lig.

Urogenital peritoneum

Apex of bladder

Visceral pelvic fascia

Body of bladder

Male urethra

Left ureter

Fundus of bladder

Ampulla of ductus deferens

Prostate

B Bladder, urethra and prostate, left lateral view.

Fig. 21.11 Urethral sphincter mechanism in the male
Lateral view.

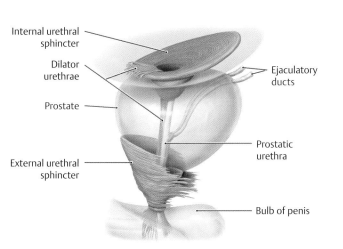

Internal urethral sphincter

Dilator urethrae

Prostate

External urethral sphincter

Ejaculatory ducts

Prostatic urethra

Bulb of penis

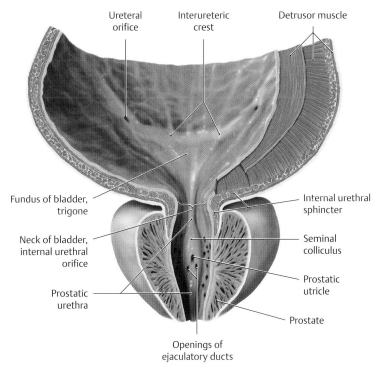

Ureteral orifice

Interureteric crest

Detrusor muscle

Fundus of bladder, trigone

Neck of bladder, internal urethral orifice

Prostatic urethra

Internal urethral sphincter

Seminal colliculus

Prostatic utricle

Prostate

Openings of ejaculatory ducts

C Trigone, urethra and prostate, coronal section, anterior view.

Overview of the Genital Organs

 The genital organs can be classified topographically (external versus internal) and functionally (**Tables 21.2 and 21.3**).

Table 21.2		Female genital organs	
	Organ		**Function**
Internal genitalia	Ovary		Germ cell and hormone production
	Uterine tube		Site of conception and transport organ for zygote
	Uterus		Organ of incubation and parturition
External genitalia	Vulva	Vagina (upper portion)	Organ of copulation and parturition
		Vagina (vestibule)	
		Labia majora and minora	Accessory copulatory organ
		Clitoris	
		Greater and lesser vestibular glands	Production of mucoid secretions
		Mons pubis	Protection of the pubic bone

Fig. 21.12 Female genital organs

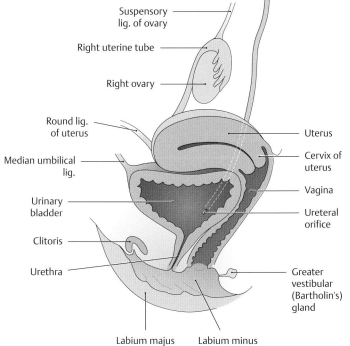

A Internal and external genitalia.

B Urogenital system. *Note:* The female urinary and genital tracts are functionally separate, though topographically close.

Table 21.3 **Male genital organs**

	Organ		Function
Internal genitalia	Testis		Germ cell and hormone production
	Epididymis		Reservoir for sperm
	Ductus deferens		Transport organ for sperm
	Accessory sex glands	Prostate	Production of secretions (semen)
		Seminal glands	
		Bulbourethral gland	
External genitalia	Penis		Copulatory and urinary organ
	Urethra		Conduit for urine and semen
	Scrotum		Protection of testis
	Coverings of the testis		

Fig. 21.13 **Male genital organs**

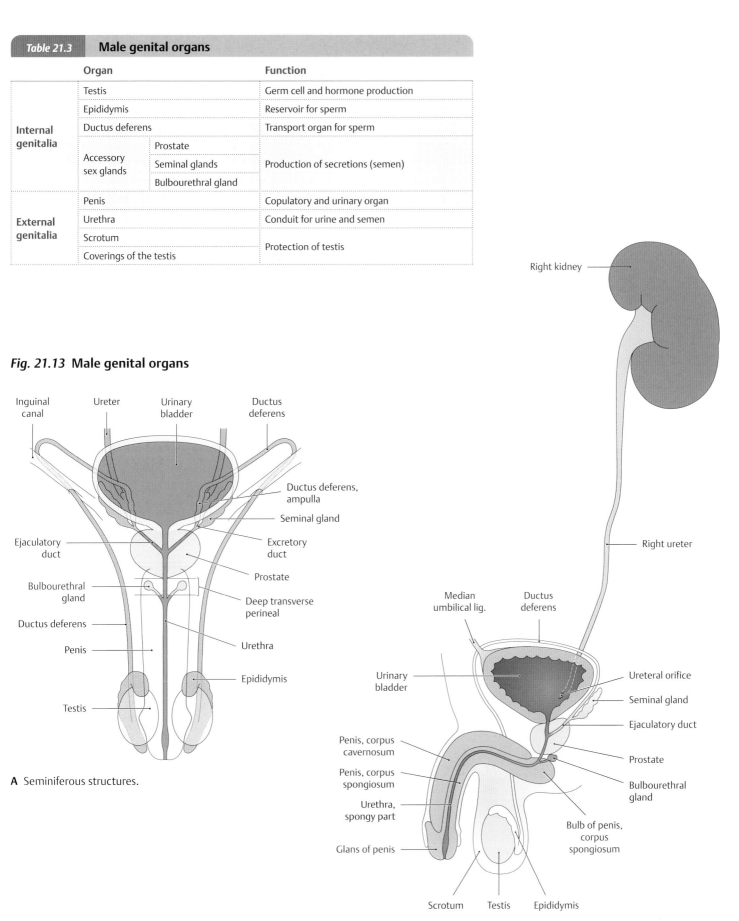

A Seminiferous structures.

B Urogenital system. *Note:* The male urethra serves as a common urinary and genital passage.

Uterus & Ovaries

Fig. 21.14 **Female internal genitalia**

The uterus and ovaries are suspended by the mesovarium and mesometrium (portions of the broad ligament of the uterus).

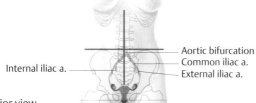

Internal iliac a.

Aortic bifurcation
Common iliac a.
External iliac a.

A Location. Anterior view.

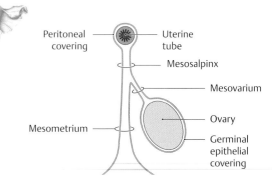

Peritoneal covering

Uterine tube

Mesosalpinx

Mesovarium

Ovary

Germinal epithelial covering

Mesometrium

B Regions of the broad ligament, sagittal section. The broad ligament of the uterus is composed of a double layer of peritoneum arranged as a combination of mesenteries: the mesosalpinx, mesovarium, and mesometrium.

Fig. 21.15 **Ovary**

Right ovary, posterior view.

Meso-varium

Mesovarial margin

Mesosalpinx

Uterine tube

Uterus, posterior surface

Lig. of ovary

Uterine pole

Follicular stigma (bulge from Graafian follicle)

Mesometrium

Vascular pole

Ovarian a. and v. (in suspensory lig. of ovary)

Medial surface

Free margin

Fig. 21.16 **Curvature of the uterus**

Midsagittal section, left lateral view. The position of the uterus can be described in terms of flexion (①) and version (②).

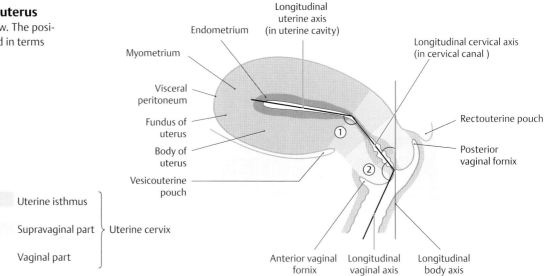

Longitudinal uterine axis (in uterine cavity)

Endometrium

Myometrium

Visceral peritoneum

Fundus of uterus

Body of uterus

Vesicouterine pouch

Longitudinal cervical axis (in cervical canal)

Rectouterine pouch

Posterior vaginal fornix

Anterior vaginal fornix

Longitudinal vaginal axis

Longitudinal body axis

① Flexion: Angle between the uterine body and isthmus.

② Version: Angle between the cervical canal and the vagina.

Uterine isthmus

Supravaginal part

Vaginal part

Uterine cervix

Fig. 21.17 **Uterus and uterine tube**

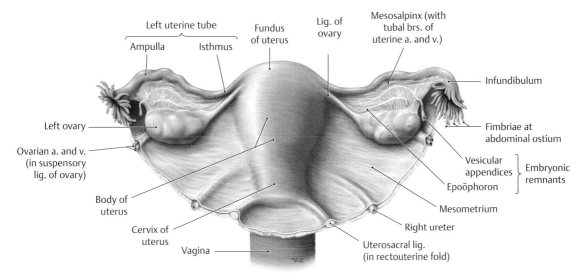

A Posterosuperior view.

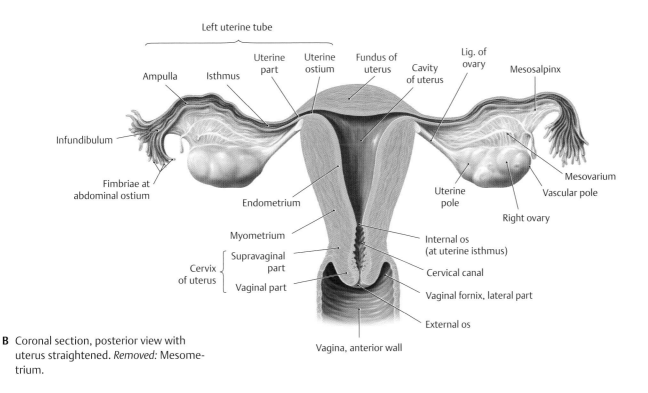

B Coronal section, posterior view with uterus straightened. *Removed:* Mesometrium.

✳ *Clinical box 21.1*

Ectopic pregnancy

After fertilization in the ampulla of the uterine tube, the ovum usually implants in the wall of the uterine cavity. However, it may become implanted at other sites (e.g., the uterine tube or even the peritoneal cavity). Tubal pregnancies, the most common type of ectopic pregnancy, pose the risk of tubal wall rupture and potentially life-threatening bleeding into the peritoneal cavity. Tubal pregnancies are promoted by adhesion of the tubal mucosa, mostly due to inflammation.

Ligaments & Fascia of the Deep Pelvis

Fig. 21.18 Ligaments of the female pelvis

Superior view. *Removed:* Peritoneum, neurovasculature, and superior portion of the bladder to demonstrate only the fascial condensations (ligaments). Deep pelvic ligaments support the uterus within the pelvic cavity and prevent uterine prolapse, the downward displacement of the uterus into the vagina.

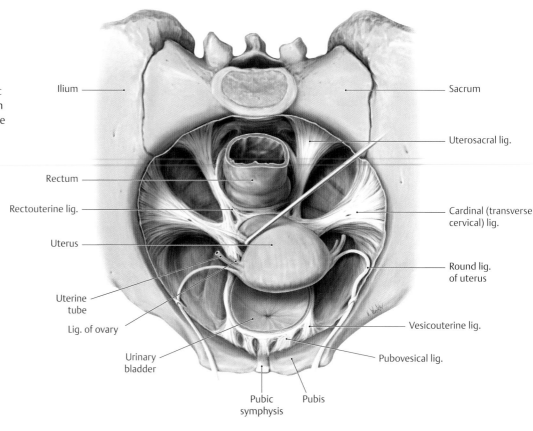

Ilium — Sacrum

Uterosacral lig.

Rectum

Rectouterine lig. — Cardinal (transverse cervical) lig.

Uterus — Round lig. of uterus

Uterine tube — Vesicouterine lig.

Lig. of ovary — Pubovesical lig.

Urinary bladder

Pubic symphysis — Pubis

Fig. 21.19 Ligaments of the deep pelvis in the female

Superior view. *Removed:* peritoneum, neurovasculature, uterus and bladder. Uterosacral ligaments and the paracolpium support, and help maintain the positions of, the cervix and vagina in the pelvis.

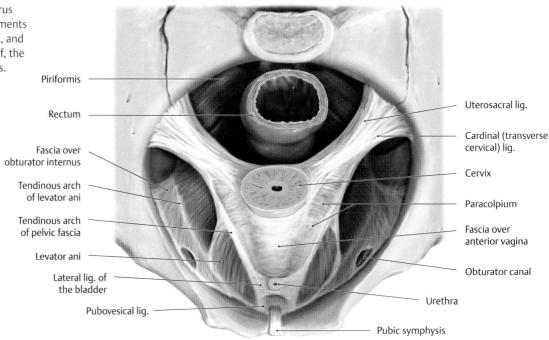

Piriformis — Uterosacral lig.

Rectum — Cardinal (transverse cervical) lig.

Fascia over obturator internus — Cervix

Tendinous arch of levator ani — Paracolpium

Tendinous arch of pelvic fascia — Fascia over anterior vagina

Levator ani — Obturator canal

Lateral lig. of the bladder — Urethra

Pubovesical lig. — Pubic symphysis

Fascia of the pelvis plays an important role in the support of pelvic viscera. On either side of the pelvic floor, where the visceral fascia of the pelvic organs is continuous with the parietal fascia of the muscular walls, thickenings called tendinous arches of the pelvic fascia are formed. In females, the paracolpium—lateral connections between the visceral fascia and the tendinous arches—suspends and supports the vagina. Pubovesical ligaments (and puboprostatic ligaments in the male) are extensions of the tendinous arches that support the bladder and prostate. Endopelvic fascia, a loose areolar (fatty) tissue that fills the spaces between pelvic viscera, condenses to form "ligaments" (cardinal ligaments, lateral ligaments of the bladder, lateral rectal ligaments; see **Fig. 21.20**) that provide passage for the ureters and neurovascular elements within the pelvis.

Fig. 21.20 Fascia and ligaments of the female pelvis

Transverse section, through cervix, superior view.

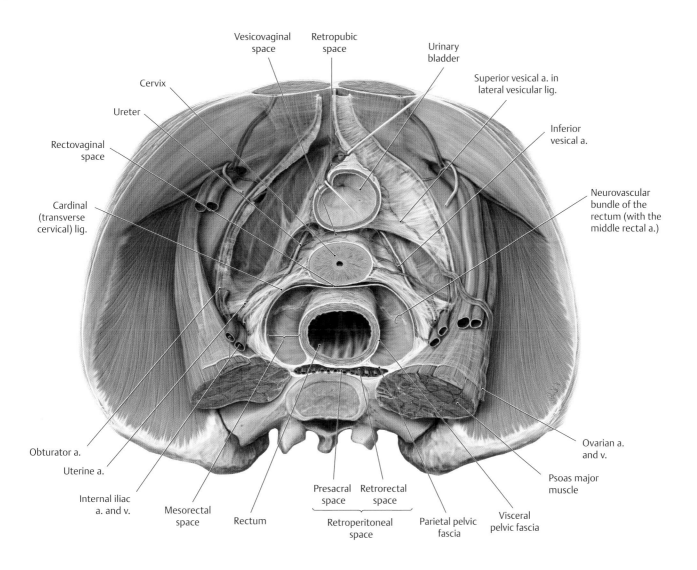

Vagina

Fig. 21.21 Location of vagina
Midsagittal section, left lateral view.

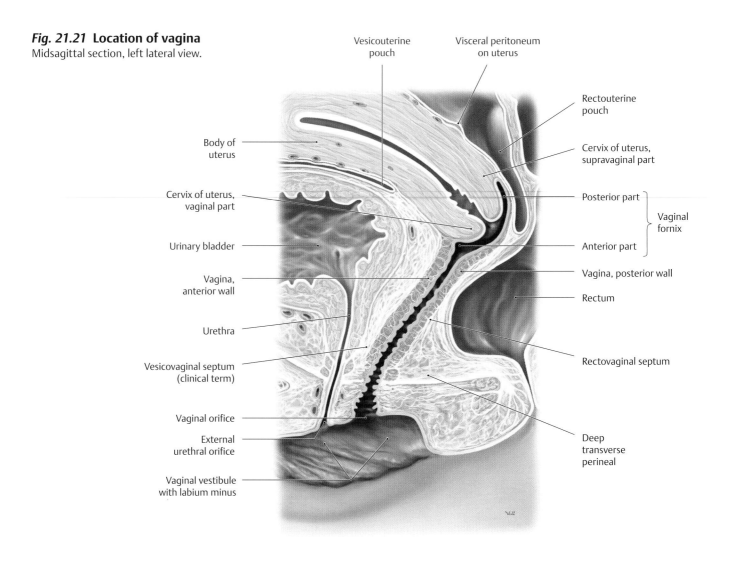

Vesicouterine pouch

Visceral peritoneum on uterus

Rectouterine pouch

Body of uterus

Cervix of uterus, supravaginal part

Cervix of uterus, vaginal part

Posterior part

Vaginal fornix

Anterior part

Urinary bladder

Vagina, anterior wall

Vagina, posterior wall

Urethra

Rectum

Vesicovaginal septum (clinical term)

Rectovaginal septum

Vaginal orifice

External urethral orifice

Deep transverse perineal

Vaginal vestibule with labium minus

Fig. 21.22 Structure of vagina
Posteriorly angled coronal section, posterior view.

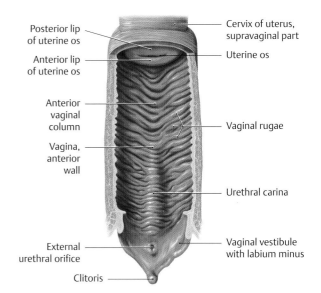

Posterior lip of uterine os

Cervix of uterus, supravaginal part

Anterior lip of uterine os

Uterine os

Anterior vaginal column

Vagina, anterior wall

Vaginal rugae

Urethral carina

External urethral orifice

Vaginal vestibule with labium minus

Clitoris

Fig. 21.23 Female genital organs: Coronal section

Anterior view. The vagina is both pelvic and perineal in location. It is also retroperitoneal.

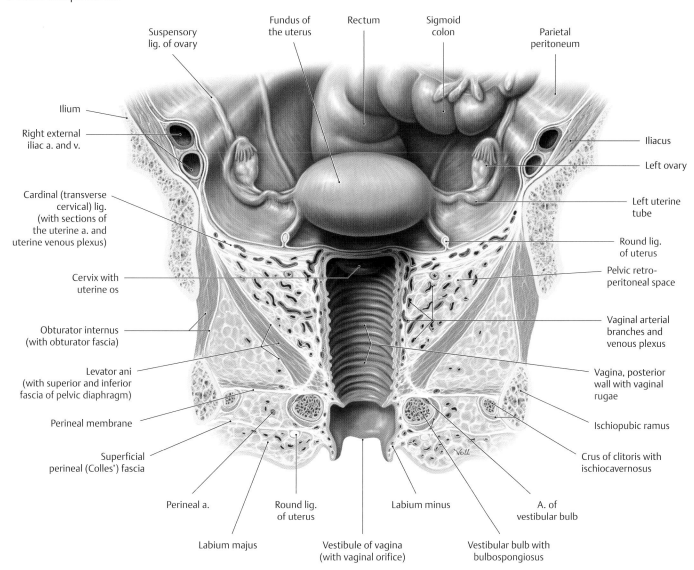

Suspensory lig. of ovary

Fundus of the uterus

Rectum

Sigmoid colon

Parietal peritoneum

Ilium

Right external iliac a. and v.

Iliacus

Left ovary

Cardinal (transverse cervical) lig. (with sections of the uterine a. and uterine venous plexus)

Left uterine tube

Round lig. of uterus

Cervix with uterine os

Pelvic retro-peritoneal space

Obturator internus (with obturator fascia)

Vaginal arterial branches and venous plexus

Levator ani (with superior and inferior fascia of pelvic diaphragm)

Vagina, posterior wall with vaginal rugae

Perineal membrane

Ischiopubic ramus

Superficial perineal (Colles') fascia

Crus of clitoris with ischiocavernosus

Perineal a.

Round lig. of uterus

Labium minus

A. of vestibular bulb

Labium majus

Vestibule of vagina (with vaginal orifice)

Vestibular bulb with bulbospongiosus

Fig. 21.24 Vagina: Location in the perineum

Inferior view.

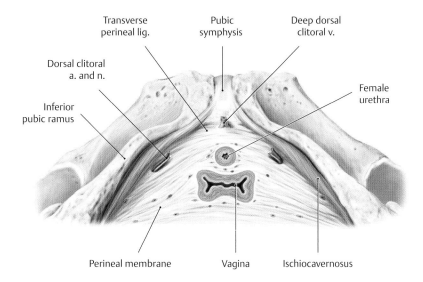

Transverse perineal lig.

Pubic symphysis

Deep dorsal clitoral v.

Dorsal clitoral a. and n.

Female urethra

Inferior pubic ramus

Perineal membrane

Vagina

Ischiocavernosus

Female External Genitalia

Fig. 21.25 **Female external genitalia**
Lithotomy position with labia minora separated.

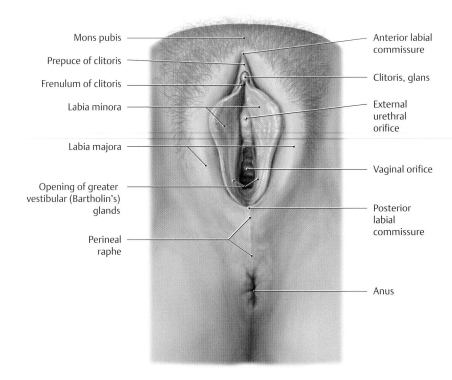

Mons pubis

Prepuce of clitoris

Frenulum of clitoris

Labia minora

Labia majora

Opening of greater
vestibular (Bartholin's)
glands

Perineal
raphe

Anterior labial
commissure

Clitoris, glans

External
urethral
orifice

Vaginal orifice

Posterior
labial
commissure

Anus

Fig. 21.26 **Vestibule and vestibular glands**
Lithotomy position with labia minora separated.

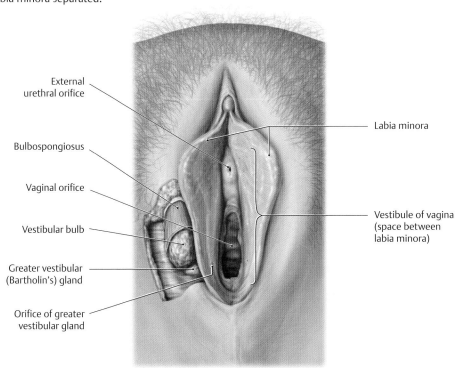

External
urethral orifice

Bulbospongiosus

Vaginal orifice

Vestibular bulb

Greater vestibular
(Bartholin's) gland

Orifice of greater
vestibular gland

Labia minora

Vestibule of vagina
(space between
labia minora)

Fig. 21.27 **Erectile tissue and muscles of the female**

Lithotomy position. *Removed:* Labia and skin. *Removed from left side:* Ischiocavernosus and bulbospongiosus muscles.

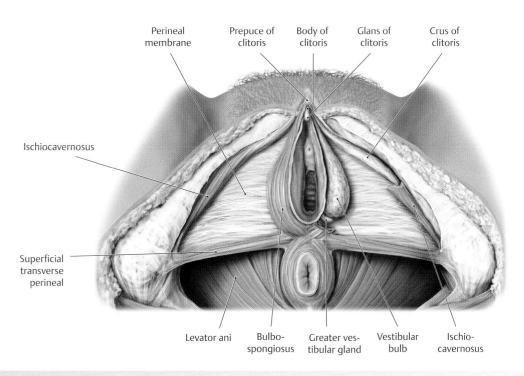

Labels (clockwise from top): Perineal membrane, Prepuce of clitoris, Body of clitoris, Glans of clitoris, Crus of clitoris, Ischiocavernosus, Superficial transverse perineal, Levator ani, Bulbo-spongiosus, Greater vestibular gland, Vestibular bulb, Ischio-cavernosus

 Clinical box 21.2

Episiotomy

Episiotomy is a common obstetric procedure used to enlarge the birth canal during the expulsive stage of labor. The procedure is generally used to expedite the delivery of a baby at risk for hypoxia during the expulsive stage. Alternately, if the perineal skin turns white (indicating diminished blood flow), there is imminent danger of perineal laceration, and an episiotomy is often performed. More lateral incisions gain more room, but they are more difficult to repair.

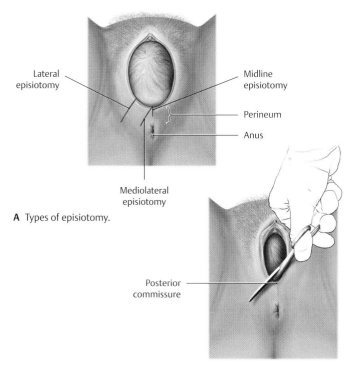

Labels: Lateral episiotomy, Midline episiotomy, Perineum, Anus, Mediolateral episiotomy, Posterior commissure

A Types of episiotomy.

B Mediolateral episiotomy at height of contraction.

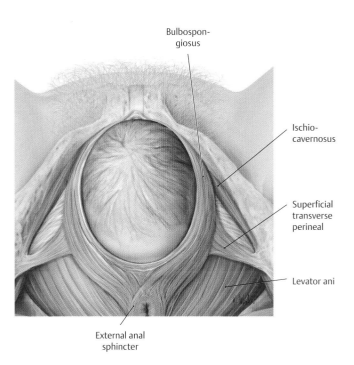

Labels: Bulbospon-giosus, Ischio-cavernosus, Superficial transverse perineal, Levator ani, External anal sphincter

C Pelvic floor with crowning of fetal head.

261

Penis, Testis & Epididymis

Fig. 21.28 **Penis**

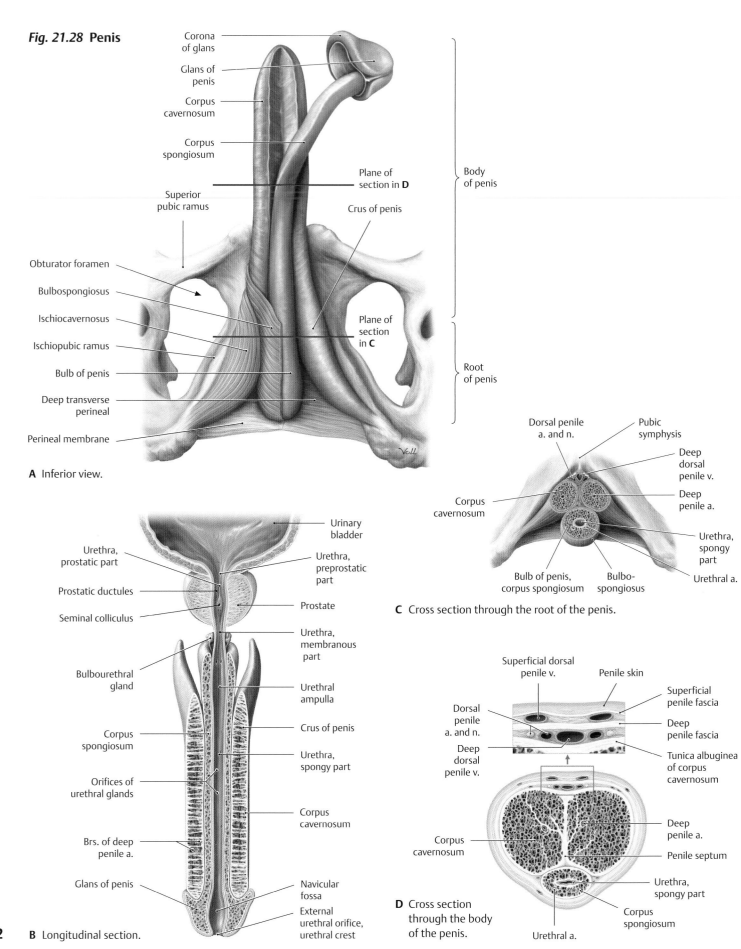

Corona of glans

Glans of penis

Corpus cavernosum

Corpus spongiosum

Superior pubic ramus

Plane of section in **D**

Crus of penis

Plane of section in **C**

Body of penis

Root of penis

Obturator foramen

Bulbospongiosus

Ischiocavernosus

Ischiopubic ramus

Bulb of penis

Deep transverse perineal

Perineal membrane

A Inferior view.

Urinary bladder

Urethra, prostatic part

Urethra, preprostatic part

Prostatic ductules

Seminal colliculus

Prostate

Bulbourethral gland

Urethra, membranous part

Urethral ampulla

Corpus spongiosum

Crus of penis

Urethra, spongy part

Orifices of urethral glands

Corpus cavernosum

Brs. of deep penile a.

Glans of penis

Navicular fossa

External urethral orifice, urethral crest

B Longitudinal section.

Dorsal penile a. and n.

Pubic symphysis

Deep dorsal penile v.

Corpus cavernosum

Deep penile a.

Urethra, spongy part

Bulb of penis, corpus spongiosum

Bulbo-spongiosus

Urethral a.

C Cross section through the root of the penis.

Superficial dorsal penile v.

Penile skin

Dorsal penile a. and n.

Superficial penile fascia

Deep penile fascia

Deep dorsal penile v.

Tunica albuginea of corpus cavernosum

Corpus cavernosum

Deep penile a.

Penile septum

Urethra, spongy part

Corpus spongiosum

Urethral a.

D Cross section through the body of the penis.

Fig. 21.29 Testis and epididymis
Left lateral view.

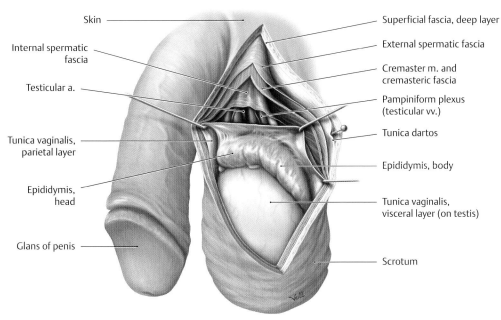

Skin — Superficial fascia, deep layer
Internal spermatic fascia — External spermatic fascia
Testicular a. — Cremaster m. and cremasteric fascia
— Pampiniform plexus (testicular vv.)
Tunica vaginalis, parietal layer — Tunica dartos
Epididymis, head — Epididymis, body
— Tunica vaginalis, visceral layer (on testis)
Glans of penis — Scrotum

A Testis and epididymis in situ.

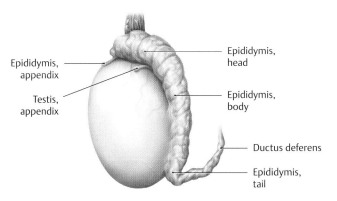

Epididymis, appendix — Epididymis, head
Testis, appendix — Epididymis, body
— Ductus deferens
— Epididymis, tail

B Surface anatomy of the testis and epididymis.

Fig. 21.30 Blood vessels of the testis
Left lateral view.

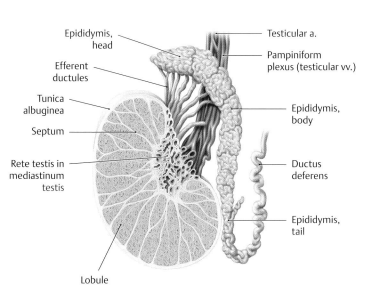

Epididymis, head — Testicular a.
Efferent ductules — Pampiniform plexus (testicular vv.)
Tunica albuginea — Epididymis, body
Septum
Rete testis in mediastinum testis — Ductus deferens
— Epididymis, tail
Lobule

C Sagittal section of the testis and epididymis.

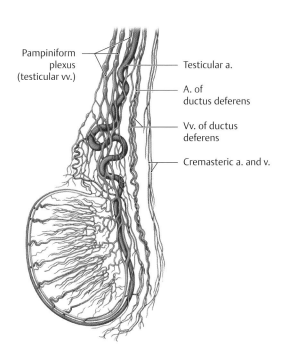

Pampiniform plexus (testicular vv.) — Testicular a.
— A. of ductus deferens
— Vv. of ductus deferens
— Cremasteric a. and v.

Male Accessory Sex Glands

 The accessory male sex glands consist of the seminal, prostate, and bulbourethral glands, which contribute fluid to the ejaculate that provides nourishment for the spermatozoa as well as neutralizes the pH of the male urethra and the vaginal environment.

Fig. 21.31 Accessory sex glands

Posterior view.
The ducts of the seminal gland and ductus deferens combine to form the ejaculatory duct.

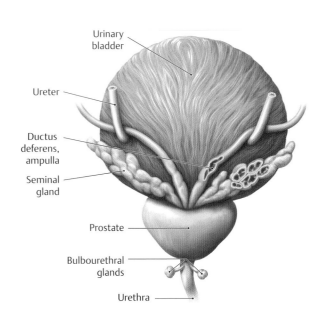

- Urinary bladder
- Ureter
- Ductus deferens, ampulla
- Seminal gland
- Prostate
- Bulbourethral glands
- Urethra

Fig. 21.32 Anatomic divisions of the prostate

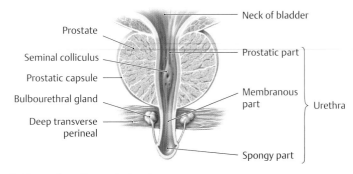

- Prostate
- Seminal colliculus
- Prostatic capsule
- Bulbourethral gland
- Deep transverse perineal
- Neck of bladder
- Prostatic part
- Membranous part
- Spongy part
- Urethra

A Coronal section, anterior view.

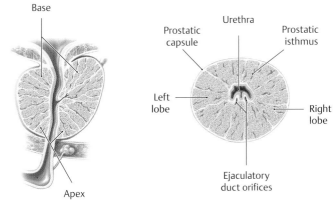

- Base
- Apex

B Sagittal section, left lateral view.

- Prostatic capsule
- Urethra
- Prostatic isthmus
- Left lobe
- Right lobe
- Ejaculatory duct orifices

C Transverse section, superior view.

Fig. 21.33 Clinical divisions of the prostate

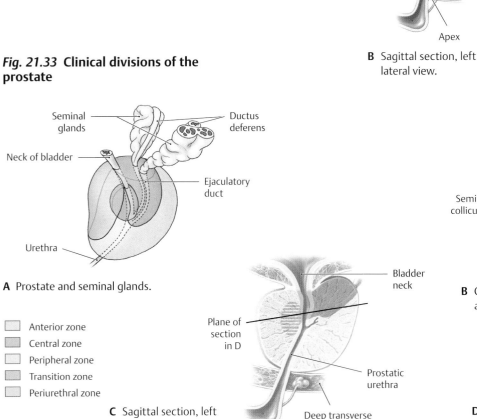

- Seminal glands
- Ductus deferens
- Neck of bladder
- Ejaculatory duct
- Urethra

A Prostate and seminal glands.

- ☐ Anterior zone
- ☐ Central zone
- ☐ Peripheral zone
- ☐ Transition zone
- ☐ Periurethral zone

- Plane of section in D
- Bladder neck
- Prostatic urethra

C Sagittal section, left lateral view.

Deep transverse perineal

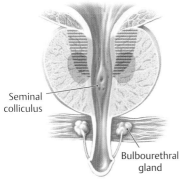

- Seminal colliculus
- Bulbourethral gland

B Coronal section, anterior view.

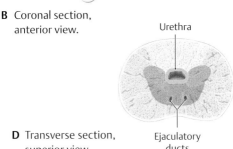

- Urethra
- Ejaculatory ducts

D Transverse section, superior view.

Fig. 21.34 **Prostate in situ**

Sagittal section through the male pelvis, left lateral view.

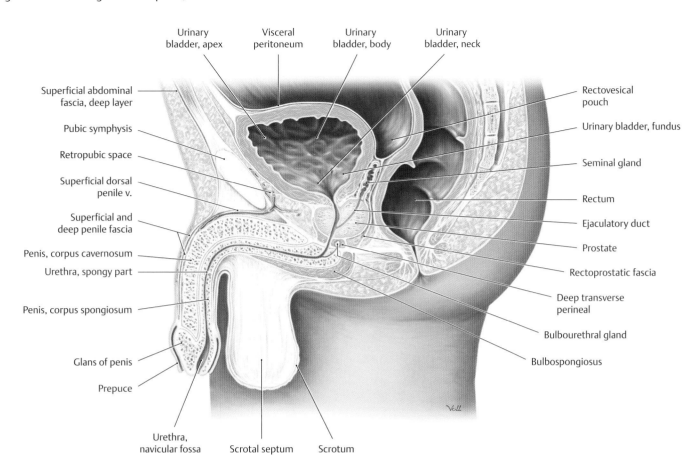

Urinary bladder, apex · Visceral peritoneum · Urinary bladder, body · Urinary bladder, neck

Superficial abdominal fascia, deep layer

Pubic symphysis

Retropubic space

Superficial dorsal penile v.

Superficial and deep penile fascia

Penis, corpus cavernosum

Urethra, spongy part

Penis, corpus spongiosum

Glans of penis

Prepuce

Urethra, navicular fossa · Scrotal septum · Scrotum

Rectovesical pouch

Urinary bladder, fundus

Seminal gland

Rectum

Ejaculatory duct

Prostate

Rectoprostatic fascia

Deep transverse perineal

Bulbourethral gland

Bulbospongiosus

 Clinical box 21.3

Prostatic carcinoma and hypertrophy

Prostatic carcinoma is one of the most common malignant tumors in older men, often growing at a subcapsular location (deep to the prostatic capsule) in the peripheral zone of the prostate. Unlike benign prostatic hyperplasia, which begins in the central part of the gland, prostatic carcinoma does not cause urinary outflow obstruction in its early stages. Being in the peripheral zone, the tumor is palpable as a firm mass through the anterior wall of the rectum during rectal examination.

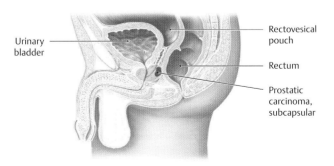

Urinary bladder

Rectovesical pouch

Rectum

Prostatic carcinoma, subcapsular

A Most common site of prostatic carcinoma.

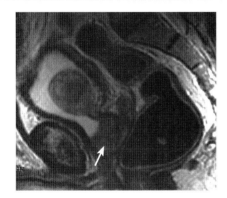

B Prostatic carcinoma (*arrow*) with bladder infiltration.

In certain prostate diseases, especially cancer, increased amounts of a protein, prostate-specific antigen or PSA, appear in the blood. This protein can be measured by a simple blood test.

Arteries & Veins of the Pelvis

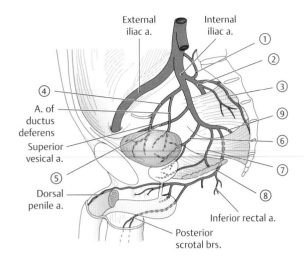

A Male pelvis.

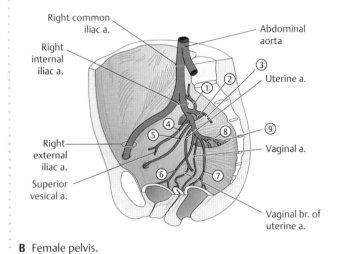

B Female pelvis.

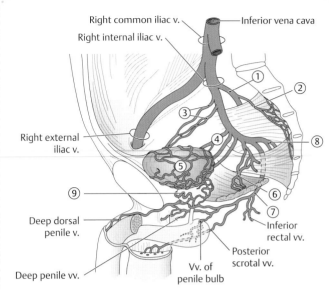

A Male pelvis.

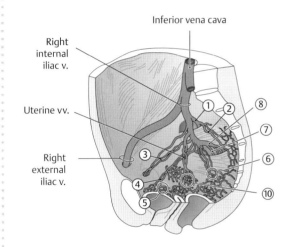

B Female pelvis.

Table 22.1	Branches of the internal iliac artery

The internal iliac artery gives off five parietal (pelvic wall) and four visceral (pelvic organs) branches.* Parietal branches are shown in italics.

Branches		
①	*Iliolumbar a.*	
②	*Superior gluteal a.*	
③	*Lateral sacral a.*	
④	Umbilical a.	A. of ductus deferens
		Superior vesical a.
⑤	*Obturator a.*	
⑥	Inferior vesical a.	
⑦	Middle rectal a.	
⑧	Internal pudendal a.	Inferior rectal a.
		Dorsal penile a.
		Posterior scrotal aa.
⑨	*Inferior gluteal a.*	

* In the female pelvis, the uterine and vaginal arteries arise directly from the anterior division of the internal iliac artery.

Table 22.2	Venous drainage of the pelvis

Tributaries	
①	Superior gluteal v.
②	Lateral sacral v.
③	Obturator vv.
④	Vesical vv.
⑤	Vesical venous plexus
⑥	Middle rectal vv. (rectal venous plexus) (also superior and inferior rectal vv., not shown)
⑦	Internal pudendal v.
⑧	Inferior gluteal vv.
⑨	Prostatic venous plexus
⑩	Uterine and vaginal venous plexus

The male pelvis also contains veins draining the penis and scrotum.

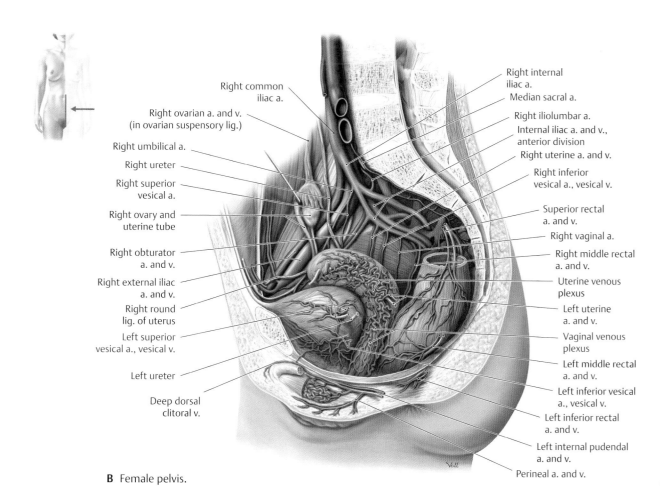

Fig. 22.1 Blood vessels of the pelvis
Idealized right hemipelvis, left lateral view.

Abdominal aorta
Inferior mesenteric a.
Left common iliac a. and v.
Umbilical a.
Right ureter
Right external iliac a. and v.
Right obturator a. and v.
Right superior vesical a. and v.
Right ductus deferens and a.
Left ureter
Left superior and inferior vesical a. and v.
Dorsal penile a., deep dorsal penile v.
Prostate
Spermatic cord

Median sacral a.
Right internal iliac a. and v.
Right iliolumbar a.
Right lateral sacral v.
Right superior gluteal a. and v.
Superior rectal a. and v. (from/to inferior mesenteric a. and v.)
Right inferior vesical a. and v.
Right middle rectal a. and v.
Seminal gland
Left middle rectal a. and v.
Left inferior rectal a. and v.
Left internal pudendal a. and v.
Perineal a. and v.

A Male pelvis.

Posterior scrotal a. and v.

Right common iliac a.
Right ovarian a. and v. (in ovarian suspensory lig.)
Right umbilical a.
Right ureter
Right superior vesical a.
Right ovary and uterine tube
Right obturator a. and v.
Right external iliac a. and v.
Right round lig. of uterus
Left superior vesical a., vesical v.
Left ureter
Deep dorsal clitoral v.

Right internal iliac a.
Median sacral a.
Right iliolumbar a.
Internal iliac a. and v., anterior division
Right uterine a. and v.
Right inferior vesical a., vesical v.
Superior rectal a. and v.
Right vaginal a.
Right middle rectal a. and v.
Uterine venous plexus
Left uterine a. and v.
Vaginal venous plexus
Left middle rectal a. and v.
Left inferior vesical a., vesical v.
Left inferior rectal a. and v.
Left internal pudendal a. and v.
Perineal a. and v.

B Female pelvis.

Arteries & Veins of the Rectum & Genitalia

Fig. 22.2 Blood vessels of the rectum

A posterior view. The main blood supply to the rectum is from the superior rectal arteries; the middle rectal arteries serve as an anastomosis between the superior and inferior rectal arteries.

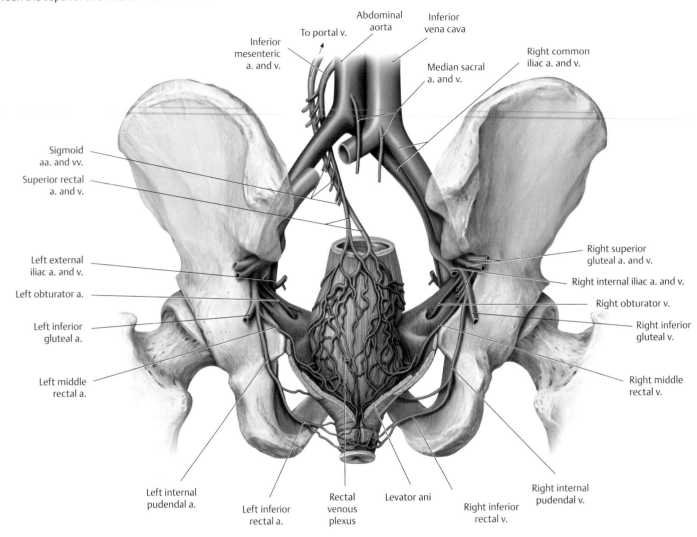

Fig. 22.3 Arterial supply of the cavernous body of the rectum (hemorrhoidal plexus)

Caudal view with patient in lithotomy position. The hemorrhoidal plexus is a permanently distended cavernous body. It's supplied by three branches of the superior rectal a. at the 3, 7, and 11 o'clock positions where they form three major cushions and four minor cushions in the area of the anal columns. These circular cavernous structures filled with blood serve as an effective continence mechanism that ensures liquid- and gas-tight closure. The sustained contraction of the muscular sphincter apparatus inhibits venous drainage, and blood is allowed to drain from the cavernous body when the sphincters relax during defecation.

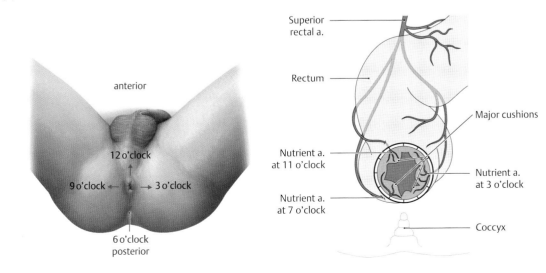

Fig. 22.4 Blood vessels of the genitalia

Anterior view.

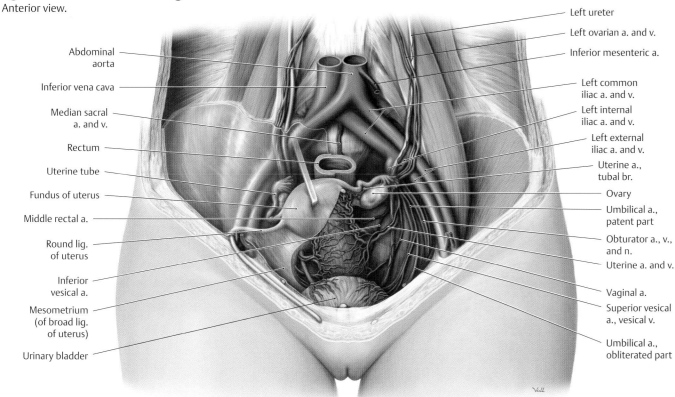

Left ureter

Left ovarian a. and v.

Inferior mesenteric a.

Abdominal aorta

Inferior vena cava

Median sacral a. and v.

Rectum

Uterine tube

Fundus of uterus

Middle rectal a.

Round lig. of uterus

Inferior vesical a.

Mesometrium (of broad lig. of uterus)

Urinary bladder

Left common iliac a. and v.

Left internal iliac a. and v.

Left external iliac a. and v.

Uterine a., tubal br.

Ovary

Umbilical a., patent part

Obturator a., v., and n.

Uterine a. and v.

Vaginal a.

Superior vesical a., vesical v.

Umbilical a., obliterated part

A Female pelvis. *Removed:* Peritoneum (left side). *Retracted:* Uterus.

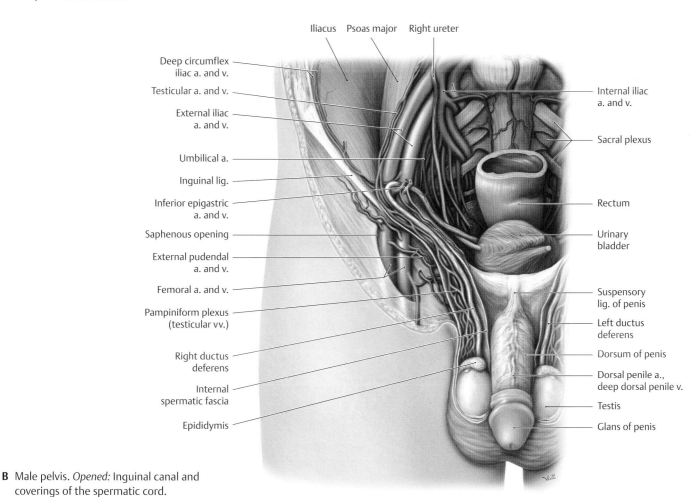

Iliacus   Psoas major   Right ureter

Deep circumflex iliac a. and v.

Testicular a. and v.

External iliac a. and v.

Umbilical a.

Inguinal lig.

Inferior epigastric a. and v.

Saphenous opening

External pudendal a. and v.

Femoral a. and v.

Pampiniform plexus (testicular vv.)

Right ductus deferens

Internal spermatic fascia

Epididymis

Internal iliac a. and v.

Sacral plexus

Rectum

Urinary bladder

Suspensory lig. of penis

Left ductus deferens

Dorsum of penis

Dorsal penile a., deep dorsal penile v.

Testis

Glans of penis

B Male pelvis. *Opened:* Inguinal canal and coverings of the spermatic cord.

269

Lymph Nodes of the Abdomen & Pelvis

Fig. 22.5 **Lymphatic drainage of the internal organs**

Lymph draining from the abdomen, pelvis, and lower limb ultimately passes through the lumbar lymph nodes (clinically, the aortic lymph nodes). (See **Table 22.3** for numbering.) The lumbar lymph nodes consist of the right lateral aortic (caval) and left lateral aortic nodes, the preaortic nodes, and the retroaortic nodes. Efferent lymph vessels from the lateral aortic lymph nodes and the retroaortic nodes form the lumbar trunks and those from the preaortic nodes form the intestinal trunks. The lumbar and intestinal trunks terminate in the cisterna chyli.

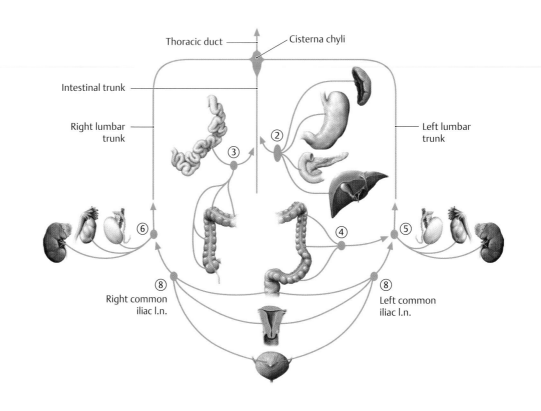

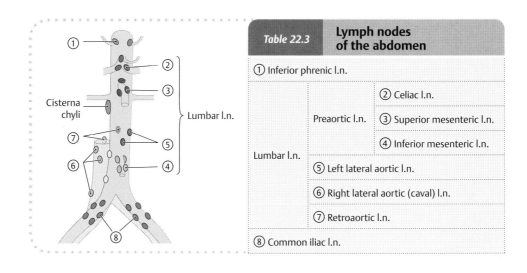

Table 22.3	Lymph nodes of the abdomen		
① Inferior phrenic l.n.			
Lumbar l.n.	Preaortic l.n.		② Celiac l.n.
			③ Superior mesenteric l.n.
			④ Inferior mesenteric l.n.
	⑤ Left lateral aortic l.n.		
	⑥ Right lateral aortic (caval) l.n.		
	⑦ Retroaortic l.n.		
⑧ Common iliac l.n.			

Fig. 22.6 Lymphatic drainage of the rectum
Anterior view.

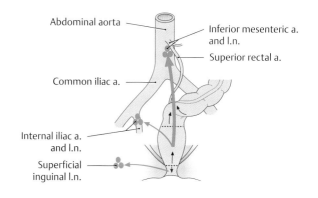

Abdominal aorta

Inferior mesenteric a. and l.n.

Superior rectal a.

Common iliac a.

Internal iliac a. and l.n.

Superficial inguinal l.n.

Fig. 22.7 Lymphatic drainage of the bladder and urethra
Anterior view.

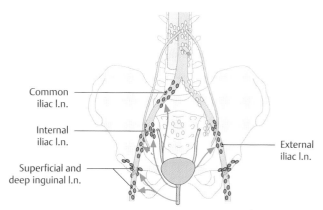

Common iliac l.n.

Internal iliac l.n.

Superficial and deep inguinal l.n.

External iliac l.n.

Fig. 22.8 Lymphatic drainage of the male genitalia
Anterior view.

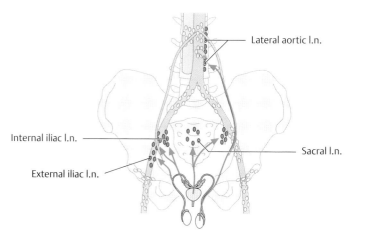

Lateral aortic l.n.

Internal iliac l.n.

External iliac l.n.

Sacral l.n.

Fig. 22.9 Lymphatic drainage of the female genitalia
Anterior view.

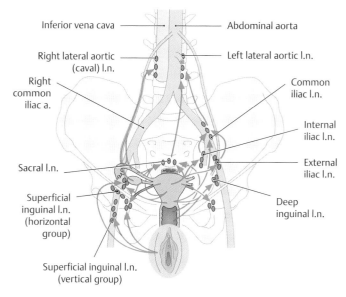

Inferior vena cava

Abdominal aorta

Right lateral aortic (caval) l.n.

Left lateral aortic l.n.

Right common iliac a.

Common iliac l.n.

Internal iliac l.n.

Sacral l.n.

External iliac l.n.

Superficial inguinal l.n. (horizontal group)

Deep inguinal l.n.

Superficial inguinal l.n. (vertical group)

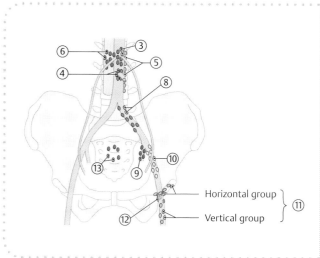

Horizontal group

Vertical group

⑪

Table 22.4	Lymph nodes of the pelvis	
Numbers continued from **Table 22.3.**		
Preaortic l.n.	③ Superior mesenteric l.n.	
	④ Inferior mesenteric l.n.	
⑤ Left lateral aortic l.n.		
⑥ Right lateral aortic (caval) l.n.		
⑧ Common iliac l.n.		
⑨ Internal iliac l.n.		
⑩ External iliac l.n.		
⑪ Superficial inguinal l.n.	Horizontal group	
	Vertical group	
⑫ Deep inguinal l.n.		
⑬ Sacral l.n.		

Lymph Nodes of the Genitalia

Fig. 22.10 Lymph nodes of the male genitalia

Anterior view. *Removed:* Gastrointestinal tract (except rectal stump) and peritoneum.

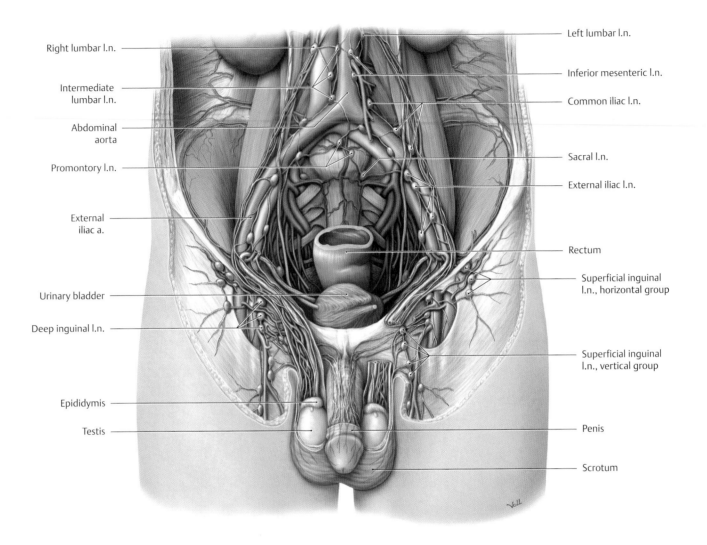

Right lumbar l.n.

Intermediate lumbar l.n.

Abdominal aorta

Promontory l.n.

External iliac a.

Urinary bladder

Deep inguinal l.n.

Epididymis

Testis

Left lumbar l.n.

Inferior mesenteric l.n.

Common iliac l.n.

Sacral l.n.

External iliac l.n.

Rectum

Superficial inguinal l.n., horizontal group

Superficial inguinal l.n., vertical group

Penis

Scrotum

Fig. 22.11 Lymph nodes of the female genitalia

Anterior view. *Removed:* Gastrointestinal tract (except rectal stump) and peritoneum. *Retracted:* Uterus.

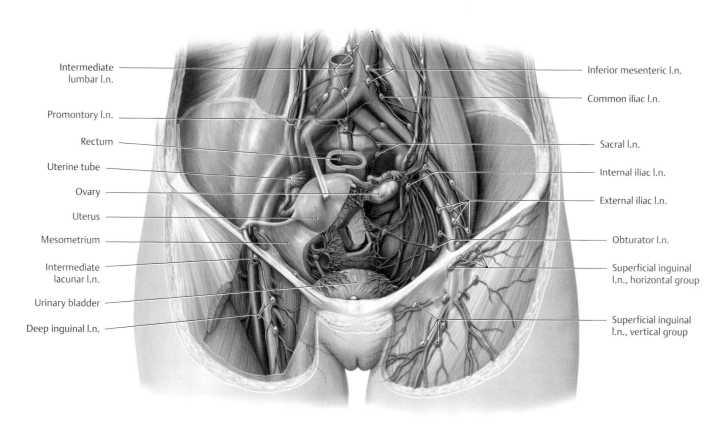

Intermediate lumbar l.n.

Promontory l.n.

Rectum

Uterine tube

Ovary

Uterus

Mesometrium

Intermediate lacunar l.n.

Urinary bladder

Deep inguinal l.n.

Inferior mesenteric l.n.

Common iliac l.n.

Sacral l.n.

Internal iliac l.n.

External iliac l.n.

Obturator l.n.

Superficial inguinal l.n., horizontal group

Superficial inguinal l.n., vertical group

Fig. 22.12 Lymphatic drainage of the pelvic organs

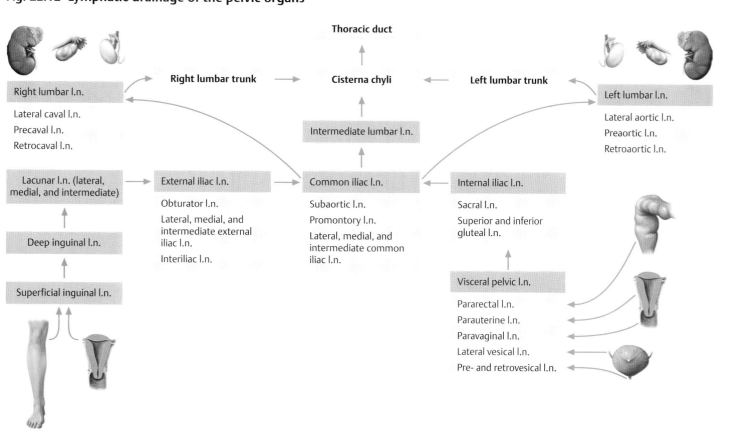

Thoracic duct

Right lumbar trunk → Cisterna chyli ← **Left lumbar trunk**

Right lumbar l.n.

Lateral caval l.n.
Precaval l.n.
Retrocaval l.n.

Left lumbar l.n.

Lateral aortic l.n.
Preaortic l.n.
Retroaortic l.n.

Intermediate lumbar l.n.

Lacunar l.n. (lateral, medial, and intermediate) → External iliac l.n. → Common iliac l.n. ← Internal iliac l.n.

Obturator l.n.

Lateral, medial, and intermediate external iliac l.n.

Interiliac l.n.

Subaortic l.n.

Promontory l.n.

Lateral, medial, and intermediate common iliac l.n.

Sacral l.n.

Superior and inferior gluteal l.n.

Deep inguinal l.n.

Superficial inguinal l.n.

Visceral pelvic l.n.

Pararectal l.n.
Parauterine l.n.
Paravaginal l.n.
Lateral vesical l.n.
Pre- and retrovesical l.n.

Autonomic Plexuses of the Pelvis

Fig. 22.13 Autonomic plexuses in the pelvis

Anterior view of the male lower abdomen. *Removed:* Peritoneum and abdominopelvic organs except kidneys.

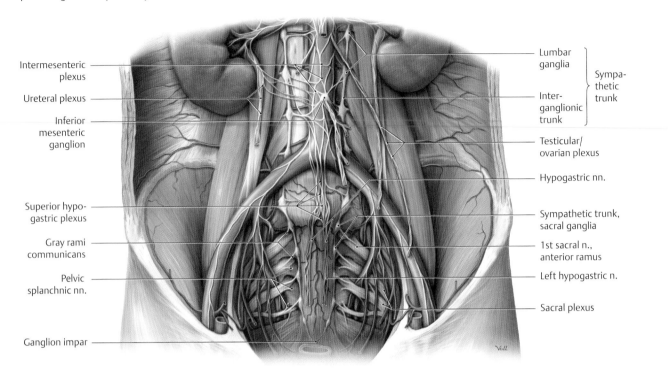

Intermesenteric plexus

Ureteral plexus

Inferior mesenteric ganglion

Superior hypogastric plexus

Gray rami communicans

Pelvic splanchnic nn.

Ganglion impar

Lumbar ganglia

Interganglionic trunk

Sympathetic trunk

Testicular/ovarian plexus

Hypogastric nn.

Sympathetic trunk, sacral ganglia

1st sacral n., anterior ramus

Left hypogastric n.

Sacral plexus

Fig. 22.14 Innervation of the urinary organs

Anterior view of the male lower abdomen and pelvis. *Removed:* Peritoneum and abdominopelvic organs except kidneys, suprarenal glands, rectal stump, and bladder. See **p. 276** for schematic of innervation of urinary organs.

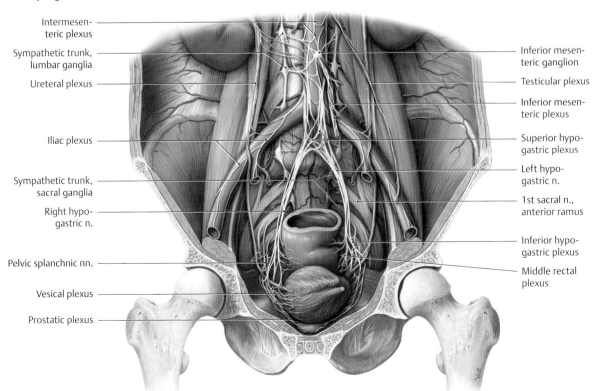

Intermesenteric plexus

Sympathetic trunk, lumbar ganglia

Ureteral plexus

Iliac plexus

Sympathetic trunk, sacral ganglia

Right hypogastric n.

Pelvic splanchnic nn.

Vesical plexus

Prostatic plexus

Inferior mesenteric ganglion

Testicular plexus

Inferior mesenteric plexus

Superior hypogastric plexus

Left hypogastric n.

1st sacral n., anterior ramus

Inferior hypogastric plexus

Middle rectal plexus

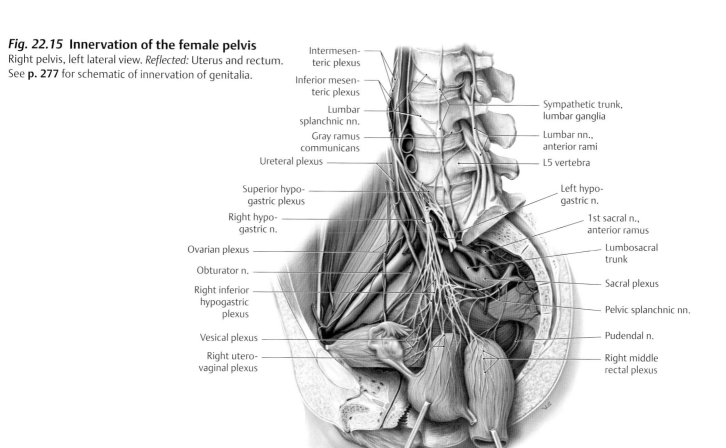

Fig. 22.15 Innervation of the female pelvis

Right pelvis, left lateral view. *Reflected:* Uterus and rectum.
See **p. 277** for schematic of innervation of genitalia.

Intermesen-
teric plexus

Inferior mesen-
teric plexus

Lumbar
splanchnic nn.

Gray ramus
communicans

Ureteral plexus

Superior hypo-
gastric plexus

Right hypo-
gastric n.

Ovarian plexus

Obturator n.

Right inferior
hypogastric
plexus

Vesical plexus

Right utero-
vaginal plexus

Sympathetic trunk,
lumbar ganglia

Lumbar nn.,
anterior rami

L5 vertebra

Left hypo-
gastric n.

1st sacral n.,
anterior ramus

Lumbosacral
trunk

Sacral plexus

Pelvic splanchnic nn.

Pudendal n.

Right middle
rectal plexus

Fig. 22.16 Innervation of the male pelvis

Right pelvis, left lateral view. See **p. 277** for schematic
of innervation of genitalia.

Intermesen-
teric plexus

Inferior mesen-
teric plexus

Lumbar
splanchnic nn.

Gray ramus
communicans

Ureteral plexus

Superior hypo-
gastric plexus

Right hypo-
gastric n.

Iliac plexus

Obturator n.

Deferential
plexus

Seminal gland

Vesical plexus

Prostatic plexus

Cavernous
nn. of penis

Dorsal n.
of the penis

Posterior
scrotal nn.

Sympathetic trunk,
lumbar ganglia

Lumbar nn.,
anterior rami

L5 vertebra

Lumbosacral
trunk

Left hypogastric n.

Pelvic splanchnic nn.

Middle
rectal plexus

Pudendal n.

Inferior rectal
plexus

Inferior rectal nn.

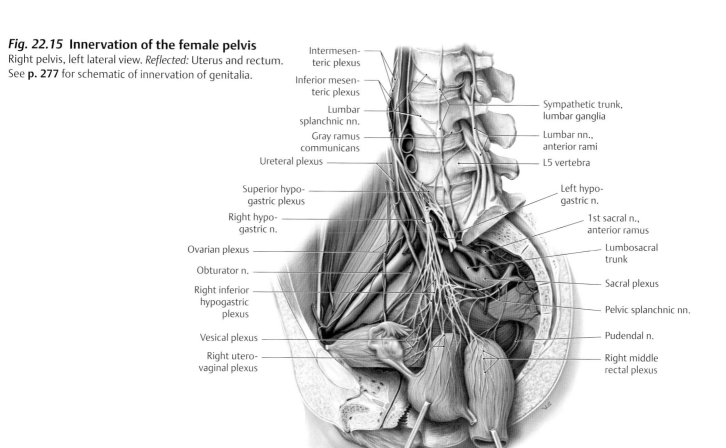

Autonomic Innervation: Urinary & Genital Organs & Rectum

Fig. 22.17 Autonomic innervation of the urinary organs

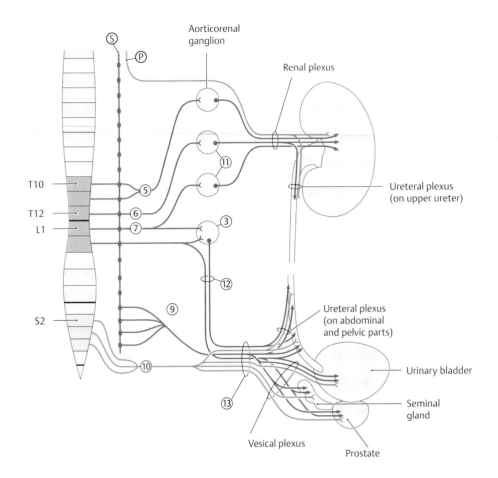

— Sympathetic fibers
— Parasympathetic fibers

Numbering continued from **p. 211.**	
Ⓢ	Sympathetic trunk
Ⓟ	Posterior vagal trunk (from right vagus n.)
③	Inferior mesenteric ganglion
⑤	Lesser splanchnic n. (T10–T11)
⑥	Least splanchnic n. (T12)
⑦	Lumbar splanchnic nn. (L1–L2)
⑨	Sacral splanchnic nn. (from 1st to 3rd sacral ganglia)
⑩	Pelvic splanchnic nn. (S2–S4)
⑪	Renal ganglia
⑫	Superior hypogastric plexus
⑬	Inferior hypogastric plexus

Labels in figure: Aorticorenal ganglion; Renal plexus; Ureteral plexus (on upper ureter); Ureteral plexus (on abdominal and pelvic parts); Urinary bladder; Seminal gland; Prostate; Vesical plexus; T10; T12; L1; S2.

✳ Clinical box 22.1

Referred pain from the internal organs

The convergence of somatic and visceral afferent fibers to a common level of the spinal cord confuses the relationship between the perceived and actual sites of pain, a phenomenon known as referred pain. Pain impulses from a particular organ are consistently projected to the same well-defined skin area.

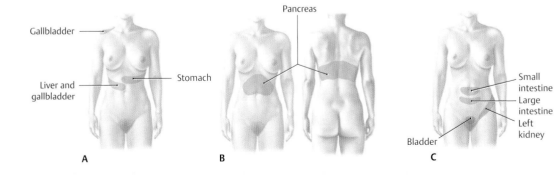
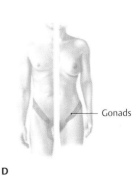

Labels: Gallbladder; Liver and gallbladder; Stomach; Pancreas; Small intestine; Large intestine; Left kidney; Bladder; Gonads.

A   B   C   D

Fig. 22.18 Autonomic innervation of the genitalia

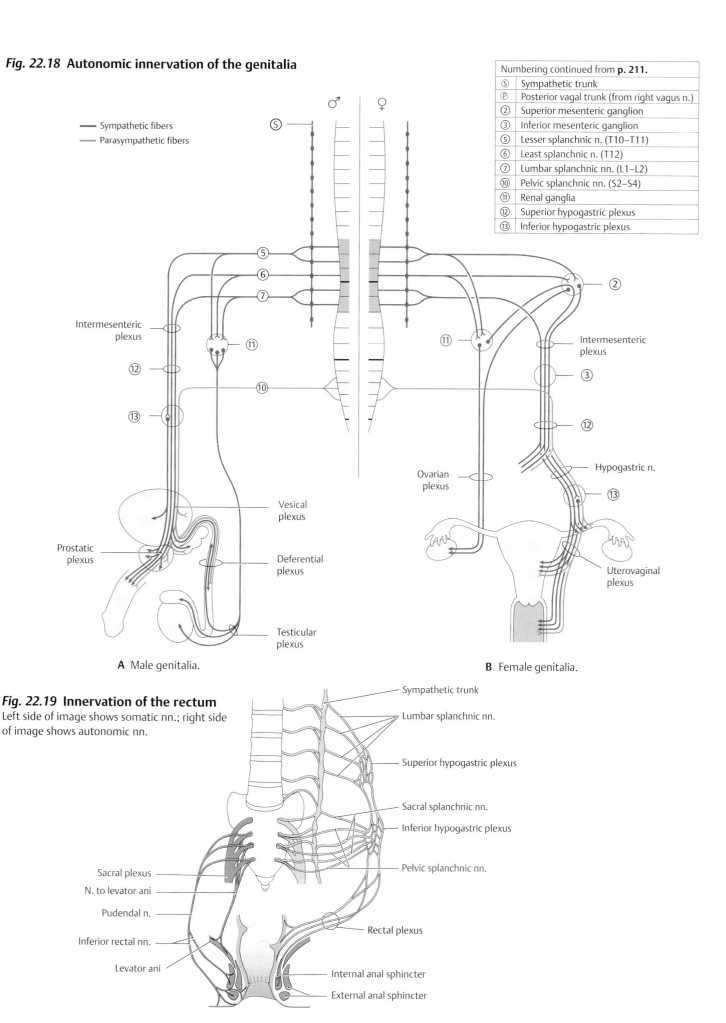

Sympathetic fibers
Parasympathetic fibers

	Numbering continued from **p. 211.**
Ⓢ	Sympathetic trunk
Ⓟ	Posterior vagal trunk (from right vagus n.)
②	Superior mesenteric ganglion
③	Inferior mesenteric ganglion
⑤	Lesser splanchnic n. (T10–T11)
⑥	Least splanchnic n. (T12)
⑦	Lumbar splanchnic nn. (L1–L2)
⑩	Pelvic splanchnic nn. (S2–S4)
⑪	Renal ganglia
⑫	Superior hypogastric plexus
⑬	Inferior hypogastric plexus

Intermesenteric plexus

Vesical plexus

Prostatic plexus

Deferential plexus

Testicular plexus

Intermesenteric plexus

Ovarian plexus

Hypogastric n.

Uterovaginal plexus

A Male genitalia.

B Female genitalia.

Fig. 22.19 Innervation of the rectum

Left side of image shows somatic nn.; right side of image shows autonomic nn.

Sympathetic trunk

Lumbar splanchnic nn.

Superior hypogastric plexus

Sacral splanchnic nn.

Inferior hypogastric plexus

Pelvic splanchnic nn.

Sacral plexus

N. to levator ani

Pudendal n.

Inferior rectal nn.

Levator ani

Rectal plexus

Internal anal sphincter

External anal sphincter

277

Neurovasculature of the Female Perineum & Genitalia

***Fig. 22.20* Nerves of the female perineum and genitalia**

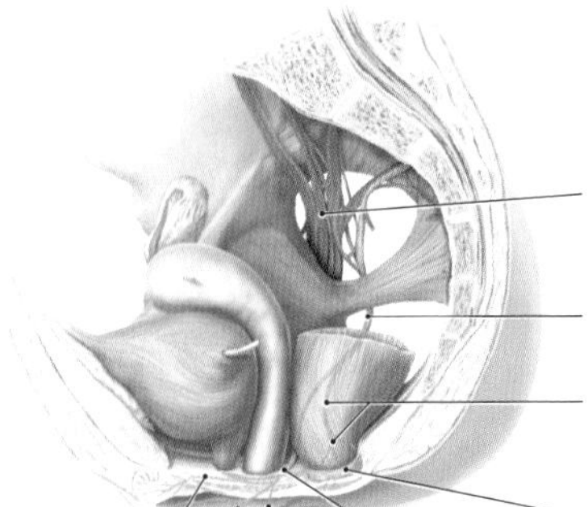

Sacral plexus

Pudendal n.

Inferior rectal nn.

External anal sphincter

Dorsal clitoral n.

Posterior labial nn.

Perineal nn.

A Nerve supply to the female external genitalia. Lesser pelvis, left lateral view.

Ilioinguinal n. and genitofemoral n., genital br. and labial br.

Pudendal n.

Posterior femoral cutaneous n.

Middle clunial nn.

Superior clunial nn.

Inferior clunial nn.

Anococcygeal nn.

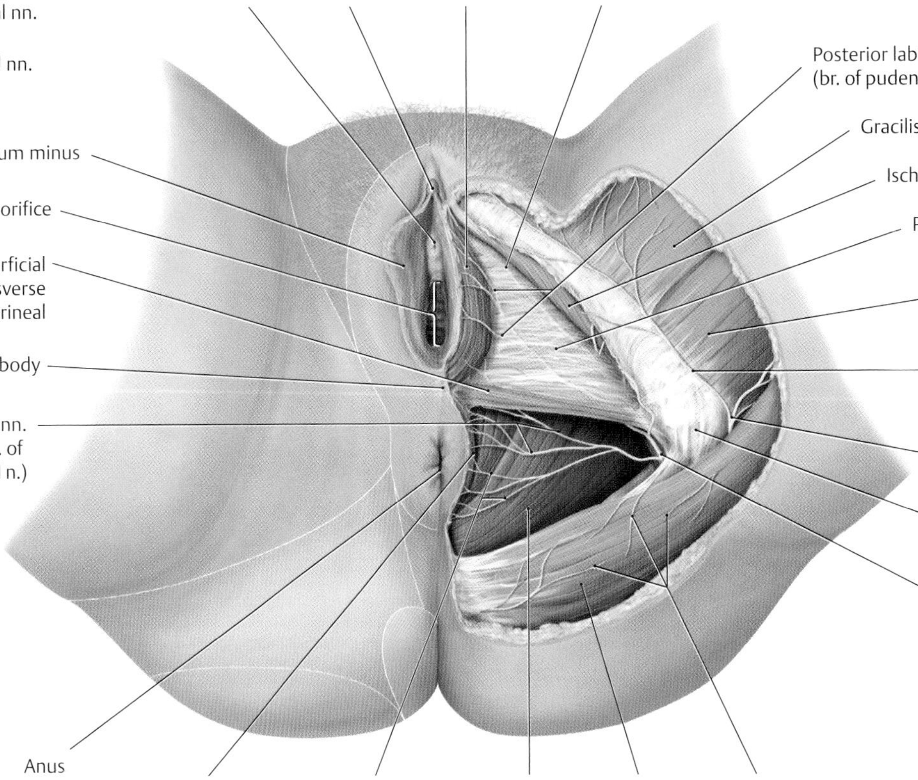

External urethral orifice

Glans of clitoris

Bulbo-spongiosus

Dorsal clitoral n. (br. of pudendal n.)

Posterior labial nn. (br. of pudendal n.)

Gracilis

Ischiocavernosus

Perineal membrane

Adductor magnus

Posterior femoral cutaneous n., perineal brs.

Posterior femoral cutaneous n.

Ischial tuberosity

Pudendal n.

Labium minus

Vaginal orifice

Superficial transverse perineal

Perineal body

Perineal nn. (brs. of pudendal n.)

Anus

External anal sphincter

Inferior rectal nn. (brs. of pudendal n.)

Levator ani

Gluteus maximus

Inferior clunial nn.

B Sensory innervation of the female perineum. Lithotomy position.

Fig. 22.21 Blood vessels of the female external genitalia

Inferior view.

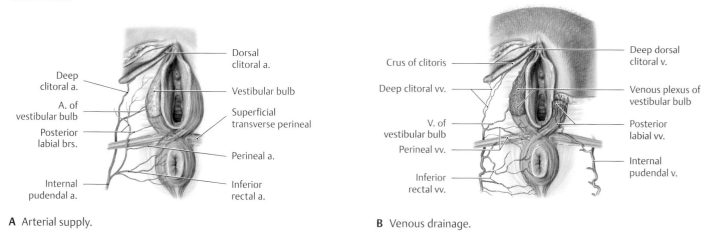

A Arterial supply.

B Venous drainage.

Fig. 22.22 Neurovasculature of the female perineum

Lithotomy position. *Removed from left side*: Bulbospongiosus and ischiocavernosus.

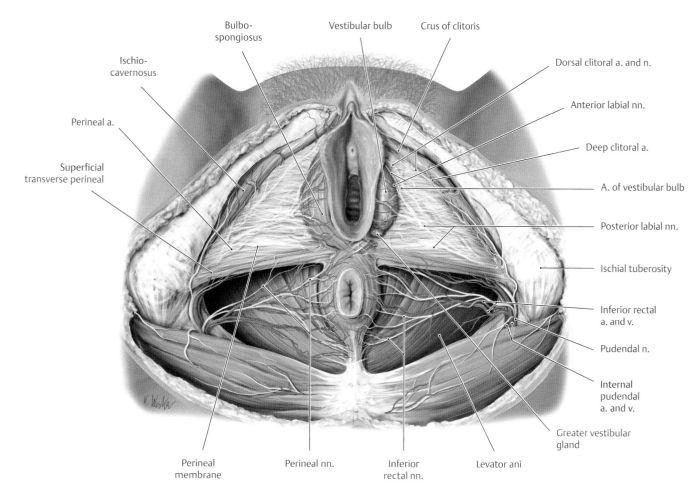

Neurovasculature of the Male Perineum & Genitalia

Fig. 22.23 Neurovasculature of the male genitalia
Left lateral view.

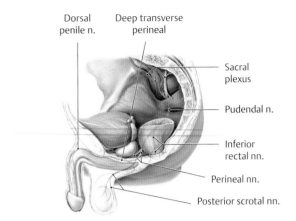

Dorsal penile n.
Deep transverse perineal
Sacral plexus
Pudendal n.
Inferior rectal nn.
Perineal nn.
Posterior scrotal nn.

A Nerve supply.

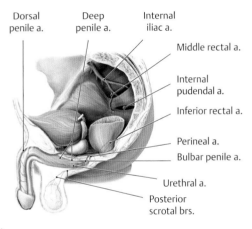

Dorsal penile a.
Deep penile a.
Internal iliac a.
Middle rectal a.
Internal pudendal a.
Inferior rectal a.
Perineal a.
Bulbar penile a.
Urethral a.
Posterior scrotal brs.

B Arterial supply.

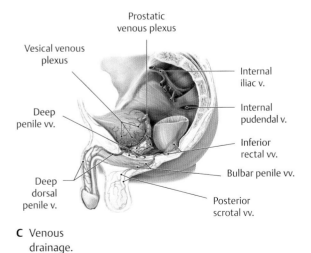

Prostatic venous plexus
Vesical venous plexus
Internal iliac v.
Internal pudendal v.
Inferior rectal vv.
Deep penile vv.
Deep dorsal penile v.
Bulbar penile vv.
Posterior scrotal vv.

C Venous drainage.

Fig. 22.24 Neurovasculature of the penis and scrotum

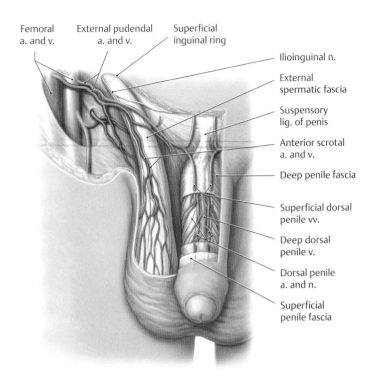

Femoral a. and v.
External pudendal a. and v.
Superficial inguinal ring
Ilioinguinal n.
External spermatic fascia
Suspensory lig. of penis
Anterior scrotal a. and v.
Deep penile fascia
Superficial dorsal penile vv.
Deep dorsal penile v.
Dorsal penile a. and n.
Superficial penile fascia

A Anterior view. *Partially removed:* Skin and fascia.

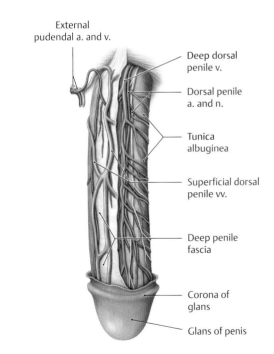

External pudendal a. and v.
Deep dorsal penile v.
Dorsal penile a. and n.
Tunica albuginea
Superficial dorsal penile vv.
Deep penile fascia
Corona of glans
Glans of penis

B Dorsal vasculature of the penis.
Removed from left side: Deep penile fascia.

Fig. 22.25 Nerves of the male perineum and genitalia

Lithotomy position.

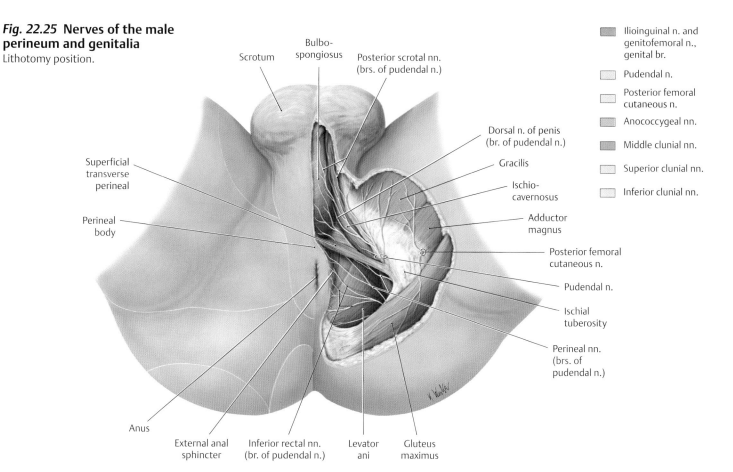

Legend:
- Ilioinguinal n. and genitofemoral n., genital br.
- Pudendal n.
- Posterior femoral cutaneous n.
- Anococcygeal nn.
- Middle clunial nn.
- Superior clunial nn.
- Inferior clunial nn.

Labels: Scrotum; Bulbo-spongiosus; Posterior scrotal nn. (brs. of pudendal n.); Dorsal n. of penis (br. of pudendal n.); Gracilis; Ischio-cavernosus; Adductor magnus; Posterior femoral cutaneous n.; Pudendal n.; Ischial tuberosity; Perineal nn. (brs. of pudendal n.); Superficial transverse perineal; Perineal body; Anus; External anal sphincter; Inferior rectal nn. (br. of pudendal n.); Levator ani; Gluteus maximus

Fig. 22.26 Neurovasculature of the male perineum

Lithotomy position. *Removed from left side*: Perineal membrane, bulbospongiosus, and root of penis.

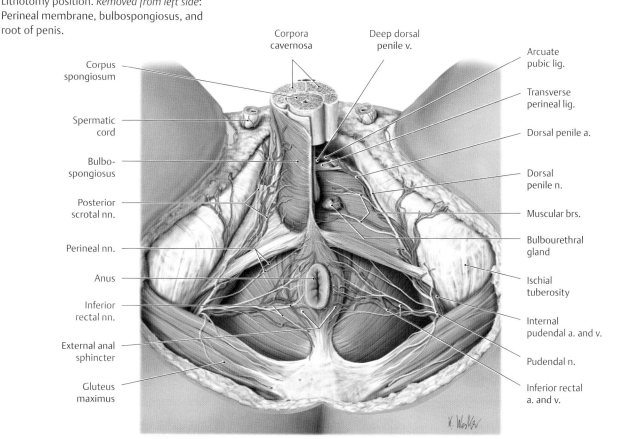

Labels: Corpora cavernosa; Deep dorsal penile v.; Corpus spongiosum; Spermatic cord; Bulbo-spongiosus; Posterior scrotal nn.; Perineal nn.; Anus; Inferior rectal nn.; External anal sphincter; Gluteus maximus; Arcuate pubic lig.; Transverse perineal lig.; Dorsal penile a.; Dorsal penile n.; Muscular brs.; Bulbourethral gland; Ischial tuberosity; Internal pudendal a. and v.; Pudendal n.; Inferior rectal a. and v.

Sectional Anatomy of the Pelvis & Perineum

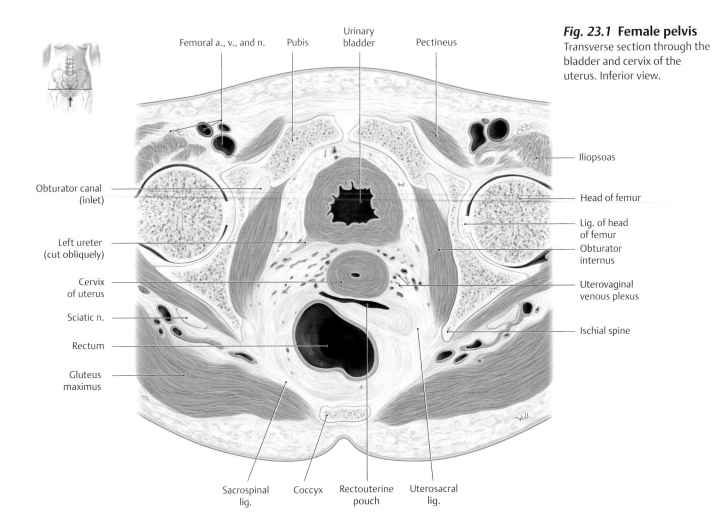

Fig. 23.1 Female pelvis
Transverse section through the bladder and cervix of the uterus. Inferior view.

Femoral a., v., and n.
Pubis
Urinary bladder
Pectineus

Obturator canal (inlet)
Left ureter (cut obliquely)
Cervix of uterus
Sciatic n.
Rectum
Gluteus maximus

Iliopsoas
Head of femur
Lig. of head of femur
Obturator internus
Uterovaginal venous plexus
Ischial spine

Sacrospinal lig.
Coccyx
Rectouterine pouch
Uterosacral lig.

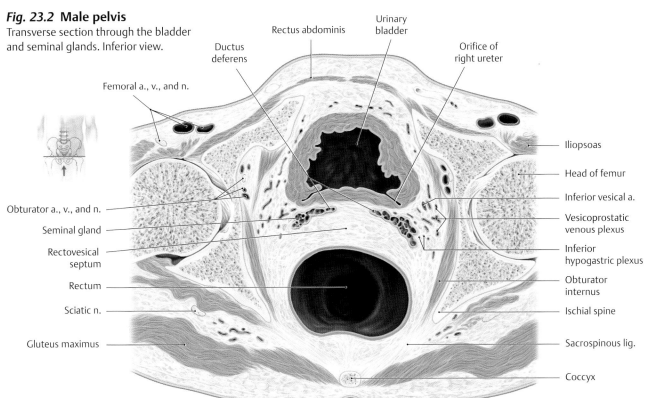

Fig. 23.2 Male pelvis
Transverse section through the bladder and seminal glands. Inferior view.

Rectus abdominis
Urinary bladder
Ductus deferens
Orifice of right ureter

Femoral a., v., and n.

Obturator a., v., and n.
Seminal gland
Rectovesical septum
Rectum
Sciatic n.
Gluteus maximus

Iliopsoas
Head of femur
Inferior vesical a.
Vesicoprostatic venous plexus
Inferior hypogastric plexus
Obturator internus
Ischial spine
Sacrospinous lig.
Coccyx

Fig. 23.3 Male pelvis

Transverse section through the prostate gland and anal canal. Inferior view.

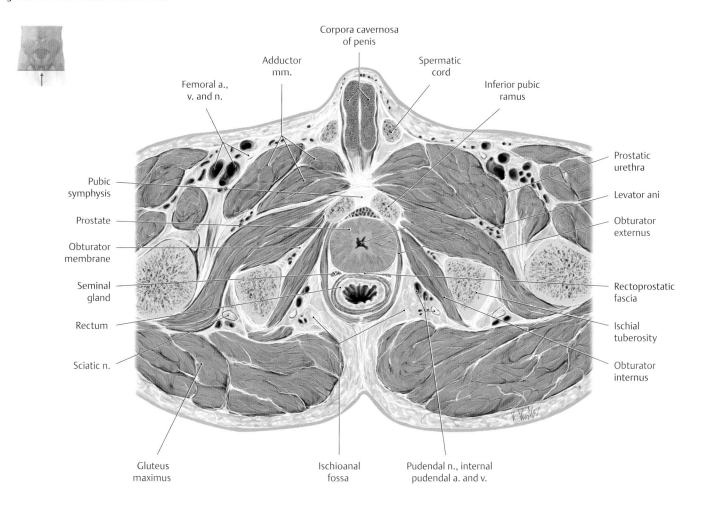

Corpora cavernosa of penis

Adductor mm.

Spermatic cord

Inferior pubic ramus

Femoral a., v. and n.

Prostatic urethra

Pubic symphysis

Levator ani

Prostate

Obturator externus

Obturator membrane

Rectoprostatic fascia

Seminal gland

Ischial tuberosity

Rectum

Obturator internus

Sciatic n.

Gluteus maximus

Ischioanal fossa

Pudendal n., internal pudendal a. and v.

Radiographic Anatomy of the Female Pelvis

Fig. 23.4 **MRI of the female pelvis**

Transverse section, inferior view.
(from Hamm, B. et al.: MRT von Abdomen und Becken, 2. Aufl. Thieme, Stuttgart 2006). The image shows the low-signal intensity cervical stroma (arrows), which surrounds the narrow high-signal intensity cervical canal.

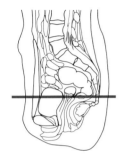

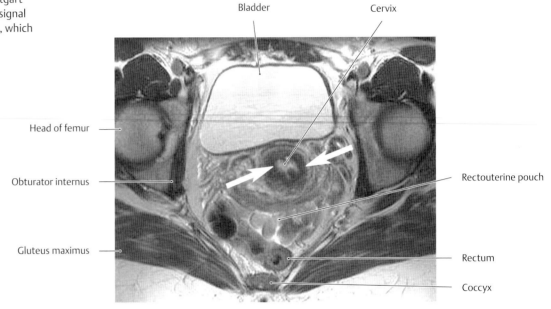

Bladder — Cervix — Head of femur — Obturator internus — Rectouterine pouch — Gluteus maximus — Rectum — Coccyx

Fig. 23.5 **MRI of the Female Pelvis**

Transverse section, inferior view.

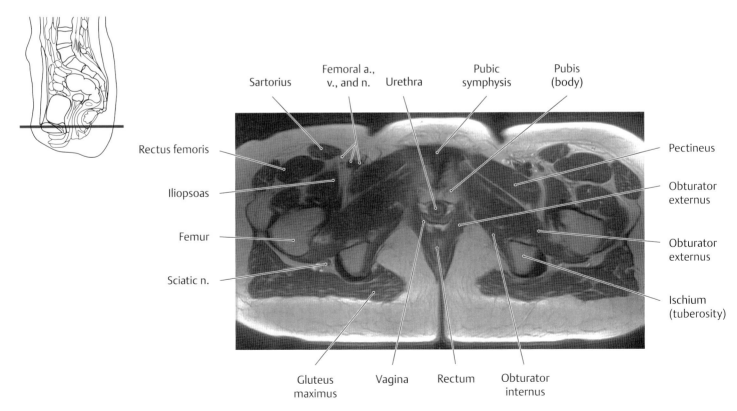

Sartorius — Femoral a., v., and n. — Urethra — Pubic symphysis — Pubis (body) — Rectus femoris — Pectineus — Iliopsoas — Obturator externus — Femur — Obturator externus — Sciatic n. — Ischium (tuberosity) — Gluteus maximus — Vagina — Rectum — Obturator internus

Fig. 23.6 MRI of the female pelvis

Sagittal section, left lateral view.
(from Hamm, B. et al.: MRT von Abdomen und Becken, 2. Aufl. Thieme, Stuttgart 2006). The image shows the uterus in the first half of the menstrual cycle (proliferative phase) with narrow endometrium and relatively low-signal intensity of the mymoetrium.

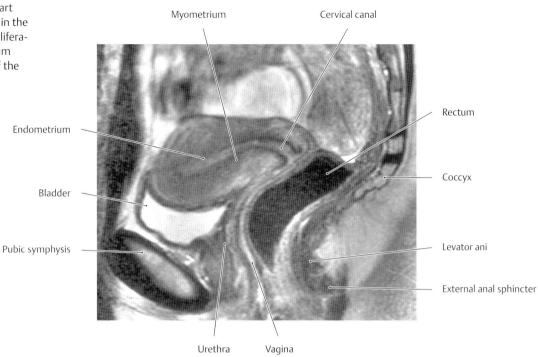

Myometrium

Cervical canal

Rectum

Coccyx

Levator ani

External anal sphincter

Endometrium

Bladder

Pubic symphysis

Urethra   Vagina

Fig. 23.7 MRI of the female pelvis

Coronal section, anterior view.

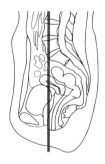

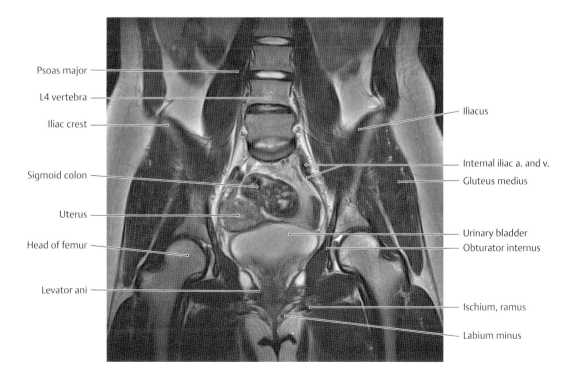

Psoas major

L4 vertebra

Iliac crest

Sigmoid colon

Uterus

Head of femur

Levator ani

Iliacus

Internal iliac a. and v.

Gluteus medius

Urinary bladder

Obturator internus

Ischium, ramus

Labium minus

Radiographic Anatomy of the Male Pelvis

Fig. 23.8 **MRI of the male pelvis**
Sagittal section, left lateral view.

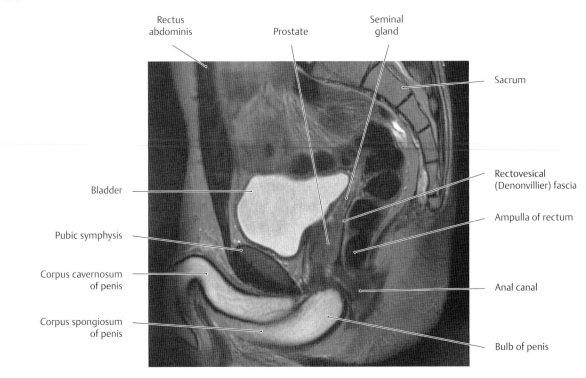

- Rectus abdominis
- Prostate
- Seminal gland
- Sacrum
- Bladder
- Rectovesical (Denonvillier) fascia
- Pubic symphysis
- Ampulla of rectum
- Corpus cavernosum of penis
- Anal canal
- Corpus spongiosum of penis
- Bulb of penis

Fig. 23.9 **MRI of the testes**
Coronal section, anterior view.

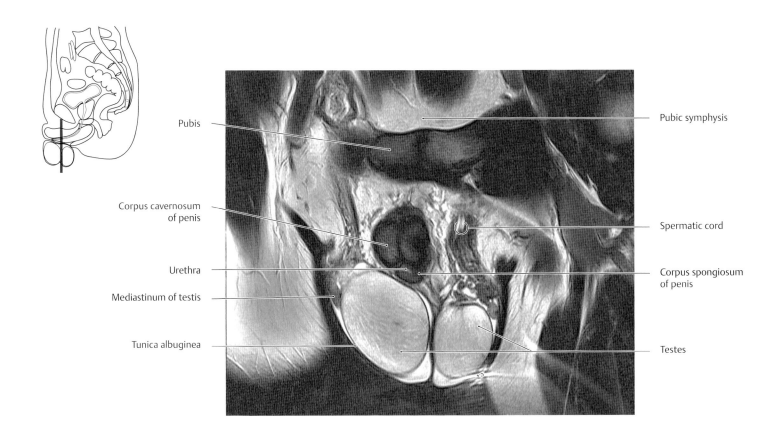

- Pubis
- Pubic symphysis
- Corpus cavernosum of penis
- Spermatic cord
- Urethra
- Corpus spongiosum of penis
- Mediastinum of testis
- Tunica albuginea
- Testes

Fig. 23.10 MRI of the prostate
Coronal section, anterior view.

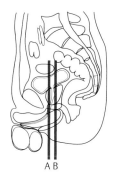

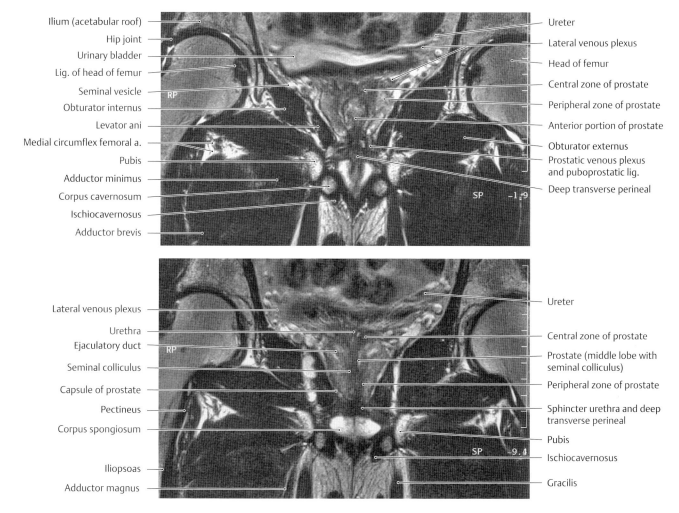

A

Ilium (acetabular roof)
Hip joint
Urinary bladder
Lig. of head of femur
Seminal vesicle
Obturator internus
Levator ani
Medial circumflex femoral a.
Pubis
Adductor minimus
Corpus cavernosum
Ischiocavernosus
Adductor brevis

Ureter
Lateral venous plexus
Head of femur
Central zone of prostate
Peripheral zone of prostate
Anterior portion of prostate
Obturator externus
Prostatic venous plexus and puboprostatic lig.
Deep transverse perineal

RP

SP   -1.9

B

Lateral venous plexus
Urethra
Ejaculatory duct
Seminal colliculus
Capsule of prostate
Pectineus
Corpus spongiosum
Iliopsoas
Adductor magnus

Ureter
Central zone of prostate
Prostate (middle lobe with seminal colliculus)
Peripheral zone of prostate
Sphincter urethra and deep transverse perineal
Pubis
Ischiocavernosus
Gracilis

RP

SP   -9.4

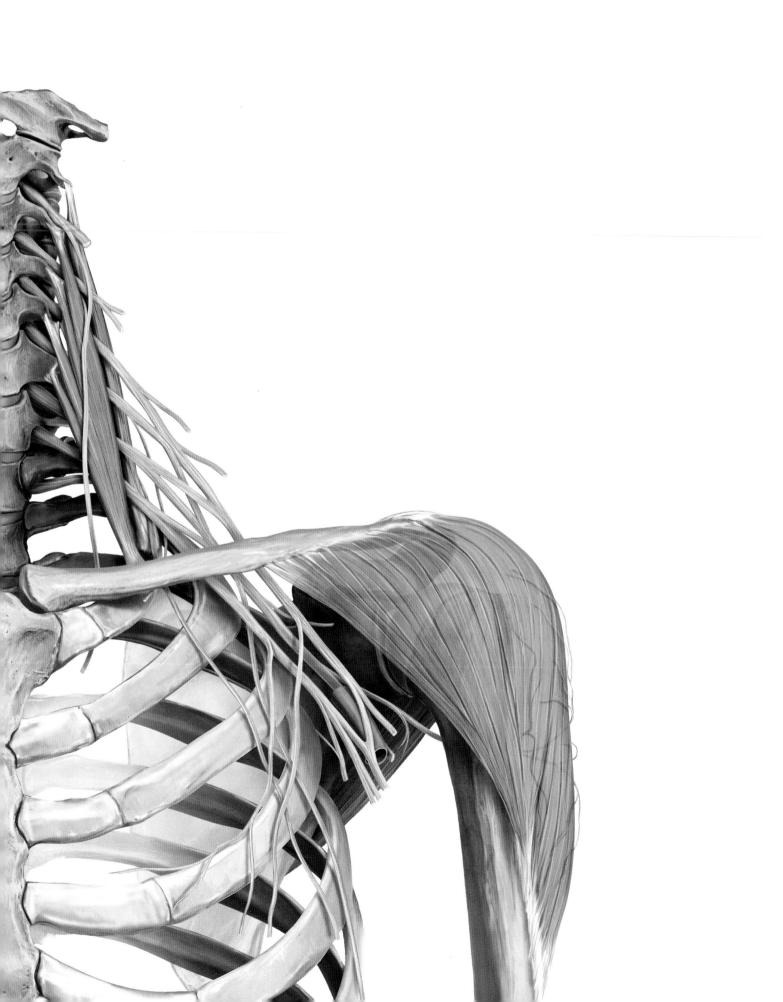

Upper Limb

Surface Anatomy

Fig. 24.1 Regions of the upper limb

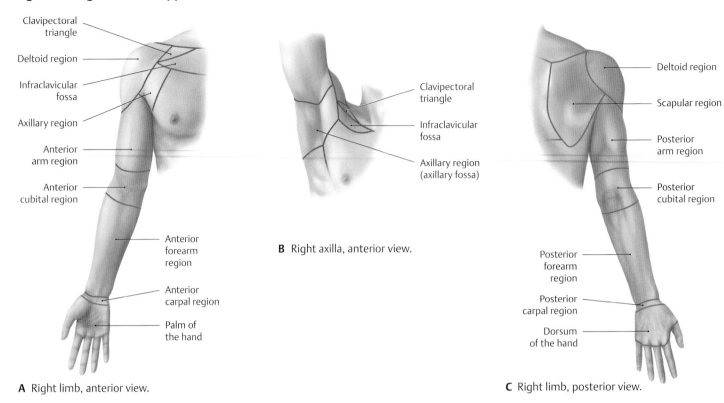

Clavipectoral triangle
Deltoid region
Infraclavicular fossa
Axillary region
Anterior arm region
Anterior cubital region
Anterior forearm region
Anterior carpal region
Palm of the hand

A Right limb, anterior view.

Clavipectoral triangle
Infraclavicular fossa
Axillary region (axillary fossa)

B Right axilla, anterior view.

Deltoid region
Scapular region
Posterior arm region
Posterior cubital region
Posterior forearm region
Posterior carpal region
Dorsum of the hand

C Right limb, posterior view.

Fig. 24.2 Palpable musculature of the upper limb

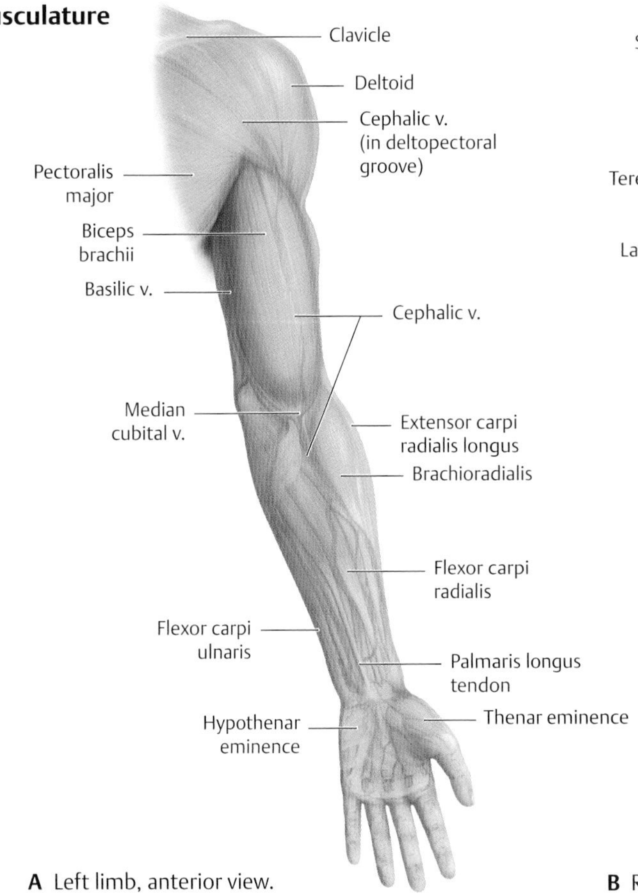

Clavicle
Deltoid
Cephalic v. (in deltopectoral groove)
Pectoralis major
Biceps brachii
Basilic v.
Cephalic v.
Median cubital v.
Extensor carpi radialis longus
Brachioradialis
Flexor carpi radialis
Flexor carpi ulnaris
Palmaris longus tendon
Hypothenar eminence
Thenar eminence

A Left limb, anterior view.

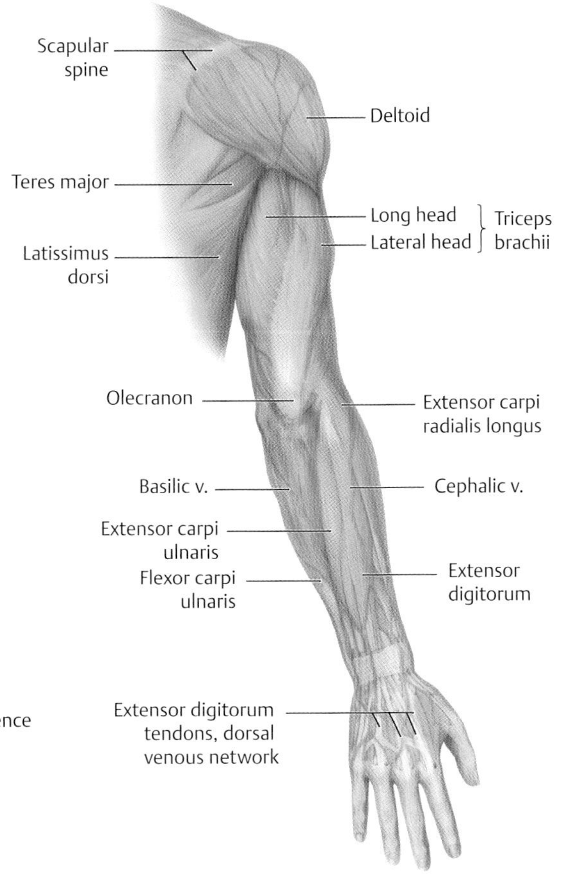

Scapular spine
Deltoid
Teres major
Long head ⎫ Triceps
Lateral head ⎭ brachii
Latissimus dorsi
Olecranon
Extensor carpi radialis longus
Basilic v.
Cephalic v.
Extensor carpi ulnaris
Flexor carpi ulnaris
Extensor digitorum
Extensor digitorum tendons, dorsal venous network

B Right limb, posterior view.

Fig. 24.3 **Palpable bony prominences of the upper limb**

Except for the lunate and trapezoid bones, all of the bones in the upper limb are palpable to some degree through the skin and soft tissues.

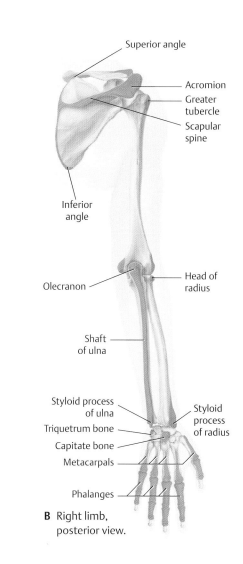
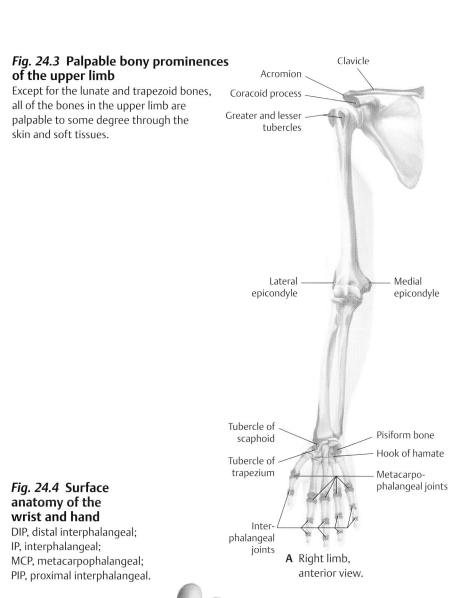

Clavicle

Acromion

Coracoid process

Greater and lesser tubercles

Superior angle

Acromion

Greater tubercle

Scapular spine

Inferior angle

Lateral epicondyle

Medial epicondyle

Olecranon

Head of radius

Shaft of ulna

Tubercle of scaphoid

Pisiform bone

Hook of hamate

Tubercle of trapezium

Metacarpo-phalangeal joints

Inter-phalangeal joints

Styloid process of ulna

Triquetrum bone

Capitate bone

Metacarpals

Phalanges

Styloid process of radius

A Right limb, anterior view.

B Right limb, posterior view.

Fig. 24.4 **Surface anatomy of the wrist and hand**

DIP, distal interphalangeal; IP, interphalangeal; MCP, metacarpophalangeal; PIP, proximal interphalangeal.

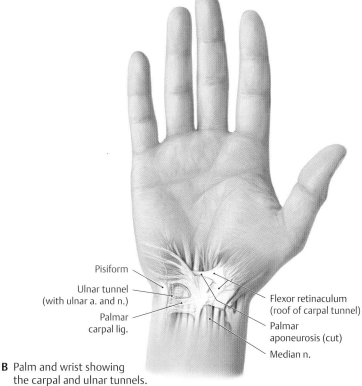

DIP joint crease

PIP joint crease

MCP joint crease

IP joint crease

MCP joint crease

Thenar eminence

Thenar crease ("life line")

Distal transverse crease

Proximal trans-verse crease

Middle crease

Hypothenar eminence

Distal wrist crease

Proximal wrist crease

Left palm and wrist.

Pisiform

Ulnar tunnel (with ulnar a. and n.)

Palmar carpal lig.

Flexor retinaculum (roof of carpal tunnel)

Palmar aponeurosis (cut)

Median n.

B Palm and wrist showing the carpal and ulnar tunnels.

Bones of the Upper Limb

Fig. 25.1 Bones of the upper limb

Right limb. The upper limb is subdivided into three regions: arm, forearm, and hand. The shoulder girdle (clavicle and scapula) joins the upper limb to the thorax at the sternoclavicular joint.

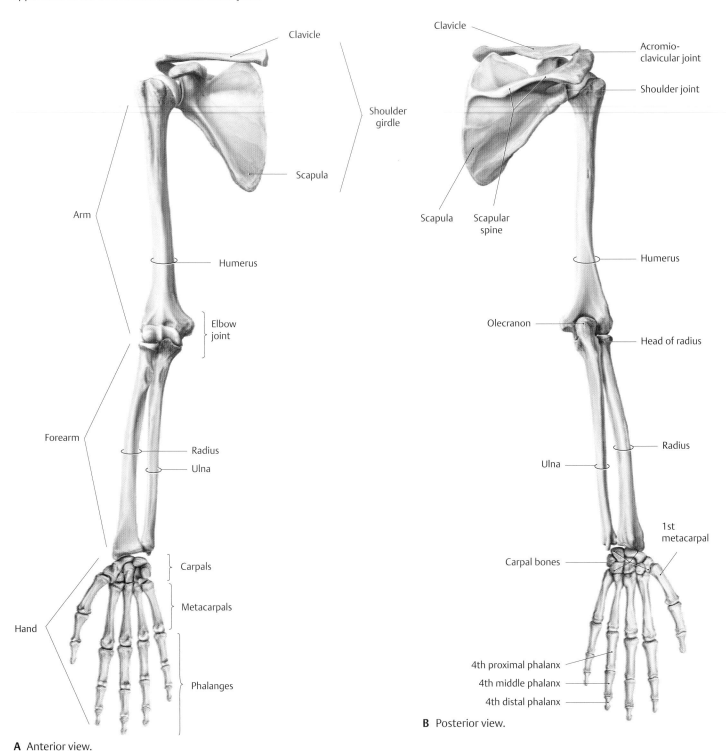

A Anterior view.

B Posterior view.

Fig. 25.2 Bones of the shoulder girdle in normal relation to those of the trunk

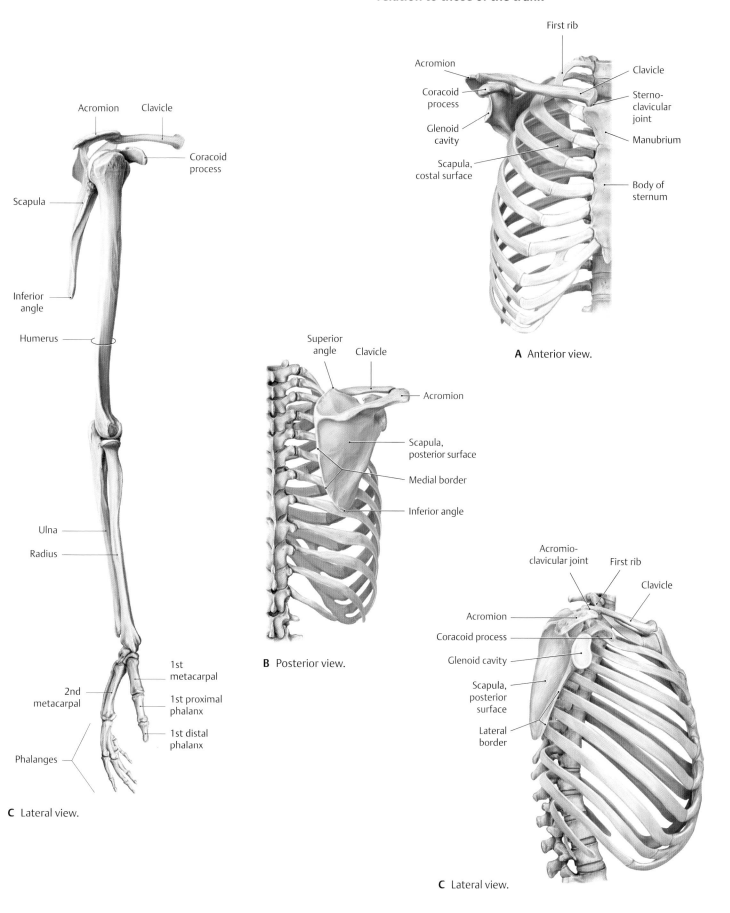

A Anterior view.

B Posterior view.

C Lateral view.

C Lateral view.

Clavicle & Scapula

 The shoulder girdle (clavicle and scapula) connects the bones of the upper limb to the thoracic cage. Whereas the pelvic girdle (paired hip bones) is firmly integrated into the axial skeleton (see **pp. 228–229**), the shoulder girdle is extremely mobile.

Fig. 25.3 **Clavicle**

Right clavicle. The S-shaped clavicle is visible and palpable along its entire length (generally 12 to 15 cm). Its medial end articulates with the sternum at the sternoclavicular joint (see **p. 299**). Its lateral end articulates with the scapula at the acromioclavicular joint (see **p. 299**).

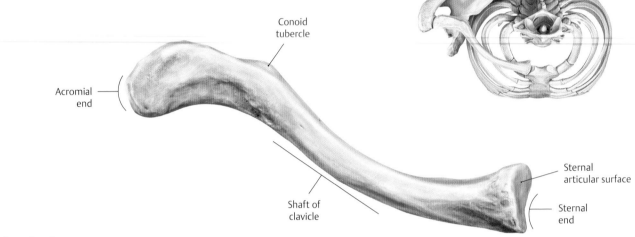

Conoid tubercle

Acromial end

Sternal articular surface

Shaft of clavicle

Sternal end

A Superior view.

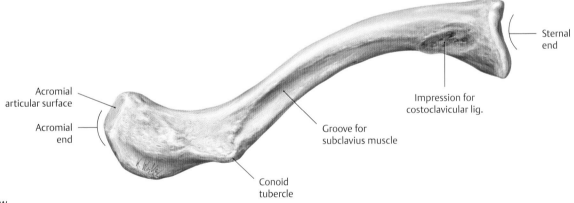

Sternal end

Acromial articular surface

Acromial end

Conoid tubercle

Groove for subclavius muscle

Impression for costoclavicular lig.

B Inferior view.

✦ *Clinical box 25.1*

Scapular foramen

The superior transverse ligament of the scapula (see **Fig. 25.13, p. 301**) may become ossified, transforming the scapular notch into an anomalous bony canal, the scapular foramen. This can lead to compression of the suprascapular nerve as it passes through the canal (see **p. 377**).

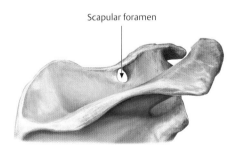

Scapular foramen

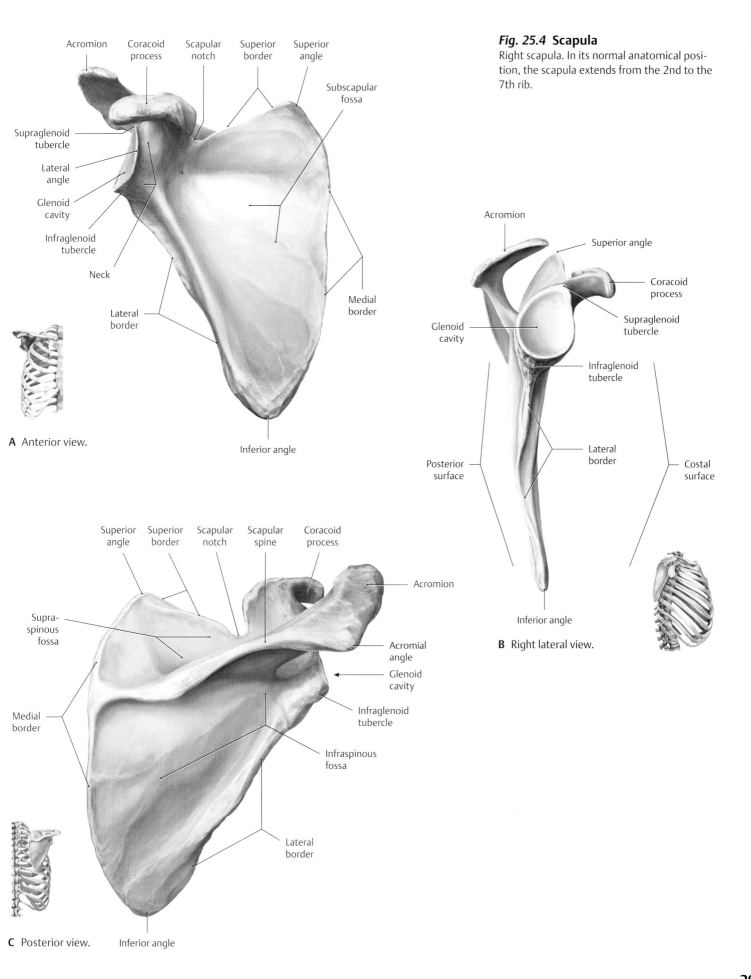

Fig. 25.4 Scapula

Right scapula. In its normal anatomical position, the scapula extends from the 2nd to the 7th rib.

Acromion
Coracoid process
Scapular notch
Superior border
Superior angle
Subscapular fossa
Supraglenoid tubercle
Lateral angle
Glenoid cavity
Infraglenoid tubercle
Neck
Lateral border
Medial border

A Anterior view.

Inferior angle

Acromion
Superior angle
Coracoid process
Supraglenoid tubercle
Glenoid cavity
Infraglenoid tubercle
Posterior surface
Lateral border
Costal surface
Inferior angle

B Right lateral view.

Superior angle
Superior border
Scapular notch
Scapular spine
Coracoid process
Acromion
Supra-spinous fossa
Acromial angle
Glenoid cavity
Infraglenoid tubercle
Medial border
Infraspinous fossa
Lateral border
Inferior angle

C Posterior view.

Humerus

Fig. 25.5 **Humerus**

Right humerus. The head of the humerus articulates with the scapula at the glenohumeral joint (see **p. 300**). The capitulum and trochlea of the humerus articulate with the radius and ulna, respectively, at the elbow (cubital) joint (see **p. 322**).

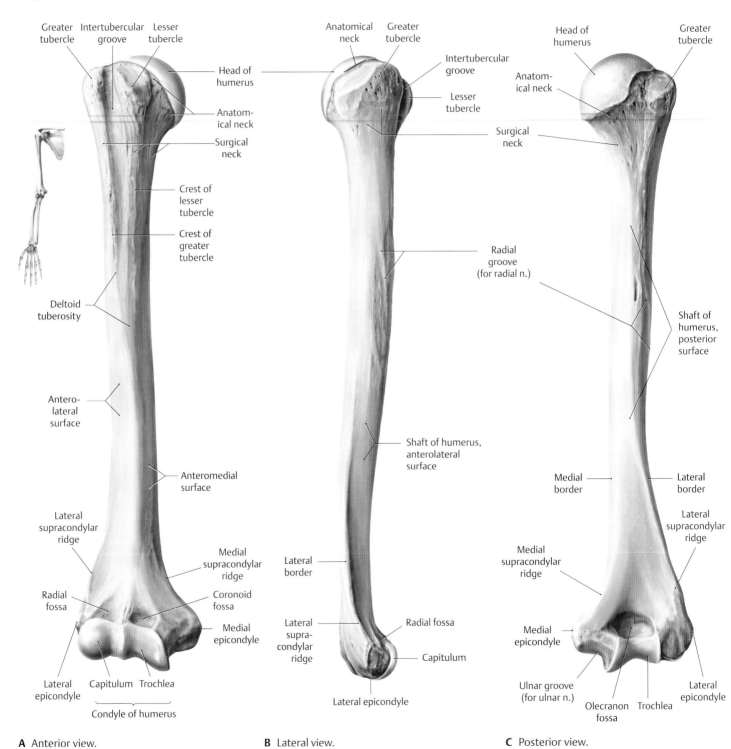

A Anterior view.

B Lateral view.

C Posterior view.

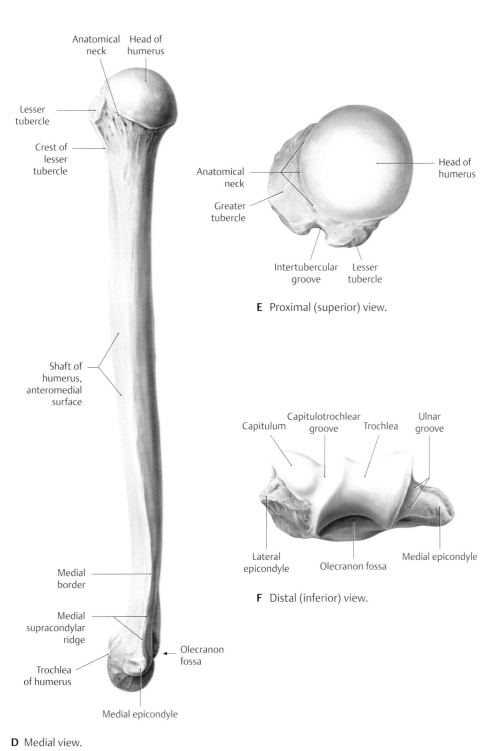

Anatomical neck
Head of humerus
Lesser tubercle
Crest of lesser tubercle

Shaft of humerus, anteromedial surface

Medial border

Medial supracondylar ridge

Olecranon fossa

Trochlea of humerus

Medial epicondyle

D Medial view.

Anatomical neck

Greater tubercle

Head of humerus

Intertubercular groove

Lesser tubercle

E Proximal (superior) view.

Capitulum
Capitulotrochlear groove
Trochlea
Ulnar groove

Lateral epicondyle
Olecranon fossa
Medial epicondyle

F Distal (inferior) view.

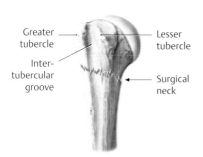

Clinical box 25.2

Fractures of the humerus
Anterior view. Fractures of the proximal humerus are very common and occur predominantly in older patients who sustain a fall onto the outstretched arm or directly onto the shoulder. Three main types are distinguished.

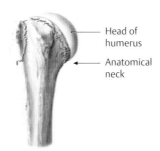

Greater tubercle

Lesser tubercle

Inter-tubercular groove

Surgical neck

A Extra-articular fracture.

Head of humerus

Anatomical neck

B Intra-articular fracture.

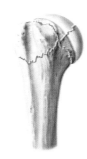

C Comminuted fracture.

Extra-articular fractures and intra-articular fractures are often accompanied by injuries of the blood vessels that supply the humeral head (anterior and posterior circumflex humeral arteries), with an associated risk of post-traumatic avascular necrosis.

Fractures of the humeral shaft and distal humerus are frequently associated with damage to the radial nerve.

Joints of the Shoulder

***Fig. 25.6* Joints of the shoulder: Overview**
Right shoulder, anterior view.

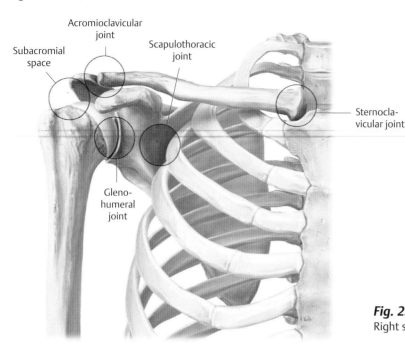

- Subacromial space
- Acromioclavicular joint
- Scapulothoracic joint
- Sternocla-vicular joint
- Gleno-humeral joint

***Fig. 25.7* Joints of the shoulder girdle**
Right side, superior view.

- Acromioclavicular joint (with acromio-clavicular lig.)
- Coraco-acromial lig.
- Glenohumeral joint
- Scapulothoracic joint
- Posterior sternoclavicular lig.
- Sternoclavicular joint (with anterior sternoclavicular lig.)

***Fig. 25.8* Scapulothoracic joint**
Right side, superior view. In all movements of the shoulder girdle, the scapula glides on a curved surface of loose connective tissue between the serratus anterior and the subscapularis muscles. This surface can be considered a scapulothoracic joint.

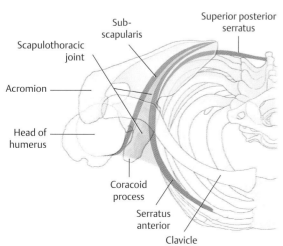
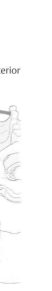

- Sub-scapularis
- Superior posterior serratus
- Scapulothoracic joint
- Acromion
- Head of humerus
- Coracoid process
- Serratus anterior
- Clavicle

Fig. 25.9 Sternoclavicular joint

Anterior view with sternum coronally sectioned (left). *Note:* A fibrocartilaginous articular disk compensates for the mismatch of surfaces between the two saddle-shaped articular facets of the clavicle and the manubrium.

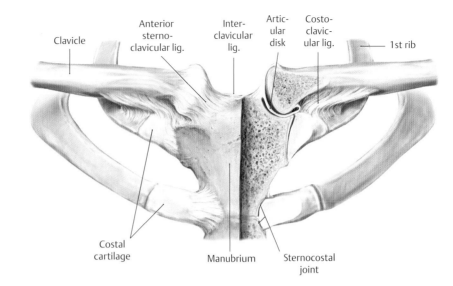

Clavicle — Anterior sterno-clavicular lig. — Inter-clavicular lig. — Artic-ular disk — Costo-clavic-ular lig. — 1st rib

Costal cartilage — Manubrium — Sternocostal joint

Fig. 25.10 Acromioclavicular joint

Anterior view. The acromioclavicular joint is a plane joint. Because the articulating surfaces are flat, they must be held in place by strong ligaments, greatly limiting the mobility of the joint.

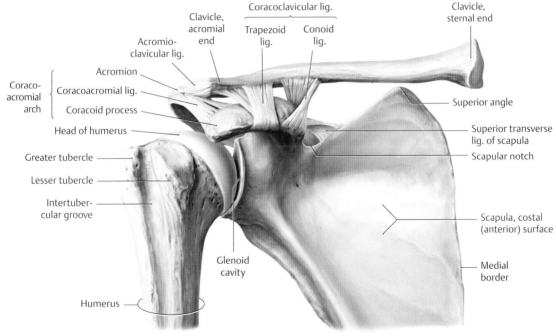

Clavicle, acromial end — Coracoclavicular lig. — Trapezoid lig. — Conoid lig. — Clavicle, sternal end

Acromio-clavicular lig. — Acromion — Coracoacromial lig. — Coracoid process — Head of humerus — Coraco-acromial arch

Greater tubercle — Lesser tubercle — Intertuber-cular groove

Superior angle — Superior transverse lig. of scapula — Scapular notch

Glenoid cavity — Scapula, costal (anterior) surface — Medial border

Humerus

 Clinical box 25.3

Injuries of the acromioclavicular joint

A fall onto the outstretched arm or shoulder frequently causes dislocation of the acromioclavicular joint and damage to the coracoclavicular ligaments.

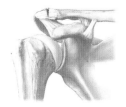

A Stretching of acromio-clavicular ligaments.

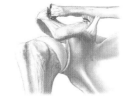

B Rupture of acromioclavicular ligament.

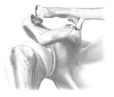

C Complete dislocation of acromioclavicular joint. Note rupture of acromioclavicular and coracoclavicular ligaments.

Joints of the Shoulder: Glenohumeral Joint

Fig. 25.11 Glenohumeral joint: Bony elements
Right shoulder.

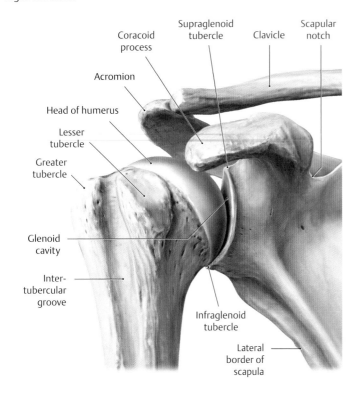

A Anterior view.

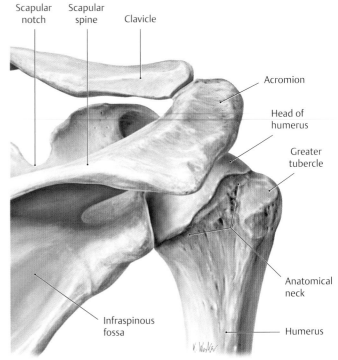

B Posterior view.

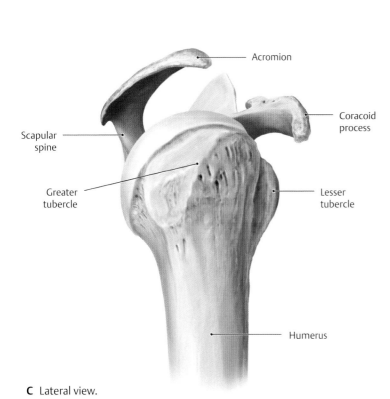

C Lateral view.

Fig. 25.12 Glenohumeral joint cavity

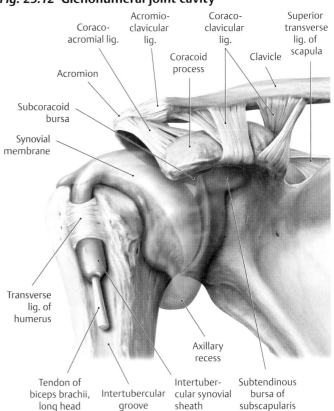

Fig. 25.13 Glenohumeral joint: Capsule and ligaments

Right shoulder.

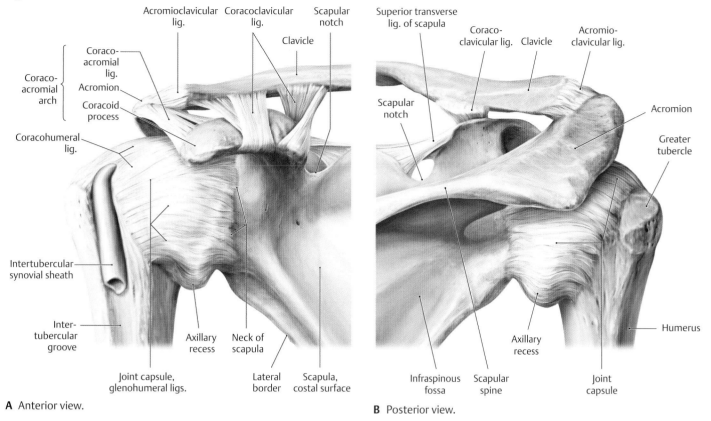

A Anterior view.

B Posterior view.

Fig. 25.14 Ligaments reinforcing capsule

Schematic representation of the ligaments reinforcing the capsule after removal of the humeral head. Right shoulder.

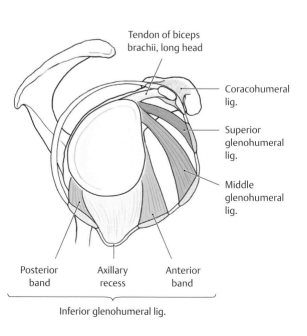

A Lateral view.

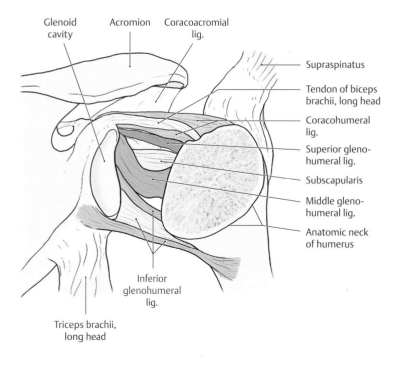

B Posterior view.

Subacromial Space & Bursae

Fig. 25.15 **Subacromial space**
Right shoulder.

Fig. 25.16 **Subacromial bursa and glenoid cavity**
Right shoulder, lateral view of sagittal section with humerus removed.

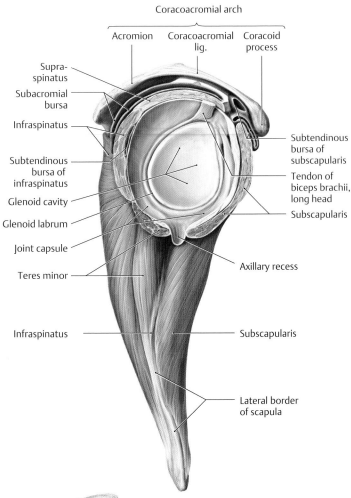

Coracoacromial arch

Acromion Coracoacromial lig. Coracoid process

Subacromial bursa

Subdeltoid bursa

Infraspinatus

Teres minor

Humerus

Subtendinous bursa of subscapularis

Greater tubercle

Transverse lig. of humerus

Intertubercular tendon sheath

Biceps brachii, short head

Biceps brachii, long head

A Lateral view.

Coracoacromial arch

Acromion Coracoacromial lig. Coracoid process

Supraspinatus

Subacromial bursa

Infraspinatus

Subtendinous bursa of infraspinatus

Glenoid cavity

Glenoid labrum

Joint capsule

Teres minor

Infraspinatus

Subtendinous bursa of subscapularis

Tendon of biceps brachii, long head

Subscapularis

Axillary recess

Subscapularis

Lateral border of scapula

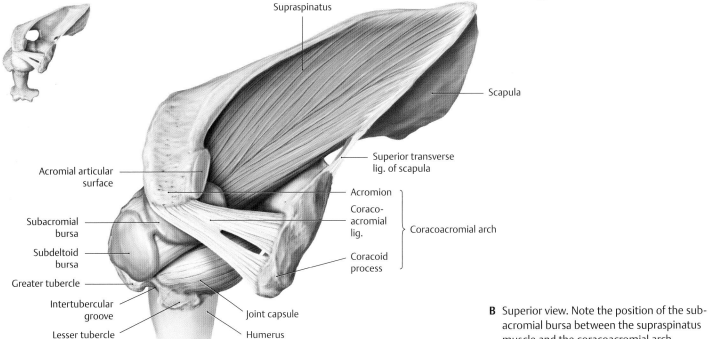

Supraspinatus

Scapula

Acromial articular surface

Superior transverse lig. of scapula

Acromion

Coraco-acromial lig.

Coracoid process

Coracoacromial arch

Subacromial bursa

Subdeltoid bursa

Greater tubercle

Intertubercular groove

Lesser tubercle

Joint capsule

Humerus

B Superior view. Note the position of the subacromial bursa between the supraspinatus muscle and the coracoacromial arch.

Fig. 25.17 **Subacromial and subdeltoid bursae**

Right shoulder, anterior view.

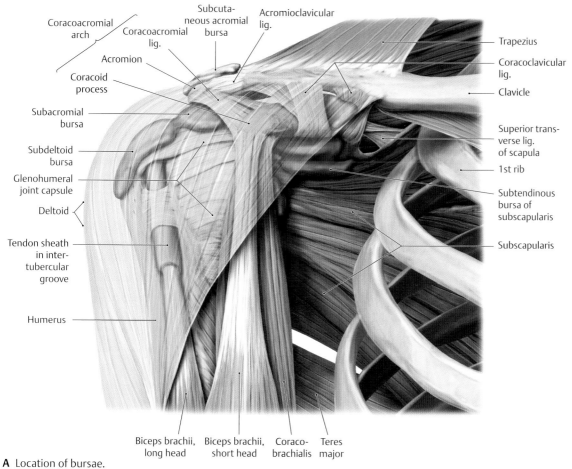

A Location of bursae.

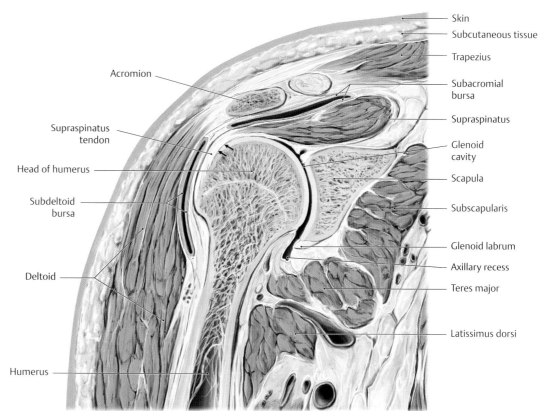

B Coronal section. The arrows are pointing at the supraspinatus tendon, which is frequently injured in a "rotator cuff tear" (for rotator cuff, see **p. 312**).

Anterior Muscles of the Shoulder & Arm (I)

Fig. 25.18 **Anterior muscles of the shoulder and arm**
Right side, anterior view. Muscle origins are shown in red,
insertions in blue.

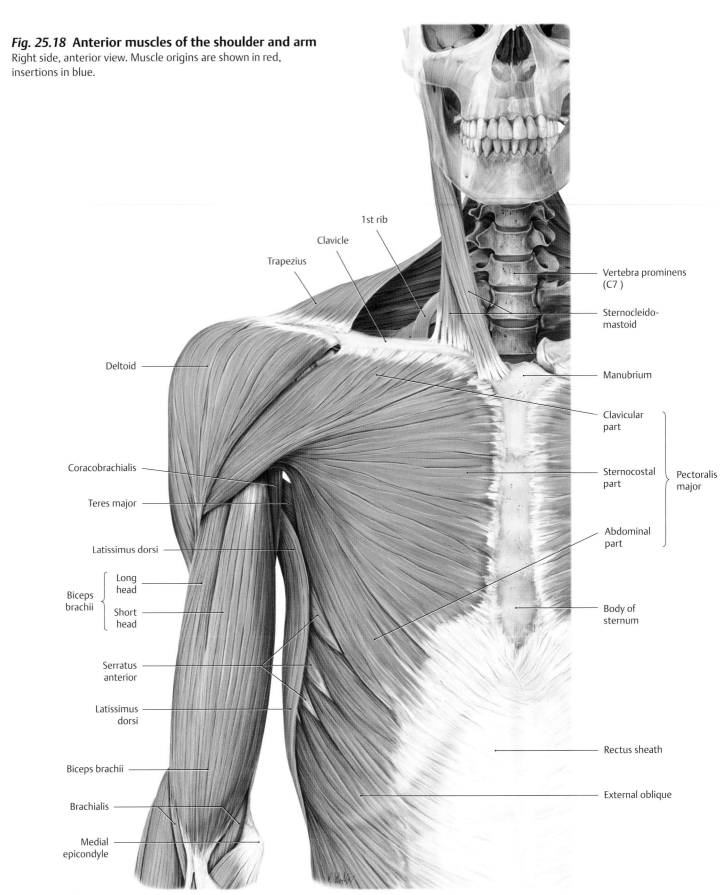

1st rib

Clavicle

Trapezius

Vertebra prominens
(C7)

Sternocleido-
mastoid

Deltoid

Manubrium

Clavicular
part

Coracobrachialis

Sternocostal
part

Pectoralis
major

Teres major

Abdominal
part

Latissimus dorsi

Long
head

Biceps
brachii

Short
head

Body of
sternum

Serratus
anterior

Latissimus
dorsi

Rectus sheath

Biceps brachii

External oblique

Brachialis

Medial
epicondyle

A Superficial dissection.

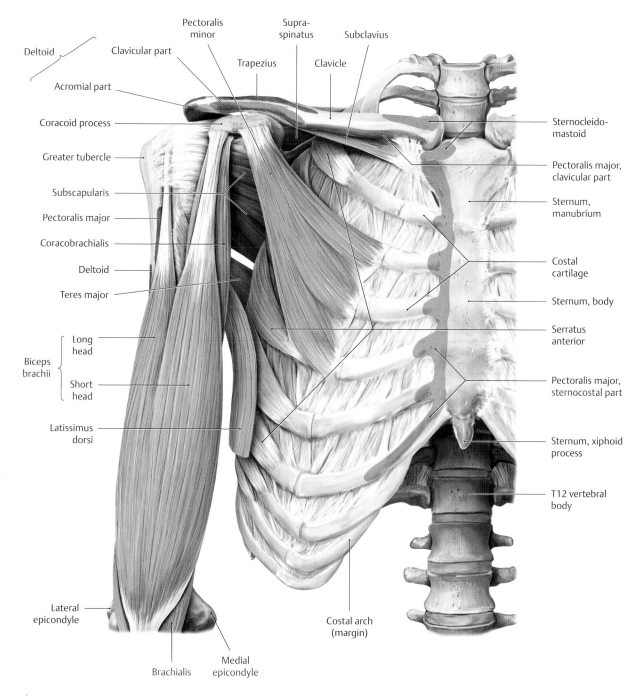

Deltoid

Clavicular part

Acromial part

Coracoid process

Greater tubercle

Subscapularis

Pectoralis major

Coracobrachialis

Deltoid

Teres major

Biceps brachii — Long head / Short head

Latissimus dorsi

Lateral epicondyle

Brachialis

Medial epicondyle

Pectoralis minor

Supra-spinatus

Trapezius

Clavicle

Subclavius

Sternocleido-mastoid

Pectoralis major, clavicular part

Sternum, manubrium

Costal cartilage

Sternum, body

Serratus anterior

Pectoralis major, sternocostal part

Sternum, xiphoid process

T12 vertebral body

Costal arch (margin)

B Deep dissection. *Removed:* Sternocleidomastoid, trapezius, pectoralis major, deltoid, and external oblique muscles.

Anterior Muscles of the Shoulder & Arm (II)

Fig. 25.19 **Anterior muscles of the shoulder and arm: Dissection**

Right arm, anterior view. Muscle origins are shown in red, insertions in blue.

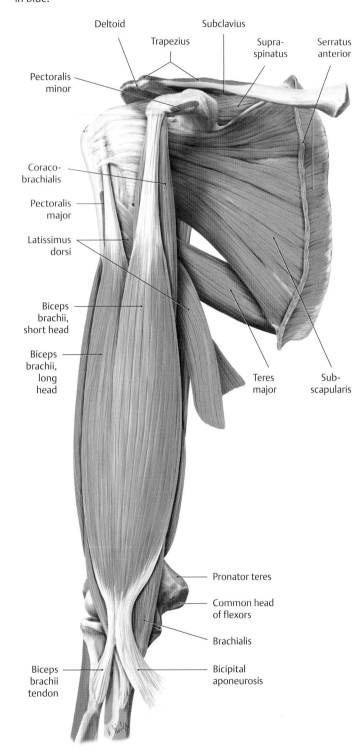

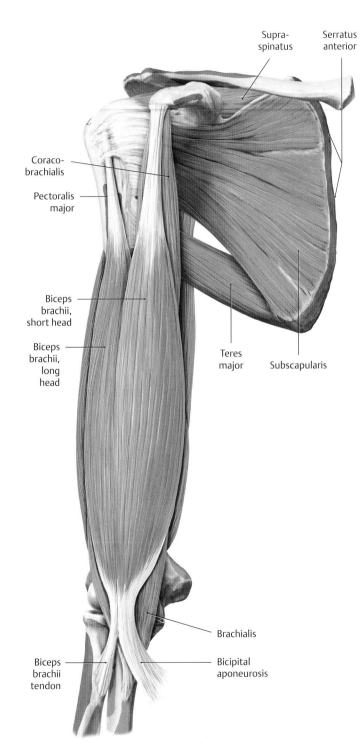

A *Removed:* Thoracic skeleton. *Partially removed:* Latissimus dorsi and serratus anterior.

B *Removed:* Latissimus dorsi and serratus anterior.

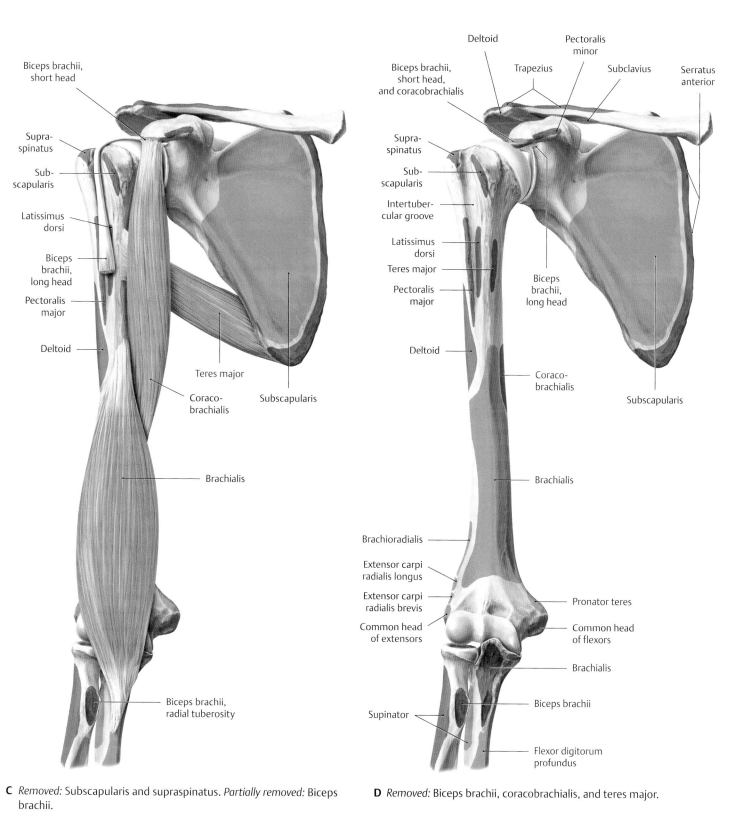

Biceps brachii, short head

Supra-spinatus

Sub-scapularis

Latissimus dorsi

Biceps brachii, long head

Pectoralis major

Deltoid

Teres major

Coraco-brachialis

Subscapularis

Brachialis

Biceps brachii, radial tuberosity

Deltoid

Pectoralis minor

Biceps brachii, short head, and coracobrachialis

Trapezius

Subclavius

Serratus anterior

Supra-spinatus

Sub-scapularis

Intertuber-cular groove

Latissimus dorsi

Teres major

Pectoralis major

Biceps brachii, long head

Deltoid

Coraco-brachialis

Subscapularis

Brachialis

Brachioradialis

Extensor carpi radialis longus

Extensor carpi radialis brevis

Common head of extensors

Pronator teres

Common head of flexors

Brachialis

Biceps brachii

Supinator

Flexor digitorum profundus

C *Removed:* Subscapularis and supraspinatus. *Partially removed:* Biceps brachii.

D *Removed:* Biceps brachii, coracobrachialis, and teres major.

307

Posterior Muscles of the Shoulder & Arm (I)

Fig. 25.20 **Posterior muscles of the shoulder and arm**
Right side, posterior view.

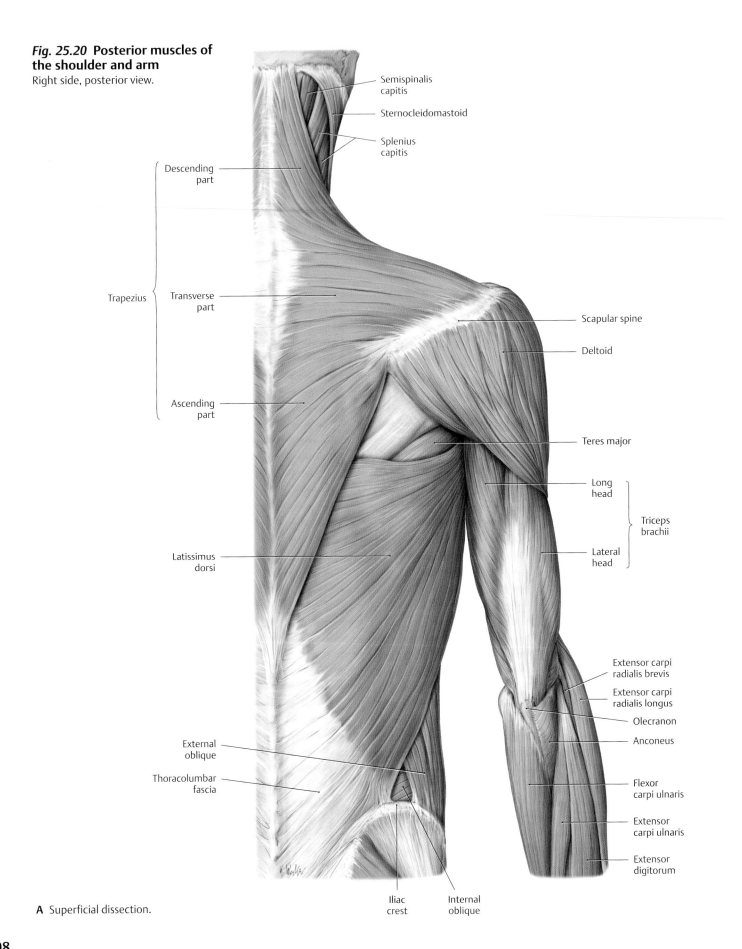

Semispinalis capitis

Sternocleidomastoid

Splenius capitis

Descending part

Transverse part

Trapezius

Ascending part

Scapular spine

Deltoid

Teres major

Long head

Triceps brachii

Lateral head

Latissimus dorsi

Extensor carpi radialis brevis

Extensor carpi radialis longus

Olecranon

Anconeus

External oblique

Thoracolumbar fascia

Flexor carpi ulnaris

Extensor carpi ulnaris

Extensor digitorum

Iliac crest

Internal oblique

A Superficial dissection.

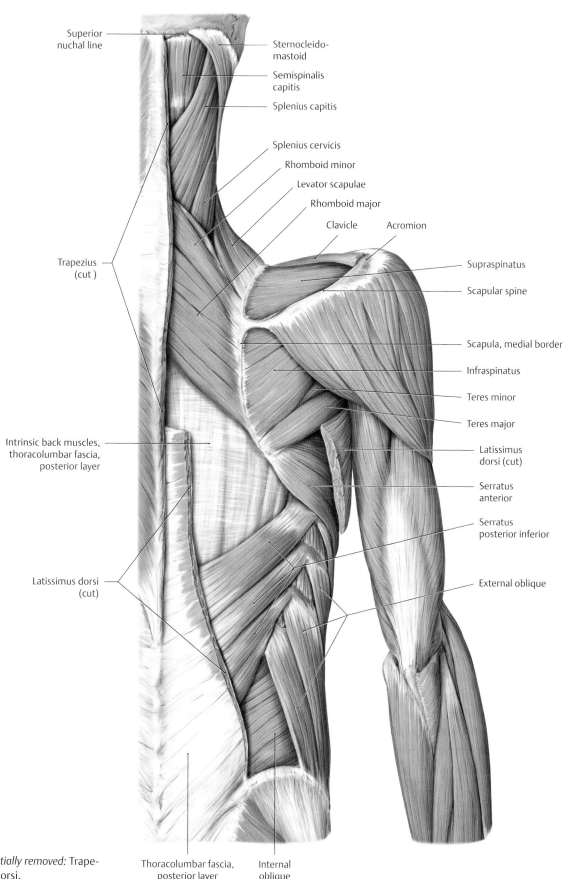

Superior
nuchal line

Sternocleido-
mastoid

Semispinalis
capitis

Splenius capitis

Splenius cervicis

Rhomboid minor

Levator scapulae

Rhomboid major

Clavicle   Acromion

Supraspinatus

Scapular spine

Trapezius
(cut)

Scapula, medial border

Infraspinatus

Teres minor

Teres major

Intrinsic back muscles,
thoracolumbar fascia,
posterior layer

Latissimus
dorsi (cut)

Serratus
anterior

Serratus
posterior inferior

Latissimus dorsi
(cut)

External oblique

Thoracolumbar fascia,
posterior layer

Internal
oblique

B Deep dissection. *Partially removed:* Trapezius and latissimus dorsi.

Posterior Muscles of the Shoulder & Arm (II)

***Fig. 25.21* Posterior muscles of the shoulder and arm: Dissection**

Right arm, posterior view. Muscle origins are shown in red, insertions in blue.

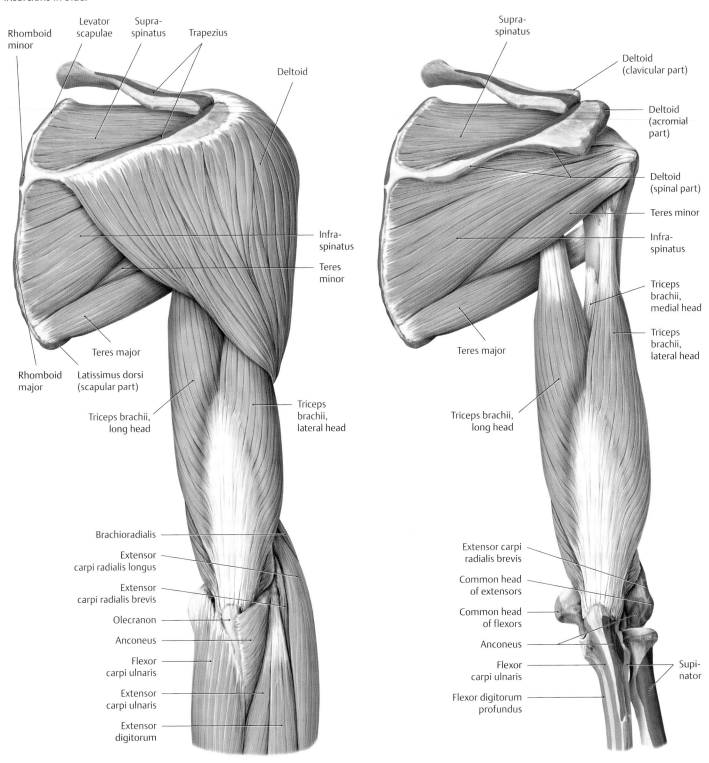

A *Removed:* Rhomboids major and minor, serratus anterior, and levator scapulae.

B *Removed:* Deltoid and forearm muscles.

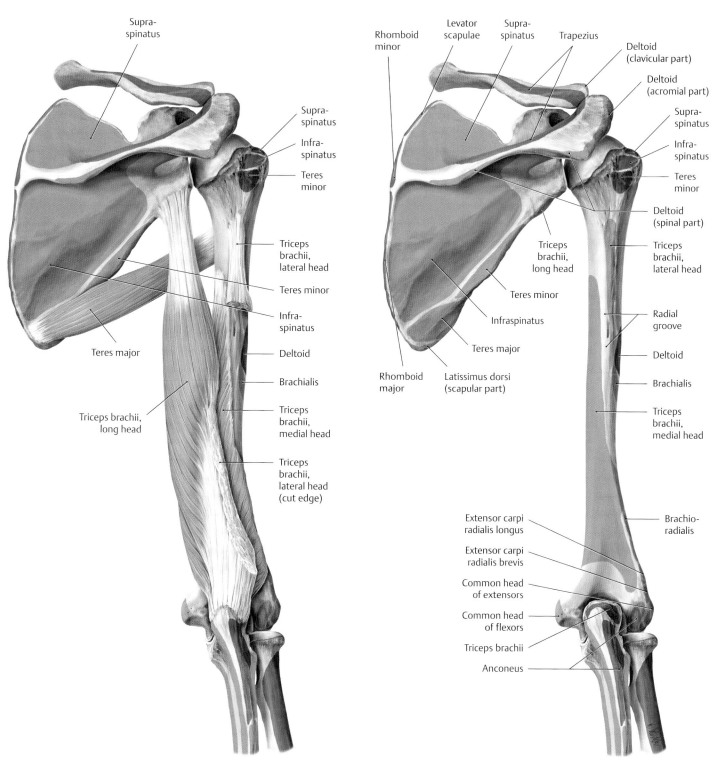

Supra-
spinatus

Supra-
spinatus

Infra-
spinatus

Teres
minor

Triceps
brachii,
lateral head

Teres minor

Infra-
spinatus

Deltoid

Brachialis

Teres major

Triceps brachii,
long head

Triceps
brachii,
medial head

Triceps
brachii,
lateral head
(cut edge)

Rhomboid
minor

Levator
scapulae

Supra-
spinatus

Trapezius

Deltoid
(clavicular part)

Deltoid
(acromial part)

Supra-
spinatus

Infra-
spinatus

Teres
minor

Deltoid
(spinal part)

Triceps
brachii,
long head

Triceps
brachii,
lateral head

Teres minor

Radial
groove

Infraspinatus

Deltoid

Teres major

Brachialis

Rhomboid
major

Latissimus dorsi
(scapular part)

Triceps
brachii,
medial head

Extensor carpi
radialis longus

Brachio-
radialis

Extensor carpi
radialis brevis

Common head
of extensors

Common head
of flexors

Triceps brachii

Anconeus

C *Removed:* Supraspinatus, infraspinatus, and teres minor. *Partially
removed:* Triceps brachii.

D *Removed:* Triceps brachii and teres major.

Muscle Facts (I)

The actions of the three parts of the deltoid muscle depend on their relationship to the position of the humerus and its axis of motion. At less than 60 degrees, the muscles act as adductors, but at greater than 60 degrees, they act as abductors. As a result, the parts of the deltoid can act antagonistically as well as synergistically.

Fig. 25.22 Deltoid
Right shoulder.

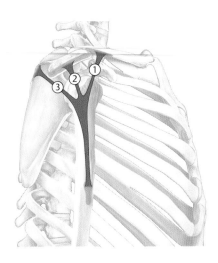

A Parts of the deltoid, right lateral view, schematic.

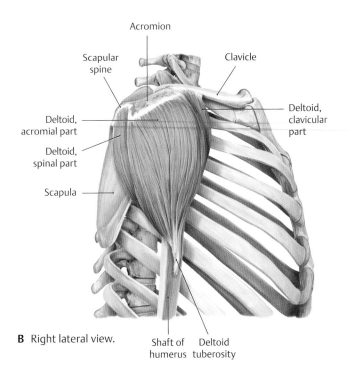

B Right lateral view.

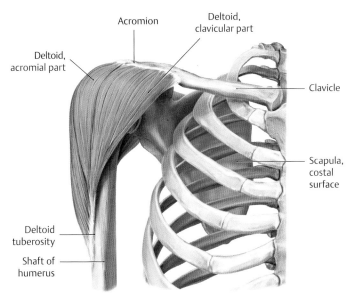

C Anterior view.

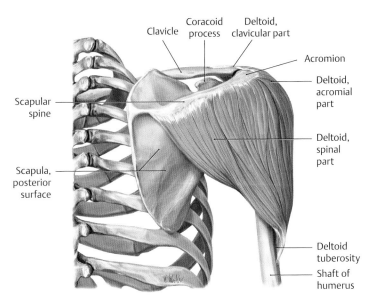

D Posterior view.

Table 25.1		Parts of the deltoid			
Muscle		**Origin**	**Insertion**	**Innervation**	**Action***
Deltoid	① Clavicular part	Lateral one third of clavicle	Humerus (deltoid tuberosity)	Axillary n. (C5, C6)	Flexion, internal rotation, adduction
	② Acromial part	Acromion			Abduction
	③ Spinal part	Scapular spine			Extension, external rotation, adduction

* Between 60 and 90 degrees of abduction, the clavicular and spinal parts assist the acromial part with abduction.

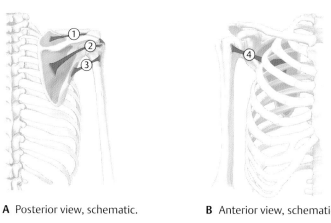

A Posterior view, schematic.   B Anterior view, schematic.

Fig. 25.23 Rotator cuff

Right shoulder. The rotator cuff consists of four muscles: supraspinatus, infraspinatus, teres minor, and subscapularis.

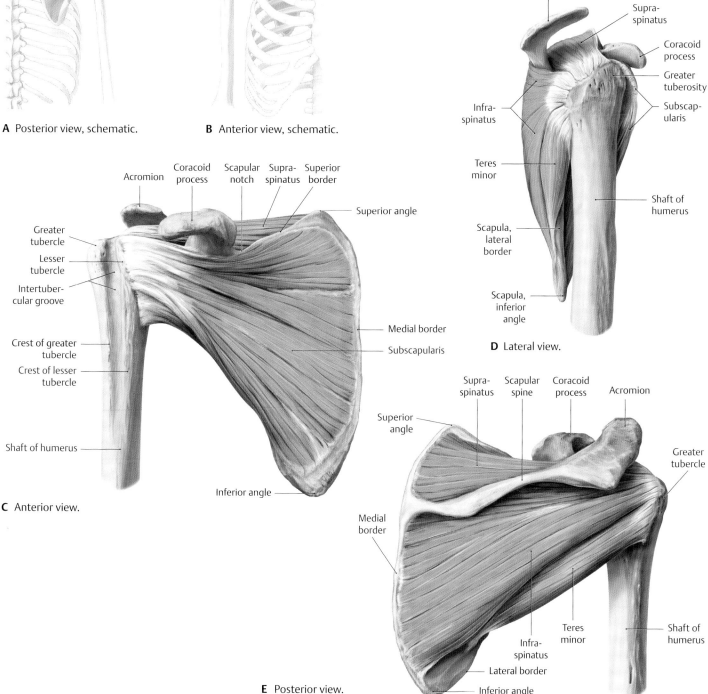

C Anterior view.
D Lateral view.
E Posterior view.

Table 25.2	Muscles of the rotator cuff				
Muscle	Origin	Insertion		Innervation	Action
① Supraspinatus		Supraspinous fossa		Suprascapular n. (C4–C6)	Abduction
② Infraspinatus		Infraspinous fossa	Humerus (greater tubercle)		External rotation
③ Teres minor	Scapula	Lateral border	Humerus	Axillary n. (C5, C6)	External rotation, weak adduction
④ Subscapularis		Subscapular fossa	Humerus (lesser tubercle)	Subscapular n. (C5, C6)	Internal rotation

313

Muscle Facts (II)

Fig. 25.24 **Pectoralis major and coracobrachialis**
Anterior view.

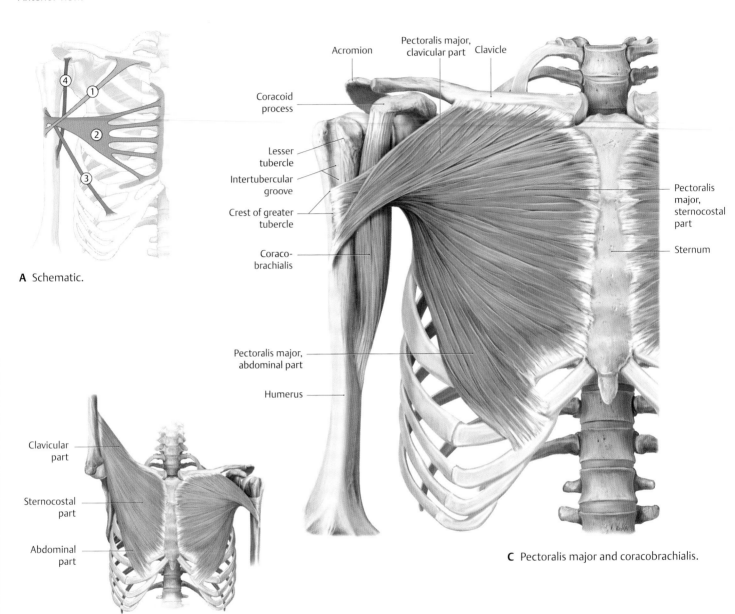

A Schematic.

B Pectoralis major in neutral position (left)
and elevation (right).

C Pectoralis major and coracobrachialis.

Table 25.3	Pectoralis major and coracobrachialis				
Muscle		**Origin**	**Insertion**	**Innervation**	**Action**
Pectoralis major	① Clavicular part	Clavicle (medial half)	Humerus (crest of greater tubercle)	Medial and lateral pectoral nn. (C5–T1)	Entire muscle: adduction, internal rotation Clavicular and sternocostal parts: flexion; assist in respiration when shoulder is fixed
	② Sternocostal part	Sternum and costal cartilages 1–6			
	③ Abdominal part	Rectus sheath (anterior layer)			
④ Coracobrachialis		Scapula (coracoid process)	Humerus (in line with crest of lesser tubercle)	Musculocutaneous nn. (C5–C7)	Flexion, adduction, internal rotation

Fig. 25.25 Subclavius and pectoralis minor

Right side, anterior view.

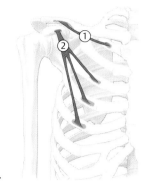

A Schematic.

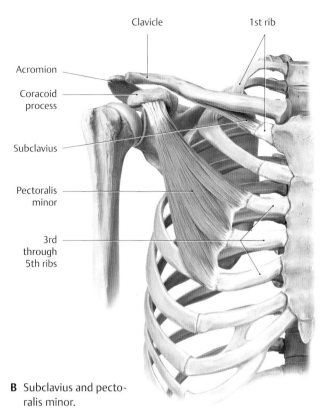

B Subclavius and pectoralis minor.

Fig. 25.26 Serratus anterior

Right lateral view.

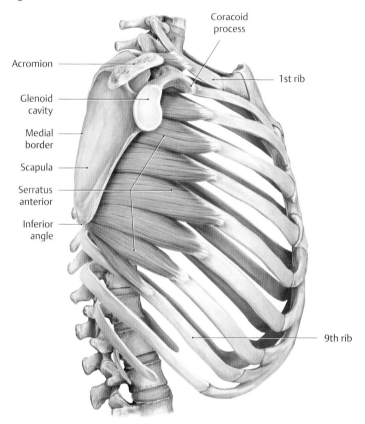

A Serratus anterior.

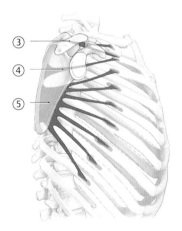

B Schematic.

Table 25.4		Subclavius, pectoralis minor, and serratus anterior			
Muscle		**Origin**	**Insertion**	**Innervation**	**Action**
① Subclavius		1st rib	Clavicle (inferior surface)	N. to subclavius (C5, C6)	Steadies the clavicle in the sternoclavicular joint
② Pectoralis minor		3rd to 5th ribs	Coracoid process	Medial pectoral n. (C8, T1)	Draws scapula downward, causing inferior angle to move posteromedially; rotates glenoid inferiorly; assists in respiration
Serratus anterior	③ Superior part	1st to 9th ribs	Scapula (costal and dorsal surfaces of superior angle)	Long thoracic n. (C5–C7)	Superior part: lowers the raised arm
	④ Intermediate part		Scapula (costal surface of medial border)		Entire muscle: draws scapula laterally forward; elevates ribs when shoulder is fixed
	⑤ Inferior part		Scapula (costal surface of medial border and costal and dorsal surfaces of inferior angle)		Inferior part: rotates inferior angle of scapula laterally forward (allows elevation of arm above 90°)

Muscle Facts (III)

Fig. 25.27 Trapezius
Posterior view.

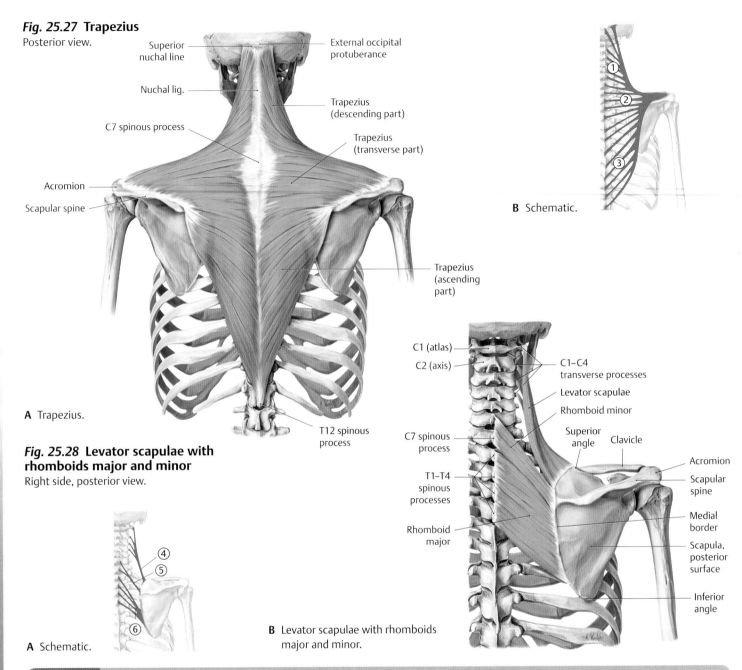

A Trapezius.

B Schematic.

Fig. 25.28 Levator scapulae with rhomboids major and minor
Right side, posterior view.

A Schematic.

B Levator scapulae with rhomboids major and minor.

Table 25.5	Trapezius, levator scapulae, and rhomboids major and minor				
Muscle		**Origin**	**Insertion**	**Innervation**	**Action**
Trapezius	① Descending part	Occipital bone; spinous processes of C1–C7	Clavicle (lateral one third)	Accessory n. (CN XI); C3–C4 of cervical plexus	Draws scapula obliquely upward; rotates glenoid cavity superiorly; tilts head to same side and rotates it to opposite
	② Transverse part	Aponeurosis at T1–T4 spinous processes	Acromion		Draws scapula medially
	③ Ascending part	Spinous processes of T5–T12	Scapular spine		Draws scapula medially downward
					Entire muscle: steadies scapula on thorax
④ Levator scapulae		Transverse processes of C1–C4	Scapula (superior angle)	Dorsal scapular n. and cervical spinal nn. (C3–C4)	Draws scapula medially upward while moving inferior angle medially; inclines neck to same side
⑤ Rhomboid minor		Spinous processes of C6, C7	Medial border of scapula above (minor) and below (major) scapular spine	Dorsal scapular n. (C4–C5)	Steadies scapula; draws scapula medially upward
⑥ Rhomboid major		Spinous processes of T1–T4 vertebrae			

CN, cranial nerve.

Fig. 25.29 Latissimus dorsi and teres major
Posterior view.

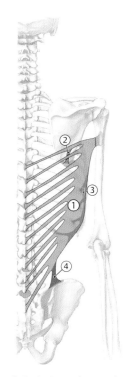

A Latissimus dorsi, schematic.

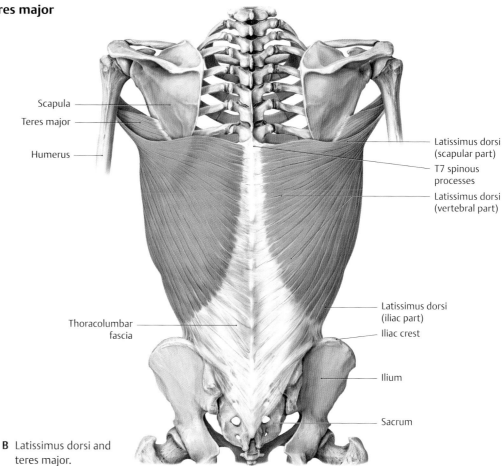

Scapula

Teres major

Humerus

Latissimus dorsi (scapular part)

T7 spinous processes

Latissimus dorsi (vertebral part)

Thoracolumbar fascia

Latissimus dorsi (iliac part)

Iliac crest

Ilium

Sacrum

B Latissimus dorsi and teres major.

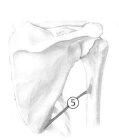

C Teres major, schematic.

D Insertion of the latissimus dorsi on the floor of the intertubercular groove and the teres major on the crest of the lesser tubercle of the humerus.

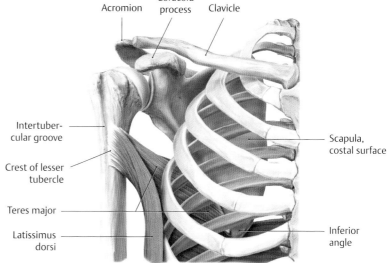

Acromion

Coracoid process

Clavicle

Intertubercular groove

Crest of lesser tubercle

Teres major

Latissimus dorsi

Scapula, costal surface

Inferior angle

Table 25.6		Latissimus dorsi and teres major			
Muscle		**Origin**	**Insertion**	**Innervation**	**Action**
Latissimus dorsi	① Vertebral part	Spinous processes of T7–T12 vertebrae; thoracolumbar fascia	Floor of the intertubercular groove of the humerus	Thoracodorsal n. (C6–C8)	Internal rotation, adduction, extension, respiration ("cough muscle")
	② Scapular part	Scapula (inferior angle)			
	③ Costal part	9th to 12th ribs			
	④ Iliac part	Iliac crest (posterior one third)			
⑤ Teres major		Scapula (inferior angle)	Crest of lesser tubercle of the humerus (anterior angle)	Lower subscapular n. (C5–C7)	Internal rotation, adduction, extension

Muscle Facts (IV)

The anterior and posterior muscles of the arm may be classified respectively as flexors and extensors relative to the movement of the elbow joint. Although the coracobrachialis is topographically part of the anterior compartment, it is functionally grouped with the muscles of the shoulder (see p. 314).

Fig. 25.30 Biceps brachii and brachialis
Right arm, anterior view.

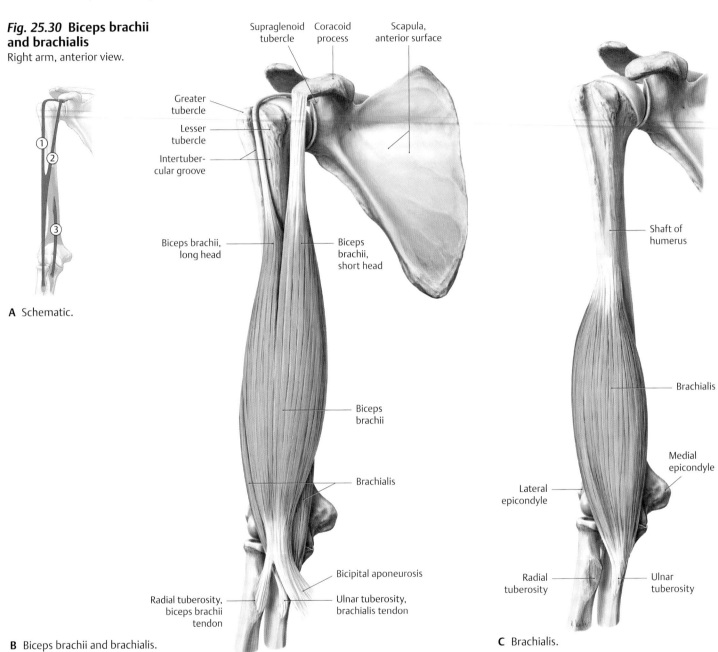

A Schematic.

B Biceps brachii and brachialis.

C Brachialis.

Table 25.7		Anterior muscles: Biceps brachii and brachialis			
Muscle		**Origin**	**Insertion**	**Innervation**	**Action**
Biceps brachii	① Long head	Supraglenoid tubercle of scapula	Radial tuberosity and bicipital aponeurosis	Musculocutaneous n. (C5–C6)	Elbow joint: flexion; supination* Shoulder joint: flexion; stabilization of humeral head during deltoid contraction; abduction and internal rotation of the humerus
	② Short head	Coracoid process of scapula			
③ Brachialis		Humerus (distal half of anterior surface)	Ulnar tuberosity	Musculocutaneous n. (C5–C6) and radial n. (C7, minor)	Flexion at the elbow joint
*Note: When the elbow is flexed, the biceps brachii acts as a powerful supinator because the lever arm is almost perpendicular to the axis of pronation/supination.					

Fig. 25.31 Triceps brachii and anconeus

Right arm, posterior view.

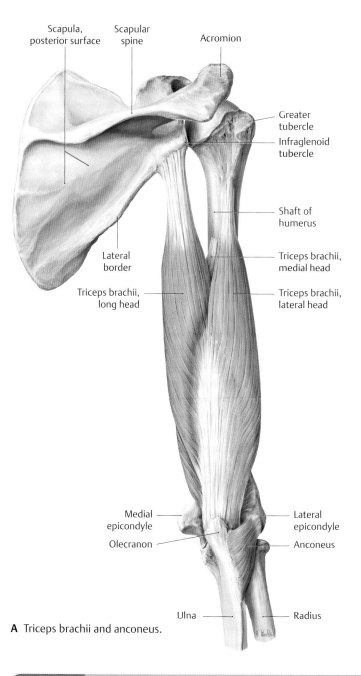

A Triceps brachii and anconeus.

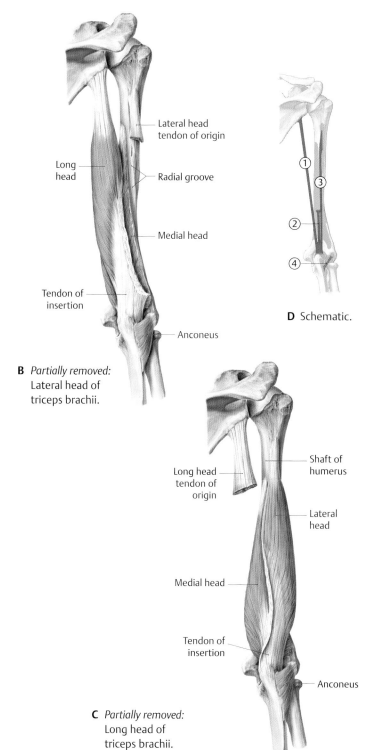

B *Partially removed:* Lateral head of triceps brachii.

D Schematic.

C *Partially removed:* Long head of triceps brachii.

Table 25.8		Posterior muscles: Triceps brachii and anconeus				
Muscle		**Origin**	**Insertion**		**Innervation**	**Action**
Triceps brachii	① Long head	Scapula (infraglenoid tubercle)	Olecranon of ulna		Radial n. (C6–C8)	Elbow joint: extension Shoulder joint, long head: extension and adduction
	② Medial head	Posterior humerus, distal to radial groove; medial intermuscular septum				
	③ Lateral head	Posterior humerus, proximal to radial groove; lateral intermuscular septum				
④ Anconeus		Lateral epicondyle of humerus (variance: posterior joint capsule)	Olecranon of ulna (radial surface)			Extends the elbow and tightens its joint

319

Radius & Ulna

Fig. 26.1 **Radius and ulna**
Right forearm.

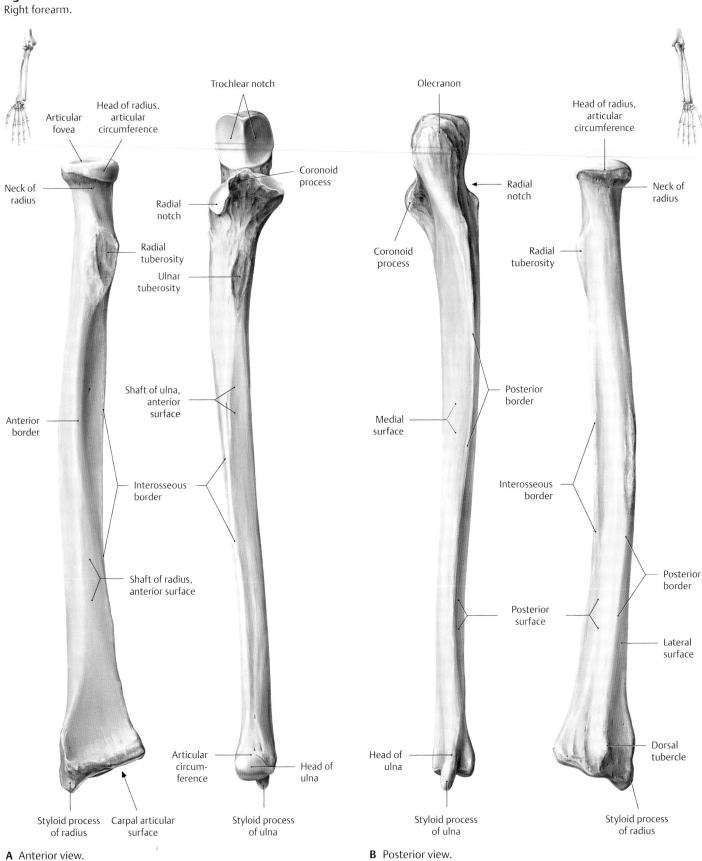

Trochlear notch

Head of radius, articular circumference

Articular fovea

Neck of radius

Coronoid process

Radial notch

Radial tuberosity

Ulnar tuberosity

Shaft of ulna, anterior surface

Anterior border

Interosseous border

Shaft of radius, anterior surface

Styloid process of radius

Carpal articular surface

Articular circum- ference

Head of ulna

Styloid process of ulna

Olecranon

Head of radius, articular circumference

Radial notch

Neck of radius

Coronoid process

Radial tuberosity

Posterior border

Medial surface

Interosseous border

Posterior surface

Posterior border

Lateral surface

Head of ulna

Dorsal tubercle

Styloid process of ulna

Styloid process of radius

A Anterior view.

B Posterior view.

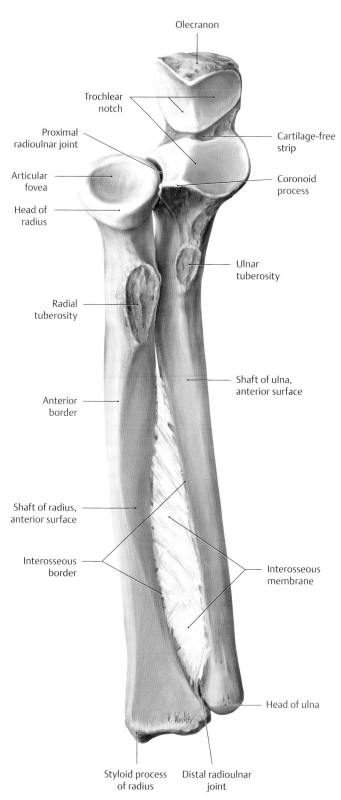

Olecranon

Trochlear notch

Proximal radioulnar joint

Articular fovea

Head of radius

Cartilage-free strip

Coronoid process

Ulnar tuberosity

Radial tuberosity

Anterior border

Shaft of ulna, anterior surface

Shaft of radius, anterior surface

Interosseous border

Interosseous membrane

Head of ulna

Styloid process of radius

Distal radioulnar joint

C Anterosuperior view.

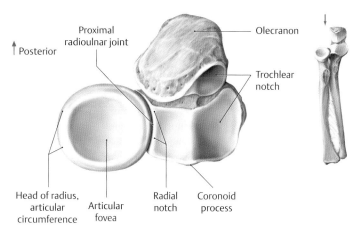

↑ Posterior

Proximal radioulnar joint

Olecranon

Trochlear notch

Head of radius, articular circumference

Articular fovea

Radial notch

Coronoid process

D Proximal view.

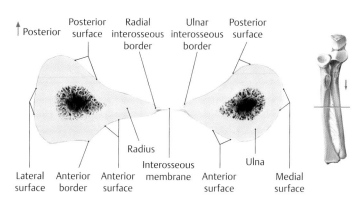

↑ Posterior

Posterior surface

Radial interosseous border

Ulnar interosseous border

Posterior surface

Lateral surface

Anterior border

Anterior surface

Radius

Interosseous membrane

Anterior surface

Ulna

Medial surface

E Transverse section, proximal view.

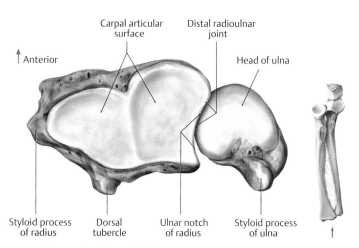

↑ Anterior

Carpal articular surface

Distal radioulnar joint

Head of ulna

Styloid process of radius

Dorsal tubercle

Ulnar notch of radius

Styloid process of ulna

F Distal arterial surfaces of radius and ulna, right forearm.

321

Elbow Joint

Fig. 26.2 Elbow (cubital) joint

Right limb. The elbow consists of three articulations between the humerus, ulna, and radius: the humeroulnar, humeroradial, and proximal radioulnar joints.

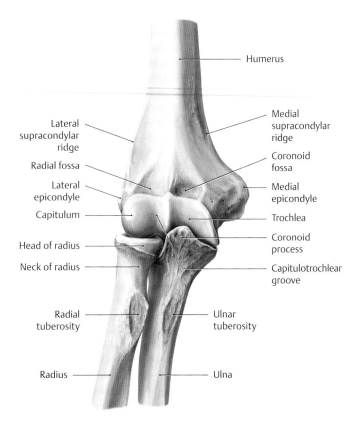

A Anterior view.

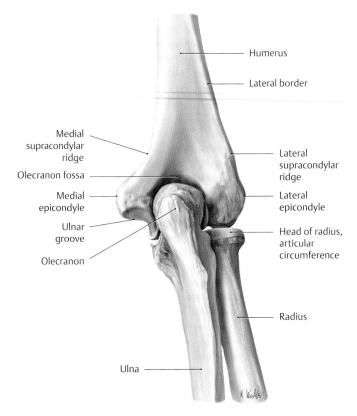

B Posterior view.

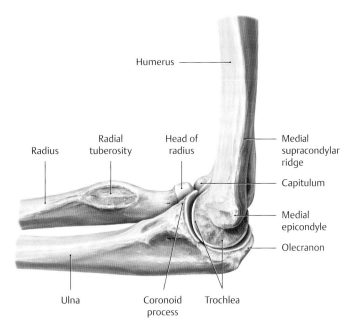

C Medial view.

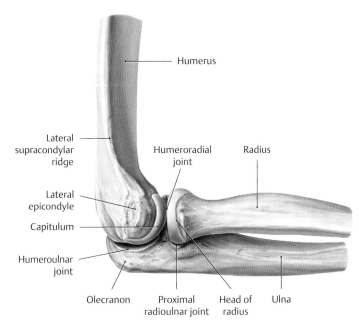

D Lateral view.

Fig. 26.3 Skeletal and soft-tissue elements of the right elbow joint

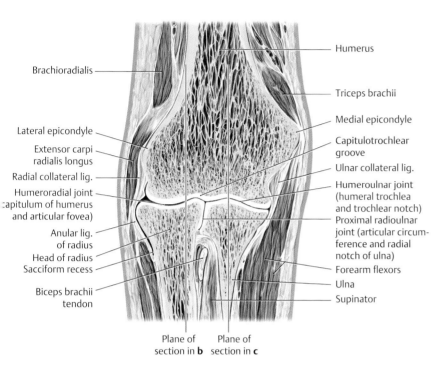

Brachioradialis

Lateral epicondyle

Extensor carpi radialis longus

Radial collateral lig.

Humeroradial joint (capitulum of humerus and articular fovea)

Anular lig. of radius

Head of radius

Sacciform recess

Biceps brachii tendon

Humerus

Triceps brachii

Medial epicondyle

Capitulotrochlear groove

Ulnar collateral lig.

Humeroulnar joint (humeral trochlea and trochlear notch)

Proximal radioulnar joint (articular circumference and radial notch of ulna)

Forearm flexors

Ulna

Supinator

Plane of section in **b**   Plane of section in **c**

A Coronal section viewed from the front (note the planes of section shown in **B** and **C**).

✱ Clinical box 26.1

Assessing elbow injuries

The fat pads between the fibrous capsule and synovial membrane are part of the normal anatomy of the elbow joint. The anterior pad is most readily seen on a sagittal MRI while the posterior pad is often hidden within the bony fossa (see **Figs. 26.3 and 29.11**). With an effusion of the joint space, the inferior edge of the anterior pad appears concave as it gets pushed superiorly by the intra-articular fluid. This causes the pad to resemble the shape of a ship's sail, thus creating a characteristic "sail sign." The alignment of the prominences in the elbow also aids in the identification of fractures and dislocations.

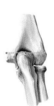

A Posterior view of extended elbow: The epicondyles and olecranon lie in a straight line.

B Medial view of flexed elbow: The epicondyles and olecranon lie in a straight line.

C Posterior view of flexed elbow: The two epicondyles and the tip of the olecranon form an equilateral triangle. Fractures and dislocations alter the shape of the triangle.

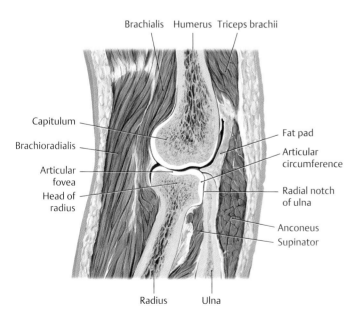

Brachialis   Humerus   Triceps brachii

Capitulum

Brachioradialis

Articular fovea

Head of radius

Fat pad

Articular circumference

Radial notch of ulna

Anconeus

Supinator

Radius   Ulna

B Sagittal section through the humeroradial joint and proximal radioulnar joint, medial view.

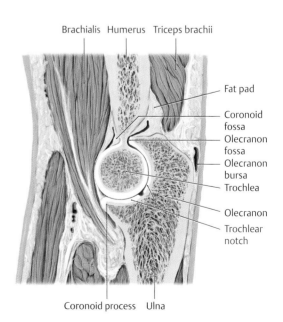

Brachialis   Humerus   Triceps brachii

Fat pad

Coronoid fossa

Olecranon fossa

Olecranon bursa

Trochlea

Olecranon

Trochlear notch

Coronoid process   Ulna

C Sagittal section through the humeroulnar joint, medial view.

Ligaments of the Elbow Joint

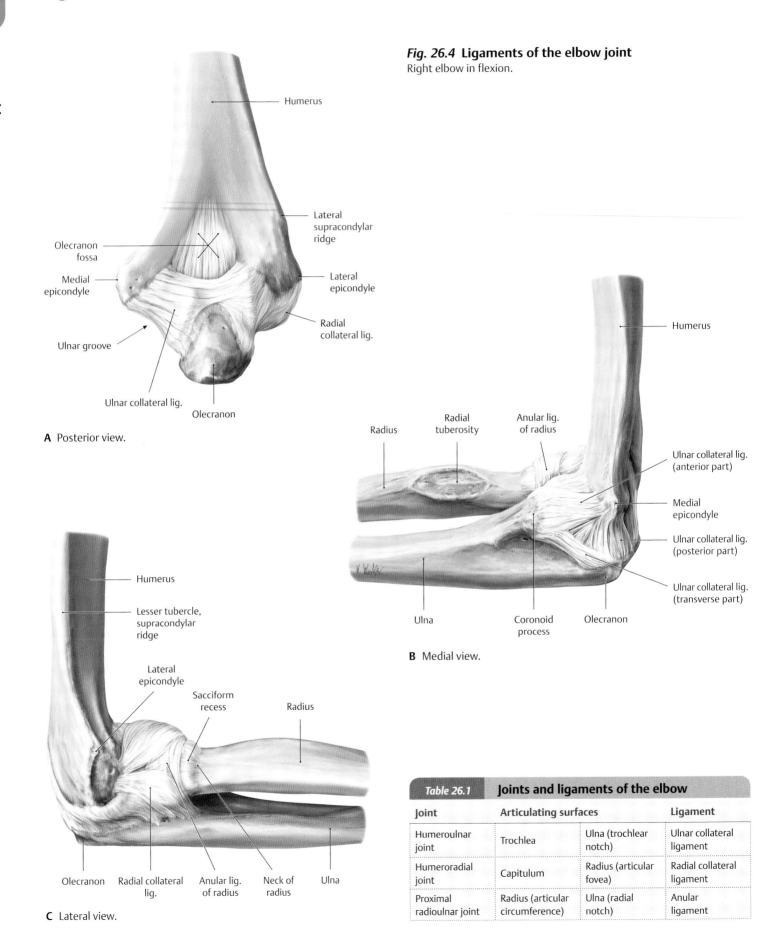

A Posterior view.

Labels in figure A:
- Humerus
- Lateral supracondylar ridge
- Olecranon fossa
- Medial epicondyle
- Lateral epicondyle
- Radial collateral lig.
- Ulnar groove
- Ulnar collateral lig.
- Olecranon

B Medial view.

Labels in figure B:
- Radius
- Radial tuberosity
- Anular lig. of radius
- Humerus
- Ulnar collateral lig. (anterior part)
- Medial epicondyle
- Ulnar collateral lig. (posterior part)
- Ulnar collateral lig. (transverse part)
- Ulna
- Coronoid process
- Olecranon

C Lateral view.

Labels in figure C:
- Humerus
- Lesser tubercle, supracondylar ridge
- Lateral epicondyle
- Sacciform recess
- Radius
- Olecranon
- Radial collateral lig.
- Anular lig. of radius
- Neck of radius
- Ulna

Fig. 26.4 **Ligaments of the elbow joint**
Right elbow in flexion.

Table 26.1	Joints and ligaments of the elbow		
Joint	**Articulating surfaces**		**Ligament**
Humeroulnar joint	Trochlea	Ulna (trochlear notch)	Ulnar collateral ligament
Humeroradial joint	Capitulum	Radius (articular fovea)	Radial collateral ligament
Proximal radioulnar joint	Radius (articular circumference)	Ulna (radial notch)	Anular ligament

Fig. 26.5 **Joint capsule of the elbow**
Right elbow in extension, anterior view.

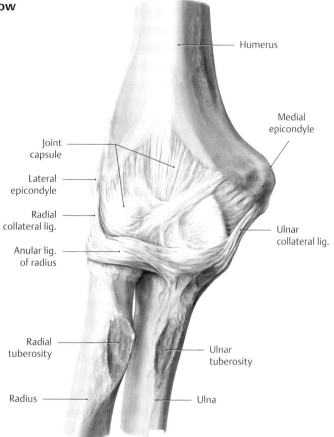

- Humerus
- Medial epicondyle
- Joint capsule
- Lateral epicondyle
- Radial collateral lig.
- Anular lig. of radius
- Ulnar collateral lig.
- Radial tuberosity
- Ulnar tuberosity
- Radius
- Ulna

A Intact joint capsule.

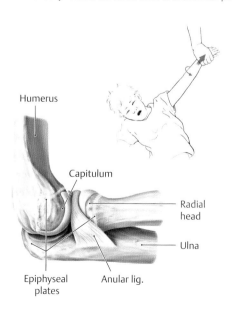
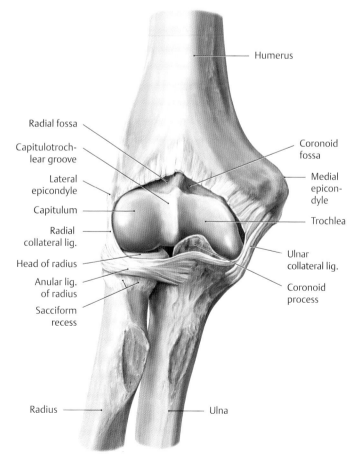

- Radial fossa
- Capitulotrochlear groove
- Lateral epicondyle
- Capitulum
- Radial collateral lig.
- Head of radius
- Anular lig. of radius
- Sacciform recess
- Humerus
- Coronoid fossa
- Medial epicondyle
- Trochlea
- Ulnar collateral lig.
- Coronoid process
- Radius
- Ulna

B Windowed joint capsule.

Radioulnar Joints

The proximal and distal radioulnar joints function together to enable pronation and supination movements of the hand. The joints are functionally linked by the interosseous membrane. The axis for pronation and supination runs obliquely from the center of the humeral capitulum through the center of the radial articular fovea down to the styloid process of the ulna.

Fig. 26.6 Supination
Right forearm, anterior view.

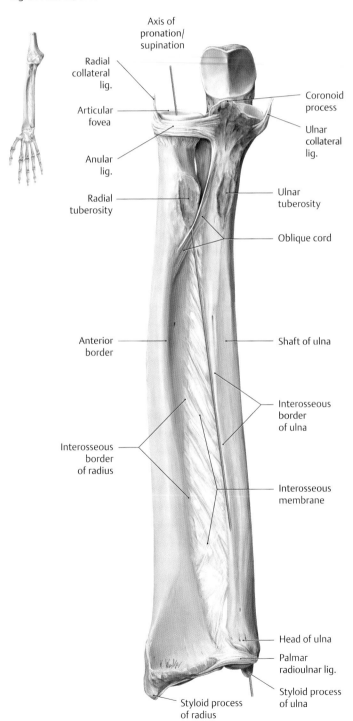

Fig. 26.7 Pronation
Right forearm, anterior view.

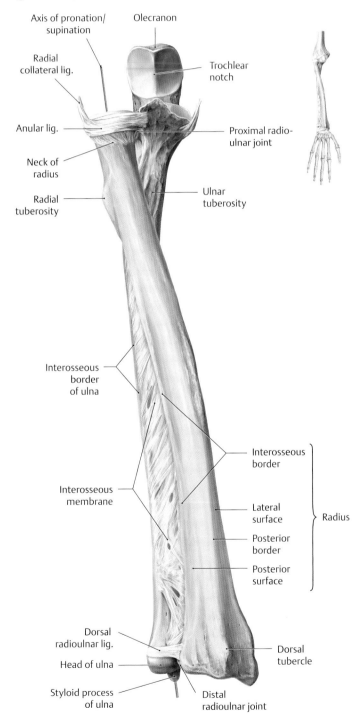

Upper Limb

Fig. 26.8 Proximal radioulnar joint

Right elbow, proximal (superior) view.

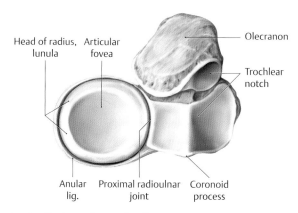

A Proximal articular surfaces of radius and ulna.

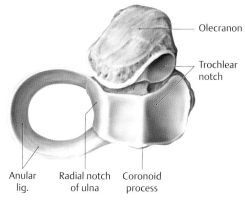

B Radius removed.

Fig. 26.9 Distal radioulnar joint rotation

Right forearm, distal view of articular surfaces of radius and ulna. The dorsal and palmar radioulnar ligaments stabilize the distal radioulnar joint.

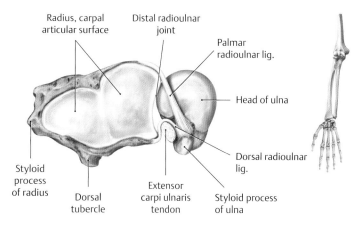

A Supination.

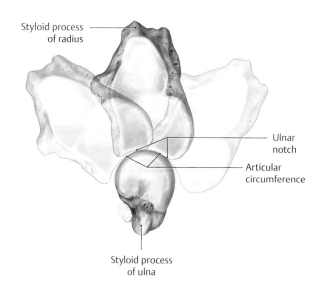

B Semipronation.

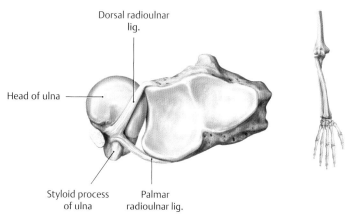

C Pronation.

Clinical box 26.3

Radius fracture

Falls onto the outstretched arm often result in fractures of the distal radius. In a Colles' fracture, the distal fragment is tilted dorsally.

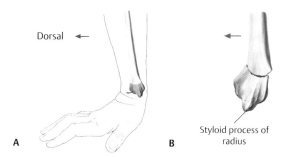

Muscles of the Forearm: Anterior Compartment

Fig. 26.10 Anterior muscles of the forearm: Dissection
Right forearm, anterior view. Muscle origins are shown in red,
insertions in blue.

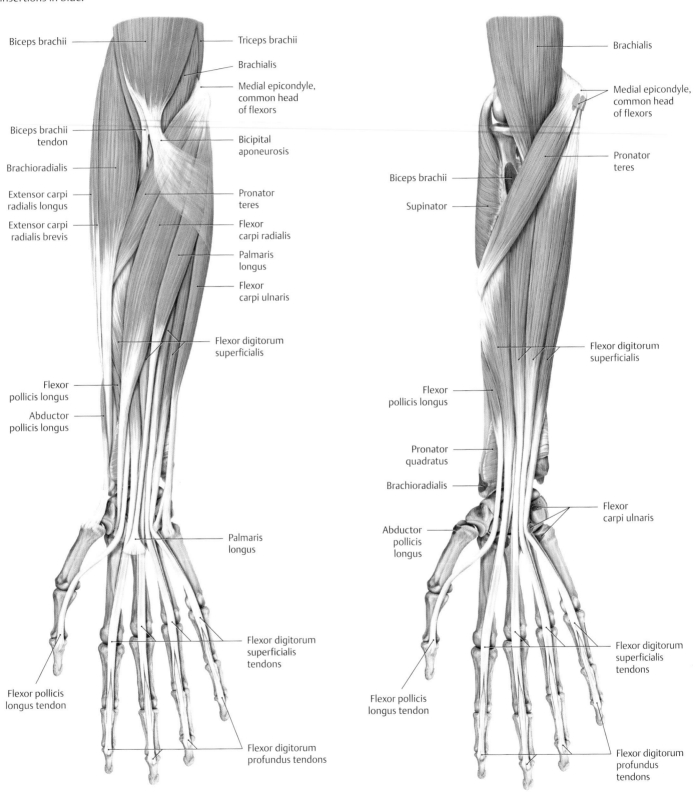

A Superficial flexors and radialis muscles.

B *Removed:* Radialis muscles (brachioradialis, extensor carpi radialis longus, and extensor carpi radialis brevis), flexor carpi radialis, flexor carpi
ulnaris, abductor pollicis longus, palmaris longus, and biceps brachii.

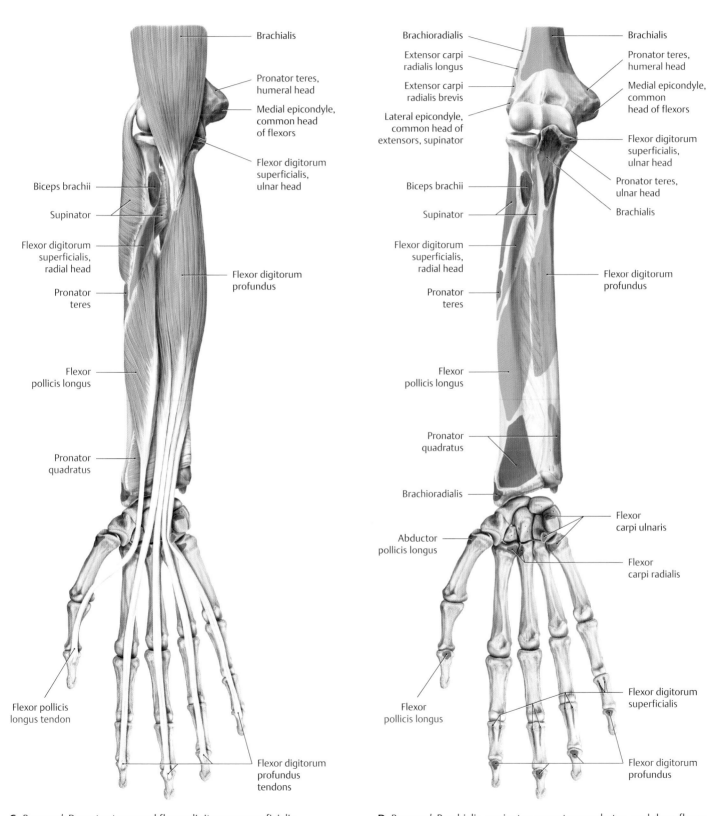

Brachialis

Pronator teres, humeral head

Medial epicondyle, common head of flexors

Flexor digitorum superficialis, ulnar head

Biceps brachii

Supinator

Flexor digitorum superficialis, radial head

Pronator teres

Flexor pollicis longus

Pronator quadratus

Flexor pollicis longus tendon

Flexor digitorum profundus

Flexor digitorum profundus tendons

Brachioradialis

Extensor carpi radialis longus

Extensor carpi radialis brevis

Lateral epicondyle, common head of extensors, supinator

Biceps brachii

Supinator

Flexor digitorum superficialis, radial head

Pronator teres

Flexor pollicis longus

Pronator quadratus

Brachioradialis

Abductor pollicis longus

Flexor pollicis longus

Brachialis

Pronator teres, humeral head

Medial epicondyle, common head of flexors

Flexor digitorum superficialis, ulnar head

Pronator teres, ulnar head

Brachialis

Flexor digitorum profundus

Flexor carpi ulnaris

Flexor carpi radialis

Flexor digitorum superficialis

Flexor digitorum profundus

C *Removed:* Pronator teres and flexor digitorum superficialis.

D *Removed:* Brachialis, supinator, pronator quadratus, and deep flexors.

329

Muscles of the Forearm: Posterior Compartment

***Fig. 26.11* Posterior muscles of the forearm: Dissection**
Right forearm, posterior view. Muscle origins are shown in red, insertions in blue.

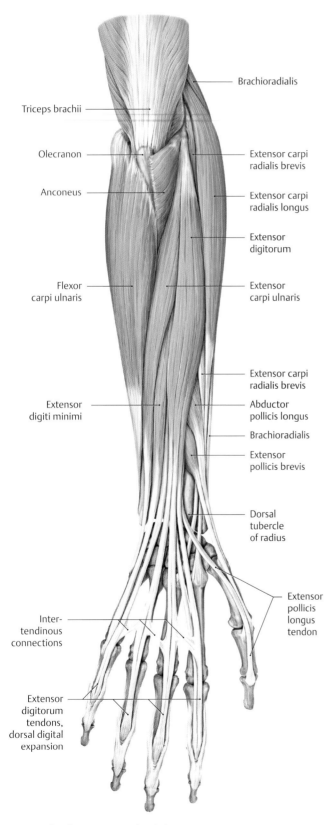

Brachioradialis

Triceps brachii

Olecranon

Anconeus

Flexor carpi ulnaris

Extensor digiti minimi

Inter-tendinous connections

Extensor digitorum tendons, dorsal digital expansion

Extensor carpi radialis brevis

Extensor carpi radialis longus

Extensor digitorum

Extensor carpi ulnaris

Extensor carpi radialis brevis

Abductor pollicis longus

Brachioradialis

Extensor pollicis brevis

Dorsal tubercle of radius

Extensor pollicis longus tendon

A Superficial extensors and radialis group.

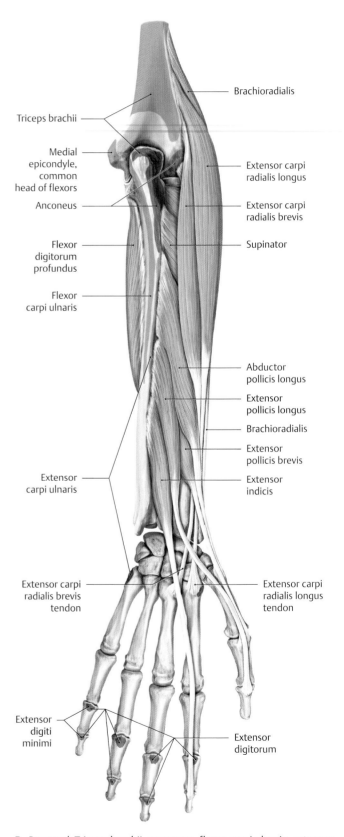

Brachioradialis

Triceps brachii

Medial epicondyle, common head of flexors

Anconeus

Flexor digitorum profundus

Flexor carpi ulnaris

Extensor carpi ulnaris

Extensor carpi radialis brevis tendon

Extensor digiti minimi

Extensor carpi radialis longus

Extensor carpi radialis brevis

Supinator

Abductor pollicis longus

Extensor pollicis longus

Brachioradialis

Extensor pollicis brevis

Extensor indicis

Extensor carpi radialis longus tendon

Extensor digitorum

B *Removed:* Triceps brachii, anconeus, flexor carpi ulnaris, extensor carpi ulnaris, and extensor digitorum.

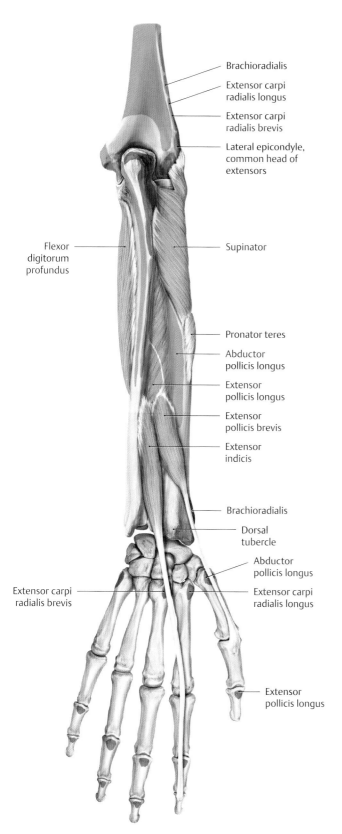

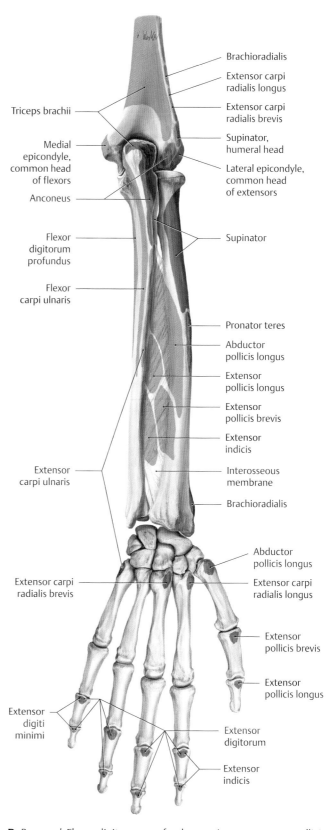

C *Removed:* Abductor pollicis longus, extensor pollicis longus, and radialis muscles.

D *Removed:* Flexor digitorum profundus, supinator, extensor pollicis brevis, and extensor indicis.

Muscle Facts (I)

Fig. 26.12 **Anterior compartment of the forearm**

Right forearm, anterior view.

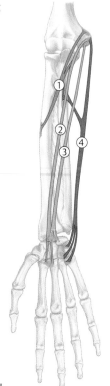
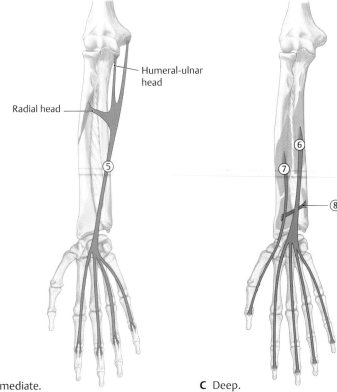

Humeral-ulnar head

Radial head

A Superficial.　　**B** Intermediate.　　**C** Deep.

Table 26.2	Anterior compartment of the forearm			
Muscle	**Origin**	**Insertion**	**Innervation**	**Action**
Superficial muscles				
① Pronator teres	Humeral head: medial epicondyle of humerus Ulnar head: coronoid process	Lateral radius (distal to supinator insertion)	Median n. (C6, C7)	Elbow: weak flexion Forearm: pronation
② Flexor carpi radialis	Medial epicondyle of humerus	Base of 2nd metacarpal (variance: base of 3rd metacarpal)		Wrist: flexion and abduction (radial deviation) of hand
③ Palmaris longus		Palmar aponeurosis	Median n. (C7, C8)	Elbow: weak flexion Wrist: flexion tightens palmar aponeurosis
④ Flexor carpi ulnaris	Humeral head: medial epicondyle Ulnar head: olecranon	Pisiform; hook of hamate; base of 5th metacarpal	Ulnar n. (C7–T1)	Wrist: flexion and adduction (ulnar deviation) of hand
Intermediate muscles				
⑤ Flexor digitorum superficialis	Humeral-ulnar head: medial epicondyle of humerus and coronoid process of ulna Radial head: upper half of anterior border of radius	Sides of middle phalanges of 2nd to 5th digits	Median n. (C8, T1)	Elbow: weak flexion Wrist, MCP, and PIP joints of 2nd to 5th digits: flexion
Deep muscles				
⑥ Flexor digitorum profundus	Ulna (proximal two thirds of flexor surface) and interosseous membrane	Distal phalanges of 2nd to 5th digits (palmar surface)	Median n. (C8, T1, radial half of fingers 2 and 3) Ulnar n. (C8, T1, ulnar half of fingers 4 and 5)	Wrist, MCP, PIP, and DIP joints of 2nd to 5th digits: flexion
⑦ Flexor pollicis longus	Radius (midanterior surface) and adjacent interosseous membrane	Distal phalanx of thumb (palmar surface)	Median n. (C8, T1)	Wrist: flexion and abduction (radial deviation) of hand Carpometacarpal joint of thumb: flexion MCP and IP joints of thumb: flexion
⑧ Pronator quadratus	Distal quarter of ulna (anterior surface)	Distal quarter of radius (anterior surface)		Hand: pronation Distal radioulnar joint: stabilization

DIP, distal interphalangeal; IP, interphalangeal; MCP, metacarpophalangeal; PIP, proximal interphalangeal.

Fig. 26.13 Anterior compartment of the forearm: Superficial and intermediate muscles

Right forearm, anterior view.

Fig. 26.14 Anterior compartment of the forearm: Deep muscles

Right forearm, anterior view.

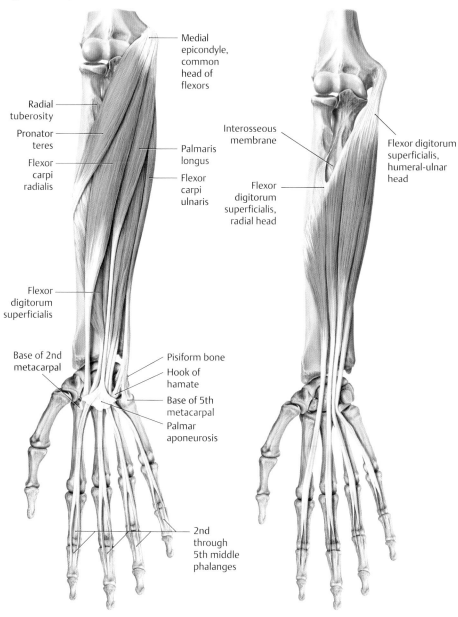

Medial epicondyle, common head of flexors

Radial tuberosity

Pronator teres

Flexor carpi radialis

Palmaris longus

Flexor carpi ulnaris

Interosseous membrane

Flexor digitorum superficialis, radial head

Flexor digitorum superficialis, humeral-ulnar head

Flexor digitorum superficialis

Base of 2nd metacarpal

Pisiform bone

Hook of hamate

Base of 5th metacarpal

Palmar aponeurosis

2nd through 5th middle phalanges

A Superficial muscles.

B Intermediate muscles.

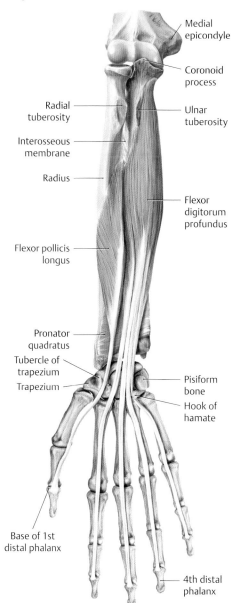

Medial epicondyle

Coronoid process

Radial tuberosity

Ulnar tuberosity

Interosseous membrane

Radius

Flexor digitorum profundus

Flexor pollicis longus

Pronator quadratus

Tubercle of trapezium

Trapezium

Pisiform bone

Hook of hamate

Base of 1st distal phalanx

4th distal phalanx

Muscle Facts (II)

Fig. 26.15 **Posterior compartment of the forearm: Radialis muscles**
Right forearm, posterior view, schematic.

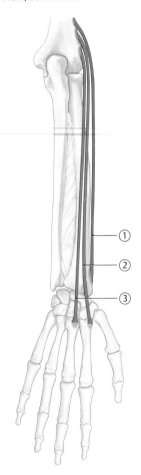

Table 26.3	**Posterior compartment of the forearm: Radialis muscles**				
Muscle	**Origin**	**Insertion**	**Innervation**	**Action**	
① Brachioradialis	Distal humerus (lateral surface), lateral intermuscular septum	Styloid process of the radius	Radial n. (C5, C6)	Elbow: flexion Forearm: semipronation	
② Extensor carpi radialis longus	Lateral supracondylar ridge of distal humerus, lateral intermuscular septum	2nd metacarpal (base)	Radial n. (C6, C7)	Elbow: weak flexion Wrist: extension and abduction	
③ Extensor carpi radialis brevis	Lateral epicondyle of humerus	3rd metacarpal (base)	Radial n. (C7, C8)		

Fig. 26.16 Posterior compartment of the forearm: Radialis muscles

Right forearm.

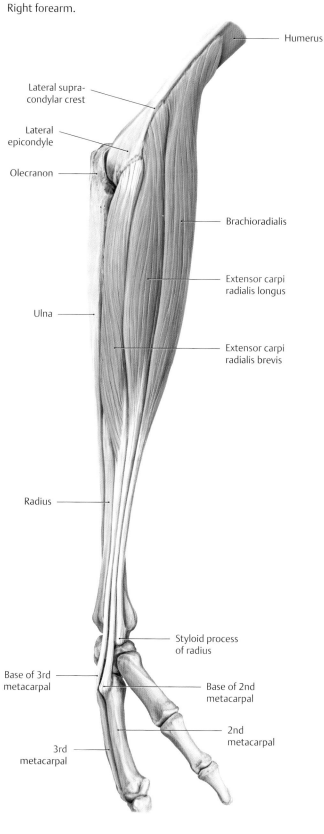

Humerus

Lateral supra-condylar crest

Lateral epicondyle

Olecranon

Brachioradialis

Extensor carpi radialis longus

Ulna

Extensor carpi radialis brevis

Radius

Styloid process of radius

Base of 3rd metacarpal

Base of 2nd metacarpal

2nd metacarpal

3rd metacarpal

A Lateral (radial) view.

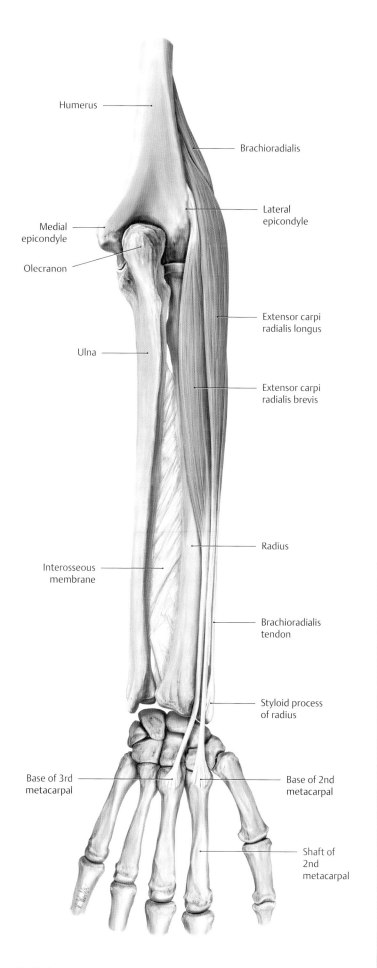

Humerus

Brachioradialis

Medial epicondyle

Lateral epicondyle

Olecranon

Extensor carpi radialis longus

Ulna

Extensor carpi radialis brevis

Radius

Interosseous membrane

Brachioradialis tendon

Styloid process of radius

Base of 3rd metacarpal

Base of 2nd metacarpal

Shaft of 2nd metacarpal

B Posterior view.

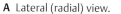

Muscle Facts (III)

Fig. 26.17 **Posterior compartment of the forearm: Superficial muscles**
Right forearm, posterior view, schematic.

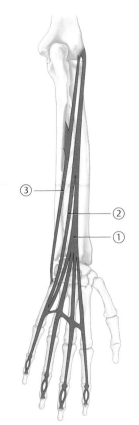

Fig. 26.18 **Posterior compartment of the forearm: Deep muscles**
Right forearm, posterior view, schematic.

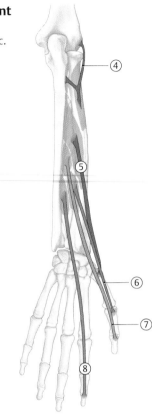

Table 26.4	Posterior compartment of the forearm			
Muscle	**Origin**	**Insertion**	**Innervation**	**Action**
Superficial muscles				
① Extensor digitorum	Common head (lateral epicondyle of humerus)	Dorsal digital expansion of 2nd to 5th digits	Radial n. (C7, C8)	Wrist: extension MCP, PIP, and DIP joints of 2nd to 5th digits: extension/abduction of fingers
② Extensor digiti minimi		Dorsal digital expansion of 5th digit		Wrist: extension, ulnar abduction of hand MCP, PIP, and DIP joints of 5th digit: extension and abduction of 5th digit
③ Extensor carpi ulnaris	Common head (lateral epicondyle of humerus) Ulnar head (dorsal surface)	Base of 5th metacarpal		Wrist: extension, adduction (ulnar deviation) of hand
Deep muscles				
④ Supinator	Olecranon, lateral epicondyle of humerus, radial collateral ligament, annular ligament of radius	Radius (between radial tuberosity and insertion of pronator teres)	Radial n. (C6, C7)	Radioulnar joints: supination
⑤ Abductor pollicis longus	Radius and ulna (dorsal surfaces, interosseous membrane)	Base of 1st metacarpal	Radial n. (C7, C8)	Radiocarpal joint: abduction of the hand Carpometacarpal joint of thumb: abduction
⑥ Extensor pollicis brevis	Radius (posterior surface) and interosseous membrane	Base of proximal phalanx of thumb		Radiocarpal joint: abduction (radial deviation) of hand Carpometacarpal and MCP joints of thumb: extension
⑦ Extensor pollicis longus	Ulna (posterior surface) and interosseous membrane	Base of distal phalanx of thumb		Wrist: extension and abduction (radial deviation) of hand Carpometacarpal joint of thumb: adduction MCP and IP joints of thumb: extension
⑧ Extensor indicis	Ulna (posterior surface) and interosseous membrane	Posterior digital extension of 2nd digit		Wrist: extension MCP, PIP, and DIP joints of 2nd digit: extension

DIP, distal interphalangeal; IP, interphalangeal; MCP, metacarpophalangeal; PIP, proximal interphalangeal.

Fig. 26.19 Posterior compartment of the forearm: Superficial and deep muscles

Right forearm, posterior view.

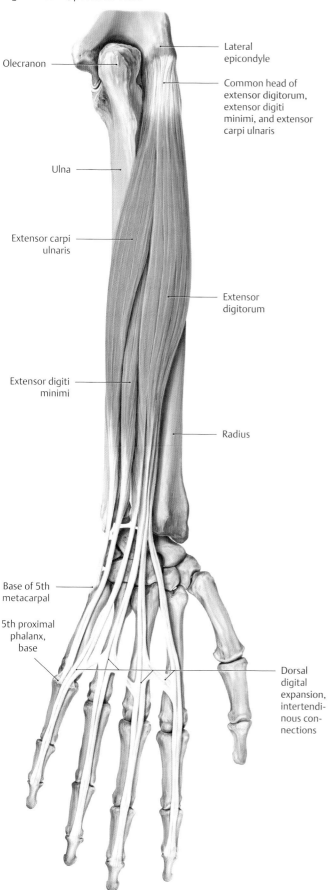

A Superficial extensors.

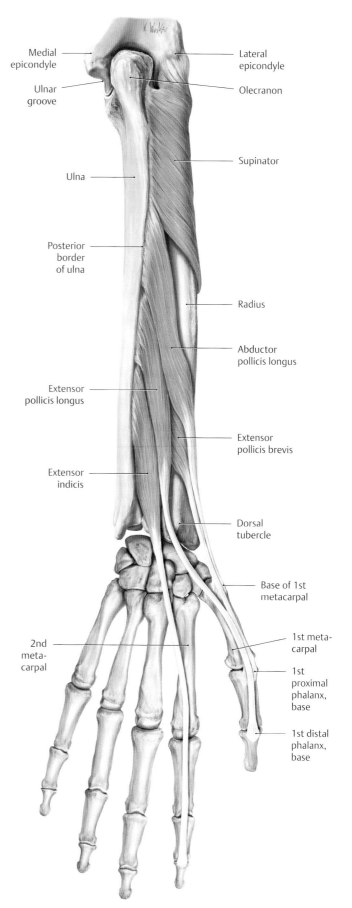

B Deep extensors with supinator.

Bones of the Wrist & Hand

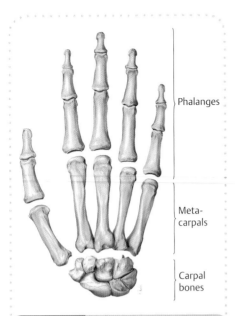

Phalanges

Meta-
carpals

Carpal
bones

Table 27.1	Bones of the wrist and hand	
Phalanges	1st to 5th proximal phalanges	
	2nd to 5th middle phalanges*	
	1st to 5th distal phalanges	
Metacarpal bones	1st to 5th metacarpals	
Carpal bones	Trapezium	Scaphoid
	Trapezoid	Lunate
	Capitate	Triquetrum
	Hamate	Pisiform

*There are only four middle phalanges (the thumb has only a proximal and a distal phalanx).

***Fig. 27.1* Dorsal view**
Right hand.

2nd distal phalanx

2nd middle phalanx

2nd proximal phalanx

1st metacarpal

Trapezoid

Trapezium

Scaphoid

Styloid process
of radius

Radius

Capitate

Hamate

Triquetrum

Lunate

Styloid process
of ulna

Ulna

Fig. 27.2 Palmar view
Right hand.

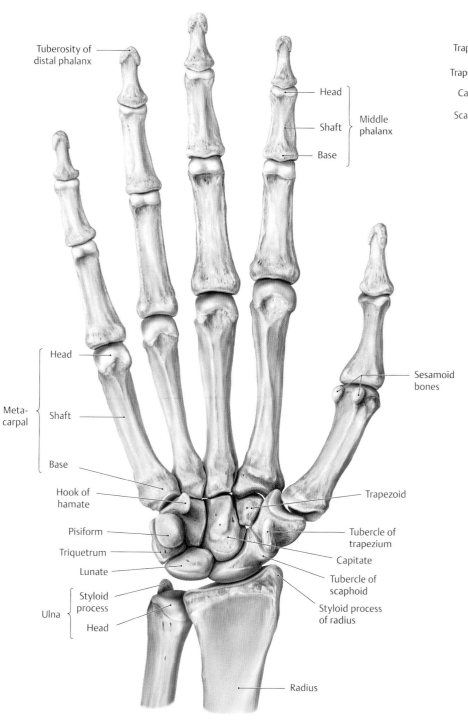

- Tuberosity of distal phalanx
- Head
- Shaft — Middle phalanx
- Base
- Head
- Meta-carpal { Shaft
- Base
- Hook of hamate
- Pisiform
- Triquetrum
- Lunate
- Ulna { Styloid process
- Head
- Sesamoid bones
- Trapezoid
- Tubercle of trapezium
- Capitate
- Tubercle of scaphoid
- Styloid process of radius
- Radius

Fig. 27.3 Radiograph of the wrist
Anteroposterior view of left limb.

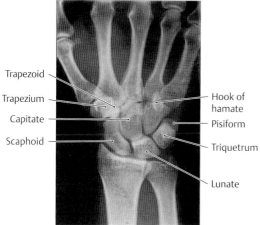

- Trapezoid
- Trapezium
- Capitate
- Scaphoid
- Hook of hamate
- Pisiform
- Triquetrum
- Lunate

Clinical box 27.1

Scaphoid Fractures
Scaphoid fractures are the most common carpal bone fractures, generally occurring at the narrowed waist between the proximal and distal poles (**A**, right scaphoid red line; **B**, white arrow). Because blood supply to the scaphoid is transmitted via the distal segment, fractures at the waist can compromise the supply to the proximal segment, often resulting in nonunion and avascular necrosis.

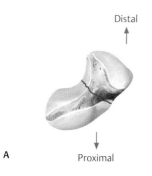

Distal

Proximal

A

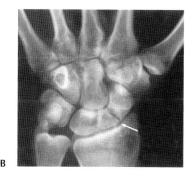

B

The Carpal Bones

Fig. 27.4 Carpal bones of the right wrist

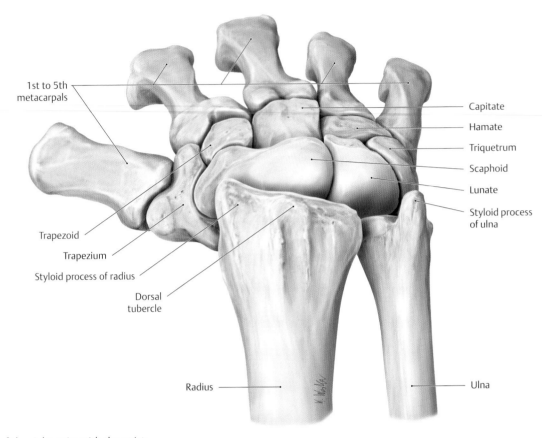

1st to 5th metacarpals

Capitate

Hamate

Triquetrum

Scaphoid

Lunate

Styloid process of ulna

Trapezoid

Trapezium

Styloid process of radius

Dorsal tubercle

Radius

Ulna

A Carpal bones of the right wrist with the wrist in flexion, proximal view.

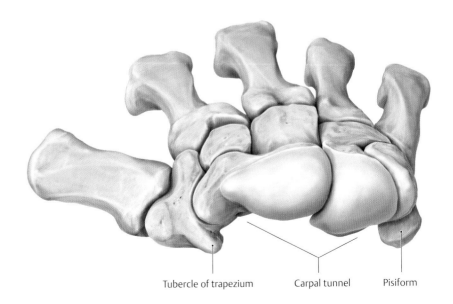

Tubercle of trapezium

Carpal tunnel

Pisiform

B Carpal and metacarpal bones of the right wrist with radius and ulna removed, proximal view.

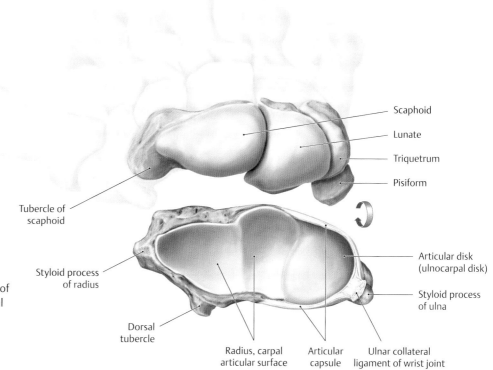

C Articular surfaces of the radiocarpal joint of the right wrist. The proximal row of carpal bones is shown from the proximal view. The articular surfaces of the radius and ulna, and the articular disk (ulnocarpal disk) are shown from the distal view.

Scaphoid

Lunate

Triquetrum

Pisiform

Tubercle of scaphoid

Styloid process of radius

Dorsal tubercle

Radius, carpal articular surface

Articular capsule

Ulnar collateral ligament of wrist joint

Articular disk (ulnocarpal disk)

Styloid process of ulna

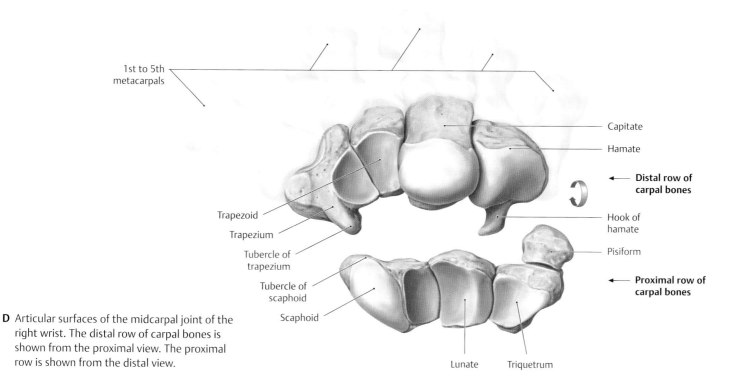

1st to 5th metacarpals

Capitate

Hamate

Distal row of carpal bones

Trapezoid

Trapezium

Tubercle of trapezium

Hook of hamate

Pisiform

Proximal row of carpal bones

Tubercle of scaphoid

Scaphoid

D Articular surfaces of the midcarpal joint of the right wrist. The distal row of carpal bones is shown from the proximal view. The proximal row is shown from the distal view.

Lunate   Triquetrum

Joints of the Wrist & Hand

Fig. 27.5 Joints of the wrist and hand

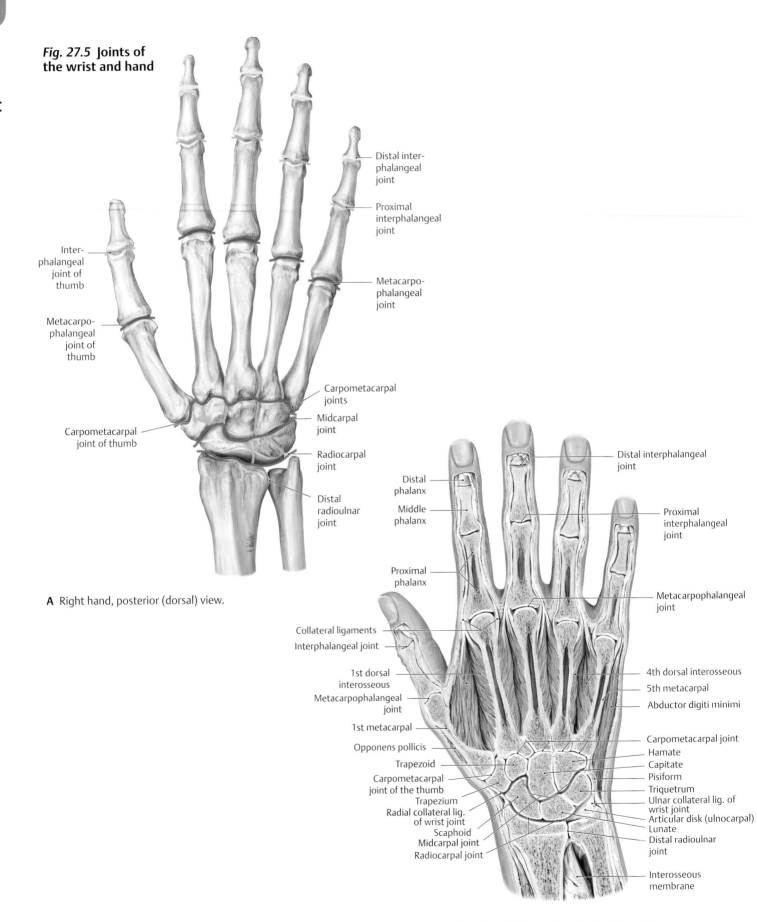

Distal inter-
phalangeal
joint

Proximal
interphalangeal
joint

Metacarpo-
phalangeal
joint

Inter-
phalangeal
joint of
thumb

Metacarpo-
phalangeal
joint of
thumb

Carpometacarpal
joint of thumb

Carpometacarpal
joints

Midcarpal
joint

Radiocarpal
joint

Distal
radioulnar
joint

A Right hand, posterior (dorsal) view.

Distal interphalangeal
joint

Distal
phalanx

Middle
phalanx

Proximal
interphalangeal
joint

Proximal
phalanx

Metacarpophalangeal
joint

Collateral ligaments

Interphalangeal joint

1st dorsal
interosseous

Metacarpophalangeal
joint

1st metacarpal

Opponens pollicis

Trapezoid

Carpometacarpal
joint of the thumb

Trapezium

Radial collateral lig.
of wrist joint

Scaphoid

Midcarpal joint

Radiocarpal joint

4th dorsal interosseous

5th metacarpal

Abductor digiti minimi

Carpometacarpal joint

Hamate

Capitate

Pisiform

Triquetrum

Ulnar collateral lig. of
wrist joint

Articular disk (ulnocarpal)

Lunate

Distal radioulnar
joint

Interosseous
membrane

B Coronal section. Right hand, posterior (dorsal) view.

Fig. 27.6 Carpometacarpal joint of the thumb

Right hand, radial view. The 1st metacarpal bone has been moved slightly distally to expose the articular surface of the trapezium. Two cardinal axes of motion are shown here: (**a**) abduction/adduction and (**b**) flexion/extension.

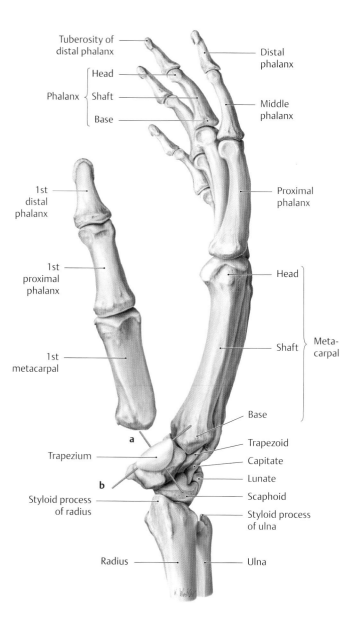

Tuberosity of distal phalanx

Head

Phalanx { Shaft

Base

Distal phalanx

Middle phalanx

1st distal phalanx

Proximal phalanx

1st proximal phalanx

Head

1st metacarpal

Shaft } Metacarpal

Base

Trapezoid

Trapezium

Capitate

Lunate

Scaphoid

Styloid process of radius

Styloid process of ulna

Radius

Ulna

Fig. 27.7 Movements of the carpometacarpal joint of the thumb

Right hand, Palmar view.

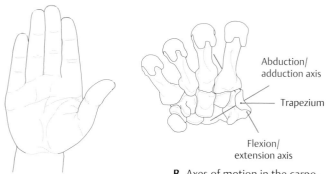

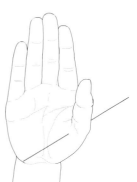
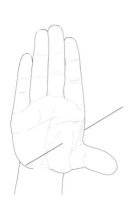

A The neutral (0°) position.

Abduction/adduction axis

Trapezium

Flexion/extension axis

B Axes of motion in the carpometacarpal joint of the thumb.

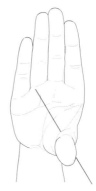
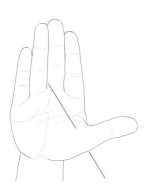

C Adduction.

D Abduction.

E Flexion.

F Extension.

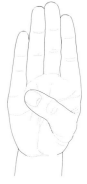

G Opposition.

Ligaments of the Hand

Fig. 27.8 Ligaments of the hand
Right hand.

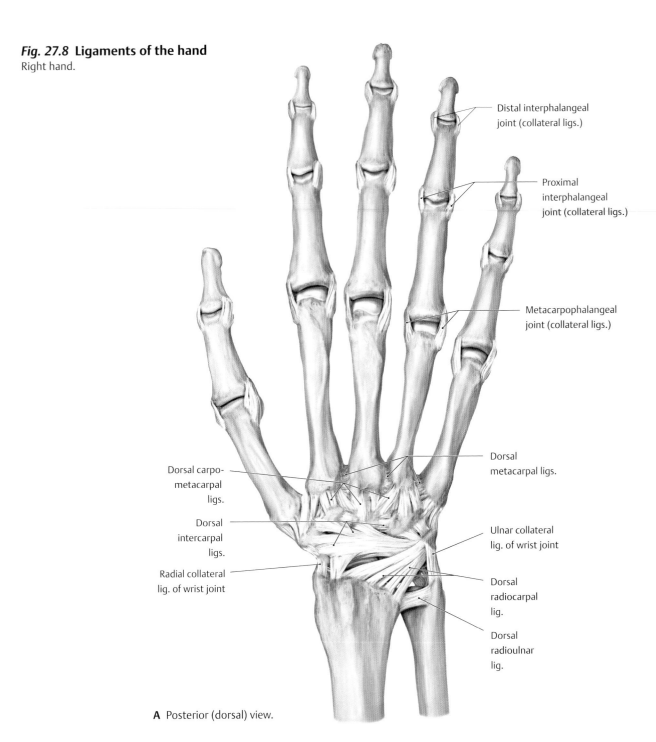

Distal interphalangeal
joint (collateral ligs.)

Proximal
interphalangeal
joint (collateral ligs.)

Metacarpophalangeal
joint (collateral ligs.)

Dorsal carpo-
metacarpal
ligs.

Dorsal
intercarpal
ligs.

Radial collateral
lig. of wrist joint

Dorsal
metacarpal ligs.

Ulnar collateral
lig. of wrist joint

Dorsal
radiocarpal
lig.

Dorsal
radioulnar
lig.

A Posterior (dorsal) view.

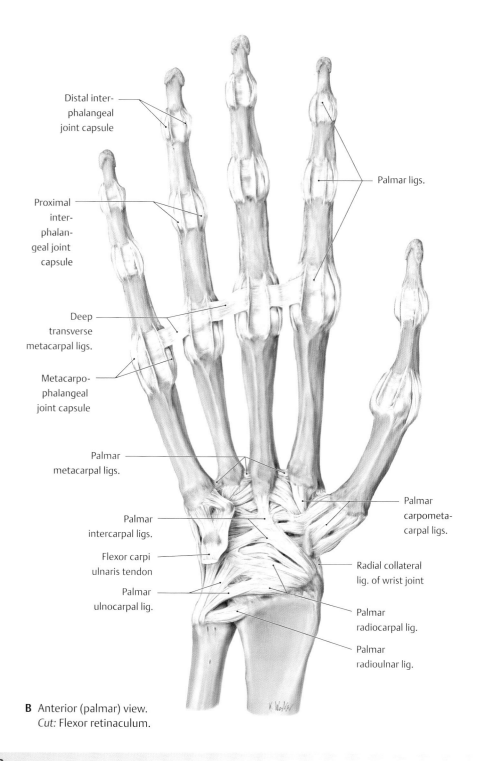

Distal inter-
phalangeal
joint capsule

Palmar ligs.

Proximal
inter-
phalan-
geal joint
capsule

Deep
transverse
metacarpal ligs.

Metacarpo-
phalangeal
joint capsule

Palmar
metacarpal ligs.

Palmar
intercarpal ligs.

Flexor carpi
ulnaris tendon

Palmar
ulnocarpal lig.

Palmar
carpometa-
carpal ligs.

Radial collateral
lig. of wrist joint

Palmar
radiocarpal lig.

Palmar
radioulnar lig.

B Anterior (palmar) view.
Cut: Flexor retinaculum.

 Clinical box 27.2

Functional position of the hand

The anatomic position of the hand, in which the palm is flat, the fingers are extended, and the forearm is supinated (palm facing forward), differs from the normal relaxed position of the hand. At rest, the forearm is in mid-supination/pronation (palm facing the body), the wrist is slightly extended, the fingers form an arcade of flexion, and the thumb is in the neutral position. Postoperative immobilization of the hand (by a cast or splint) fixes the fingers in flexion and the wrist in extension to prevent shortening of the ligaments and to maintain the ability of the hand to assume normal resting position.

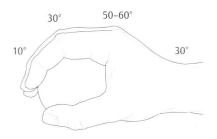

Ligaments and Compartments of the Wrist

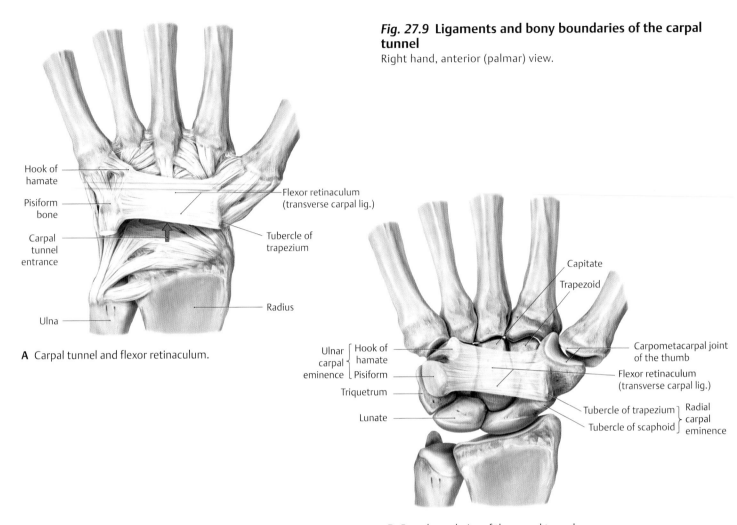

Fig. 27.9 Ligaments and bony boundaries of the carpal tunnel
Right hand, anterior (palmar) view.

A Carpal tunnel and flexor retinaculum.

B Bony boundaries of the carpal tunnel.

Fig. 27.10 Carpal tunnel

Right hand, transverse section. The contents of the carpal tunnel are discussed on **p. 396**. See **p. 387** for the ulnar tunnel and palmar carpal ligament.

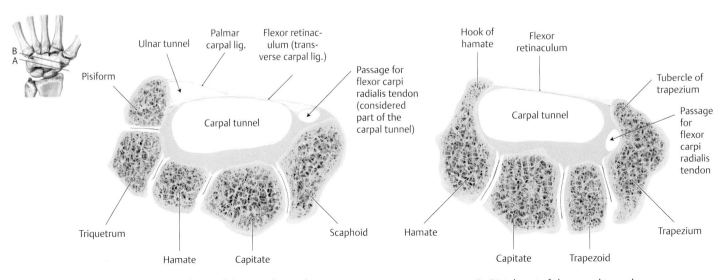

A Proximal part of the carpal tunnel.

B Distal part of the carpal tunnel.

Fig. 27.11 Ulnocarpal complex

Right hand. The ulnocarpal complex (triangular fibrocartilage complex) consists of ligaments and disks that connect the distal ulna, distal radioulnar joint, and the proximal carpal row.

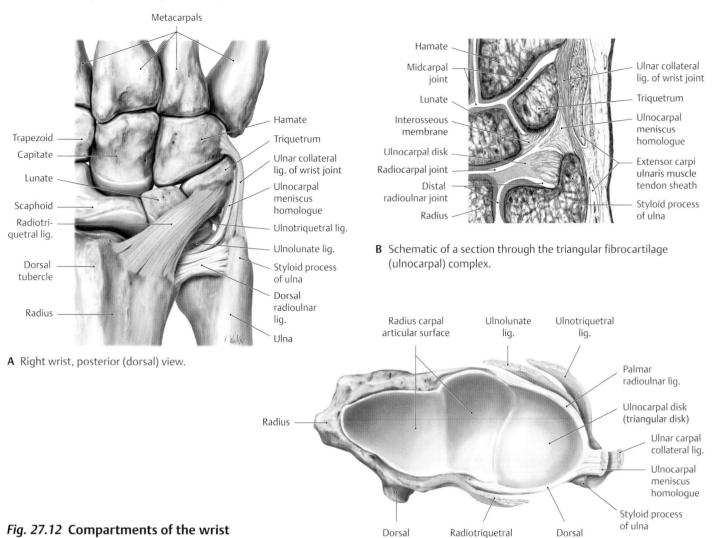

A Right wrist, posterior (dorsal) view.

B Schematic of a section through the triangular fibrocartilage (ulnocarpal) complex.

C Right wrist, distal view.

Fig. 27.12 Compartments of the wrist

Right wrist, posterior view, schematic. Interosseous ligaments and the ulnocarpal disk divide the interarticular space into compartments.

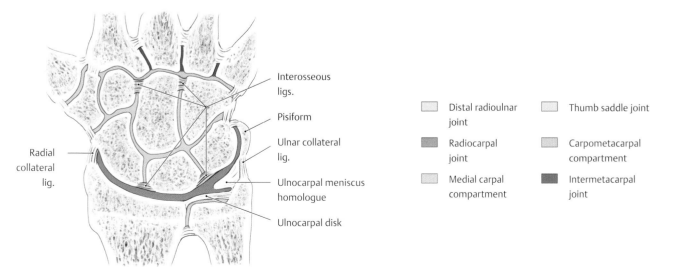

Distal radioulnar joint

Thumb saddle joint

Radiocarpal joint

Carpometacarpal compartment

Medial carpal compartment

Intermetacarpal joint

Ligaments of the Fingers

Fig. 27.13 Ligaments of the fingers: Lateral view

Right middle finger. Joint capsules, ligaments, and digital tendon sheaths. The outer fibrous layer of the tendon sheaths (stratum fibrosum) is strengthened by the anular and cruciform ligaments, which also bind the sheaths to the palmar surface of the phalanx and prevent palmar deviation of the sheaths during flexion.

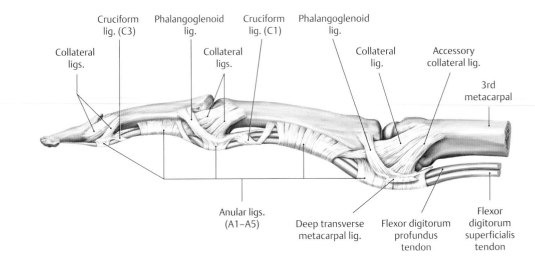

Fig. 27.14 Ligaments during extension and flexion of fingers: Lateral view

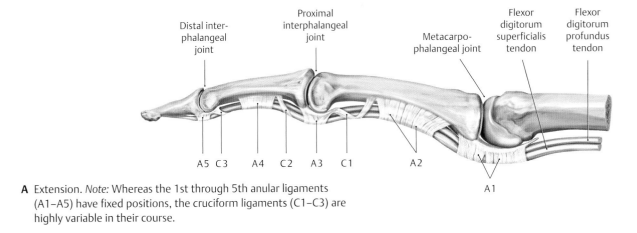

A Extension. *Note:* Whereas the 1st through 5th anular ligaments (A1–A5) have fixed positions, the cruciform ligaments (C1–C3) are highly variable in their course.

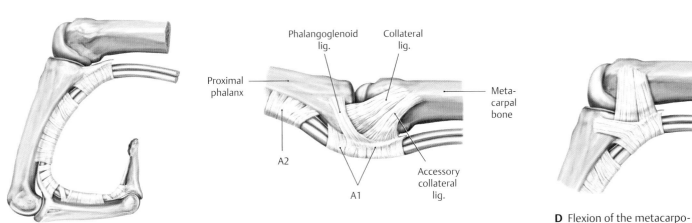

B Flexion.

C Extension of the metacarpophalangeal joint. *Note:* The collateral ligament is lax.

D Flexion of the metacarpophalangeal joint. *Note:* The collateral ligament is taut.

Fig. 27.15 Ligaments of the fingers: Anterior (palmar) view
Right middle finger.

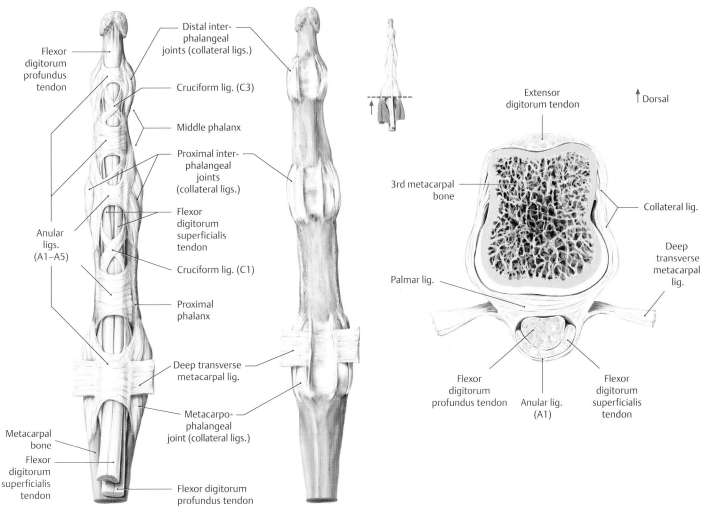

Flexor digitorum profundus tendon

Distal inter-phalangeal joints (collateral ligs.)

Cruciform lig. (C3)

Middle phalanx

Proximal inter-phalangeal joints (collateral ligs.)

Flexor digitorum superficialis tendon

Cruciform lig. (C1)

Proximal phalanx

Anular ligs. (A1–A5)

Deep transverse metacarpal lig.

Metacarpal bone

Flexor digitorum superficialis tendon

Metacarpo-phalangeal joint (collateral ligs.)

Flexor digitorum profundus tendon

A Superficial ligaments.

B Deep ligaments with digital tendon sheath removed.

Fig. 27.16 Third metacarpal: Transverse section
Proximal view.

Extensor digitorum tendon

↑ Dorsal

3rd metacarpal bone

Collateral lig.

Deep transverse metacarpal lig.

Palmar lig.

Flexor digitorum profundus tendon

Anular lig. (A1)

Flexor digitorum superficialis tendon

Fig. 27.17 Fingertip: Longitudinal section
The palmar articular surfaces of the phalanges are enlarged proximally at the joints by the palmar ligament. This fibrocartilaginous plate, also known as the volar plate, forms the floor of the digital tendon sheaths.

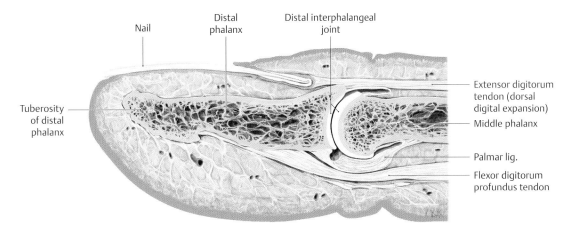

Nail

Distal phalanx

Distal interphalangeal joint

Extensor digitorum tendon (dorsal digital expansion)

Middle phalanx

Palmar lig.

Flexor digitorum profundus tendon

Tuberosity of distal phalanx

349

Muscles of the Hand: Superficial & Middle Layers

Fig. 27.18 Intrinsic muscles of the hand: Superficial and middle layers
Right hand, palmar surface.

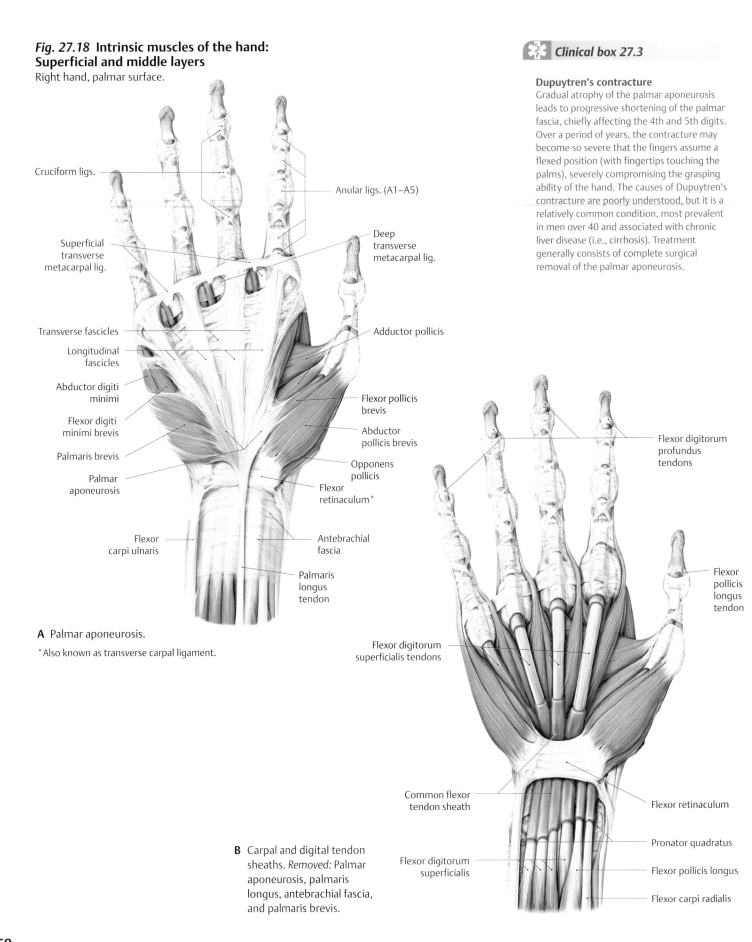

Cruciform ligs.

Anular ligs. (A1–A5)

Superficial transverse metacarpal lig.

Deep transverse metacarpal lig.

Transverse fascicles

Adductor pollicis

Longitudinal fascicles

Abductor digiti minimi

Flexor pollicis brevis

Flexor digiti minimi brevis

Abductor pollicis brevis

Palmaris brevis

Opponens pollicis

Palmar aponeurosis

Flexor retinaculum*

Flexor carpi ulnaris

Antebrachial fascia

Palmaris longus tendon

A Palmar aponeurosis.

*Also known as transverse carpal ligament.

Flexor digitorum profundus tendons

Flexor pollicis longus tendon

Flexor digitorum superficialis tendons

Common flexor tendon sheath

Flexor retinaculum

Pronator quadratus

B Carpal and digital tendon sheaths. *Removed:* Palmar aponeurosis, palmaris longus, antebrachial fascia, and palmaris brevis.

Flexor digitorum superficialis

Flexor pollicis longus

Flexor carpi radialis

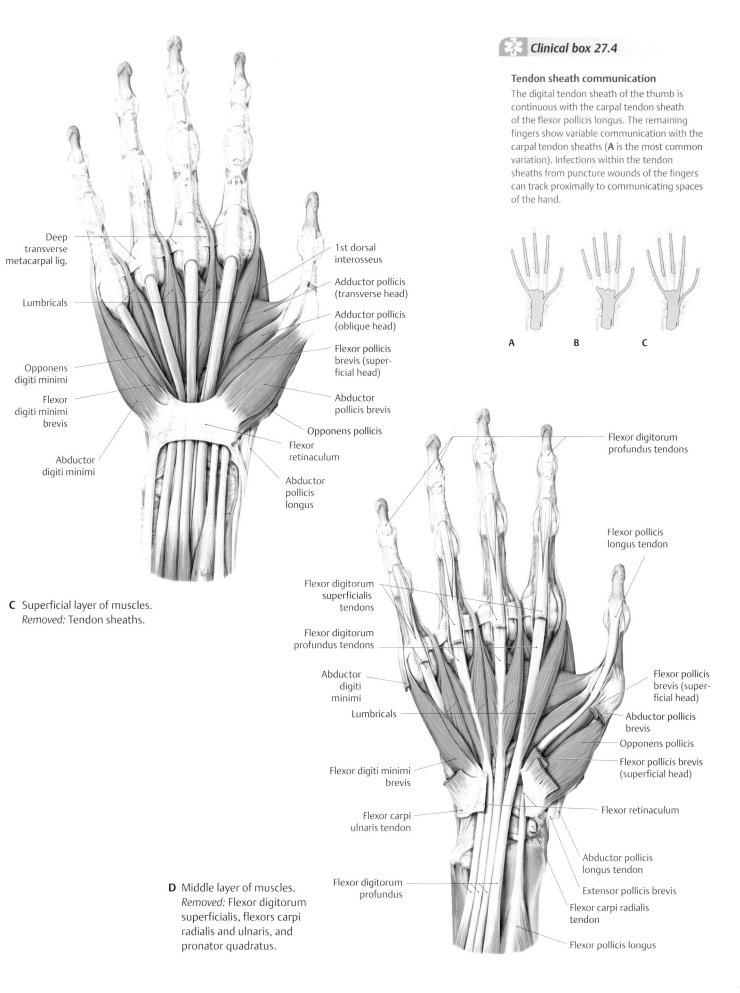

Deep transverse metacarpal lig.

Lumbricals

Opponens digiti minimi

Flexor digiti minimi brevis

Abductor digiti minimi

1st dorsal interosseus

Adductor pollicis (transverse head)

Adductor pollicis (oblique head)

Flexor pollicis brevis (superficial head)

Abductor pollicis brevis

Opponens pollicis

Flexor retinaculum

Abductor pollicis longus

C Superficial layer of muscles.
Removed: Tendon sheaths.

Clinical box 27.4

Tendon sheath communication

The digital tendon sheath of the thumb is continuous with the carpal tendon sheath of the flexor pollicis longus. The remaining fingers show variable communication with the carpal tendon sheaths (**A** is the most common variation). Infections within the tendon sheaths from puncture wounds of the fingers can track proximally to communicating spaces of the hand.

A   **B**   **C**

Flexor digitorum profundus tendons

Flexor digitorum superficialis tendons

Flexor digitorum profundus tendons

Abductor digiti minimi

Lumbricals

Flexor digiti minimi brevis

Flexor carpi ulnaris tendon

Flexor digitorum profundus

Flexor pollicis longus tendon

Flexor pollicis brevis (superficial head)

Abductor pollicis brevis

Opponens pollicis

Flexor pollicis brevis (superficial head)

Flexor retinaculum

Abductor pollicis longus tendon

Extensor pollicis brevis

Flexor carpi radialis tendon

Flexor pollicis longus

D Middle layer of muscles.
Removed: Flexor digitorum superficialis, flexors carpi radialis and ulnaris, and pronator quadratus.

Muscles of the Hand: Middle & Deep Layers

**Fig. 27.19 Intrinsic muscles of the hand:
Middle and deep layers**
Right hand, palmar surface.

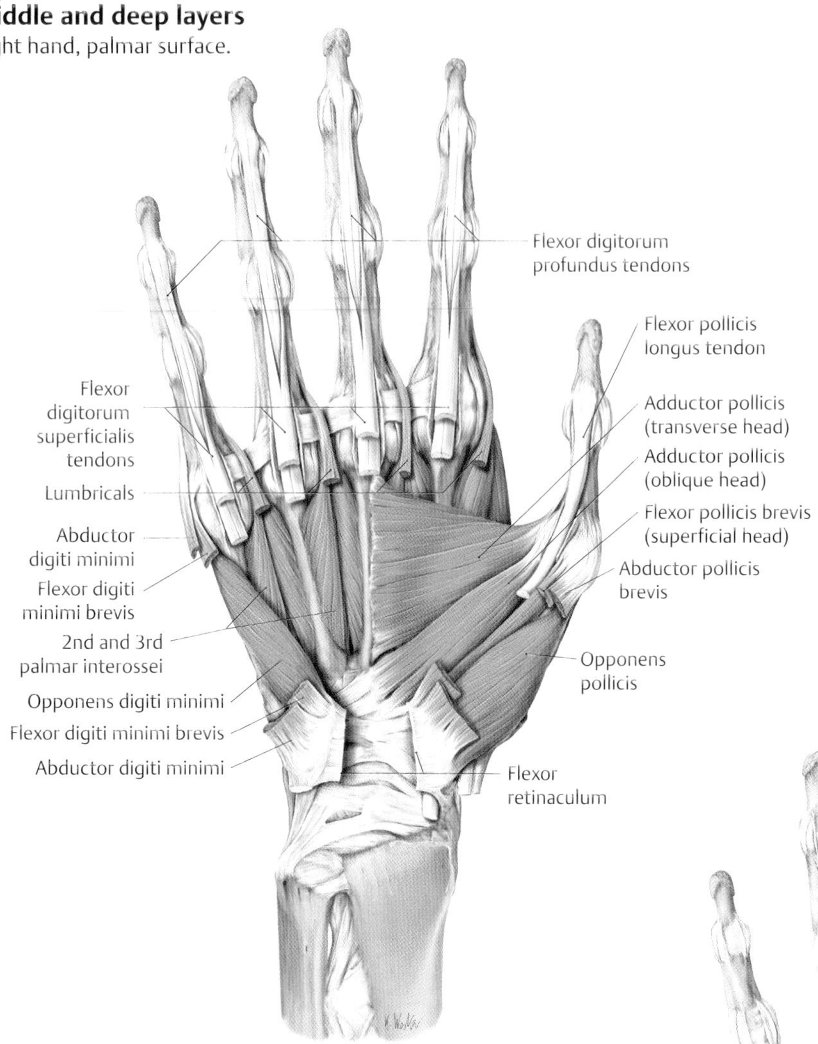

Flexor digitorum
profundus tendons

Flexor
digitorum
superficialis
tendons

Lumbricals

Abductor
digiti minimi

Flexor digiti
minimi brevis

2nd and 3rd
palmar interossei

Opponens digiti minimi

Flexor digiti minimi brevis

Abductor digiti minimi

Flexor pollicis
longus tendon

Adductor pollicis
(transverse head)

Adductor pollicis
(oblique head)

Flexor pollicis brevis
(superficial head)

Abductor pollicis
brevis

Opponens
pollicis

Flexor
retinaculum

A Middle layer of muscles. *Cut:* Flexor digitorum
profundus, lumbricals, flexor pollicis longus,
and flexor digiti minimi brevis.

Palmar ligs.

1st through
4th dorsal
interossei

Opponens digiti minimi

1st through 3rd
palmar interossei

Flexor carpi
ulnaris tendon

Adductor pollicis

Flexor pollicis brevis
(superficial head)

Flexor pollicis brevis
(deep head)

Opponens pollicis

Abductor pollicis
longus tendon

Extensor pollicis brevis

Flexor carpi
radialis tendon

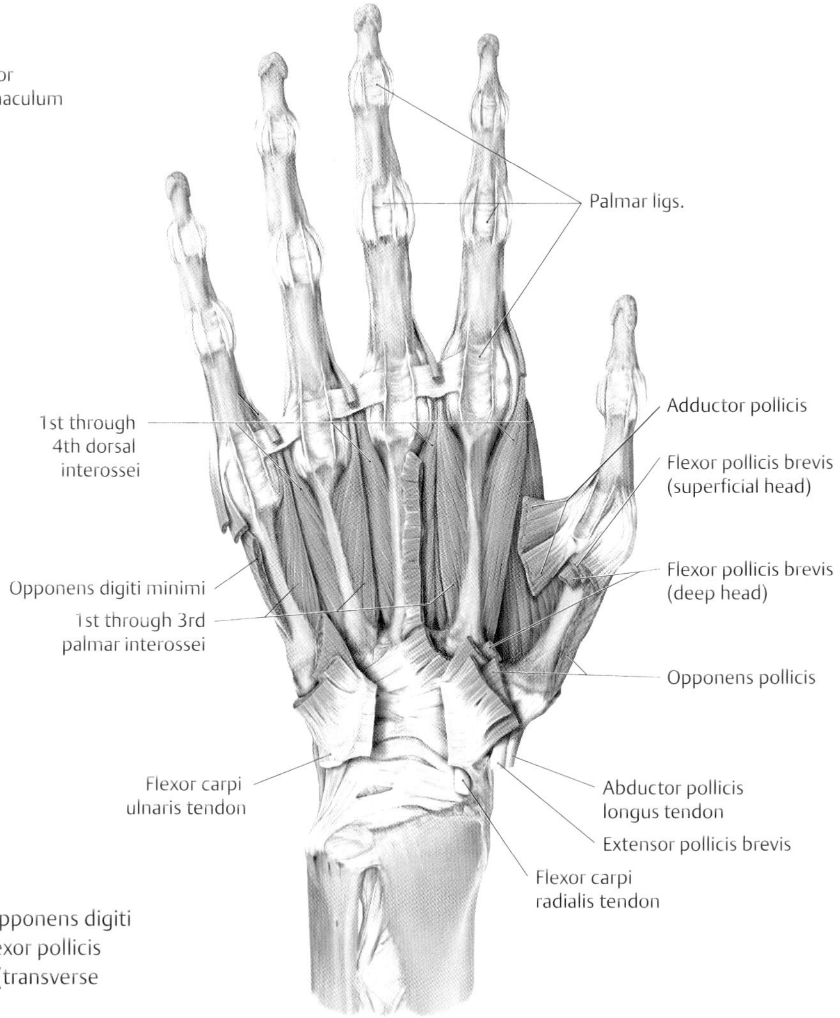

B Deep layer of muscles. *Cut:* Opponens digiti
minimi, opponens pollicis, flexor pollicis
brevis, and adductor pollicis (transverse
and oblique heads).

Fig. 27.20 Origins and insertions of muscles of the hand

Right hand. Muscle origins shown in red, insertions in blue.

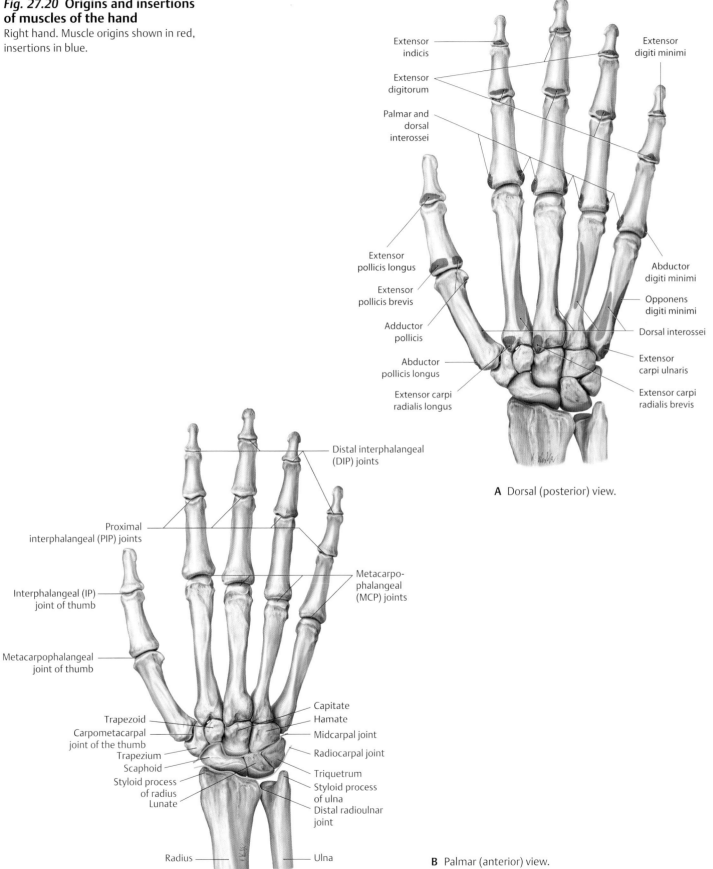

Extensor indicis

Extensor digitorum

Palmar and dorsal interossei

Extensor pollicis longus

Extensor pollicis brevis

Adductor pollicis

Abductor pollicis longus

Extensor carpi radialis longus

Extensor digiti minimi

Abductor digiti minimi

Opponens digiti minimi

Dorsal interossei

Extensor carpi ulnaris

Extensor carpi radialis brevis

A Dorsal (posterior) view.

Distal interphalangeal (DIP) joints

Proximal interphalangeal (PIP) joints

Interphalangeal (IP) joint of thumb

Metacarpophalangeal joint of thumb

Metacarpophalangeal (MCP) joints

Trapezoid

Carpometacarpal joint of the thumb

Trapezium

Scaphoid

Styloid process of radius

Lunate

Capitate

Hamate

Midcarpal joint

Radiocarpal joint

Triquetrum

Styloid process of ulna

Distal radioulnar joint

Radius

Ulna

B Palmar (anterior) view.

Dorsum of the Hand

Fig. 27.21 Extensor retinaculum and dorsal carpal tendon sheaths

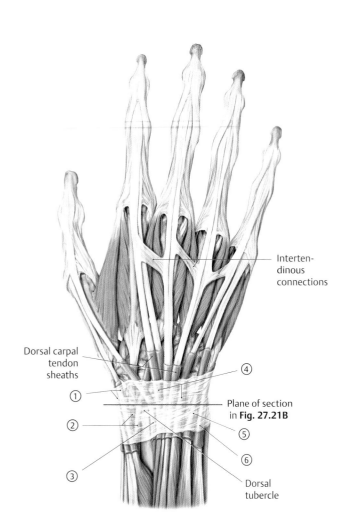

A Right hand, posterior (dorsal) view.

Intertendinous connections

Dorsal carpal tendon sheaths

① ② ③

④

Plane of section in **Fig. 27.21B**

⑤

⑥

Dorsal tubercle

Fig. 27.22 Muscles and tendons of the dorsum
Right hand, posterior (dorsal) view.

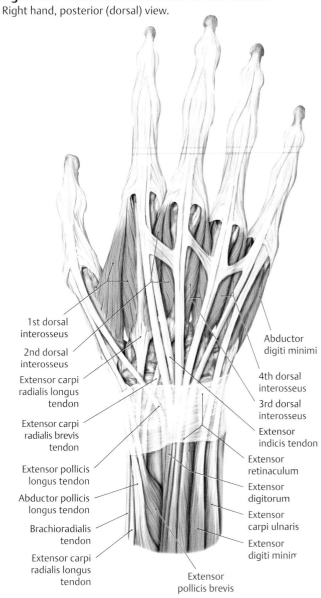

1st dorsal interosseus

2nd dorsal interosseus

Extensor carpi radialis longus tendon

Extensor carpi radialis brevis tendon

Extensor pollicis longus tendon

Abductor pollicis longus tendon

Brachioradialis tendon

Extensor carpi radialis longus tendon

Abductor digiti minimi

4th dorsal interosseus

3rd dorsal interosseus

Extensor indicis tendon

Extensor retinaculum

Extensor digitorum

Extensor carpi ulnaris

Extensor digiti minim

Extensor pollicis brevis

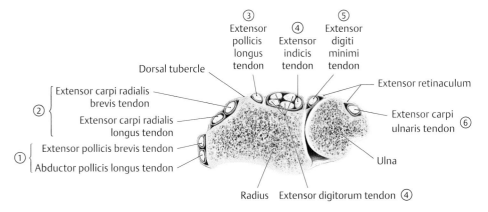

③ Extensor pollicis longus tendon

④ Extensor indicis tendon

⑤ Extensor digiti minimi tendon

Dorsal tubercle

Extensor carpi radialis brevis tendon

② Extensor carpi radialis longus tendon

Extensor pollicis brevis tendon

① Abductor pollicis longus tendon

Extensor retinaculum

Extensor carpi ulnaris tendon ⑥

Ulna

Radius   Extensor digitorum tendon ④

B Posterior (dorsal) compartments, proximal view of section in **Fig. 27.21A.**

Table 27.2	Dorsal compartments for extensor tendons
①	Abductor pollicis longus
	Extensor pollicis brevis
②	Extensor carpi radialis longus
	Extensor carpi radialis brevis
③	Extensor pollicis longus
④	Extensor digitorum
	Extensor indicis
⑤	Extensor digiti minimi
⑥	Extensor carpi ulnaris

Fig. 27.23 Dorsal digital expansion

Right hand, middle finger. The dorsal digital expansion permits the long digital flexors and the short muscles of the hand to act on all three finger joints.

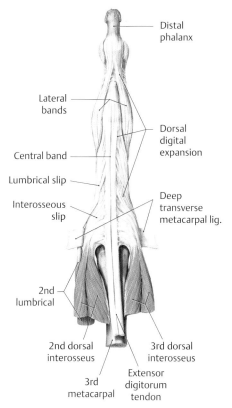

A Posterior view.

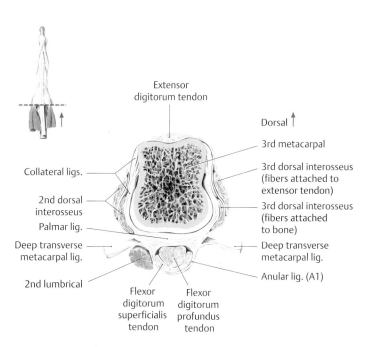

B Cross section through 3rd metacarpal head, proximal view.

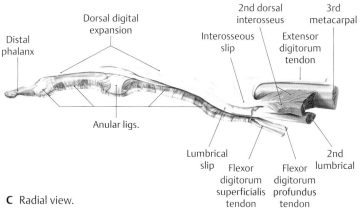

C Radial view.

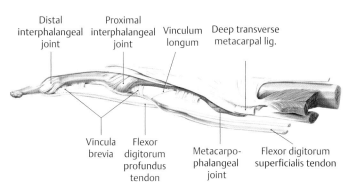

D Radial view with common tendon sheath of flexor digitorum superficialis and profundus opened.

Muscle Facts (I)

 The intrinsic muscles of the hand are divided into three groups: the thenar, hypothenar, and metacarpal muscles (see **p. 358**).

The thenar muscles are responsible for movement of the thumb, while the hypothenar muscles move the 5th digit.

Table 27.3	Thenar muscles					
Muscle	**Origin**	**Insertion**		**Innervation**		**Action**
① Adductor pollicis	Transverse head: 3rd metacarpal (palmar surface)	Thumb (base of proximal phalanx) via the ulnar sesamoid	Via the ulnar sesamoid	Ulnar n. (C8, T1)		CMC joint of thumb: adduction MCP joint of thumb: flexion
	Oblique head: capitate bone, 2nd and 3rd metacarpals (bases)					
② Abductor pollicis brevis	Scaphoid bone and trapezium, flexor retinaculum	Thumb (base of proximal phalanx) via the radial sesamoid	Via the radial sesamoid	Median n. (C8, T1)	C8, T1	CMC joint of thumb: abduction
③ Flexor pollicis brevis	Superficial head: flexor retinaculum			Superficial head: median n. (C8, T1)		CMC joint of thumb: flexion
	Deep head: capitate bone, trapezium			Deep head: ulnar n. (C8, T1)		
④ Opponens pollicis	Trapezium	1st metacarpal (radial border)		Median n. (C8, T1)		CMC joint of thumb: opposition

CMC, carpometacarpal; MCP, metacarpophalangeal.

Fig. 27.24 **Thenar and hypothenar muscles**
Right hand, palmar (anterior) view, schematic.

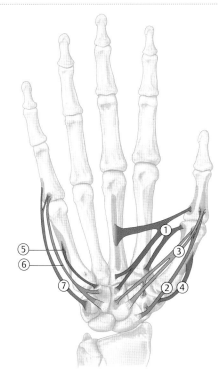

Table 27.4	Hypothenar muscles				
Muscle	**Origin**	**Insertion**		**Innervation**	**Action**
⑤ Opponens digiti minimi	Hook of hamate, flexor retinaculum	5th metacarpal (ulnar border)		Ulnar n. (C8, T1)	Draws metacarpal in palmar direction (opposition)
⑥ Flexor digiti minimi brevis		5th proximal phalanx (base)			MCP joint of little finger: flexion
⑦ Abductor digiti minimi	Pisiform bone	5th proximal phalanx (ulnar base) and dorsal digital expansion of 5th digit			MCP joint of little finger: flexion and abduction of little finger PIP and DIP joints of little finger: extension
Palmaris brevis	Palmar aponeurosis (ulnar border)	Skin of hypothenar eminence			Tightens the palmar aponeurosis (protective function)

DIP, distal interphalangeal; MCP, metacarpophalangeal; PIP, proximal interphalangeal.

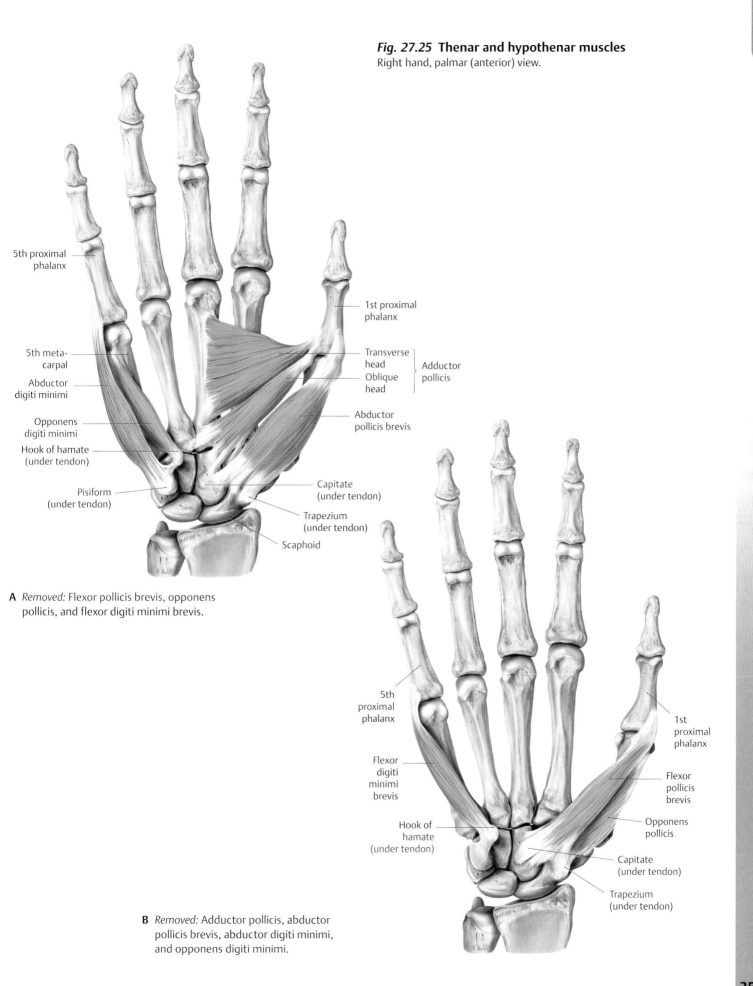

Fig. 27.25 Thenar and hypothenar muscles
Right hand, palmar (anterior) view.

5th proximal phalanx

5th meta-carpal

Abductor digiti minimi

Opponens digiti minimi

Hook of hamate (under tendon)

Pisiform (under tendon)

1st proximal phalanx

Transverse head
Oblique head
} Adductor pollicis

Abductor pollicis brevis

Capitate (under tendon)

Trapezium (under tendon)

Scaphoid

A *Removed:* Flexor pollicis brevis, opponens pollicis, and flexor digiti minimi brevis.

5th proximal phalanx

Flexor digiti minimi brevis

Hook of hamate (under tendon)

1st proximal phalanx

Flexor pollicis brevis

Opponens pollicis

Capitate (under tendon)

Trapezium (under tendon)

B *Removed:* Adductor pollicis, abductor pollicis brevis, abductor digiti minimi, and opponens digiti minimi.

Muscle Facts (II)

 The metacarpal muscles of the hand consist of the lumbricals and interossei. They are responsible for the movement of the digits (with the hypothenars, which act on the 5th digit).

Fig. 27.26 **Metacarpal muscles of the hand**
Right hand, palmar view, schematic.

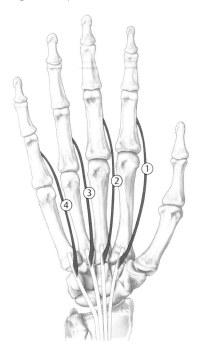

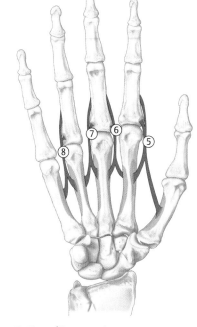

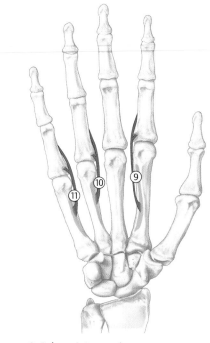

A Lumbricals.　　　　**B** Dorsal interossei.　　　　**C** Palmar interossei.

Table 27.5	Metacarpal muscles				
Muscle group	**Muscle**	**Origin**	**Insertion**	**Innervation**	**Action**
Lumbricals	① 1st	Tendons of flexor digitorum profundus (radial sides)	2nd digit (dde)	Median n. (C8, T1)	2nd to 5th digits: • MCP joints: flexion • Proximal and distal IP joints: extension
	② 2nd		3rd digit (dde)		
	③ 3rd	Tendons of flexor digitorum profundus (bipennate from medial and lateral sides)	4th digit (dde)		
	④ 4th		5th digit (dde)		
Dorsal interossei	⑤ 1st	1st and 2nd metacarpals (adjacent sides, two heads)	2nd digit (dde) 2nd proximal phalanx (radial side)	Ulnar n. (C8, T1)	2nd to 4th digits: • MCP joints: flexion • Proximal and distal IP joints: extension and abduction from 3rd digit
	⑥ 2nd	2nd and 3rd metacarpals (adjacent sides, two heads)	3rd digit (dde) 3rd proximal phalanx (radial side)		
	⑦ 3rd	3rd and 4th metacarpals (adjacent sides, two heads)	3rd digit (dde) 3rd proximal phalanx (ulnar side)		
	⑧ 4th	4th and 5th metacarpals (adjacent sides, two heads)	4th digit (dde) 4th proximal phalanx (ulnar side)		
Palmar interossei	⑨ 1st	2nd metacarpal (ulnar side)	2nd digit (dde) 2nd proximal phalanx (base)		2nd, 4th, and 5th digits: • MCP joints: flexion • Proximal and distal IP joints: extension and adduction toward 3rd digit
	⑩ 2nd	4th metacarpal (radial side)	4th digit (dde) 4th proximal phalanx (base)		
	⑪ 3rd	5th metacarpal (radial side)	5th digit (dde) 5th proximal phalanx (base)		

dde, dorsal digital expansion; IP, interphalangeal; MCP, metacarpophalangeal.

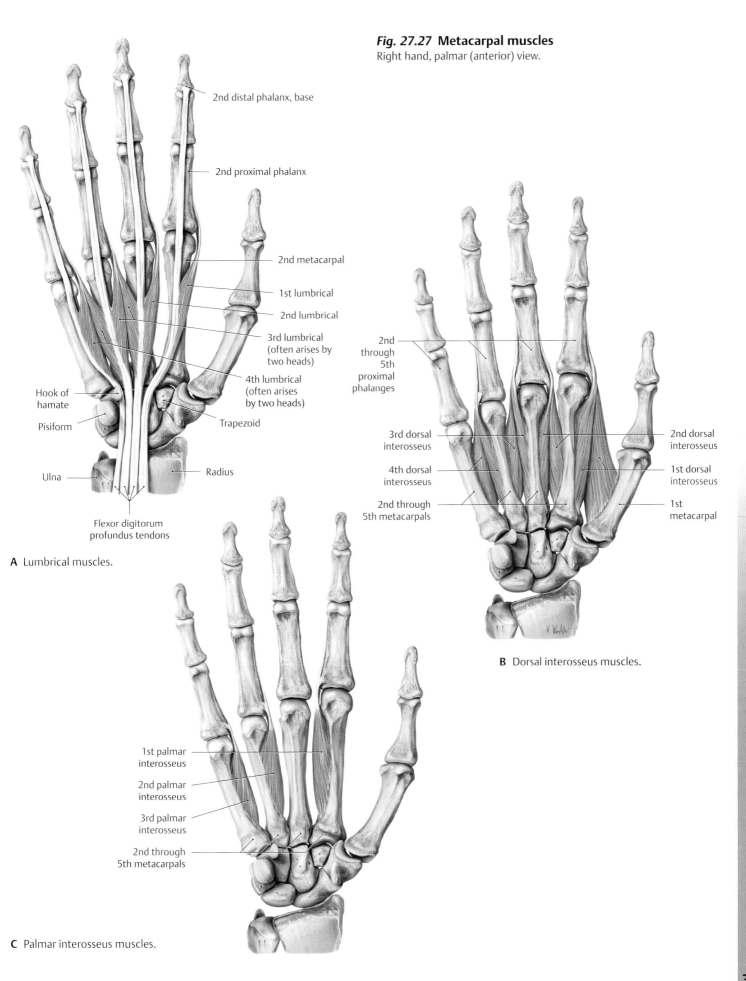

Fig. 27.27 Metacarpal muscles
Right hand, palmar (anterior) view.

2nd distal phalanx, base

2nd proximal phalanx

2nd metacarpal

1st lumbrical

2nd lumbrical

3rd lumbrical
(often arises by
two heads)

4th lumbrical
(often arises
by two heads)

Hook of
hamate

Pisiform

Trapezoid

Ulna

Radius

Flexor digitorum
profundus tendons

A Lumbrical muscles.

2nd
through
5th
proximal
phalanges

3rd dorsal
interosseus

4th dorsal
interosseus

2nd through
5th metacarpals

2nd dorsal
interosseus

1st dorsal
interosseus

1st
metacarpal

B Dorsal interosseus muscles.

1st palmar
interosseus

2nd palmar
interosseus

3rd palmar
interosseus

2nd through
5th metacarpals

C Palmar interosseus muscles.

Arteries of the Upper Limb

Fig. 28.1 Arteries of the upper limb
Right limb, anterior view.

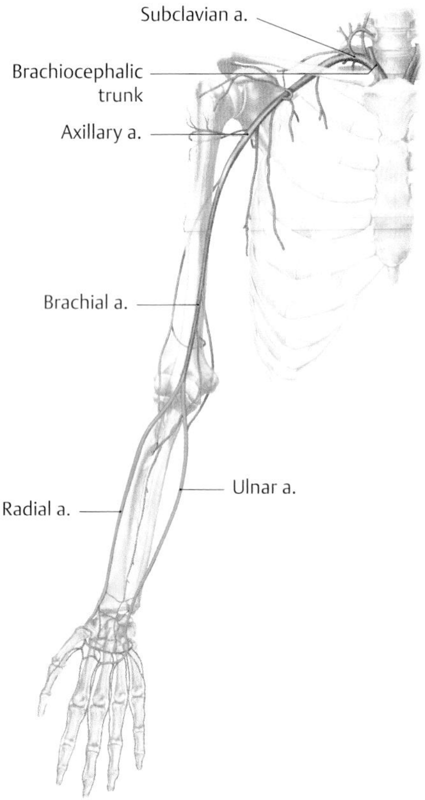

Subclavian a.
Brachiocephalic trunk
Axillary a.
Brachial a.
Radial a.
Ulnar a.

A Main arterial segments.

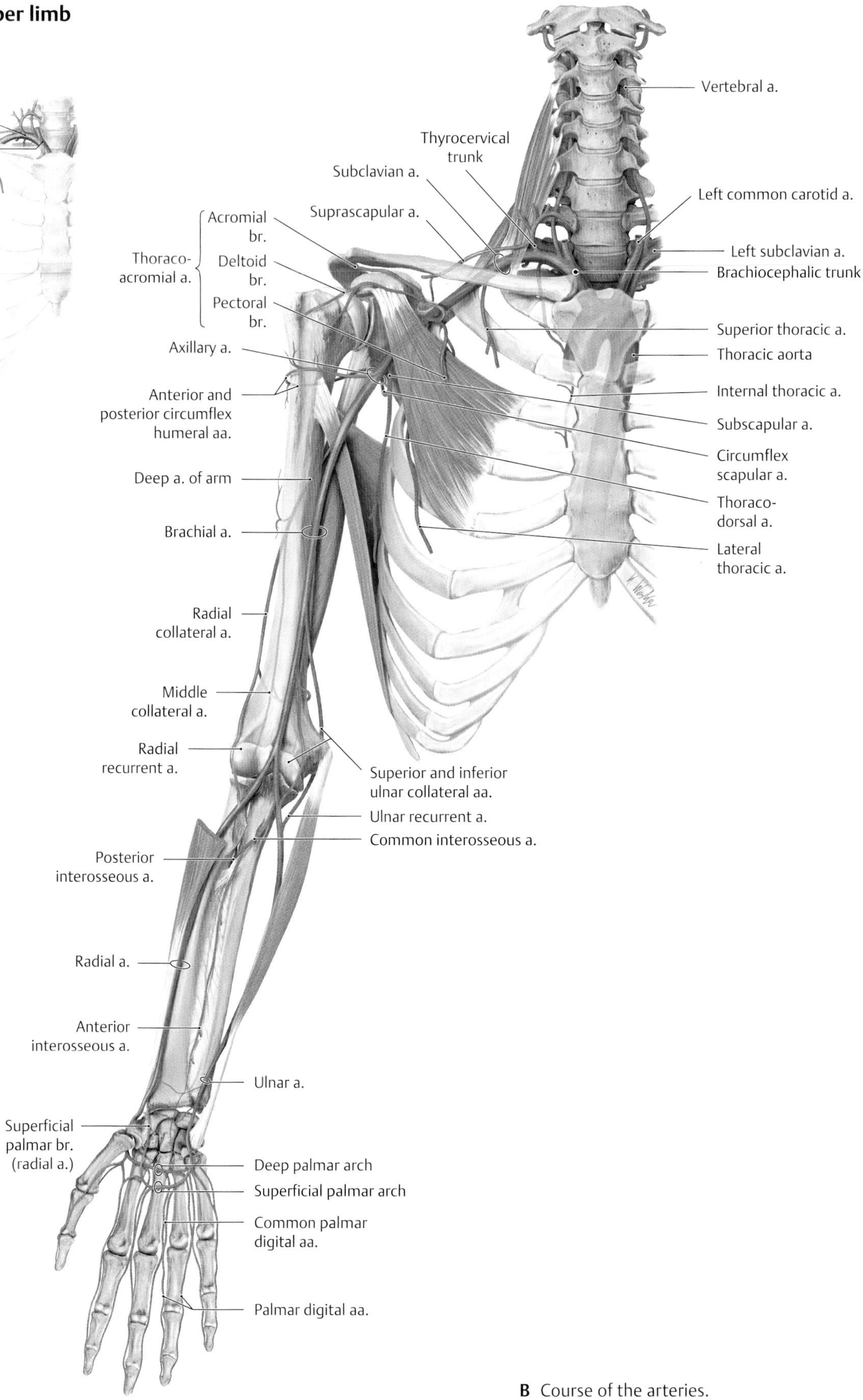

Acromial br.
Thoraco-acromial a.
Deltoid br.
Pectoral br.
Axillary a.
Anterior and posterior circumflex humeral aa.
Deep a. of arm
Brachial a.
Radial collateral a.
Middle collateral a.
Radial recurrent a.
Posterior interosseous a.
Radial a.
Anterior interosseous a.
Superficial palmar br. (radial a.)

Thyrocervical trunk
Subclavian a.
Suprascapular a.

Vertebral a.
Left common carotid a.
Left subclavian a.
Brachiocephalic trunk
Superior thoracic a.
Thoracic aorta
Internal thoracic a.
Subscapular a.
Circumflex scapular a.
Thoraco-dorsal a.
Lateral thoracic a.

Superior and inferior ulnar collateral aa.
Ulnar recurrent a.
Common interosseous a.

Ulnar a.
Deep palmar arch
Superficial palmar arch
Common palmar digital aa.
Palmar digital aa.

B Course of the arteries.

Fig. 28.2 **Branches of the subclavian artery**

Right side, anterior view.

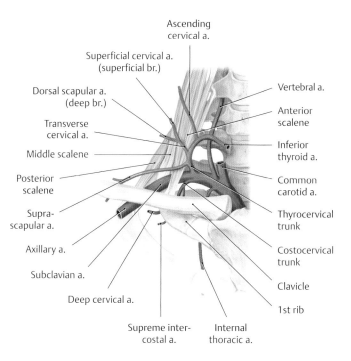

Ascending cervical a.

Superficial cervical a. (superficial br.)

Dorsal scapular a. (deep br.)

Transverse cervical a.

Middle scalene

Posterior scalene

Supra-scapular a.

Axillary a.

Subclavian a.

Deep cervical a.

Supreme inter-costal a.

Internal thoracic a.

Vertebral a.

Anterior scalene

Inferior thyroid a.

Common carotid a.

Thyrocervical trunk

Costocervical trunk

Clavicle

1st rib

Fig. 28.3 **Scapular arcade**

Right side, posterior view.

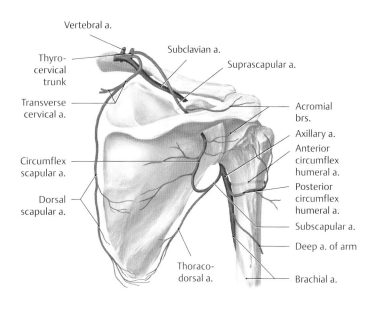

Vertebral a.

Thyro-cervical trunk

Transverse cervical a.

Circumflex scapular a.

Dorsal scapular a.

Thoraco-dorsal a.

Subclavian a.

Suprascapular a.

Acromial brs.

Axillary a.

Anterior circumflex humeral a.

Posterior circumflex humeral a.

Subscapular a.

Deep a. of arm

Brachial a.

Fig. 28.4 **Arteries of the forearm and hand**

Right limb. The ulnar and radial arteries are interconnected by the superficial and deep palmar arches, the perforating branches, and the dorsal carpal network.

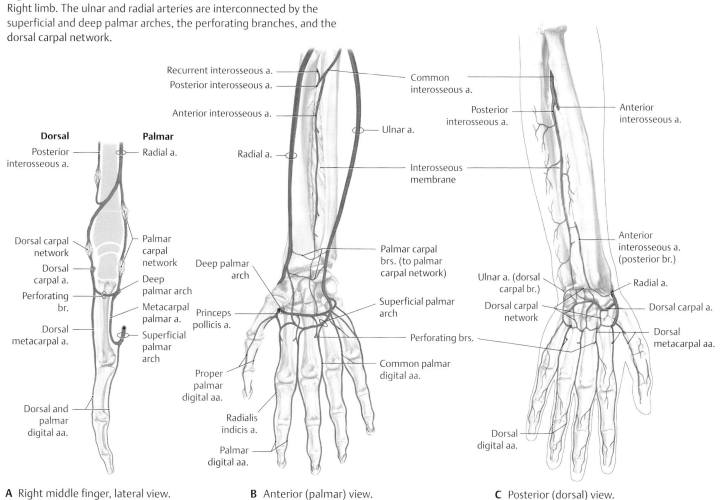

Recurrent interosseous a.

Posterior interosseous a.

Anterior interosseous a.

Dorsal

Posterior interosseous a.

Dorsal carpal network

Dorsal carpal a.

Perforating br.

Dorsal metacarpal a.

Dorsal and palmar digital aa.

A Right middle finger, lateral view.

Palmar

Radial a.

Palmar carpal network

Deep palmar arch

Metacarpal palmar a.

Superficial palmar arch

Radial a.

Deep palmar arch

Princeps pollicis a.

Proper palmar digital aa.

Radialis indicis a.

Palmar digital aa.

Common interosseous a.

Ulnar a.

Interosseous membrane

Palmar carpal brs. (to palmar carpal network)

Superficial palmar arch

Perforating brs.

Common palmar digital aa.

B Anterior (palmar) view.

Posterior interosseous a.

Ulnar a. (dorsal carpal br.)

Dorsal carpal network

Dorsal digital aa.

Anterior interosseous a.

Anterior interosseous a. (posterior br.)

Radial a.

Dorsal carpal a.

Dorsal metacarpal aa.

C Posterior (dorsal) view.

361

Veins & Lymphatics of the Upper Limb

Fig. 28.5 Veins of the upper limb
Right limb, anterior view.

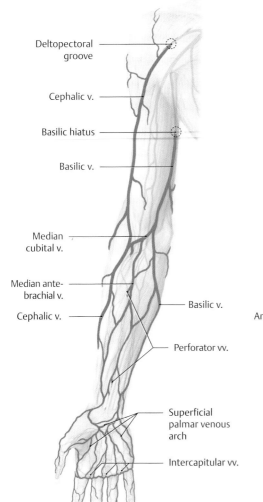

Deltopectoral groove

Cephalic v.

Basilic hiatus

Basilic v.

Median cubital v.

Median ante-brachial v.

Cephalic v.

Perforator vv.

Superficial palmar venous arch

Intercapitular vv.

A Superficial veins.

Subclavian v.

Axillary v.

Subscapular v.

Basilic v.

Brachial vv.

Anterior inter-osseous vv.

Radial vv.

Ulnar vv.

Deep palmar venous arch

Palmar metacarpal vv.

Palmar digital vv.

B Deep veins.

Fig. 28.6 Veins of the dorsum
Right hand, posterior view.

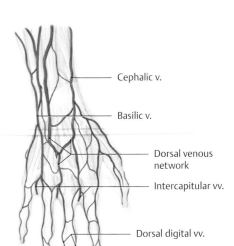

Cephalic v.

Basilic v.

Dorsal venous network

Intercapitular vv.

Dorsal digital vv.

![Clinical box icon] **Clinical box 28.1**

Venipuncture
The veins of the cubital fossa are frequently used when drawing blood. In preparation, a tourniquet is applied above the cubital fossa. This allows arterial blood to flow, but blocks the return of venous blood. The resulting swelling makes the veins more visible and palpable.

Fig. 28.7 Cubital fossa
Right limb, anterior view. The subcutaneous veins of the cubital fossa have a highly variable course.

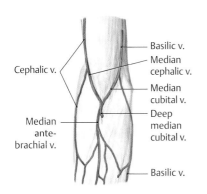

Cephalic v.

Basilic v.

Median cephalic v.

Median cubital v.

Deep median cubital v.

Median ante-brachial v.

Basilic v.

A M-shaped.

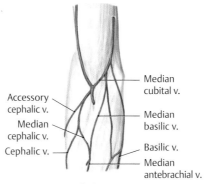

Accessory cephalic v.

Median cephalic v.

Cephalic v.

Median cubital v.

Median basilic v.

Basilic v.

Median antebrachial v.

B Accessory cephalic vein.

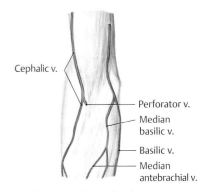

Cephalic v.

Perforator v.

Median basilic v.

Basilic v.

Median antebrachial v.

C Absent median cubital vein.

Lymph from the upper limb and breast drains to the axillary lymph nodes. The superficial lymphatics of the upper limb lie in the subcutaneous tissue, while the deep lymphatics accompany the arteries and deep veins. Numerous anastomoses exist between the two systems.

Fig. 28.8 Lymph vessels of the upper limb
Right limb.

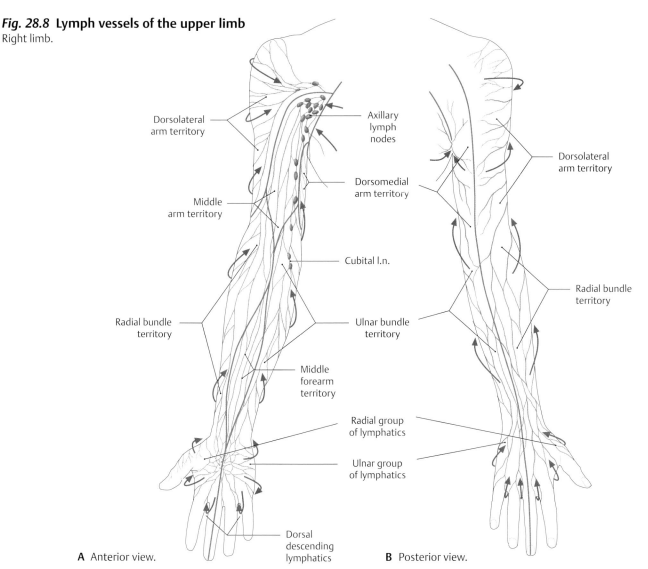

Dorsolateral arm territory

Axillary lymph nodes

Dorsomedial arm territory

Dorsolateral arm territory

Middle arm territory

Cubital l.n.

Radial bundle territory

Radial bundle territory

Ulnar bundle territory

Middle forearm territory

Radial group of lymphatics

Ulnar group of lymphatics

Dorsal descending lymphatics

A Anterior view.

B Posterior view.

Fig. 28.9 Lymphatic drainage of the hand
Right hand, radial view. Most of the hand drains to the axillary nodes via cubital nodes. However, the thumb, index finger, and dorsum of the hand drain directly.

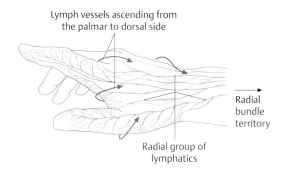

Lymph vessels ascending from the palmar to dorsal side

Radial bundle territory

Radial group of lymphatics

Fig. 28.10 Axillary lymph nodes
Right side, anterior view. For surgical purposes, the axillary lymph nodes are divided into three levels with respect to their relationship with the pectoralis minor: lateral (level I), posterior (level II), or medial (level III). They have major clinical importance in breast cancer (see **p. 77**).

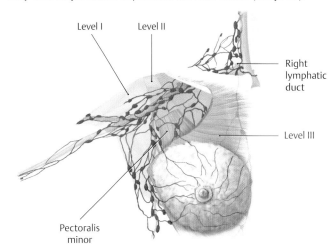

Level I

Level II

Right lymphatic duct

Level III

Pectoralis minor

Nerves of the Upper Limb: Brachial Plexus

Almost all muscles in the upper limb are innervated by the brachial plexus, which arises from spinal cord segments C5 to T1. The anterior rami of the spinal nerves give off direct branches (supraclavicular part of the brachial plexus) and merge to form three trunks, six divisions (three anterior and three posterior), and three cords. The infraclavicular part of the brachial plexus consists of short branches that arise directly from the cords and long (terminal) branches that traverse the limb.

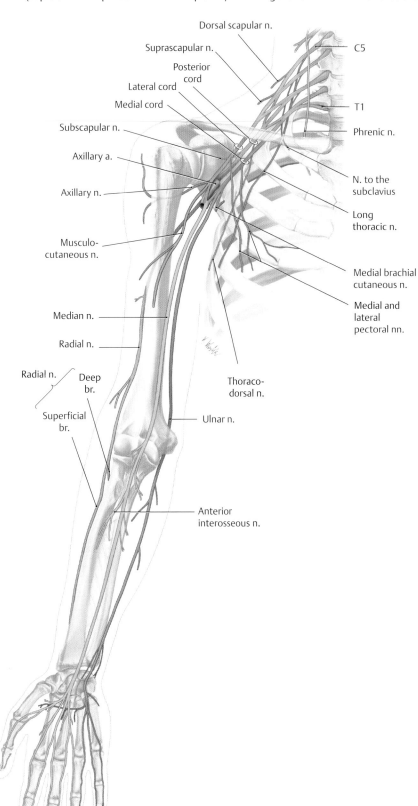

Dorsal scapular n.
Suprascapular n.
Posterior cord
Lateral cord
Medial cord
Subscapular n.
Axillary a.
Axillary n.
Musculo-cutaneous n.
Median n.
Radial n.
Radial n.
Deep br.
Superficial br.
C5
T1
Phrenic n.
N. to the subclavius
Long thoracic n.
Medial brachial cutaneous n.
Medial and lateral pectoral nn.
Thoraco-dorsal n.
Ulnar n.
Anterior interosseous n.

Table 28.1	Nerves of the brachial plexus			
Supraclavicular part				
Direct branches from the anterior rami or plexus trunks				
		Dorsal scapular n.		C4–C5
		Suprascapular n.		C4–C6
		N. to the subclavius		C5–C6
		Long thoracic n.		C5–C7
Infraclavicular part				
Short and long branches from the plexus cords				
	Lateral cord	Lateral pectoral n.		C5–C7
		Musculocutaneous n.		
		Median n.	Lateral root	C6–C7
			Medial root	
	Medial cord	Medial pectoral n.		C8–T1
		Medial antebrachial cutaneous n.		
		Medial brachial cutaneous n.		T1
		Ulnar n.		C7–T1
	Posterior cord	Upper subscapular n.		C5–C6
		Thoracodorsal n.		C6–C8
		Lower subscapular n.		C5–C6
		Axillary n.		
		Radial n.		C5–T1

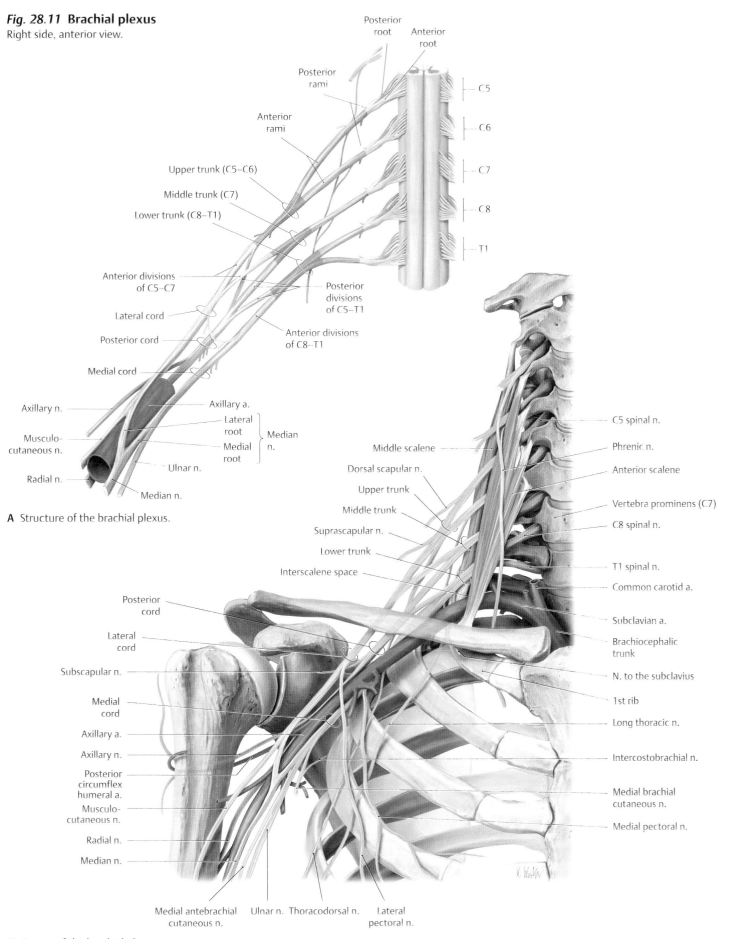

Fig. 28.11 **Brachial plexus**
Right side, anterior view.

Posterior
root
Anterior
root

Posterior
rami

Anterior
rami

C5

C6

C7

C8

T1

Upper trunk (C5–C6)

Middle trunk (C7)

Lower trunk (C8–T1)

Anterior divisions
of C5–C7

Posterior
divisions
of C5–T1

Lateral cord

Anterior divisions
of C8–T1

Posterior cord

Medial cord

Axillary n.

Axillary a.

Musculo-
cutaneous n.

Lateral
root

Medial
root

Median
n.

Radial n.

Ulnar n.

Median n.

A Structure of the brachial plexus.

Middle scalene

C5 spinal n.

Dorsal scapular n.

Phrenic n.

Upper trunk

Anterior scalene

Middle trunk

Suprascapular n.

Vertebra prominens (C7)

Lower trunk

C8 spinal n.

Interscalene space

T1 spinal n.

Common carotid a.

Posterior
cord

Subclavian a.

Lateral
cord

Brachiocephalic
trunk

Subscapular n.

N. to the subclavius

Medial
cord

1st rib

Axillary a.

Long thoracic n.

Axillary n.

Posterior
circumflex
humeral a.

Intercostobrachial n.

Musculo-
cutaneous n.

Medial brachial
cutaneous n.

Radial n.

Medial pectoral n.

Median n.

Medial antebrachial
cutaneous n.

Ulnar n.   Thoracodorsal n.

Lateral
pectoral n.

B Course of the brachial plexus,
stretched for clarity.

Supraclavicular Branches & Posterior Cord

Fig. 28.12 Supraclavicular branches
Right shoulder.

The supraclavicular branches of the brachial plexus arise directly from the plexus roots (anterior rami of the spinal nerves) or from the plexus trunks in the lateral cervical triangle.

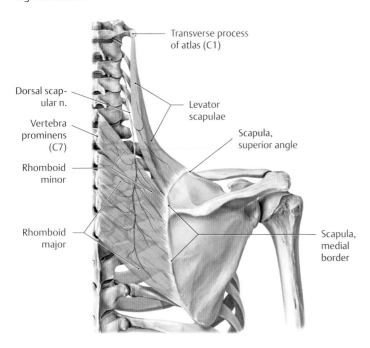

A Dorsal scapular nerve. Posterior view.

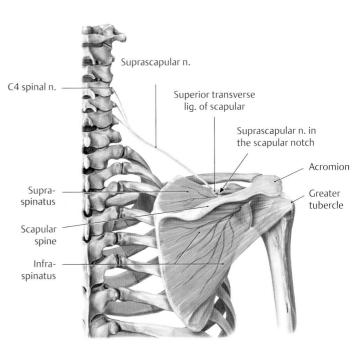

B Suprascapular nerve. Posterior view.

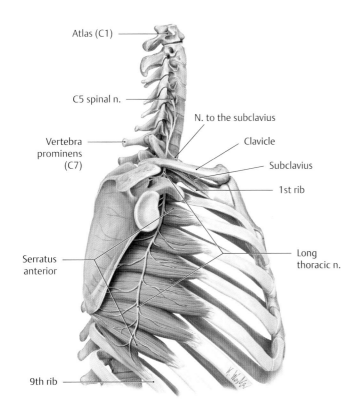

C Long thoracic nerve and nerve to the sub-clavius. Right lateral view.

Table 28.2	Supraclavicular branches	
Nerve	**Level**	**Innervated muscle**
Dorsal scapular n.	C4–C5	Levator scapulae Rhomboids major and minor
Suprascapular n.	C4–C6	Supraspinatus Infraspinatus
N. to the subclavius	C5–C6	Subclavius
Long thoracic n.	C5–C7	Serratus anterior

Fig. 28.13 Posterior cord: Short branches
Right shoulder.

 The posterior cord gives off three short branches (arising at the level of the plexus cords) and two long branches (terminal nerves, see pp. 368–369).

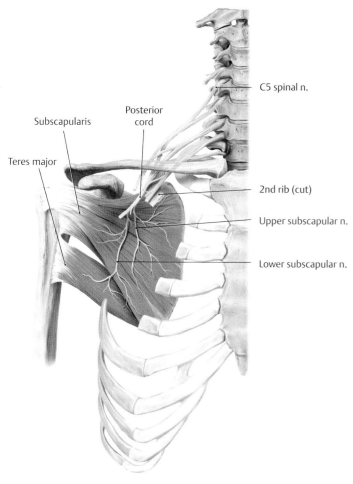

A Subscapular nerves. Anterior view.

Labels in figure A:
- Subscapularis
- Posterior cord
- Teres major
- C5 spinal n.
- 2nd rib (cut)
- Upper subscapular n.
- Lower subscapular n.

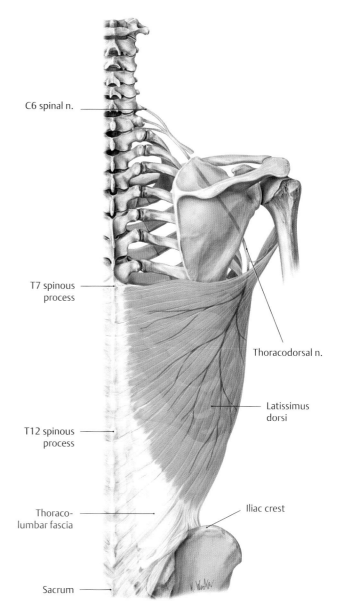

B Thoracodorsal nerve. Posterior view.

Labels in figure B:
- C6 spinal n.
- T7 spinous process
- T12 spinous process
- Thoraco-lumbar fascia
- Sacrum
- Thoracodorsal n.
- Latissimus dorsi
- Iliac crest

Table 28.3	Branches of the posterior cord	
Nerve	**Level**	**Innervated muscle**
Short branches		
Upper subscapular n.	C5–C6	Subscapularis
Lower subscapular n.		Subscapularis Teres major
Thoracodorsal n.	C6–C8	Latissimus dorsi
Long (terminal) branches		
Axillary n.	C5–C6	See **p. 368**
Radial n.	C5–T1	See **p. 369**

Posterior Cord: Axillary & Radial Nerves

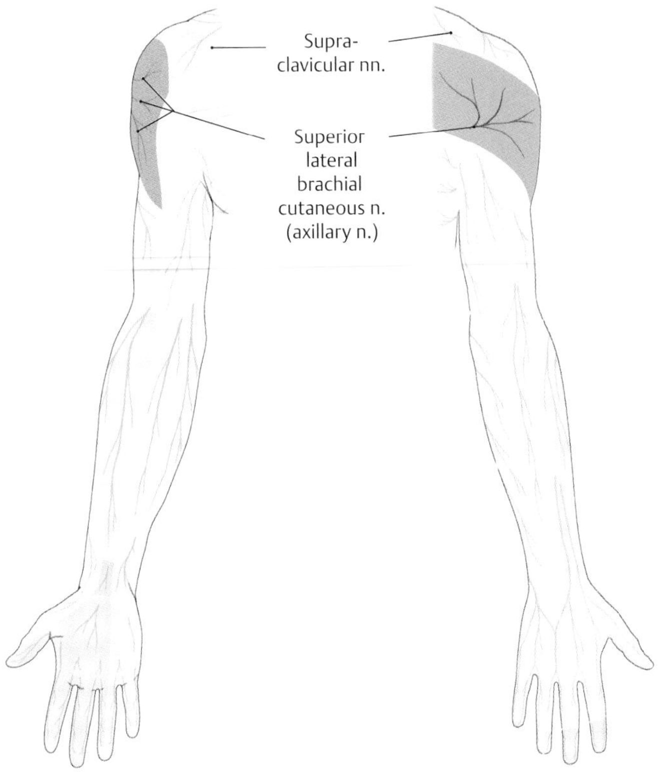

Fig. 28.14 Axillary nerve: Cutaneous distribution
Right limb.

Supra-clavicular nn.

Superior lateral brachial cutaneous n. (axillary n.)

A Anterior view.

B Posterior view.

The axillary nerve may be damaged in a fracture of the surgical neck of the humerus. This results in limited ability to abduct the arm and may cause a loss of profile of the shoulder.

Fig. 28.15 Axillary nerve
Right side, anterior view, stretched for clarity.

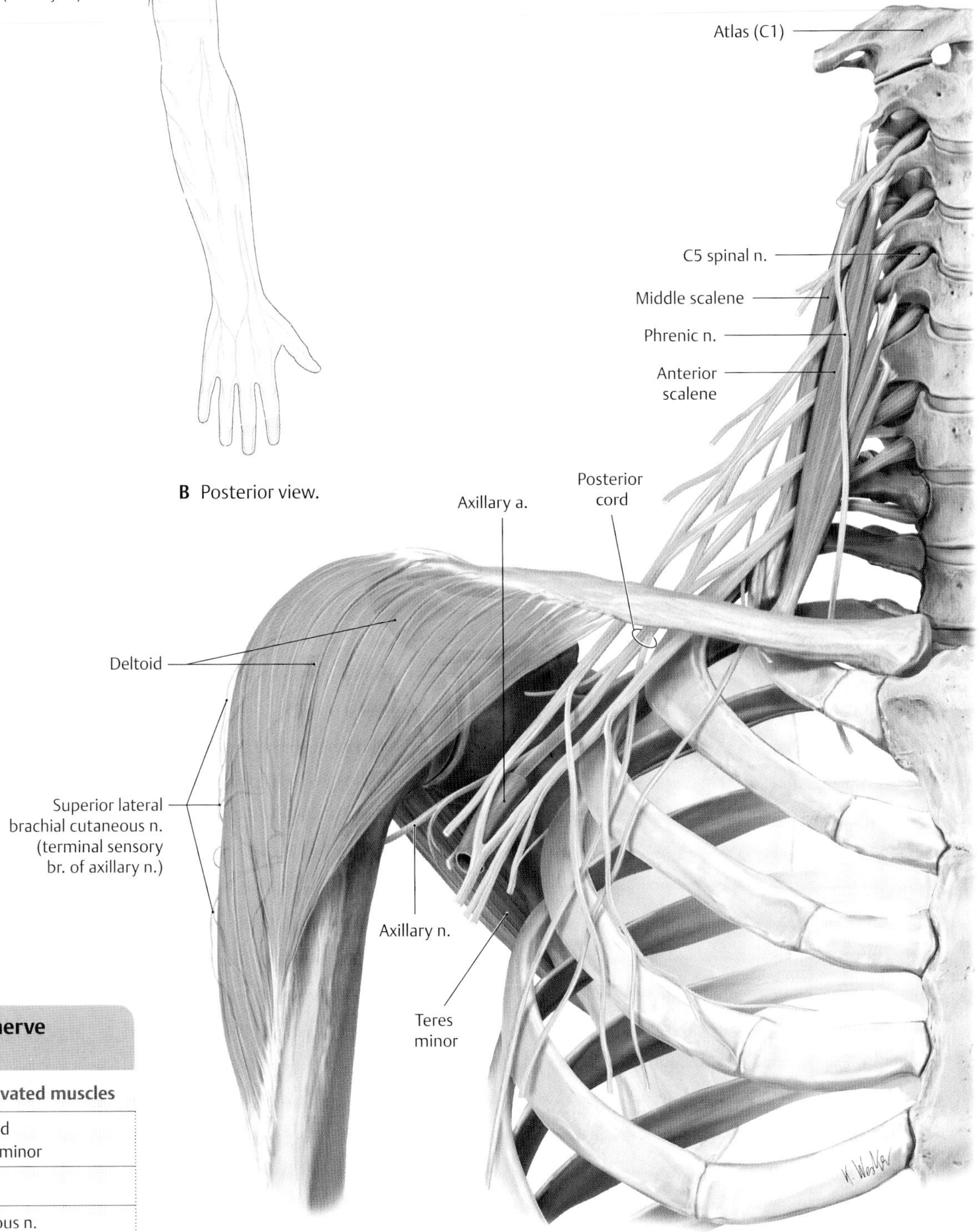

Atlas (C1)

C5 spinal n.

Middle scalene

Phrenic n.

Anterior scalene

Posterior cord

Axillary a.

Deltoid

Superior lateral brachial cutaneous n. (terminal sensory br. of axillary n.)

Axillary n.

Teres minor

Table 28.4	Axillary nerve (C5–C6)	
Motor branches	**Innervated muscles**	
Muscular brs.	Deltoid Teres minor	
Sensory branch		
Superior lateral brachial cutaneous n.		

Fig. 28.16 Radial nerve: Cutaneous distribution

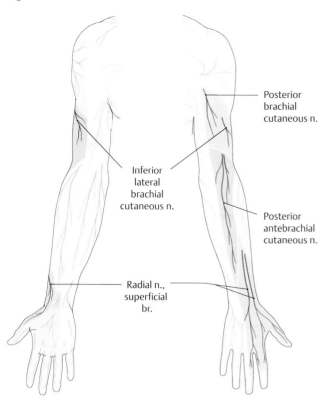

Posterior brachial cutaneous n.

Inferior lateral brachial cutaneous n.

Posterior antebrachial cutaneous n.

Radial n., superficial br.

A Anterior view.   **B** Posterior view.

Table 28.5	Radial nerve (C5–T1)
Motor branches	**Innervated muscles**
Muscular brs.	Brachialis (partial)
	Triceps brachii
	Anconeus
	Brachioradialis
	Extensors carpi radialis longus and brevis
Deep br. (terminal br.: posterior interosseous n.)	Supinator
	Extensor digitorum
	Extensor digiti minimi
	Extensor carpi ulnaris
	Extensors pollicis brevis and longus
	Extensor indicis
	Abductor pollicis longus
Sensory branches	
Articular brs. from radial n.: Capsule of the shoulder joint	
Articular brs. from posterior interosseous n.: Joint capsule of the wrist and four radial metacarpophalangeal joints	
Posterior brachial cutaneous n.	
Inferior lateral brachial cutaneous n.	
Posterior antebrachial cutaneous n.	
Superficial brs.	Dorsal digital nn.
	Ulnar communicating br.

Fig. 28.17 Radial nerve
Right limb, anterior view with forearm pronated.

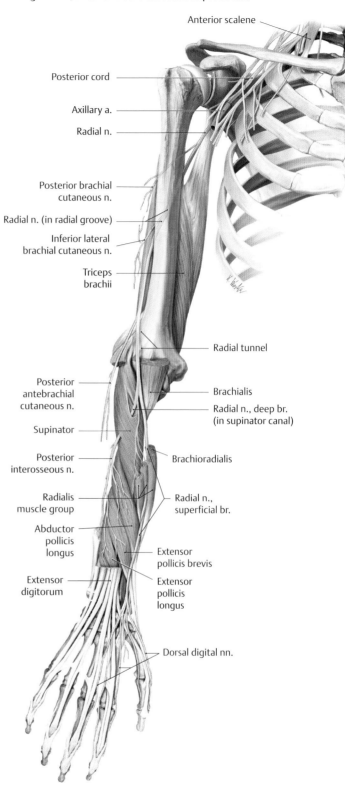

Anterior scalene

Posterior cord

Axillary a.

Radial n.

Posterior brachial cutaneous n.

Radial n. (in radial groove)

Inferior lateral brachial cutaneous n.

Triceps brachii

Radial tunnel

Brachialis

Radial n., deep br. (in supinator canal)

Posterior antebrachial cutaneous n.

Supinator

Brachioradialis

Posterior interosseous n.

Radialis muscle group

Radial n., superficial br.

Abductor pollicis longus

Extensor pollicis brevis

Extensor digitorum

Extensor pollicis longus

Dorsal digital nn.

Clinical box 28.3

Chronic radial nerve compression in the axilla (e.g., due to extended/improper crutch use) may cause loss of sensation or motor function in the hand, forearm, and posterior arm. More distal injuries (e.g., during anesthesia) affect fewer muscles, potentially resulting in wrist drop with intact triceps brachii function.

Medial & Lateral Cords

The medial and lateral cords give off four short branches. The intercostobrachial nerves are included with the short branches of the brachial plexus, although they are actually the cutaneous branches of the 2nd and 3rd intercostal nerves.

Table 28.6	Branches of the medial and lateral cords		
Nerve	**Level**	**Cord**	**Innervated muscle**
Short branches			
Lateral pectoral n.	C5–C7	Lateral cord	Pectoralis major
Medial pectoral n.	C8–T1		Pectoralis major and minor
Medial brachial cutaneous n.	T1	Medial cord	— (sensory brs., do not innervate any muscles)
Medial antebrachial cutaneous n.	C8–T1		
Intercostobrachial nn.	T2–T3		
Long (terminal) branches			
Musculocutaneous n.	C5–C7	Lateral cord	Coracobrachialis Biceps brachii Brachialis
Median n.	C6–T1	Medial cord	See **p. 372**
Ulnar n.	C7–T1		See **p. 373**

Fig. 28.19 Short branches of medial and lateral cords: Cutaneous distribution

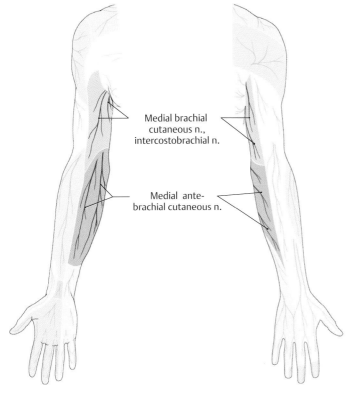

A Anterior view. **B** Posterior view.

Fig. 28.18 Medial and lateral cords: Short branches

Right side, anterior view.

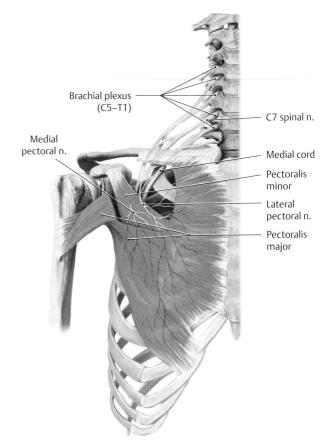

A Medial and lateral pectoral nerves.

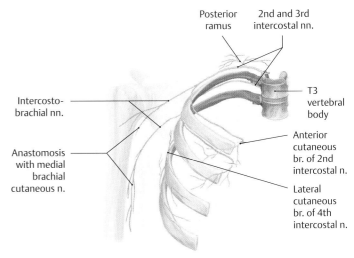

B Intercostobrachial nerves.

Fig. 28.20 Musculocutaneous nerve
Right limb, anterior view.

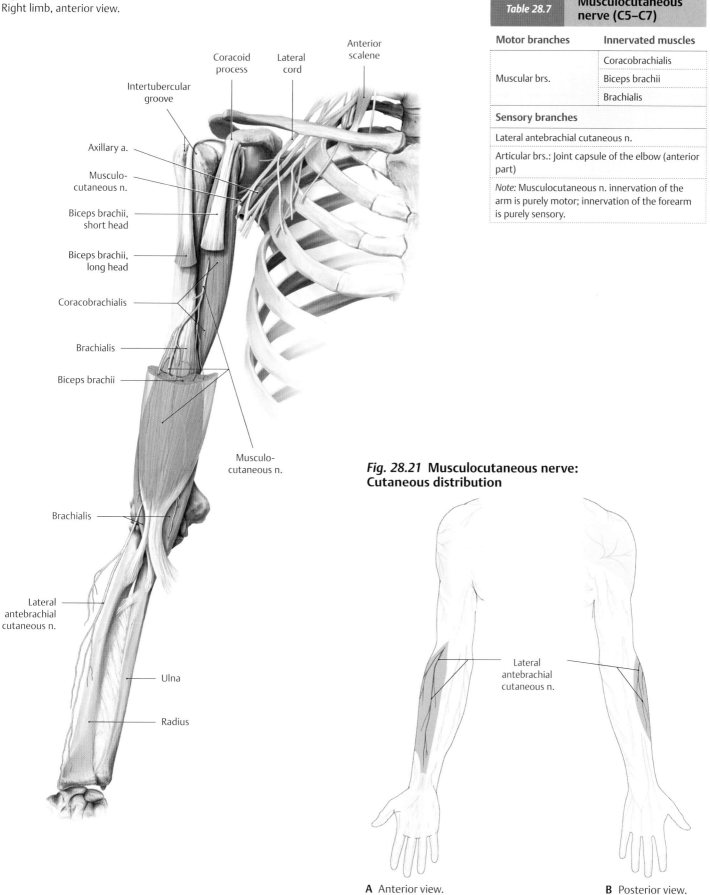

Table 28.7	Musculocutaneous nerve (C5–C7)
Motor branches	**Innervated muscles**
Muscular brs.	Coracobrachialis
	Biceps brachii
	Brachialis
Sensory branches	
Lateral antebrachial cutaneous n.	
Articular brs.: Joint capsule of the elbow (anterior part)	
Note: Musculocutaneous n. innervation of the arm is purely motor; innervation of the forearm is purely sensory.	

Fig. 28.21 Musculocutaneous nerve: Cutaneous distribution

A Anterior view.

B Posterior view.

Median & Ulnar Nerves

The median nerve is a terminal branch arising from both the medial and the lateral cords. The ulnar nerve arises exclusively from the medial cord.

Fig. 28.22 **Median nerve**
Right limb, anterior view.

Anterior scalene
Lateral cord
Medial cord
Axillary a.
Lateral root
Median n. {
Medial root
Median n.
Humeral epicondyle
Articular br.
Pronator teres, humeral head
Flexor carpi radialis
Pronator teres, ulnar head
Palmaris longus
Flexor digitorum superficialis
Anterior interosseous n.
Flexor digitorum profundus
Flexor pollicis longus
Pronator quadratus
Thenar muscular br.
Median n., palmar br.
Flexor retinaculum
Common palmar digital nn.
1st and 2nd lumbricals
Proper palmar digital nn.

Fig. 28.23 **Median nerve: Cutaneous distribution**

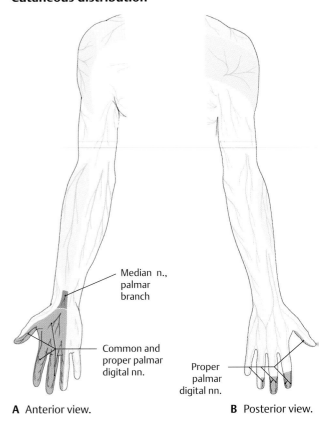

Median n., palmar branch
Common and proper palmar digital nn.
Proper palmar digital nn.

A Anterior view. **B** Posterior view.

Clinical box 28.4

Median nerve injury caused by fracture/ dislocation of the elbow joint may result in compromised grasping ability and sensory loss in the fingertips (see **Fig. 28.23** for territories). See also carpal tunnel syndrome (**p. 387**).

Table 28.8	Median nerve (C6–T1)	
Motor branches	**Innervated muscles**	
Direct muscular brs.	Pronator teres	
	Flexor carpi radialis	
	Palmaris longus	
	Flexor digitorum superficialis	
Muscular brs. from anterior interosseous n.	Pronator quadratus	
	Flexor pollicis longus	
	Flexor digitorum profundus (radial half)	
Thenar muscular br.	Abductor pollicis brevis	
	Flexor pollicis brevis (superficial head)	
	Opponens pollicis	
Muscular brs. from common palmar digital nn.	1st and 2nd lumbricals	
Sensory branches		
Articular brs.: Capsules of the elbow and wrist joints		
Palmar br. of median n. (thenar eminence)		
Communicating br. to ulnar n.		
Common palmar digital nn.		
Proper palmar digital nn.		

Fig. 28.24 Ulnar nerve: Cutaneous distribution

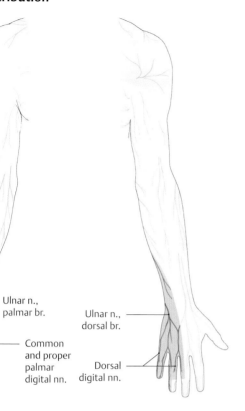

A Anterior view.　　　　**B** Posterior view.

Ulnar n., palmar br.

Common and proper palmar digital nn.

Ulnar n., dorsal br.

Dorsal digital nn.

Fig. 28.25 Ulnar nerve
Right limb, anterior view.

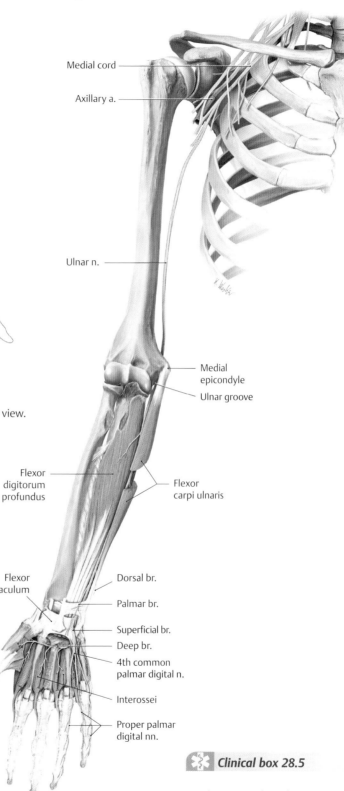

Medial cord

Axillary a.

Ulnar n.

Medial epicondyle

Ulnar groove

Flexor digitorum profundus

Flexor carpi ulnaris

Flexor retinaculum

Dorsal br.

Palmar br.

Superficial br.

Deep br.

4th common palmar digital n.

Interossei

Proper palmar digital nn.

Table 28.9	Ulnar nerve (C7–T1)
Motor branches	**Innervated muscles**
Direct muscular brs.	Flexor carpi ulnaris
	Flexor digitorum profundus (ulnar half)
Muscular br. from superior ulnar n.	Palmaris brevis
Muscular brs. from deep ulnar n.	Abductor digiti minimi
	Flexor digiti minimi brevis
	Opponens digiti minimi
	3rd and 4th lumbricals
	Palmar and dorsal interosseous muscles
	Adductor pollicis
	Flexor pollicis brevis (deep head)
Sensory branches	
Articular brs.: Capsules of the elbow, carpal, and metacarpophalangeal joints	
Dorsal br. (terminal brs.: dorsal digital nn.)	
Palmar br.	
Proper palmar digital n. (from superficial br.)	
Common palmar digital n. (from superficial br.; terminal brs.: proper palmar digital nn.)	

Clinical box 28.5

Ulnar nerve palsy is the most common peripheral nerve damage. The ulnar nerve is most vulnerable to trauma or chronic compression in the elbow joint and ulnar tunnel (see **p. 387**). Nerve damage causes "clawing" of the hand and atrophy of the interossei. Sensory losses are often limited to the 5th digit.

Superficial Veins & Nerves of the Upper Limb

Fig. 28.26 Superficial cutaneous veins and nerves of the upper limb

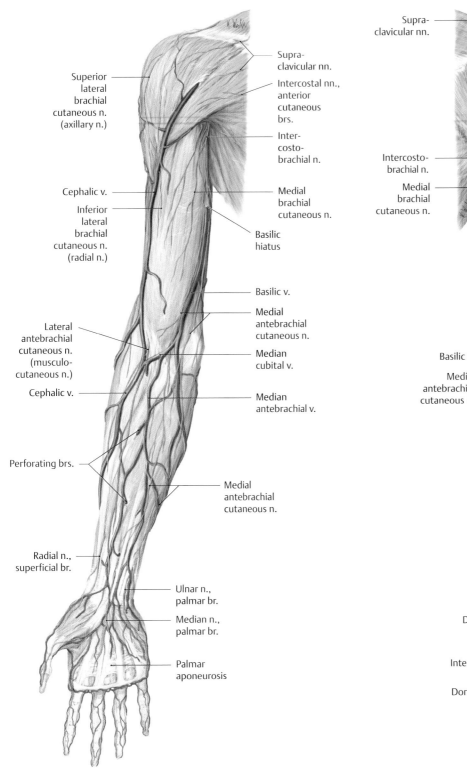

Superior lateral brachial cutaneous n. (axillary n.)

Supra-clavicular nn.

Intercostal nn., anterior cutaneous brs.

Inter-costo-brachial n.

Cephalic v.

Medial brachial cutaneous n.

Inferior lateral brachial cutaneous n. (radial n.)

Basilic hiatus

Basilic v.

Medial antebrachial cutaneous n.

Median cubital v.

Lateral antebrachial cutaneous n. (musculo-cutaneous n.)

Cephalic v.

Median antebrachial v.

Perforating brs.

Medial antebrachial cutaneous n.

Radial n., superficial br.

Ulnar n., palmar br.

Median n., palmar br.

Palmar aponeurosis

A Anterior view. See **pp. 388–389** for nerves of the palm.

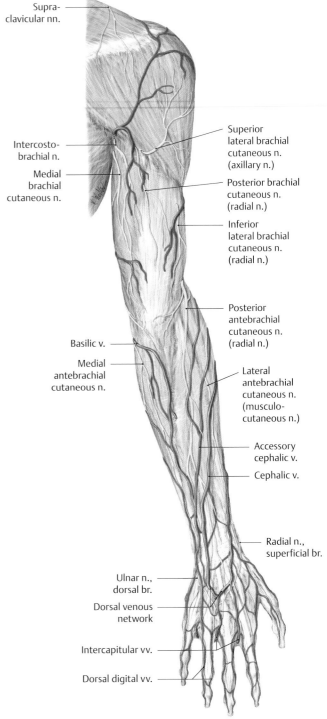

Supra-clavicular nn.

Intercosto-brachial n.

Medial brachial cutaneous n.

Superior lateral brachial cutaneous n. (axillary n.)

Posterior brachial cutaneous n. (radial n.)

Inferior lateral brachial cutaneous n. (radial n.)

Posterior antebrachial cutaneous n. (radial n.)

Basilic v.

Medial antebrachial cutaneous n.

Lateral antebrachial cutaneous n. (musculo-cutaneous n.)

Accessory cephalic v.

Cephalic v.

Radial n., superficial br.

Ulnar n., dorsal br.

Dorsal venous network

Intercapitular vv.

Dorsal digital vv.

B Posterior view. See **pp. 390–391** for nerves of the dorsum.

Fig. 28.27 Cutaneous innervation of the upper limb

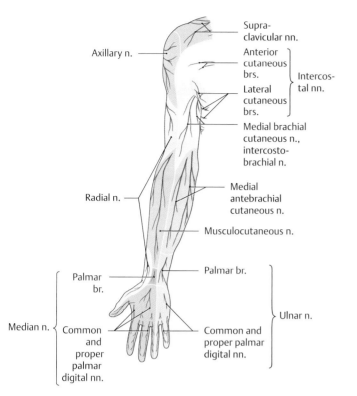

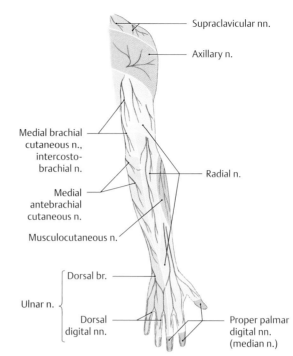

A Anterior view.

B Posterior view.

Fig. 28.28 Dermatomes of the upper limb

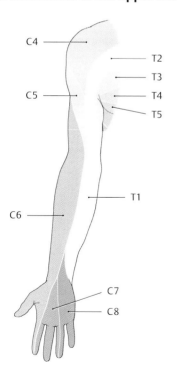

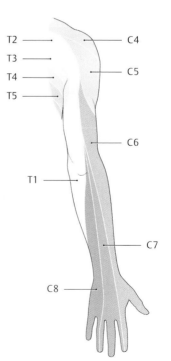

A Anterior view.

B Posterior view.

Posterior Shoulder & Arm

***Fig. 28.29* Posterior shoulder**

Right shoulder, posterior view. *Raised:* Trapezius (transverse part).
Windowed: Supraspinatus. *Revealed:* Suprascapular region.

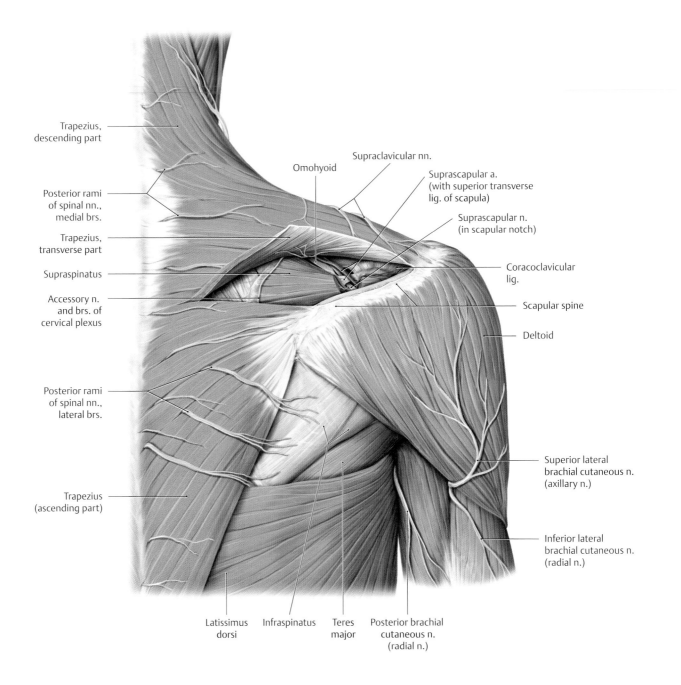

Trapezius,
descending part

Posterior rami
of spinal nn.,
medial brs.

Trapezius,
transverse part

Supraspinatus

Accessory n.
and brs. of
cervical plexus

Posterior rami
of spinal nn.,
lateral brs.

Trapezius
(ascending part)

Omohyoid

Supraclavicular nn.

Suprascapular a.
(with superior transverse
lig. of scapula)

Suprascapular n.
(in scapular notch)

Coracoclavicular
lig.

Scapular spine

Deltoid

Superior lateral
brachial cutaneous n.
(axillary n.)

Inferior lateral
brachial cutaneous n.
(radial n.)

Latissimus
dorsi

Infraspinatus

Teres
major

Posterior brachial
cutaneous n.
(radial n.)

Table 28.10 Neurovascular tracts of the scapula

Passageway	Boundaries	Transmitted structures
① Scapular notch	Superior transverse lig. of scapula, scapula	Suprascapular a. and n.
② Medial border	Scapula	Dorsal scapular a. and n.
③ Triangular space	Teres major and minor	Circumflex scapular a.
④ Triceps hiatus	Triceps brachii, humerus, teres major	Deep a. of arm and radial n.
⑤ Quadrangular space	Teres major and minor, triceps brachii, humerus	Posterior circumflex humeral a. and axillary n.

Fig. 28.30 Triangular and quadrangular spaces

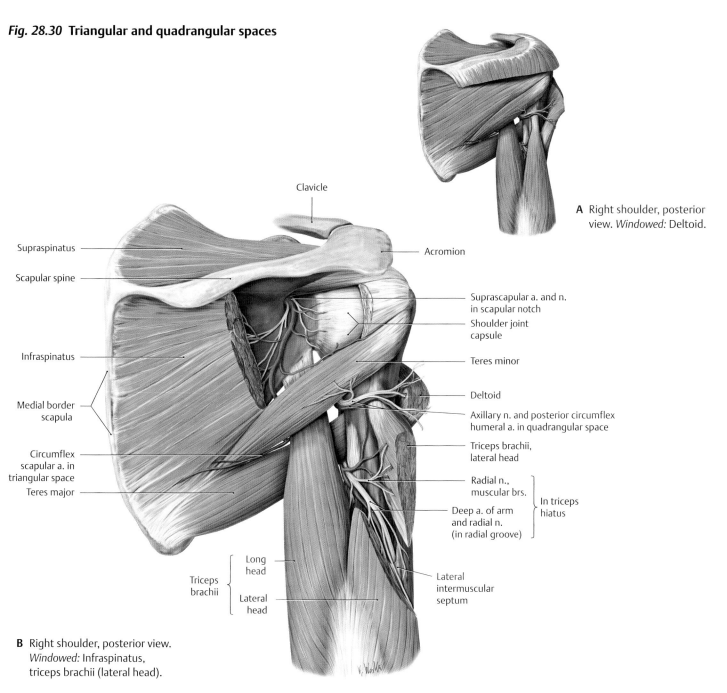

① Superior transverse lig. of scapula

Inferior transverse lig. of scapula

⑤

④

③

②

A Right shoulder, posterior view. *Windowed:* Deltoid.

Clavicle

Supraspinatus

Scapular spine

Acromion

Suprascapular a. and n. in scapular notch

Shoulder joint capsule

Infraspinatus

Teres minor

Medial border scapula

Deltoid

Axillary n. and posterior circumflex humeral a. in quadrangular space

Circumflex scapular a. in triangular space

Triceps brachii, lateral head

Teres major

Radial n., muscular brs.

In triceps hiatus

Deep a. of arm and radial n. (in radial groove)

Triceps brachii — Long head, Lateral head

Lateral intermuscular septum

B Right shoulder, posterior view. *Windowed:* Infraspinatus, triceps brachii (lateral head).

Anterior Shoulder

Fig. 28.31 Anterior shoulder: Superficial dissection
Right shoulder.

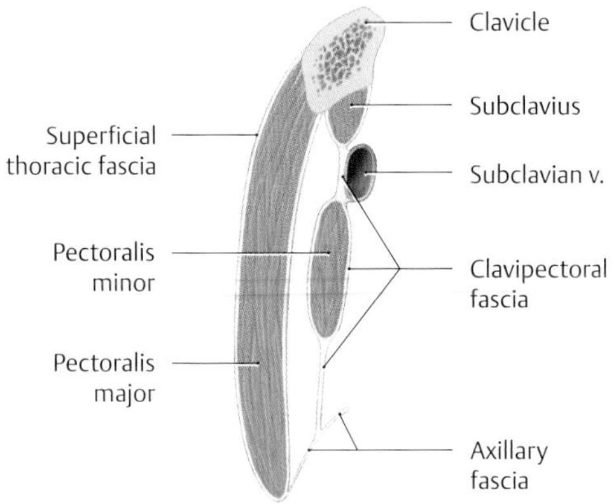
Clavicle
Subclavius
Superficial thoracic fascia
Subclavian v.
Pectoralis minor
Clavipectoral fascia
Pectoralis major
Axillary fascia

A Sagittal section through anterior wall.

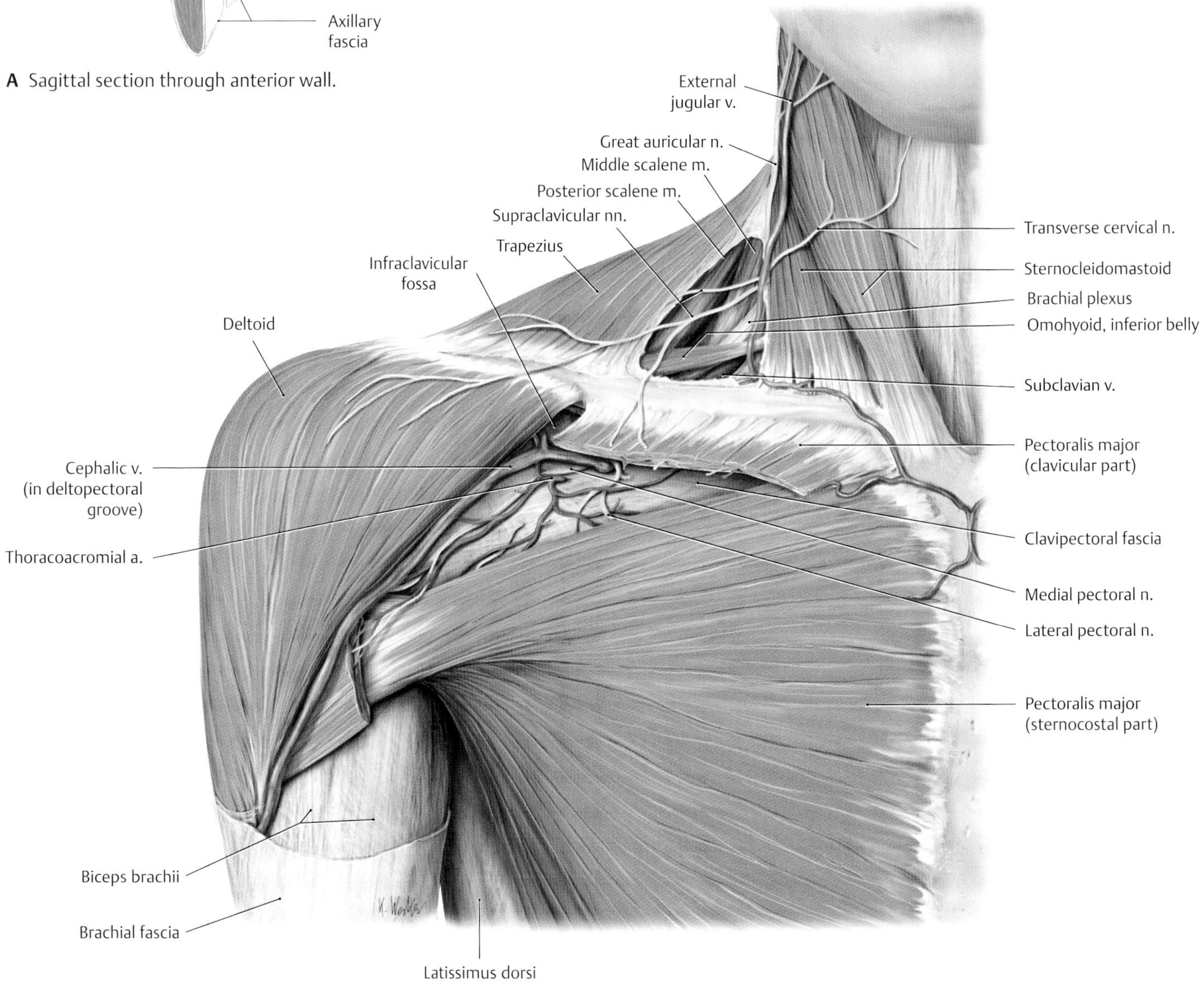
External jugular v.
Great auricular n.
Middle scalene m.
Posterior scalene m.
Supraclavicular nn.
Trapezius
Infraclavicular fossa
Deltoid
Transverse cervical n.
Sternocleidomastoid
Brachial plexus
Omohyoid, inferior belly
Subclavian v.
Pectoralis major (clavicular part)
Cephalic v. (in deltopectoral groove)
Clavipectoral fascia
Thoracoacromial a.
Medial pectoral n.
Lateral pectoral n.
Pectoralis major (sternocostal part)
Biceps brachii
Brachial fascia
Latissimus dorsi

B Anterior view. *Removed:* Platysma, muscle fasciae, superficial layer of cervical fascia, and pectoralis major (clavicular part). *Revealed:* Clavipectoral triangle.

Fig. 28.32 Shoulder: Transverse section

Right shoulder, inferior view.

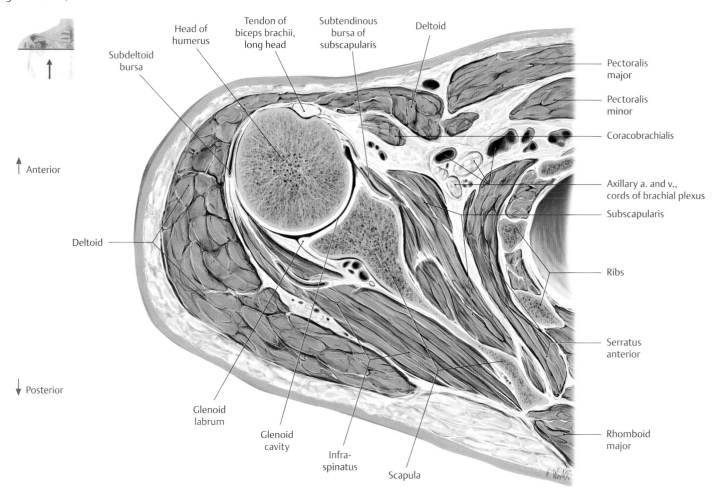

- Head of humerus
- Subdeltoid bursa
- Tendon of biceps brachii, long head
- Subtendinous bursa of subscapularis
- Deltoid
- Pectoralis major
- Pectoralis minor
- Coracobrachialis
- Axillary a. and v., cords of brachial plexus
- Subscapularis
- Ribs
- Anterior
- Deltoid
- Serratus anterior
- Posterior
- Glenoid labrum
- Glenoid cavity
- Infra-spinatus
- Scapula
- Rhomboid major

Fig. 28.33 Anterior shoulder: Deep dissection

Right limb, anterior view. *Removed:* Sternocleidomastoid, omohyoid, and pectoralis major. This dissection reveals the neurovascular contents of the lateral cervical triangle (see p. 642) and axilla (see pp. 380–381).

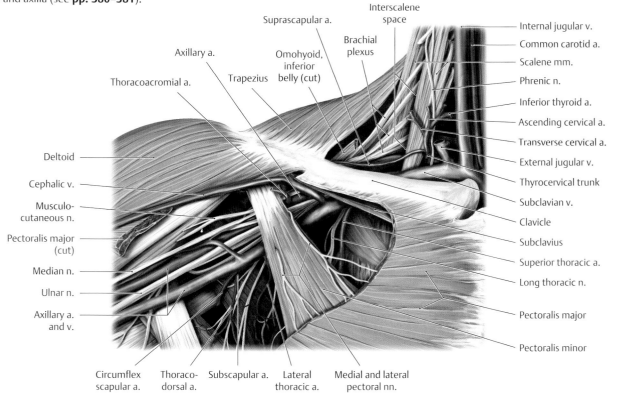

- Suprascapular a.
- Interscalene space
- Axillary a.
- Omohyoid, inferior belly (cut)
- Brachial plexus
- Internal jugular v.
- Common carotid a.
- Thoracoacromial a.
- Trapezius
- Scalene mm.
- Phrenic n.
- Inferior thyroid a.
- Ascending cervical a.
- Transverse cervical a.
- External jugular v.
- Deltoid
- Thyrocervical trunk
- Cephalic v.
- Subclavian v.
- Musculo-cutaneous n.
- Clavicle
- Pectoralis major (cut)
- Subclavius
- Superior thoracic a.
- Median n.
- Long thoracic n.
- Ulnar n.
- Axillary a. and v.
- Pectoralis major
- Pectoralis minor
- Circumflex scapular a.
- Thoraco-dorsal a.
- Subscapular a.
- Lateral thoracic a.
- Medial and lateral pectoral nn.

Axilla

Fig. 28.34 **Axilla: Dissection**
Right shoulder, anterior view.

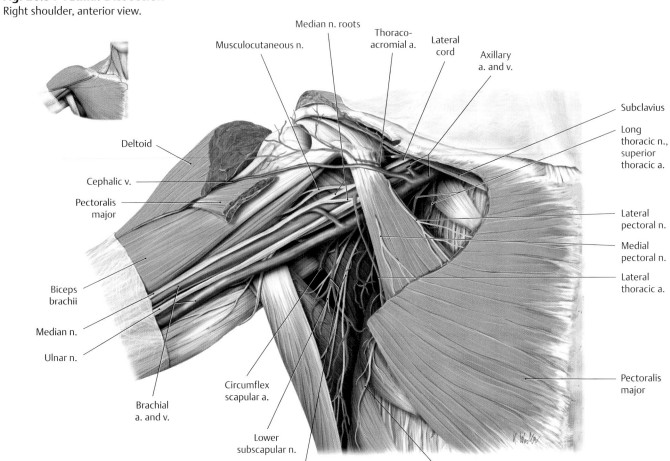

A *Removed:* Pectoralis major and clavipectoral fascia.

Table 28.11	Walls of the axilla
Anterior wall	Pectoralis major Pectoralis minor Clavipectoral fascia
Lateral wall	Intertubercular groove of humerus
Posterior wall	Subscapularis Teres major Latissimus dorsi
Medial wall	Lateral thoracic wall Serratus anterior

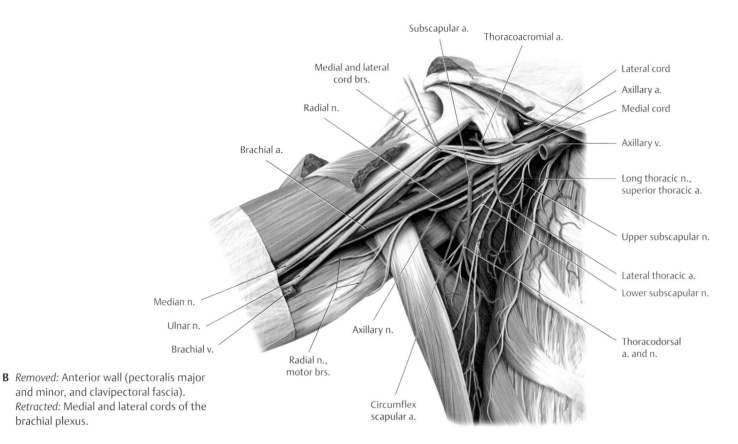

Subscapular a.

Thoracoacromial a.

Medial and lateral cord brs.

Radial n.

Brachial a.

Lateral cord

Axillary a.

Medial cord

Axillary v.

Long thoracic n., superior thoracic a.

Upper subscapular n.

Lateral thoracic a.

Lower subscapular n.

Thoracodorsal a. and n.

Median n.

Ulnar n.

Brachial v.

Radial n., motor brs.

Axillary n.

Circumflex scapular a.

B *Removed:* Anterior wall (pectoralis major and minor, and clavipectoral fascia). *Retracted:* Medial and lateral cords of the brachial plexus.

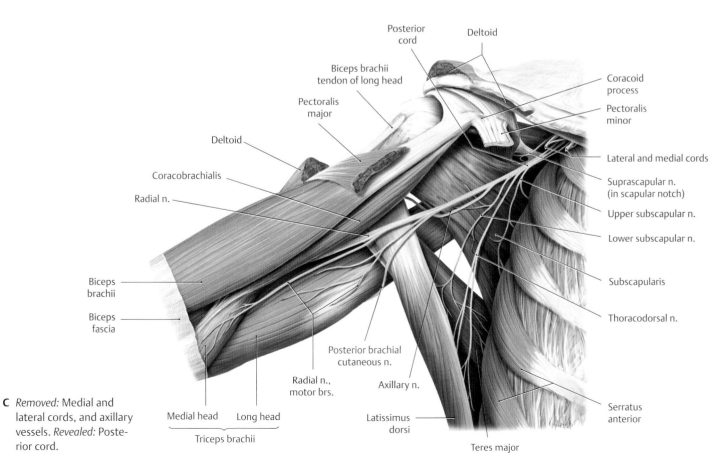

Posterior cord

Deltoid

Biceps brachii tendon of long head

Pectoralis major

Deltoid

Coracobrachialis

Radial n.

Coracoid process

Pectoralis minor

Lateral and medial cords

Suprascapular n. (in scapular notch)

Upper subscapular n.

Lower subscapular n.

Subscapularis

Thoracodorsal n.

Biceps brachii

Biceps fascia

Posterior brachial cutaneous n.

Radial n., motor brs.

Axillary n.

Serratus anterior

C *Removed:* Medial and lateral cords, and axillary vessels. *Revealed:* Posterior cord.

Medial head   Long head

Triceps brachii

Latissimus dorsi

Teres major

Anterior Arm & Cubital Region

Fig. 28.35 **Brachial region**
Right arm, anterior view. *Removed:* Deltoid, pectoralis major and minor. *Revealed:* Medial bicipital groove.

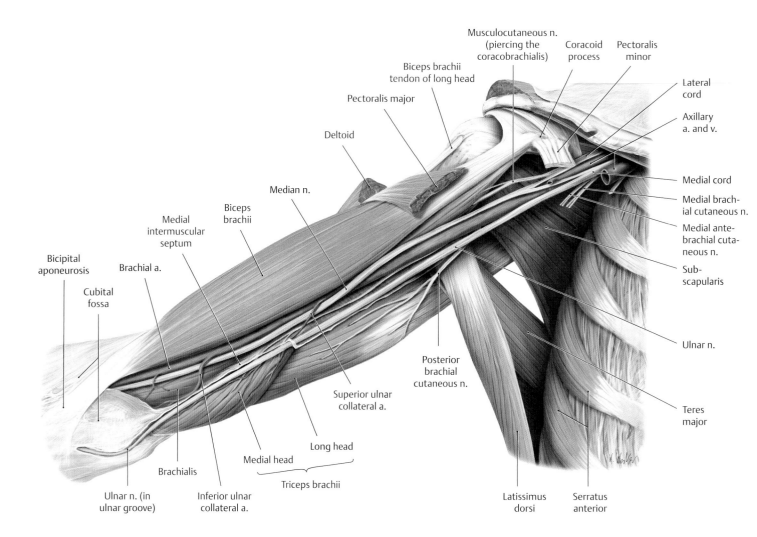

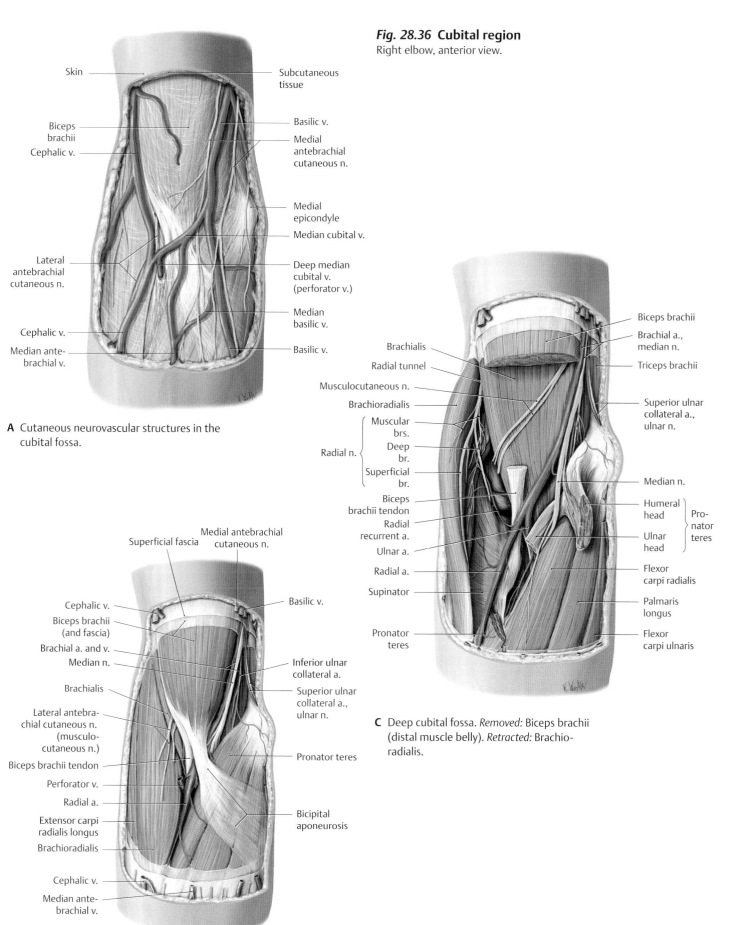

Fig. 28.36 Cubital region
Right elbow, anterior view.

A Cutaneous neurovascular structures in the cubital fossa.

Labels in A:
Skin
Biceps brachii
Cephalic v.
Lateral antebrachial cutaneous n.
Cephalic v.
Median antebrachial v.
Subcutaneous tissue
Basilic v.
Medial antebrachial cutaneous n.
Medial epicondyle
Median cubital v.
Deep median cubital v. (perforator v.)
Median basilic v.
Basilic v.

B Superficial cubital fossa. *Removed:* Fasciae and epifascial neurovascular structures.

Labels in B:
Superficial fascia
Medial antebrachial cutaneous n.
Cephalic v.
Biceps brachii (and fascia)
Brachial a. and v.
Median n.
Brachialis
Lateral antebrachial cutaneous n. (musculocutaneous n.)
Biceps brachii tendon
Perforator v.
Radial a.
Extensor carpi radialis longus
Brachioradialis
Cephalic v.
Median antebrachial v.
Basilic v.
Inferior ulnar collateral a.
Superior ulnar collateral a., ulnar n.
Pronator teres
Bicipital aponeurosis

C Deep cubital fossa. *Removed:* Biceps brachii (distal muscle belly). *Retracted:* Brachioradialis.

Labels in C:
Brachialis
Radial tunnel
Musculocutaneous n.
Brachioradialis
Radial n. { Muscular brs. / Deep br. / Superficial br. }
Biceps brachii tendon
Radial recurrent a.
Ulnar a.
Radial a.
Supinator
Pronator teres
Biceps brachii
Brachial a., median n.
Triceps brachii
Superior ulnar collateral a., ulnar n.
Median n.
Humeral head / Ulnar head } Pronator teres
Flexor carpi radialis
Palmaris longus
Flexor carpi ulnaris

383

Anterior and Posterior Forearm

***Fig. 28.37* Anterior forearm**
Right forearm, anterior view.

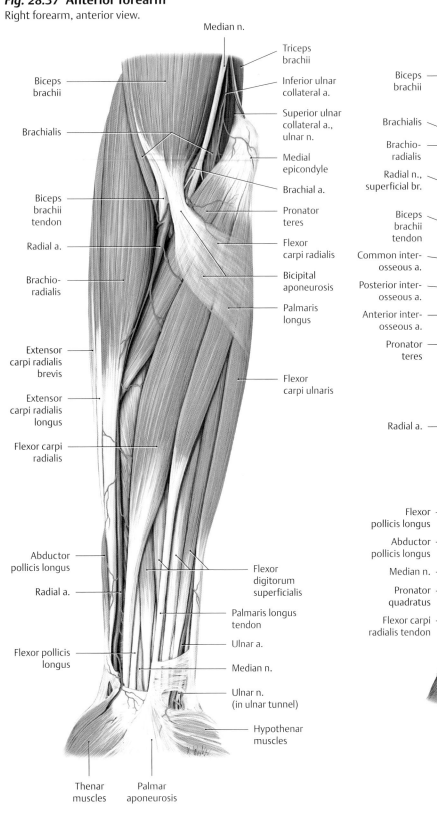

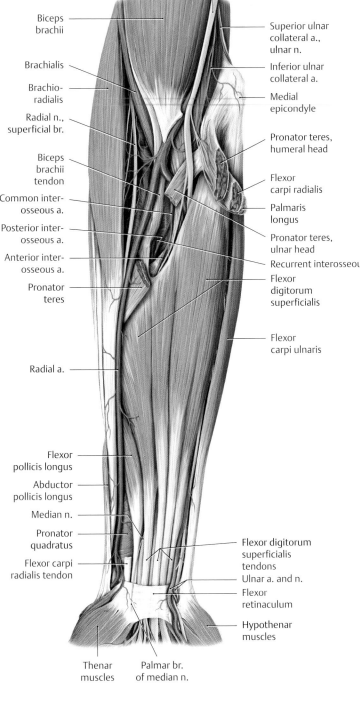

A Superficial layer. *Removed:* Fasciae and superficial neurovasculature.

B Middle layer. *Partially removed:* Superficial flexors (pronator teres, flexor digitorum superficialis, palmaris longus, and flexor carpi radialis).

Fig. 28.38 Posterior forearm

Right forearm, anterior view during pronation. *Reflected:* Anconeus and triceps brachii. *Removed:* Extensor carpi ulnaris and extensor digitorum.

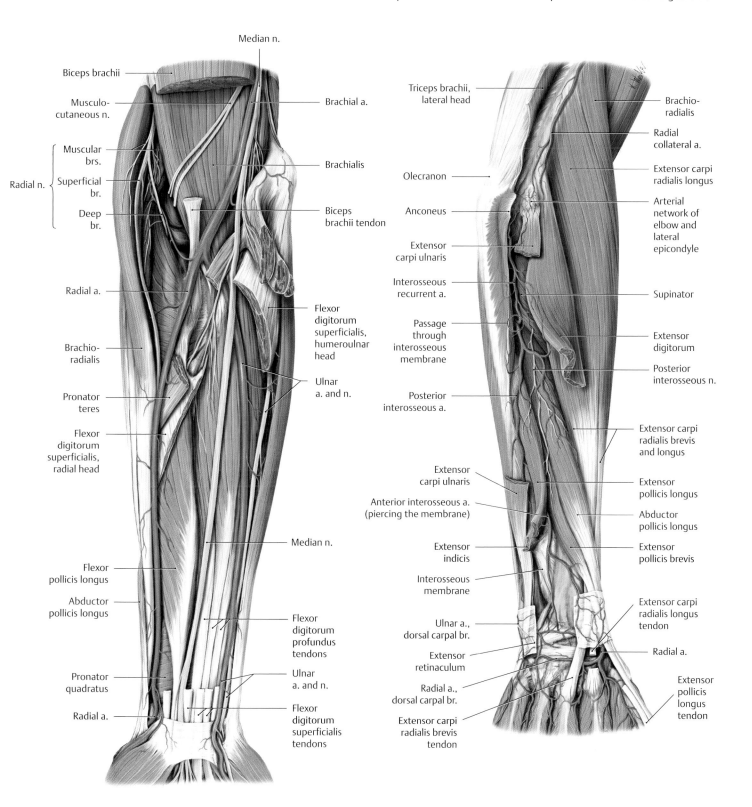

Median n.

Biceps brachii

Musculo-cutaneous n.

Radial n. { Muscular brs. / Superficial br. / Deep br.

Brachial a.

Brachialis

Biceps brachii tendon

Radial a.

Brachio-radialis

Pronator teres

Flexor digitorum superficialis, radial head

Flexor pollicis longus

Abductor pollicis longus

Pronator quadratus

Radial a.

Flexor digitorum superficialis, humeroulnar head

Ulnar a. and n.

Median n.

Flexor digitorum profundus tendons

Ulnar a. and n.

Flexor digitorum superficialis tendons

Triceps brachii, lateral head

Olecranon

Anconeus

Extensor carpi ulnaris

Interosseous recurrent a.

Passage through interosseous membrane

Posterior interosseous a.

Extensor carpi ulnaris

Anterior interosseous a. (piercing the membrane)

Extensor indicis

Interosseous membrane

Ulnar a., dorsal carpal br.

Extensor retinaculum

Radial a., dorsal carpal br.

Extensor carpi radialis brevis tendon

Brachio-radialis

Radial collateral a.

Extensor carpi radialis longus

Arterial network of elbow and lateral epicondyle

Supinator

Extensor digitorum

Posterior interosseous n.

Extensor carpi radialis brevis and longus

Extensor pollicis longus

Abductor pollicis longus

Extensor pollicis brevis

Extensor carpi radialis longus tendon

Radial a.

Extensor pollicis longus tendon

C Deep layer. *Removed:* Deep flexors.

Carpal Region

Fig. 28.39 Anterior carpal region
Right hand, anterior (palmar) view.

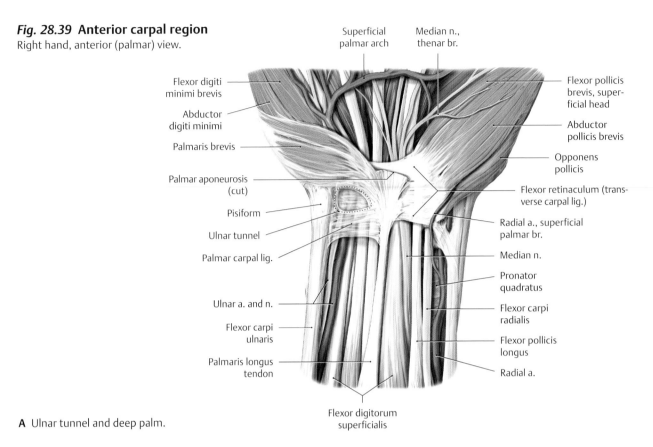

Flexor digiti minimi brevis

Abductor digiti minimi

Palmaris brevis

Palmar aponeurosis (cut)

Pisiform

Ulnar tunnel

Palmar carpal lig.

Ulnar a. and n.

Flexor carpi ulnaris

Palmaris longus tendon

Superficial palmar arch

Median n., thenar br.

Flexor pollicis brevis, superficial head

Abductor pollicis brevis

Opponens pollicis

Flexor retinaculum (transverse carpal lig.)

Radial a., superficial palmar br.

Median n.

Pronator quadratus

Flexor carpi radialis

Flexor pollicis longus

Radial a.

Flexor digitorum superficialis

A Ulnar tunnel and deep palm.

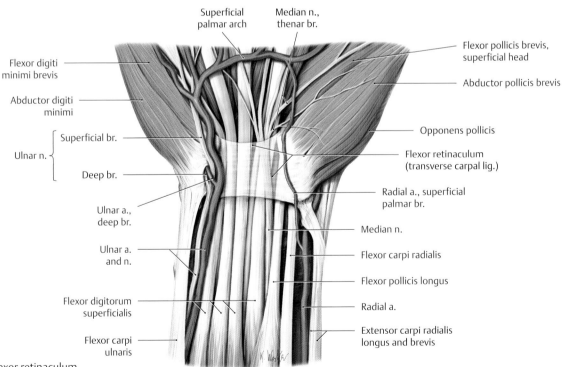

Flexor digiti minimi brevis

Abductor digiti minimi

Ulnar n. { Superficial br.

Deep br.

Ulnar a., deep br.

Ulnar a. and n.

Flexor digitorum superficialis

Flexor carpi ulnaris

Superficial palmar arch

Median n., thenar br.

Flexor pollicis brevis, superficial head

Abductor pollicis brevis

Opponens pollicis

Flexor retinaculum (transverse carpal lig.)

Radial a., superficial palmar br.

Median n.

Flexor carpi radialis

Flexor pollicis longus

Radial a.

Extensor carpi radialis longus and brevis

B Carpal tunnel with flexor retinaculum transparent. *Removed:* palmaris brevis, palmaris longus, palmar aponeurosis, and palmar carpal ligament.

Fig. 28.40 Ulnar tunnel

Right hand, anterior (palmar) view.

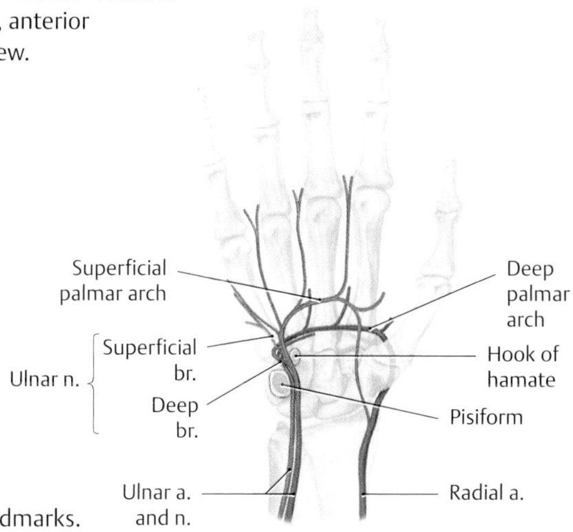

Superficial palmar arch

Deep palmar arch

Ulnar n.
- Superficial br.
- Deep br.

Hook of hamate

Pisiform

Ulnar a. and n.

Radial a.

A Bony landmarks.

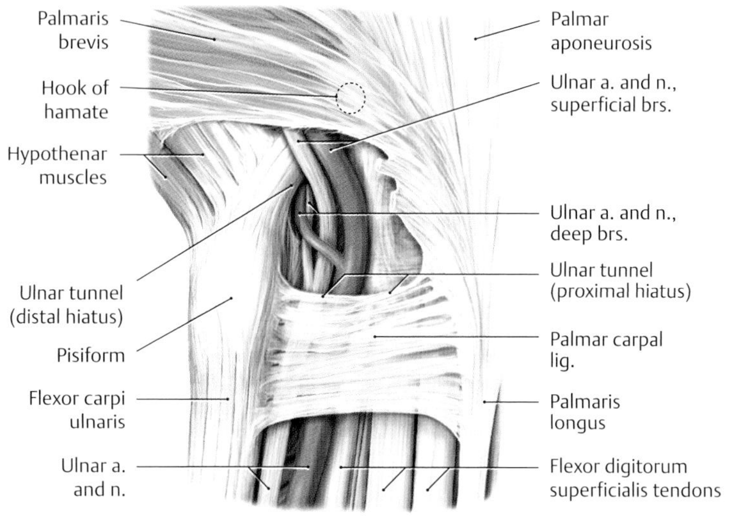

Palmaris brevis

Hook of hamate

Hypothenar muscles

Ulnar tunnel (distal hiatus)

Pisiform

Flexor carpi ulnaris

Ulnar a. and n.

Palmar aponeurosis

Ulnar a. and n., superficial brs.

Ulnar a. and n., deep brs.

Ulnar tunnel (proximal hiatus)

Palmar carpal lig.

Palmaris longus

Flexor digitorum superficialis tendons

B Apertures and walls of the ulnar tunnel.

Fig. 28.41 Carpal tunnel: Cross section

Right hand, proximal view. The tight fit of sensitive neurovascular structures with closely apposed, frequently moving tendons in the carpal tunnel often causes problems (carpal tunnel syndrome) when any of the structures swell or degenerate.

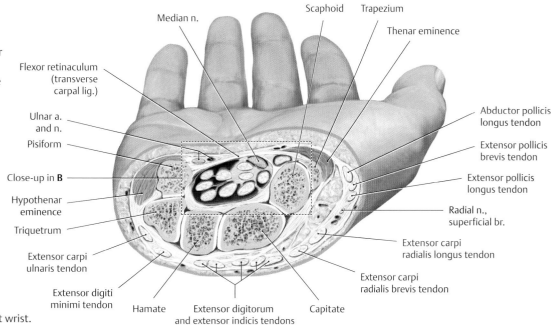

Median n.

Flexor retinaculum (transverse carpal lig.)

Ulnar a. and n.

Pisiform

Close-up in **B**

Hypothenar eminence

Triquetrum

Extensor carpi ulnaris tendon

Extensor digiti minimi tendon

Hamate

Extensor digitorum and extensor indicis tendons

Capitate

Scaphoid

Trapezium

Thenar eminence

Abductor pollicis longus tendon

Extensor pollicis brevis tendon

Extensor pollicis longus tendon

Radial n., superficial br.

Extensor carpi radialis longus tendon

Extensor carpi radialis brevis tendon

A Cross section through the right wrist.

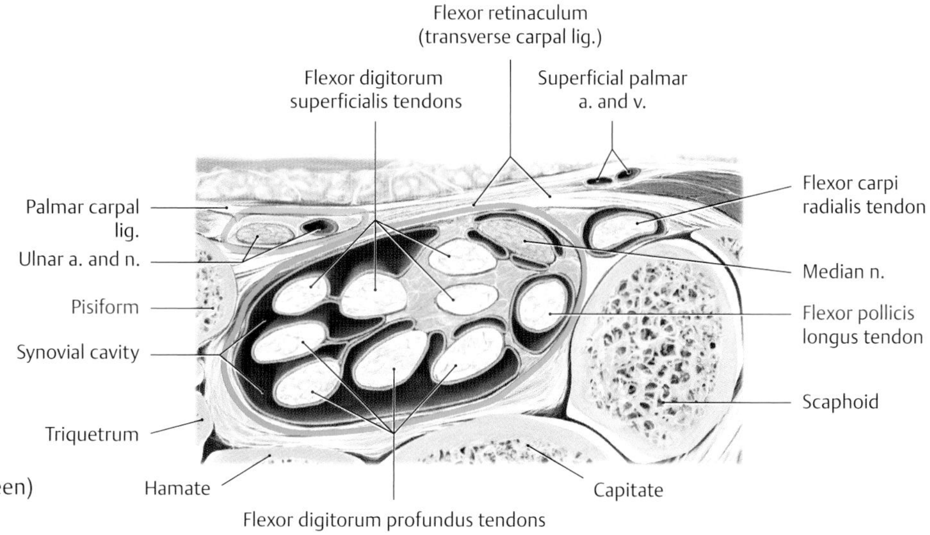

Flexor retinaculum (transverse carpal lig.)

Flexor digitorum superficialis tendons

Superficial palmar a. and v.

Palmar carpal lig.

Ulnar a. and n.

Pisiform

Synovial cavity

Triquetrum

Hamate

Flexor digitorum profundus tendons

Flexor carpi radialis tendon

Median n.

Flexor pollicis longus tendon

Scaphoid

Capitate

B Structures in the ulnar tunnel (green) and carpal tunnel (blue).

Palm of the Hand

Fig. 28.42 **Superficial neurovascular structures of the palm**
Right hand, anterior view.

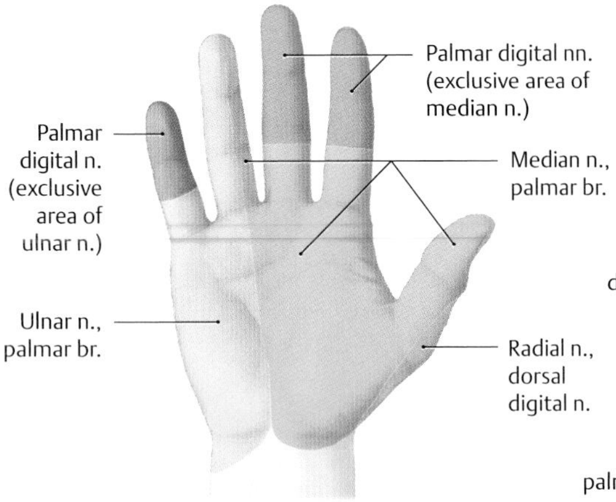

Palmar digital n. (exclusive area of ulnar n.)

Palmar digital nn. (exclusive area of median n.)

Median n., palmar br.

Ulnar n., palmar br.

Radial n., dorsal digital n.

A Sensory territories. Extensive overlap exists between adjacent areas. *Exclusive* nerve territories indicated with darker shading.

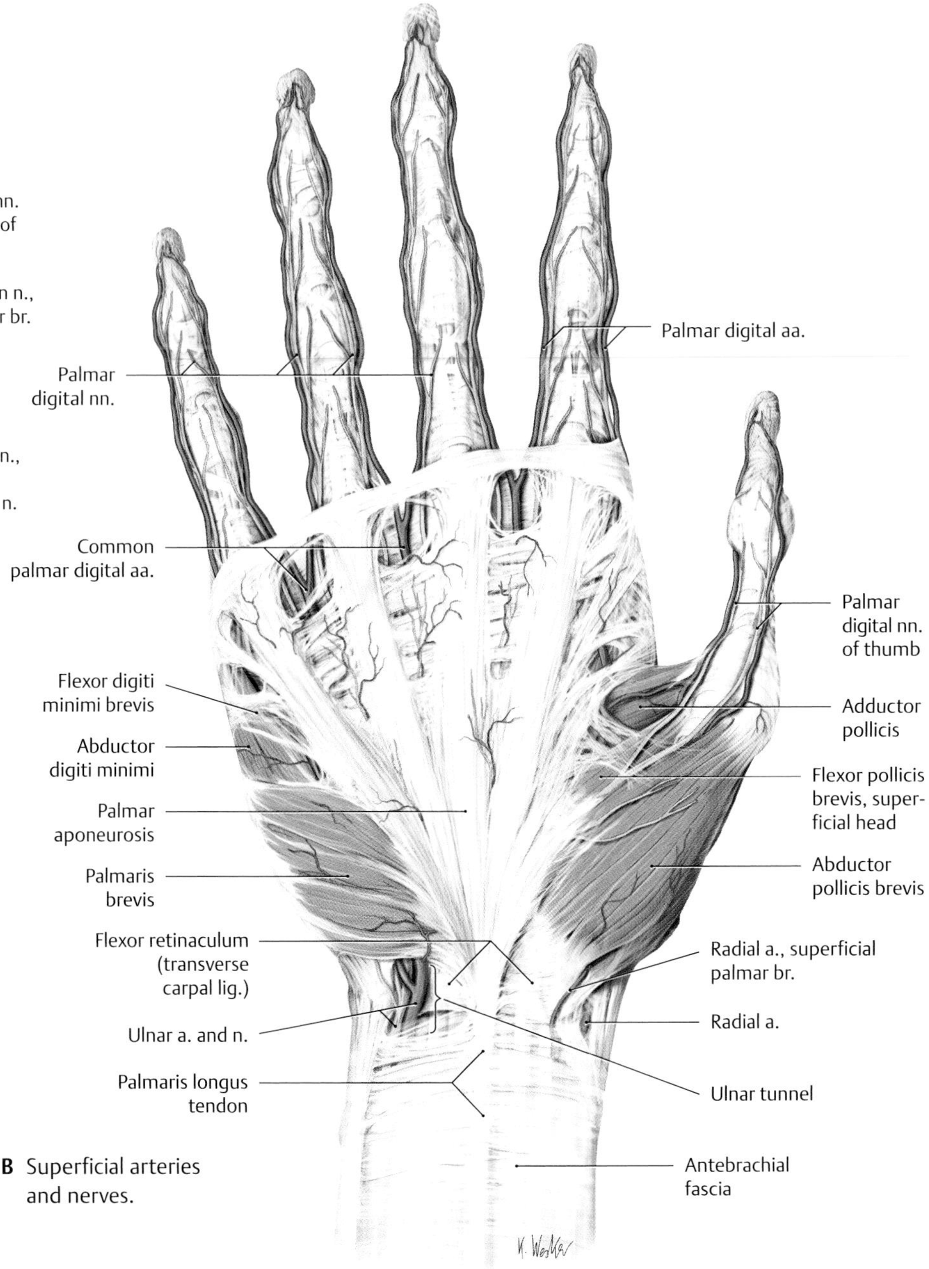

Palmar digital nn.

Palmar digital aa.

Common palmar digital aa.

Palmar digital nn. of thumb

Flexor digiti minimi brevis

Abductor digiti minimi

Palmar aponeurosis

Palmaris brevis

Flexor retinaculum (transverse carpal lig.)

Ulnar a. and n.

Palmaris longus tendon

Adductor pollicis

Flexor pollicis brevis, superficial head

Abductor pollicis brevis

Radial a., superficial palmar br.

Radial a.

Ulnar tunnel

Antebrachial fascia

B Superficial arteries and nerves.

Fig. 28.43 **Neurovasculature of the finger**
Right middle finger, lateral view.

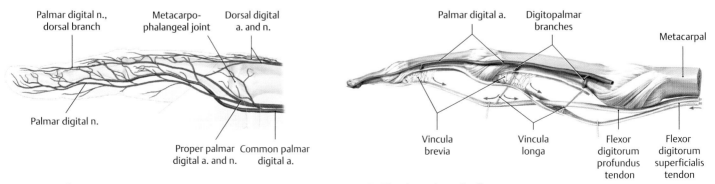

Palmar digital n., dorsal branch

Metacarpophalangeal joint

Dorsal digital a. and n.

Palmar digital n.

Proper palmar digital a. and n.

Common palmar digital a.

A Nerves and arteries.

Palmar digital a.

Digitopalmar branches

Metacarpal

Vincula brevia

Vincula longa

Flexor digitorum profundus tendon

Flexor digitorum superficialis tendon

B Blood supply to the flexor tendons in the tendon sheath.

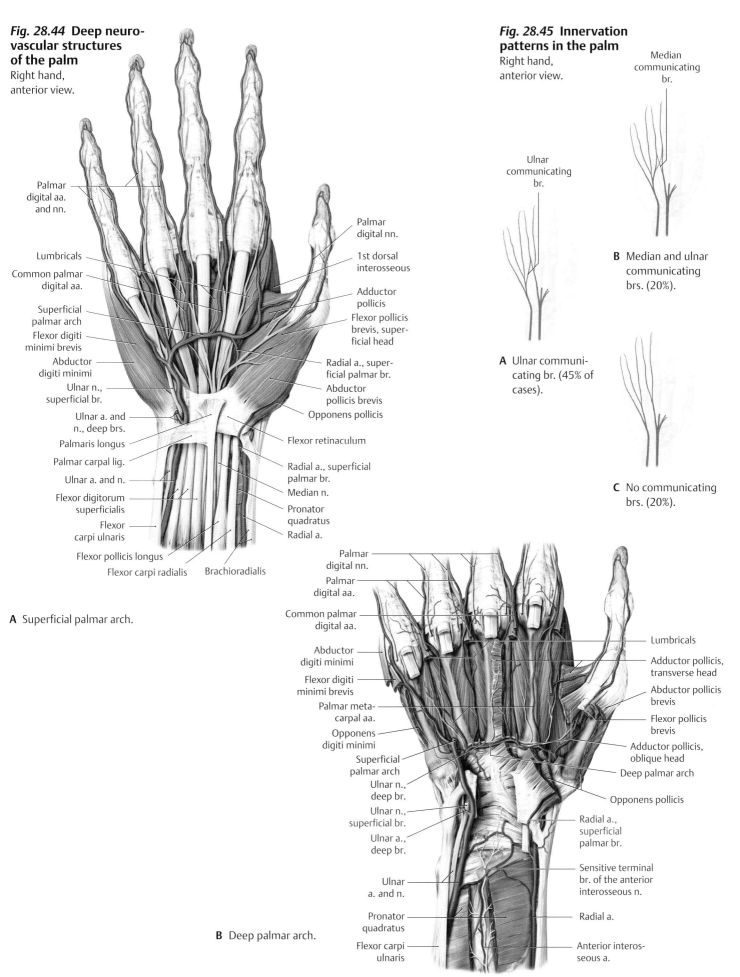

Fig. 28.44 Deep neuro-vascular structures of the palm
Right hand, anterior view.

Palmar digital aa. and nn.

Lumbricals

Common palmar digital aa.

Superficial palmar arch

Flexor digiti minimi brevis

Abductor digiti minimi

Ulnar n., superficial br.

Ulnar a. and n., deep brs.

Palmaris longus

Palmar carpal lig.

Ulnar a. and n.

Flexor digitorum superficialis

Flexor carpi ulnaris

Flexor pollicis longus

Flexor carpi radialis

Brachioradialis

Palmar digital nn.

1st dorsal interosseous

Adductor pollicis

Flexor pollicis brevis, super-ficial head

Radial a., super-ficial palmar br.

Abductor pollicis brevis

Opponens pollicis

Flexor retinaculum

Radial a., superficial palmar br.

Median n.

Pronator quadratus

Radial a.

A Superficial palmar arch.

Fig. 28.45 Innervation patterns in the palm
Right hand, anterior view.

Median communicating br.

Ulnar communicating br.

B Median and ulnar communicating brs. (20%).

A Ulnar communi-cating br. (45% of cases).

C No communicating brs. (20%).

Palmar digital nn.

Palmar digital aa.

Common palmar digital aa.

Abductor digiti minimi

Flexor digiti minimi brevis

Palmar meta-carpal aa.

Opponens digiti minimi

Superficial palmar arch

Ulnar n., deep br.

Ulnar n., superficial br.

Ulnar a., deep br.

Ulnar a. and n.

Pronator quadratus

Flexor carpi ulnaris

Lumbricals

Adductor pollicis, transverse head

Abductor pollicis brevis

Flexor pollicis brevis

Adductor pollicis, oblique head

Deep palmar arch

Opponens pollicis

Radial a., superficial palmar br.

Sensitive terminal br. of the anterior interosseous n.

Radial a.

Anterior interos-seous a.

B Deep palmar arch.

389

Dorsum of the Hand

Fig. 28.46 Cutaneous innervation of the dorsum of the hand
Right hand, posterior view.

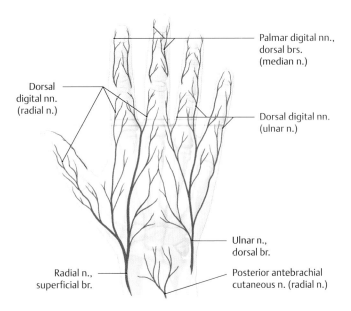

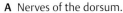

A Nerves of the dorsum.

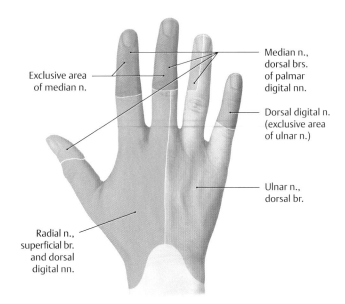

B Sensory territories. Extensive overlap exists between adjacent areas. *Exclusive* nerve territories indicated with darker shading.

Fig. 28.47 Anatomic snuffbox
Right hand, radial view. The three-sided "anatomic snuffbox" is bounded by the tendons of insertion of the abductor pollicis longus and extensors pollicis brevis and longus.

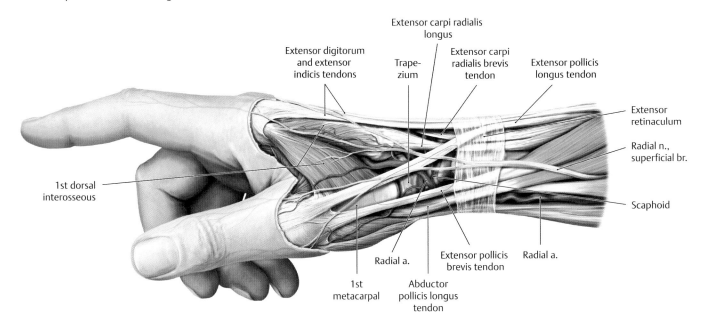

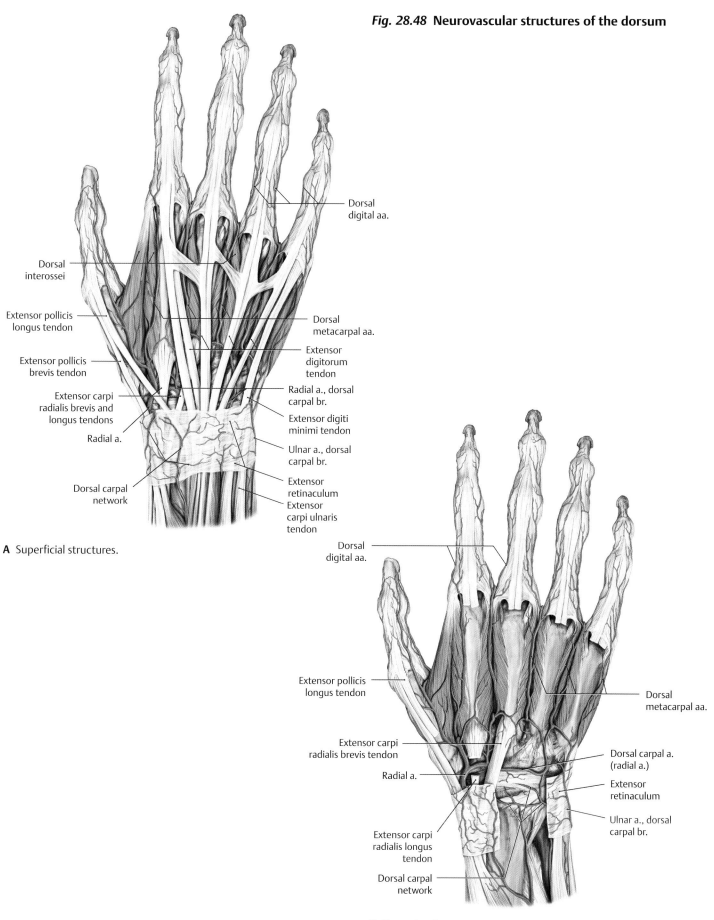

Fig. 28.48 Neurovascular structures of the dorsum

Dorsal digital aa.

Dorsal interossei

Extensor pollicis longus tendon

Dorsal metacarpal aa.

Extensor pollicis brevis tendon

Extensor digitorum tendon

Extensor carpi radialis brevis and longus tendons

Radial a., dorsal carpal br.

Radial a.

Extensor digiti minimi tendon

Ulnar a., dorsal carpal br.

Dorsal carpal network

Extensor retinaculum

Extensor carpi ulnaris tendon

A Superficial structures.

Dorsal digital aa.

Extensor pollicis longus tendon

Dorsal metacarpal aa.

Extensor carpi radialis brevis tendon

Dorsal carpal a. (radial a.)

Radial a.

Extensor retinaculum

Extensor carpi radialis longus tendon

Ulnar a., dorsal carpal br.

Dorsal carpal network

B Deep structures.

Sectional Anatomy of the Upper Limb

Fig. 29.1 **Compartments of the arm**

Right limb, transverse section, distal (inferior) view. Anterior compartment outlined in red; posterior compartment outlined in green.

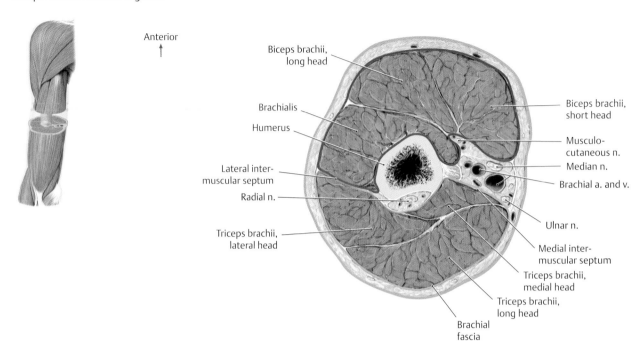

Fig. 29.2 **Compartments of the forearm**

Right limb, transverse section, distal (inferior) view. Anterior compartment outlined in red; posterior compartment outlined in green.

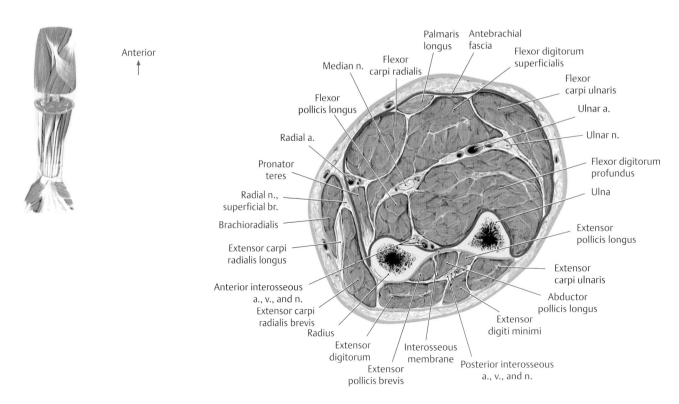

Fig. 29.3 MRI of the right arm
Transverse section, distal (inferior) view.

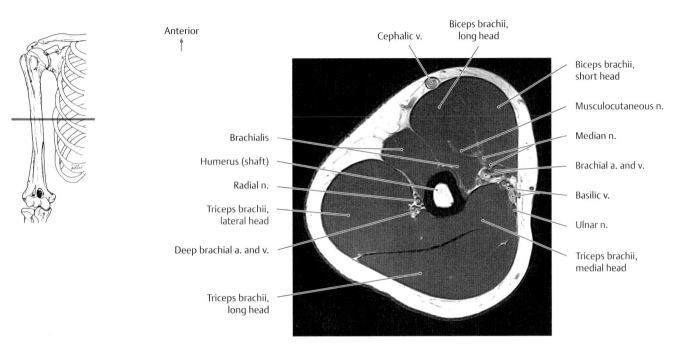

Anterior

Cephalic v.
Biceps brachii, long head
Biceps brachii, short head
Musculocutaneous n.
Median n.
Brachial a. and v.
Basilic v.
Ulnar n.
Triceps brachii, medial head

Brachialis
Humerus (shaft)
Radial n.
Triceps brachii, lateral head
Deep brachial a. and v.
Triceps brachii, long head

Fig. 29.4 MRI of the right forearm
Transverse section, distal (inferior) view.

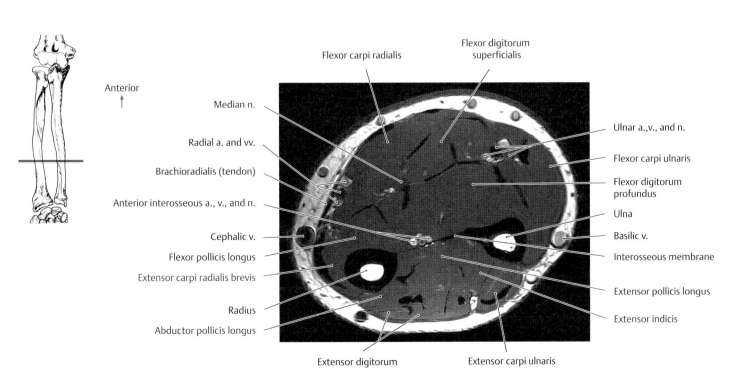

Anterior

Flexor carpi radialis
Flexor digitorum superficialis

Median n.
Radial a. and vv.
Brachioradialis (tendon)
Anterior interosseous a., v., and n.
Cephalic v.
Flexor pollicis longus
Extensor carpi radialis brevis
Radius
Abductor pollicis longus

Ulnar a.,v., and n.
Flexor carpi ulnaris
Flexor digitorum profundus
Ulna
Basilic v.
Interosseous membrane
Extensor pollicis longus
Extensor indicis

Extensor digitorum
Extensor carpi ulnaris

Radiographic Anatomy of the Upper Limb (I)

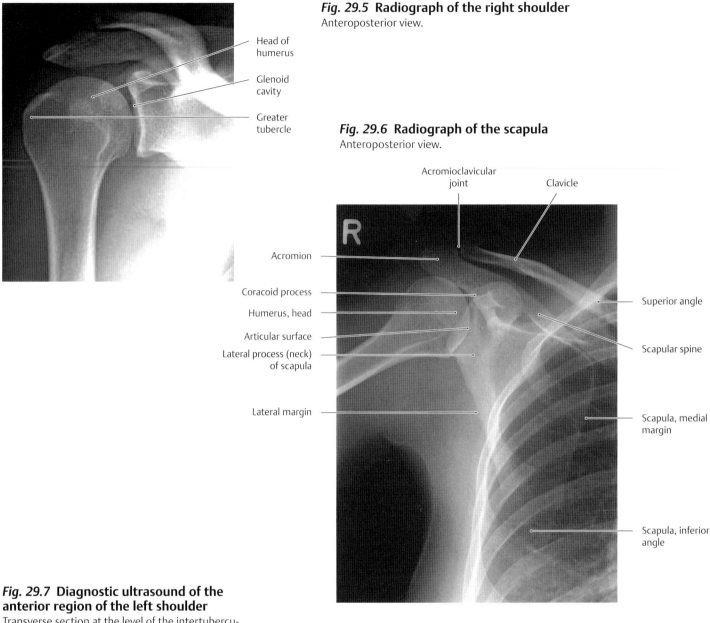

***Fig. 29.5* Radiograph of the right shoulder**
Anteroposterior view.

Head of humerus
Glenoid cavity
Greater tubercle

***Fig. 29.6* Radiograph of the scapula**
Anteroposterior view.

Acromioclavicular joint
Clavicle
Acromion
Coracoid process
Humerus, head
Articular surface
Lateral process (neck) of scapula
Lateral margin
Superior angle
Scapular spine
Scapula, medial margin
Scapula, inferior angle

***Fig. 29.7* Diagnostic ultrasound of the anterior region of the left shoulder**
Transverse section at the level of the intertubercular groove.

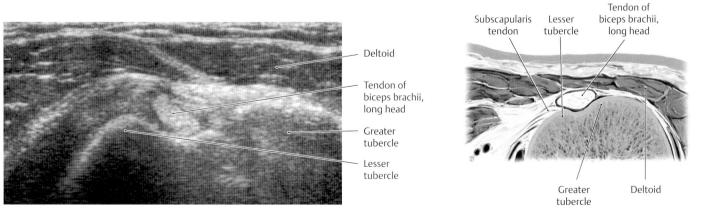

Deltoid
Tendon of biceps brachii, long head
Greater tubercle
Lesser tubercle

Subscapularis tendon
Lesser tubercle
Tendon of biceps brachii, long head
Greater tubercle
Deltoid

A Sonogram.

B Schematic of the transverse section.

Fig. 29.8 MRI of the right shoulder joint in three planes

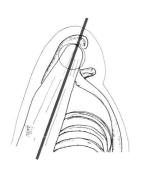

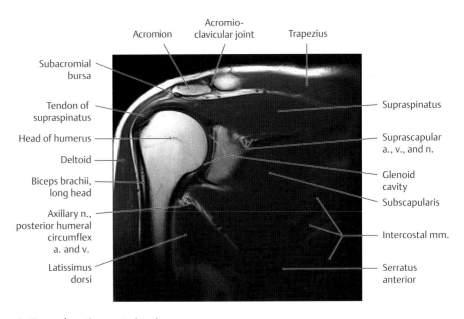

- Acromion
- Acromio-clavicular joint
- Trapezius
- Subacromial bursa
- Tendon of supraspinatus
- Head of humerus
- Deltoid
- Biceps brachii, long head
- Axillary n., posterior humeral circumflex a. and v.
- Latissimus dorsi
- Supraspinatus
- Suprascapular a., v., and n.
- Glenoid cavity
- Subscapularis
- Intercostal mm.
- Serratus anterior

A Coronal section, anterior view.

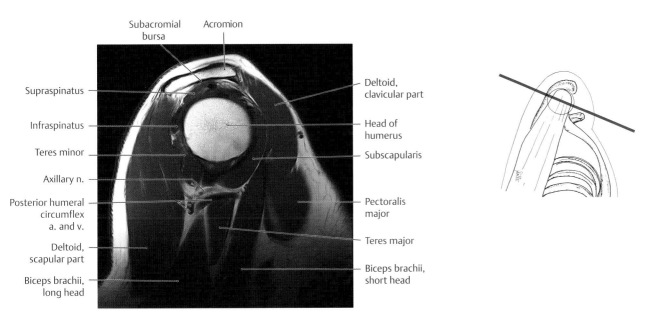

- Subacromial bursa
- Acromion
- Supraspinatus
- Infraspinatus
- Teres minor
- Axillary n.
- Posterior humeral circumflex a. and v.
- Deltoid, scapular part
- Biceps brachii, long head
- Deltoid, clavicular part
- Head of humerus
- Subscapularis
- Pectoralis major
- Teres major
- Biceps brachii, short head

B Sagittal section, lateral view.

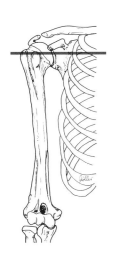

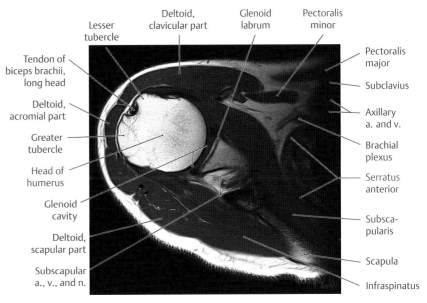

- Lesser tubercle
- Tendon of biceps brachii, long head
- Deltoid, acromial part
- Greater tubercle
- Head of humerus
- Glenoid cavity
- Deltoid, scapular part
- Subscapular a., v., and n.
- Deltoid, clavicular part
- Glenoid labrum
- Pectoralis minor
- Pectoralis major
- Subclavius
- Axillary a. and v.
- Brachial plexus
- Serratus anterior
- Subscapularis
- Scapula
- Infraspinatus

C Transverse section, inferior view.

Radiographic Anatomy of the Upper Limb (II)

Fig. 29.9 **Radiograph of the elbow**
Anteroposterior view.

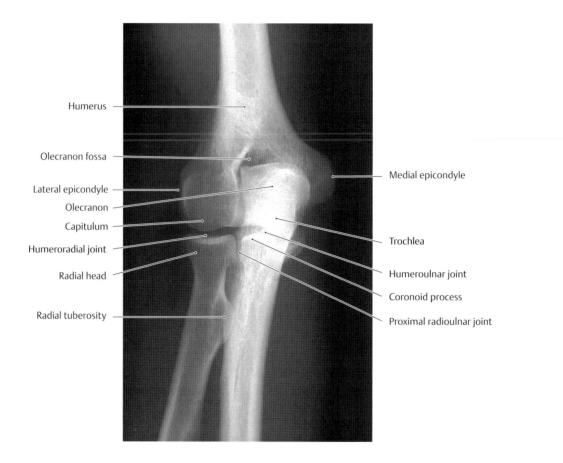

Fig. 29.10 **Radiograph of the elbow**
Lateral view.

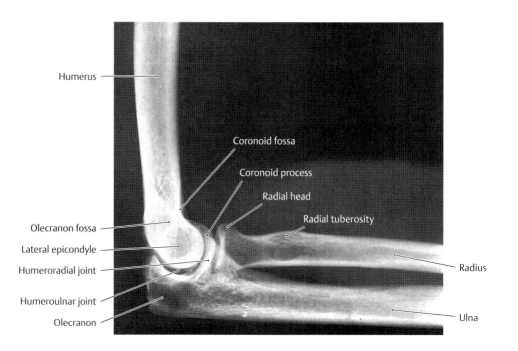

Fig. 29.11 **MRI of the elbow**

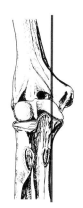

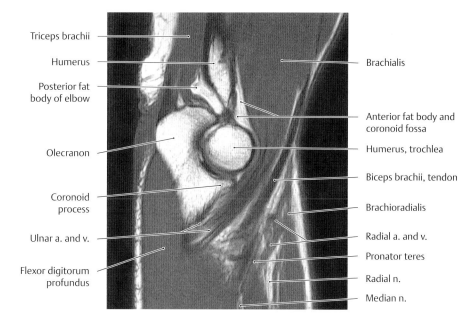

Triceps brachii

Humerus

Posterior fat body of elbow

Olecranon

Coronoid process

Ulnar a. and v.

Flexor digitorum profundus

Brachialis

Anterior fat body and coronoid fossa

Humerus, trochlea

Biceps brachii, tendon

Brachioradialis

Radial a. and v.

Pronator teres

Radial n.

Median n.

A Sagittal section through the humeroulnar joint.

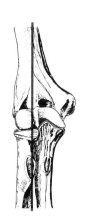

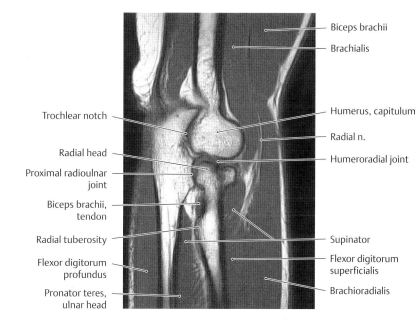

Trochlear notch

Radial head

Proximal radioulnar joint

Biceps brachii, tendon

Radial tuberosity

Flexor digitorum profundus

Pronator teres, ulnar head

Biceps brachii

Brachialis

Humerus, capitulum

Radial n.

Humeroradial joint

Supinator

Flexor digitorum superficialis

Brachioradialis

B Sagittal section through the humeroulnar and humeroradial joints.

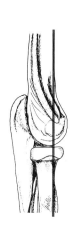

Brachioradialis

Extensor carpi radialis longus

Lateral epicondyle

Humeroradial joint

Radial head

Supinator

Radial tuberosity

Extensor digitorum

Brachialis

Medial epicondyle

Pronator teres

Medial collateral lig.

Humeroulnar joint

Ulna, coronoid process

Brachialis

Flexor carpi radialis

C Coronal section through the humeroulnar and humeroradial joints.

Radiographic Anatomy of the Upper Limb (III)

Fig. 29.12 **Radiograph of the hand**

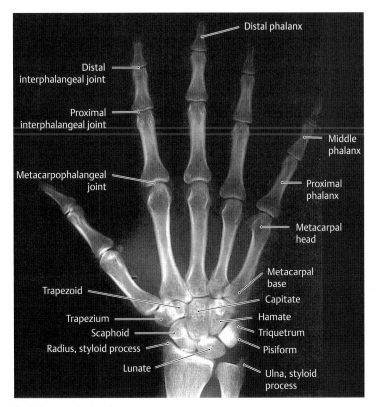
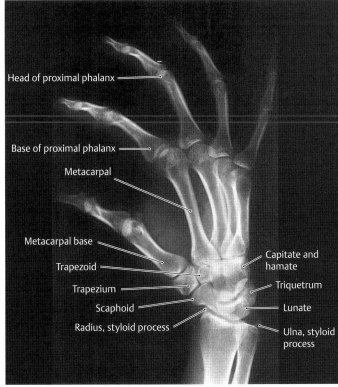

A Anteroposterior view.

B Oblique view.

Fig. 29.13 **MRI of the right wrist**
Transverse section, distal view.

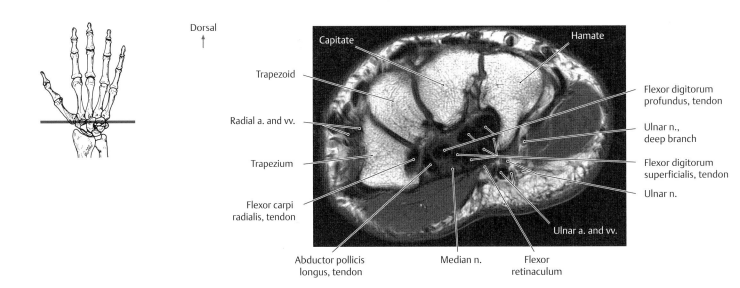

Fig. 29.14 MRI of the hand

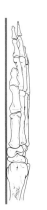

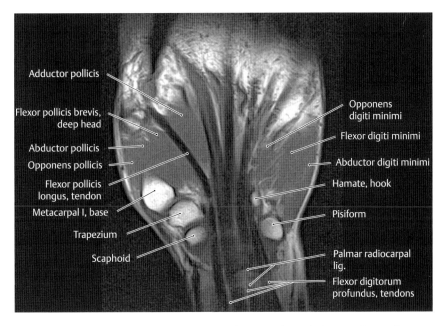

Adductor pollicis

Flexor pollicis brevis, deep head

Abductor pollicis

Opponens pollicis

Flexor pollicis longus, tendon

Metacarpal I, base

Trapezium

Scaphoid

Opponens digiti minimi

Flexor digiti minimi

Abductor digiti minimi

Hamate, hook

Pisiform

Palmar radiocarpal lig.

Flexor digitorum profundus, tendons

A Coronal section through the carpal tunnel.

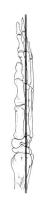

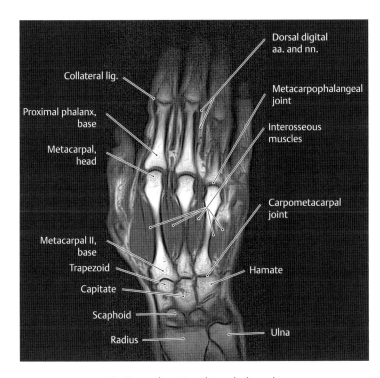

Collateral lig.

Proximal phalanx, base

Metacarpal, head

Metacarpal II, base

Trapezoid

Capitate

Scaphoid

Radius

Dorsal digital aa. and nn.

Metacarpophalangeal joint

Interosseous muscles

Carpometacarpal joint

Hamate

Ulna

B Coronal section through the palm.

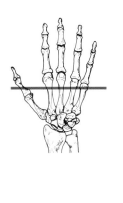

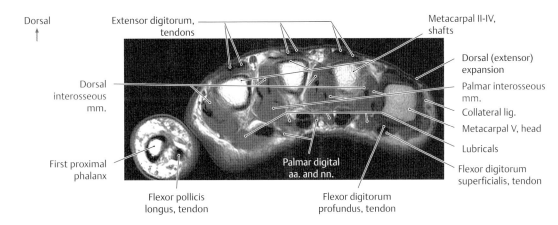

Dorsal

Extensor digitorum, tendons

Dorsal interosseous mm.

First proximal phalanx

Flexor pollicis longus, tendon

Palmar digital aa. and nn.

Flexor digitorum profundus, tendon

Metacarpal II–IV, shafts

Dorsal (extensor) expansion

Palmar interosseous mm.

Collateral lig.

Metacarpal V, head

Lubricals

Flexor digitorum superficialis, tendon

C Transverse section through the palm, distal view.

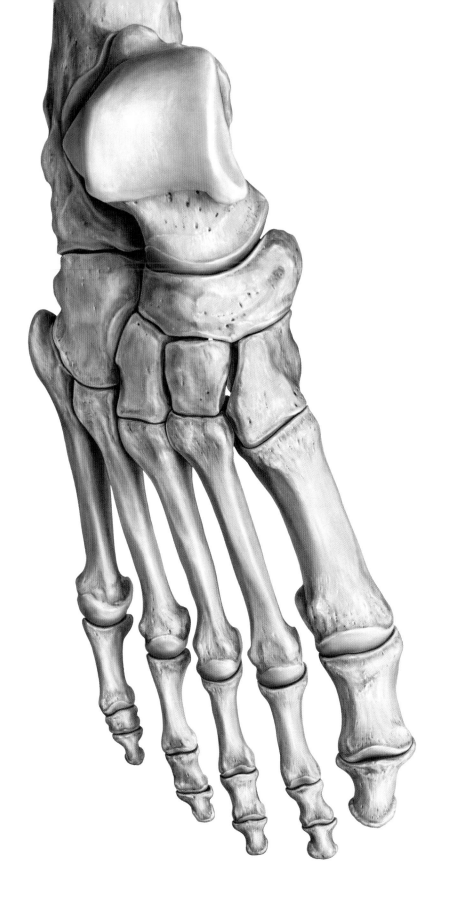

Lower Limb

Surface Anatomy

Fig. 30.1 Palpable bony prominences of the lower limb
Right limb.

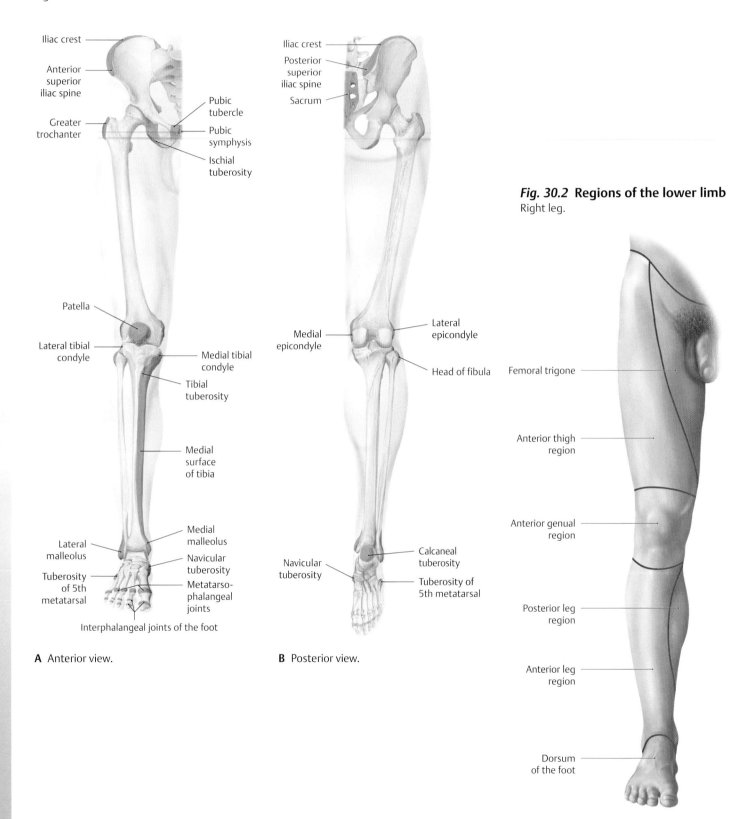

Iliac crest
Anterior superior iliac spine
Greater trochanter
Pubic tubercle
Pubic symphysis
Ischial tuberosity

Patella
Lateral tibial condyle
Medial tibial condyle
Tibial tuberosity
Medial surface of tibia

Lateral malleolus
Medial malleolus
Navicular tuberosity
Tuberosity of 5th metatarsal
Metatarso-phalangeal joints
Interphalangeal joints of the foot

A Anterior view.

Iliac crest
Posterior superior iliac spine
Sacrum

Medial epicondyle
Lateral epicondyle
Head of fibula

Navicular tuberosity
Calcaneal tuberosity
Tuberosity of 5th metatarsal

B Posterior view.

Fig. 30.2 Regions of the lower limb
Right leg.

Femoral trigone
Anterior thigh region
Anterior genual region
Posterior leg region
Anterior leg region
Dorsum of the foot

A Anterior view.

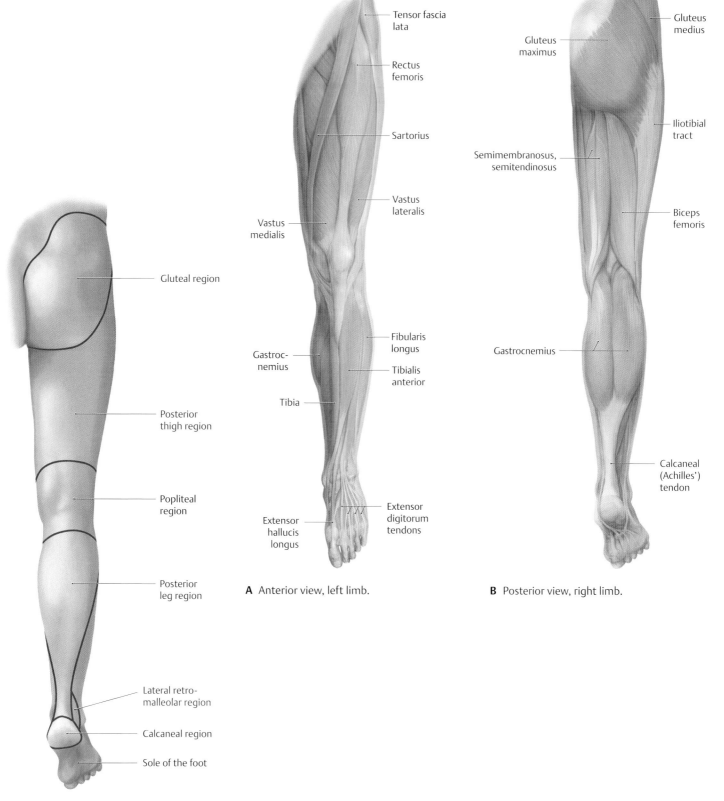

Fig. 30.3 **Palpable musculature of the lower limb**

Gluteal region

Posterior thigh region

Popliteal region

Posterior leg region

Lateral retro-malleolar region

Calcaneal region

Sole of the foot

B Posterior view.

Tensor fascia lata

Rectus femoris

Sartorius

Vastus lateralis

Vastus medialis

Fibularis longus

Gastroc-nemius

Tibialis anterior

Tibia

Extensor hallucis longus

Extensor digitorum tendons

A Anterior view, left limb.

Iliac crest

Gluteus medius

Gluteus maximus

Iliotibial tract

Semimembranosus, semitendinosus

Biceps femoris

Gastrocnemius

Calcaneal (Achilles') tendon

B Posterior view, right limb.

Lower Limb

Bones of the Lower Limb

The skeleton of the lower limb consists of a hip bone and a free limb. The paired hip bones attach to the trunk at the sacroiliac joint to form the pelvic girdle (see **p. 228**), and the free limb, divided into a thigh, leg, and foot, attaches to the pelvic girdle at the hip joint. Stability of the pelvic girdle is important in the distribution of weight from the upper body to the lower limbs.

Fig. 31.1 Bones of the lower limb

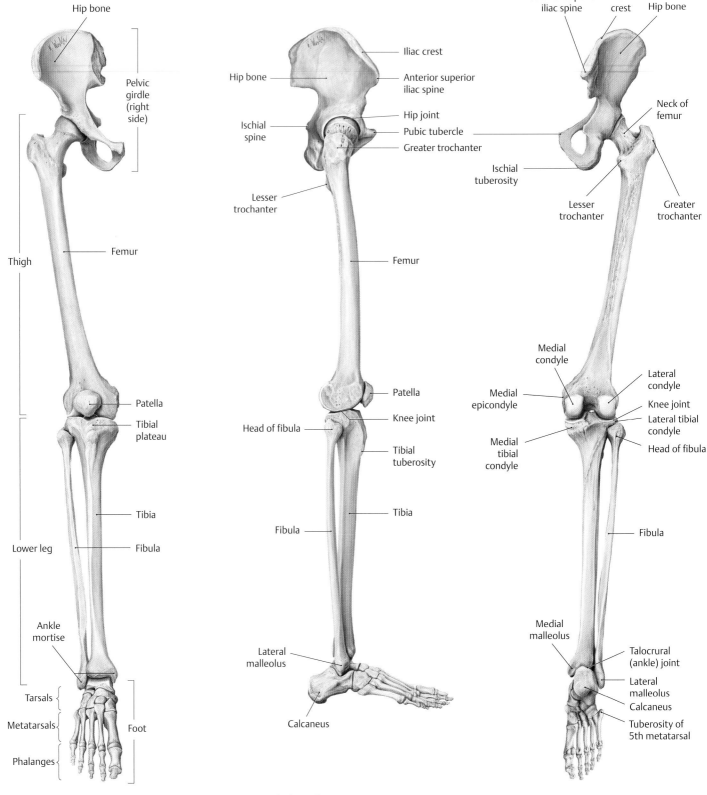

A Anterior view.

B Right lateral view.

C Posterior view.

Fig. 31.2 Line of gravity

Right lateral view. The line of gravity runs vertically from the whole-body center of gravity to the ground with characteristic points of intersection.

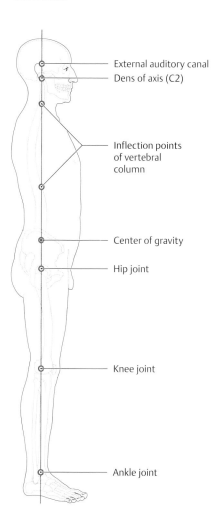

External auditory canal
Dens of axis (C2)

Inflection points of vertebral column

Center of gravity

Hip joint

Knee joint

Ankle joint

Fig. 31.3 The hip bones and their relation to bones of the trunk.

The paired hip bones and sacrum form the pelvic girdle (see **p. 228**).

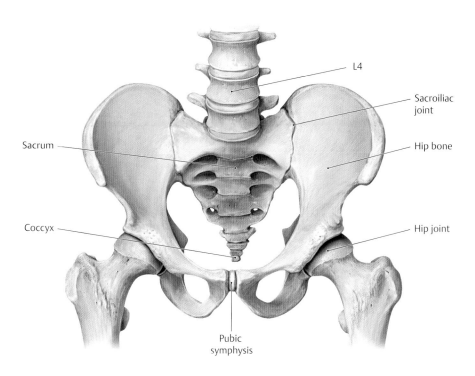

L4

Sacroiliac joint

Sacrum

Hip bone

Coccyx

Hip joint

Pubic symphysis

A Anterior view.

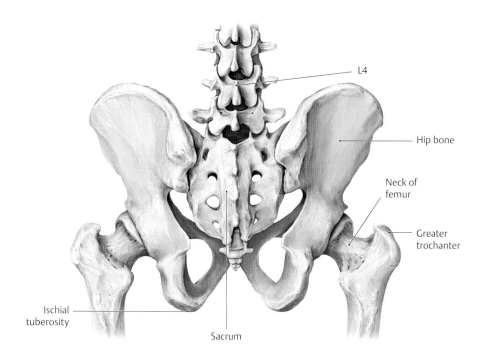

L4

Hip bone

Neck of femur

Greater trochanter

Ischial tuberosity

Sacrum

B Posterior view.

Femur

Fig. 31.4 **Right femur**

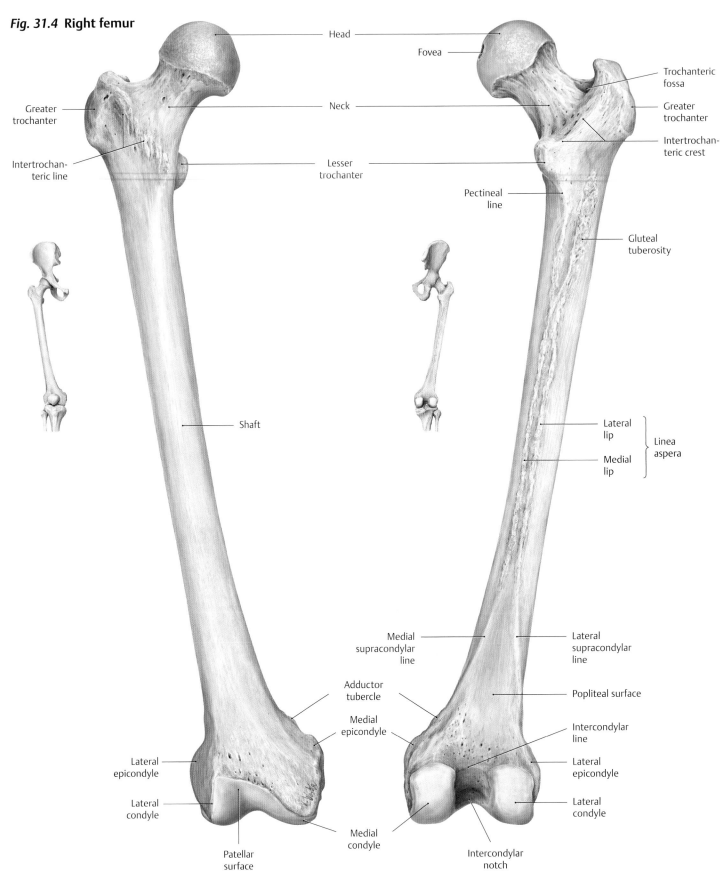

Head

Fovea

Trochanteric fossa

Greater trochanter

Greater trochanter

Neck

Intertrochanteric crest

Intertrochanteric line

Lesser trochanter

Pectineal line

Gluteal tuberosity

Shaft

Lateral lip

Linea aspera

Medial lip

Medial supracondylar line

Lateral supracondylar line

Adductor tubercle

Popliteal surface

Medial epicondyle

Intercondylar line

Lateral epicondyle

Lateral epicondyle

Lateral condyle

Lateral condyle

Patellar surface

Medial condyle

Intercondylar notch

A Anterior view.

B Posterior view.

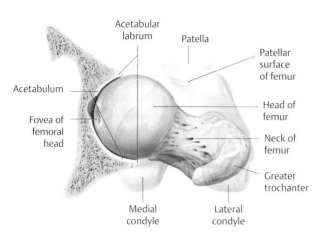

Acetabular labrum

Patella

Patellar surface of femur

Acetabulum

Fovea of femoral head

Head of femur

Neck of femur

Greater trochanter

Medial condyle

Lateral condyle

C Proximal view. The acetabulum has been sectioned in the horizontal plane.

⚕ **Clinical box 31.1**

Fractures of the femur
Femoral fractures caused by falls in patients with osteoporosis are most frequently located in the neck of the femur. Femoral shaft fractures are less frequent and are usually caused by strong trauma (e.g., a car accident).

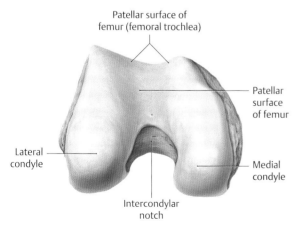

Patellar surface of femur (femoral trochlea)

Patellar surface of femur

Lateral condyle

Medial condyle

Intercondylar notch

D Distal view. See **pp. 428–429** for the knee joint.

Fig. 31.5 **Head of femur in the hip joint**
Right hip joint, superior view.

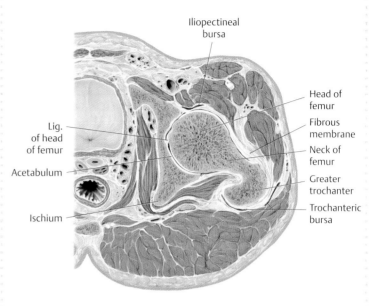

Iliopectineal bursa

Lig. of head of femur

Acetabulum

Ischium

Head of femur

Fibrous membrane

Neck of femur

Greater trochanter

Trochanteric bursa

A Transverse section.

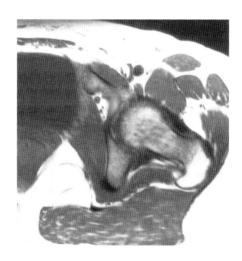

B T1-weighted MRI.

Hip Joint: Overview

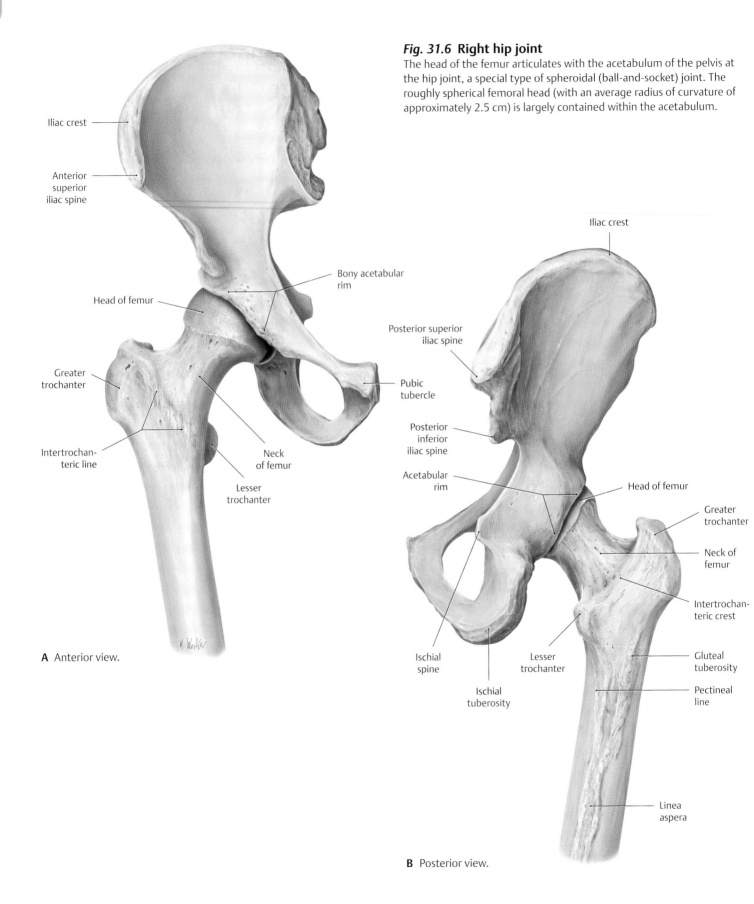

Iliac crest

Anterior
superior
iliac spine

Bony acetabular
rim

Head of femur

Greater
trochanter

Intertrochan-
teric line

Neck
of femur

Lesser
trochanter

A Anterior view.

Fig. 31.6 Right hip joint
The head of the femur articulates with the acetabulum of the pelvis at
the hip joint, a special type of spheroidal (ball-and-socket) joint. The
roughly spherical femoral head (with an average radius of curvature of
approximately 2.5 cm) is largely contained within the acetabulum.

Iliac crest

Posterior superior
iliac spine

Posterior
inferior
iliac spine

Acetabular
rim

Head of femur

Greater
trochanter

Neck of
femur

Intertrochan-
teric crest

Gluteal
tuberosity

Pectineal
line

Ischial
spine

Lesser
trochanter

Ischial
tuberosity

Linea
aspera

B Posterior view.

Fig. 31.7 Hip joint: Coronal section
Right hip joint, anterior view.

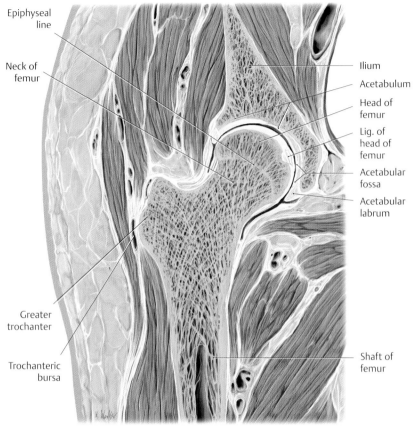

Epiphyseal line

Neck of femur

Greater trochanter

Trochanteric bursa

Ilium

Acetabulum

Head of femur

Lig. of head of femur

Acetabular fossa

Acetabular labrum

Shaft of femur

A Coronal section.

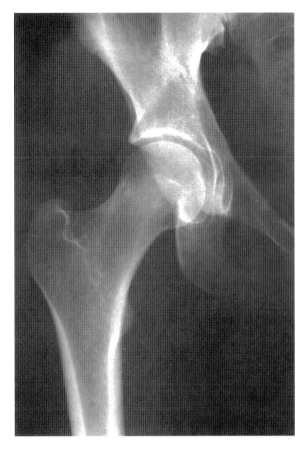

B Anteroposterior radiograph.

Clinical box 31.2

Diagnosing hip dysplasia and dislocation
Ultrasonography, the most important imaging method for screening the infant hip, is used to identify morphological changes such as hip dysplasia and dislocation. Clinically, hip dislocation presents with instability and limited abduction of the hip joint, and leg shortening with asymmetry of the gluteal folds.

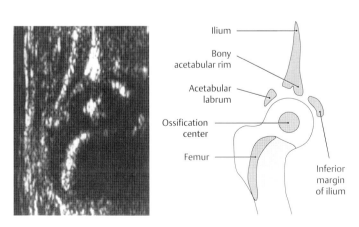

Ilium

Bony acetabular rim

Acetabular labrum

Ossification center

Femur

Inferior margin of ilium

A Normal hip joint in a 5-month-old.

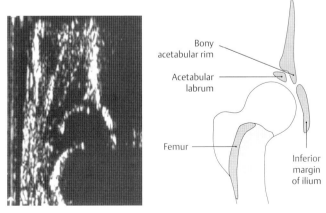

Bony acetabular rim

Acetabular labrum

Femur

Inferior margin of ilium

B Hip dislocation and dysplasia in a 3-month-old.

Hip Joint: Ligaments & Capsule

 The hip joint has three major ligaments: iliofemoral, pubofemoral, and ischiofemoral. The zona orbicularis (annular ligament) is not visible externally and encircles the femoral neck like a buttonhole.

Fig. 31.8 **Hip joint: Lateral view**
Right hip joint.

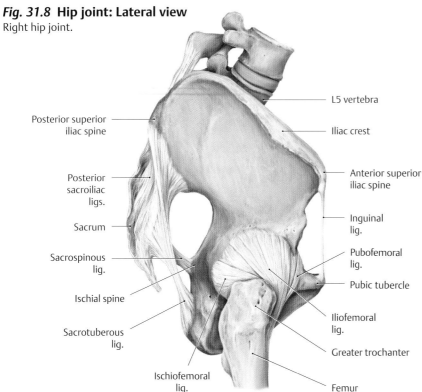

Posterior superior iliac spine

L5 vertebra

Iliac crest

Posterior sacroiliac ligs.

Sacrum

Anterior superior iliac spine

Sacrospinous lig.

Inguinal lig.

Ischial spine

Pubofemoral lig.

Sacrotuberous lig.

Pubic tubercle

Iliofemoral lig.

Greater trochanter

Ischiofemoral lig.

Femur

A Ligaments of the hip joint.

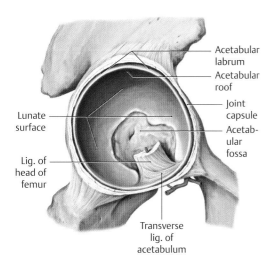

Acetabular labrum

Acetabular roof

Joint capsule

Lunate surface

Acetabular fossa

Lig. of head of femur

Transverse lig. of acetabulum

C Acetabulum of hip joint. *Note:* The ligament of the femoral head (cut) transmits branches from the obturator artery that nourish the femoral head (see **p. 467**).

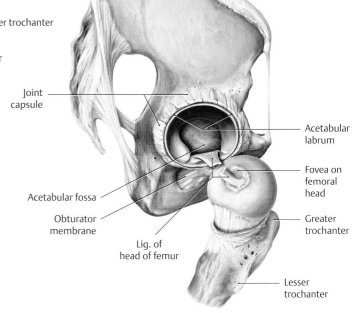

Joint capsule

Acetabular labrum

Fovea on femoral head

Acetabular fossa

Greater trochanter

Obturator membrane

Lig. of head of femur

Lesser trochanter

B Joint capsule. The capsule has been divided and the femoral head dislocated to expose the cut ligament of the head of the femur.

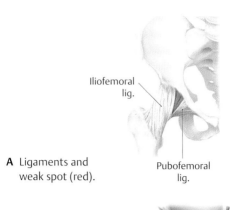

A Ligaments and weak spot (red).

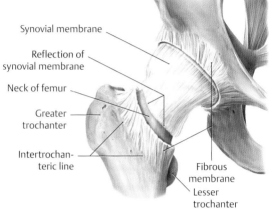

C Joint capsule. *Removed:* Fibrous membrane (at level of femoral neck). *Exposed:* Synovial membrane.

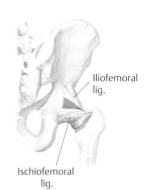

A Ligaments and weak spot (red).

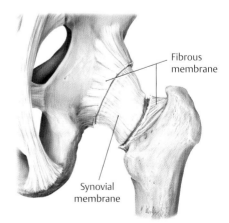

C Joint capsule.

Fig. 31.9 **Hip joint: Anterior view**
Right hip joint.

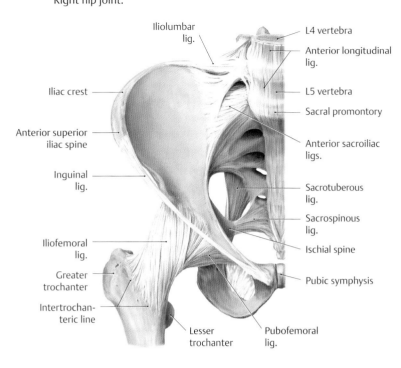

B Ligaments of the hip joint.

Fig. 31.10 **Hip Joint: Posterior view**
Right hip joint.

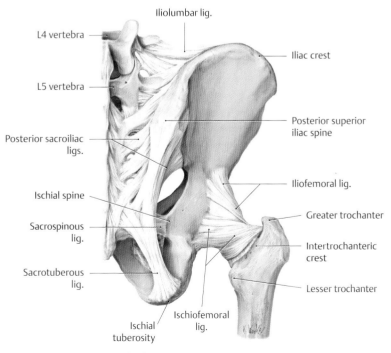

B Ligaments of the hip joint.

Fig. 31.11 Anterior muscles of the hip and thigh (I)

Right limb. Muscle origins are shown in red, insertions in blue.

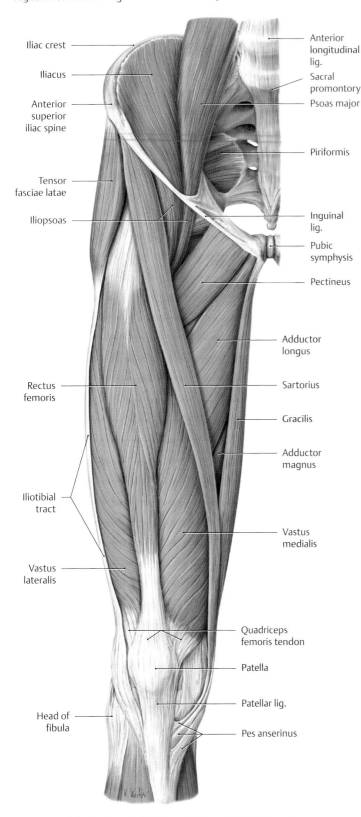

Iliac crest

Iliacus

Anterior superior iliac spine

Tensor fasciae latae

Iliopsoas

Rectus femoris

Iliotibial tract

Vastus lateralis

Head of fibula

Anterior longitudinal lig.

Sacral promontory

Psoas major

Piriformis

Inguinal lig.

Pubic symphysis

Pectineus

Adductor longus

Sartorius

Gracilis

Adductor magnus

Vastus medialis

Quadriceps femoris tendon

Patella

Patellar lig.

Pes anserinus

A *Removed:* Fascia lata of thigh (to the lateral iliotibial tract).

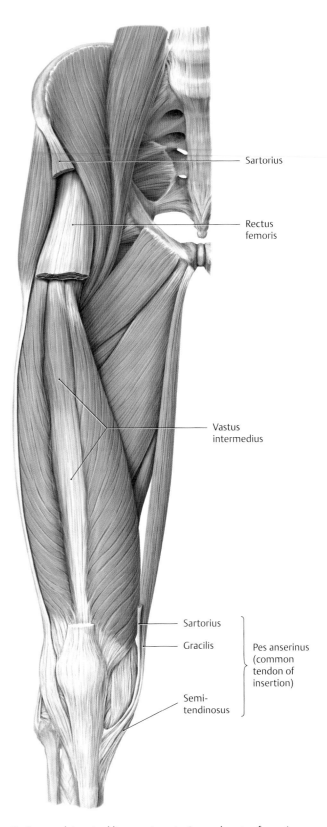

Sartorius

Rectus femoris

Vastus intermedius

Sartorius

Gracilis

Semi-tendinosus

Pes anserinus (common tendon of insertion)

B *Removed:* Inguinal ligament, sartorius and rectus femoris.

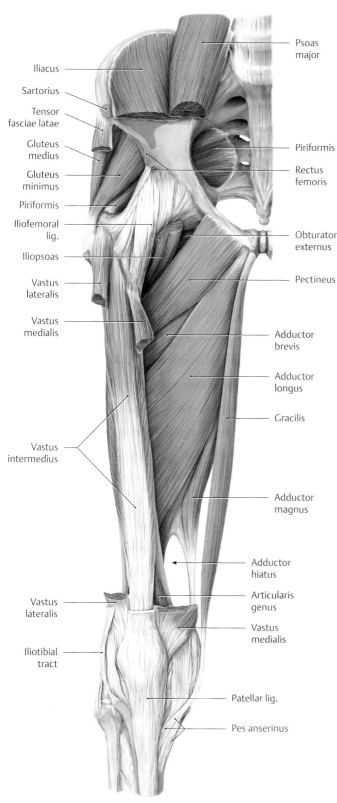

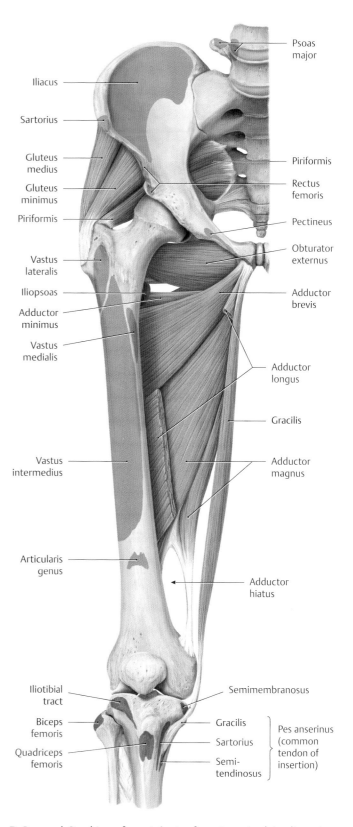

C *Removed:* Rectus femoris (completely), vastus lateralis, vastus medialis, iliopsoas, and tensor fasciae latae.

D *Removed:* Quadriceps femoris (rectus femoris, vastus lateralis, vastus medialis, vastus intermedius), iliopsoas, tensor fasciae latae, pectineus, and midportion of adductor longus.

413

Anterior Muscles of the Hip, Thigh & Gluteal Region (II)

***Fig. 31.12* Anterior muscles of the hip and thigh (II)**
Right limb. Muscle origins are shown in red, insertions in blue.

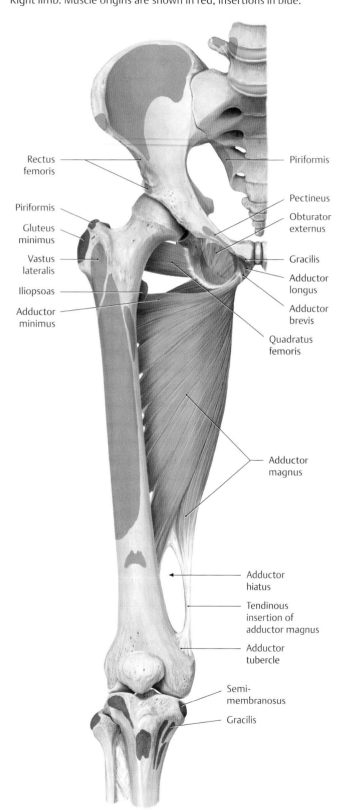

A *Removed:* Gluteus medius and minimus, piriformis, obturator externus, adductor brevis and longus, and gracilis.

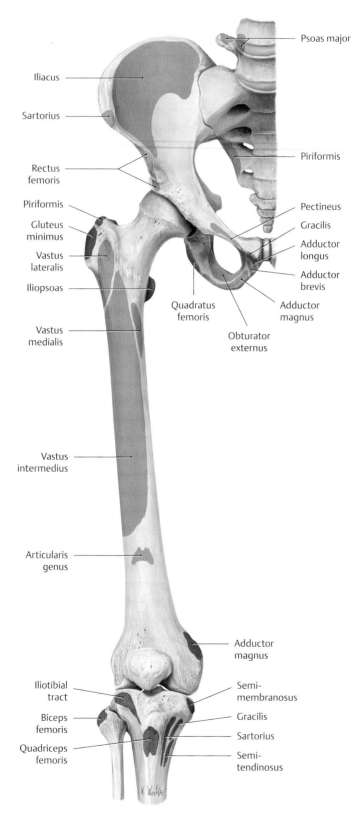

B *Removed:* All muscles.

Fig. 31.13 **Medial muscles of the hip, thigh, and gluteal region**
Midsagittal section.

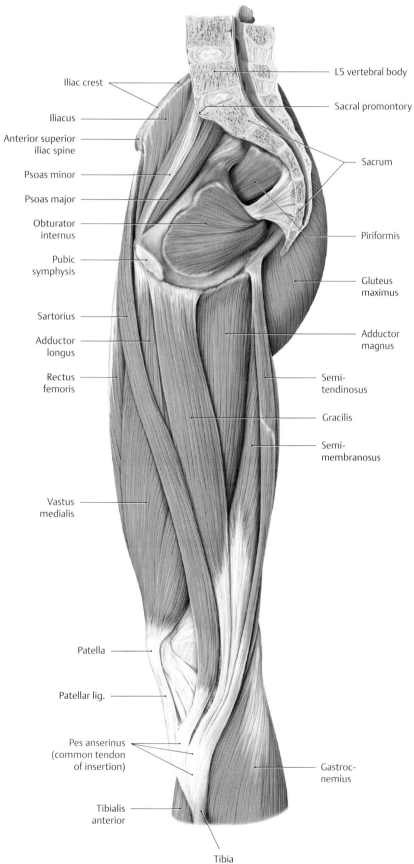

Iliac crest

Iliacus

Anterior superior
iliac spine

Psoas minor

Psoas major

Obturator
internus

Pubic
symphysis

Sartorius

Adductor
longus

Rectus
femoris

Vastus
medialis

Patella

Patellar lig.

Pes anserinus
(common tendon
of insertion)

Tibialis
anterior

Tibia

L5 vertebral body

Sacral promontory

Sacrum

Piriformis

Gluteus
maximus

Adductor
magnus

Semi-
tendinosus

Gracilis

Semi-
membranosus

Gastroc-
nemius

Posterior Muscles of the Hip, Thigh & Gluteal Region (I)

Fig. 31.14 **Posterior muscles of the hip, thigh, and gluteal region (I)**
Right limb. Muscle origins are shown in red, insertions in blue.

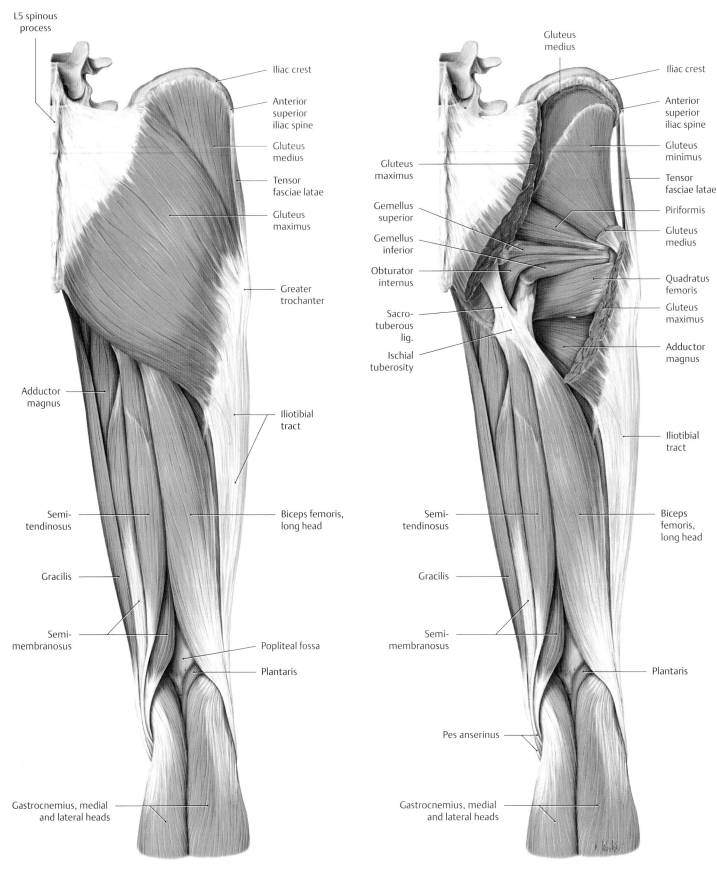

L5 spinous process

Iliac crest

Anterior superior iliac spine

Gluteus medius

Tensor fasciae latae

Gluteus maximus

Greater trochanter

Adductor magnus

Iliotibial tract

Semi-tendinosus

Biceps femoris, long head

Gracilis

Semi-membranosus

Popliteal fossa

Plantaris

Gastrocnemius, medial and lateral heads

Gluteus medius

Iliac crest

Anterior superior iliac spine

Gluteus minimus

Tensor fasciae latae

Piriformis

Gluteus medius

Gluteus maximus

Gemellus superior

Gemellus inferior

Obturator internus

Quadratus femoris

Gluteus maximus

Sacro-tuberous lig.

Ischial tuberosity

Adductor magnus

Iliotibial tract

Semi-tendinosus

Biceps femoris, long head

Gracilis

Semi-membranosus

Plantaris

Pes anserinus

Gastrocnemius, medial and lateral heads

A *Removed:* Fascia lata (to iliotibial tract).

B *Partially removed:* Gluteus maximus and medius.

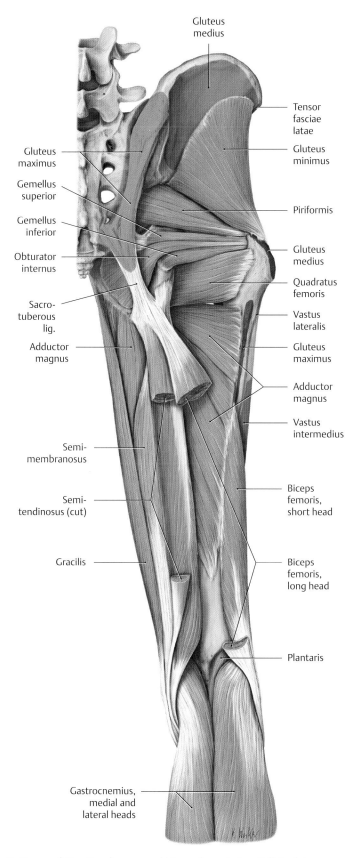

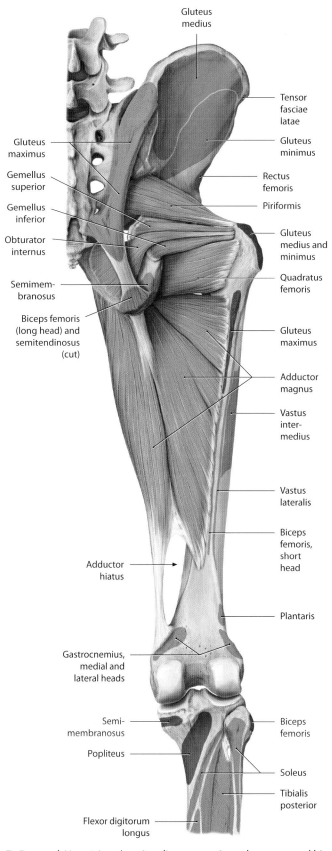

C *Removed:* Semitendinosus and biceps femoris (partially); gluteus maximus and medius (completely).

D *Removed:* Hamstrings (semitendinosus, semimembranosus, and biceps femoris), gluteus minimus, gastrocnemius, and muscles of the leg.

417

Posterior Muscles of the Hip, Thigh & Gluteal Region (II)

Fig. 31.15 Posterior muscles of the hip, thigh, and gluteal region (II)
Right limb. Muscle origins are shown in red, insertions in blue.

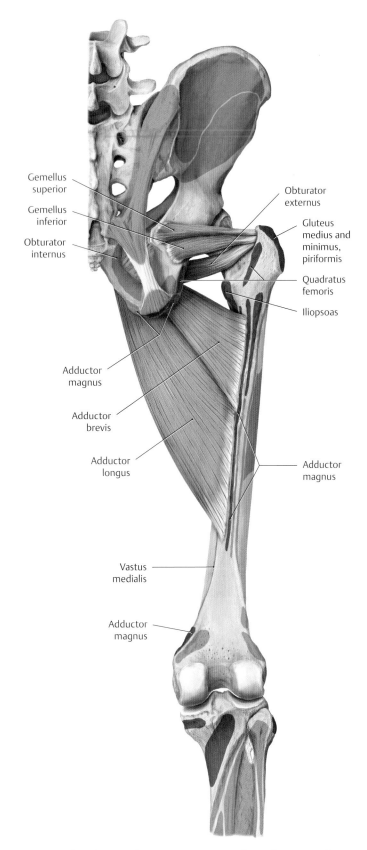

Gluteus medius

Tensor fasciae latae

Gluteus minimus

Rectus femoris

Obturator internus and externus, gemellus superior and inferior

Gluteus medius and minimus, piriformis

Quadratus femoris

Gluteus maximus

Pectineus

Vastus lateralis

Adductor brevis

Vastus intermedius

Adductor magnus

Biceps femoris, short head

Plantaris

Biceps femoris

Soleus

Tibialis posterior

Gemellus superior

Gemellus inferior

Obturator internus

Obturator externus

Gluteus medius and minimus, piriformis

Quadratus femoris

Iliopsoas

Adductor magnus

Adductor brevis

Adductor longus

Adductor magnus

Vastus medialis

Adductor magnus

Gluteus maximus

Gluteus maximus

Gemellus superior

Gemellus inferior

Obturator internus

Semimembranosus

Biceps femoris, long head and semitendinosus

Iliopsoas

Adductor magnus

Vastus medialis

Adductor longus

Adductor magnus

Gastrocnemius, medial and lateral heads

Semimembranosus

Popliteus

Flexor digitorum longus

A *Removed:* Piriformis, obturator internus, quadratus femoris, and adductor magnus.

B *Removed:* All muscles.

Fig. 31.16 Lateral muscles of the hip, thigh, and gluteal region

Note: The iliotibial tract (the thickened band of fascia lata) functions as a tension band to reduce the bending loads on the proximal femur.

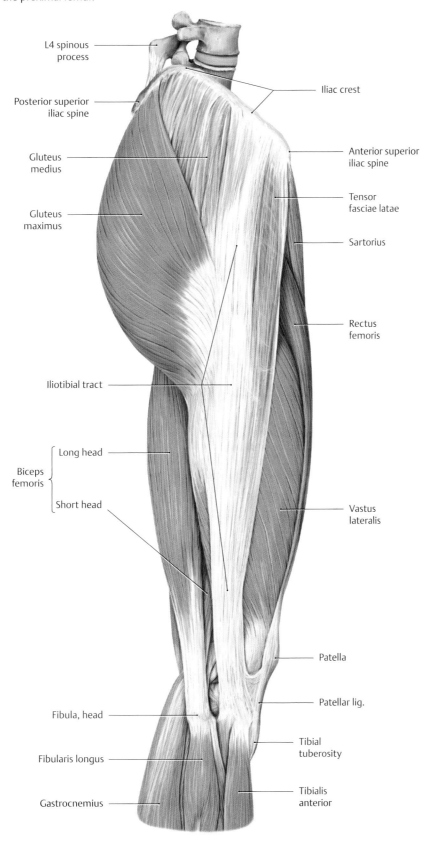

Muscle Facts (I)

| Table 31.1 | Iliopsoas muscle |

Muscles		Origin	Insertion	Innervation	Action
③ Iliopsoas	① Psoas major*	*Superficial:* T12–L4 and associated intervertebral disks (lateral surfaces) *Deep:* L1–L5 vertebrae (costal processes)	Femur (lesser trochanter)	Lumbar plexus L1, L2(L3)	• Hip joint: flexion and external rotation • Lumbar spine: *unilateral* contraction (with the femur fixed) bends the trunk laterally to the same side; *bilateral* contraction raises the trunk from the supine position
	② Iliacus	Iliac fossa		Femoral n. (L2–L3)	

* The psoas minor, present in approximately 50% of the population, is often found on the superficial surface of the psoas major (see **Fig. 31.17**). It is not a muscle of the lower limb. It originates, inserts, and exerts its action on the abdomen (see **Table 13.2, p. 148**).

Fig. 31.17 Muscles of the hip
Right side, schematic.

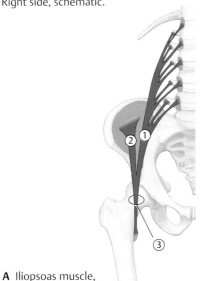

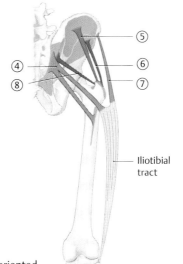

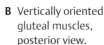

A Iliopsoas muscle, anterior view.

B Vertically oriented gluteal muscles, posterior view.

Iliotibial tract

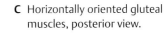

C Horizontally oriented gluteal muscles, posterior view.

| Table 31.2 | Gluteal muscles |

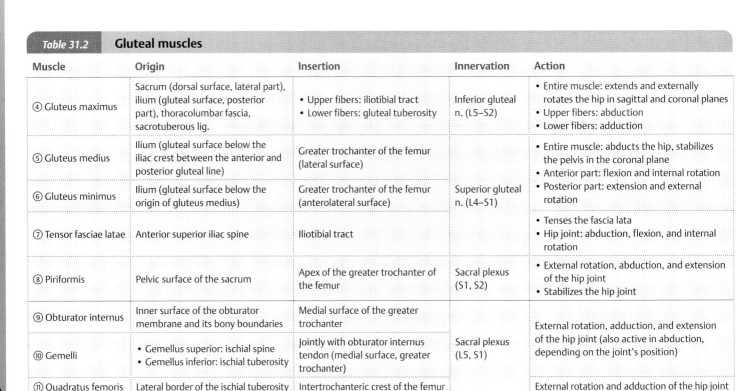

Muscle	Origin	Insertion	Innervation	Action
④ Gluteus maximus	Sacrum (dorsal surface, lateral part), ilium (gluteal surface, posterior part), thoracolumbar fascia, sacrotuberous lig.	• Upper fibers: iliotibial tract • Lower fibers: gluteal tuberosity	Inferior gluteal n. (L5–S2)	• Entire muscle: extends and externally rotates the hip in sagittal and coronal planes • Upper fibers: abduction • Lower fibers: adduction
⑤ Gluteus medius	Ilium (gluteal surface below the iliac crest between the anterior and posterior gluteal line)	Greater trochanter of the femur (lateral surface)	Superior gluteal n. (L4–S1)	• Entire muscle: abducts the hip, stabilizes the pelvis in the coronal plane • Anterior part: flexion and internal rotation • Posterior part: extension and external rotation
⑥ Gluteus minimus	Ilium (gluteal surface below the origin of gluteus medius)	Greater trochanter of the femur (anterolateral surface)		
⑦ Tensor fasciae latae	Anterior superior iliac spine	Iliotibial tract		• Tenses the fascia lata • Hip joint: abduction, flexion, and internal rotation
⑧ Piriformis	Pelvic surface of the sacrum	Apex of the greater trochanter of the femur	Sacral plexus (S1, S2)	• External rotation, abduction, and extension of the hip joint • Stabilizes the hip joint
⑨ Obturator internus	Inner surface of the obturator membrane and its bony boundaries	Medial surface of the greater trochanter	Sacral plexus (L5, S1)	External rotation, adduction, and extension of the hip joint (also active in abduction, depending on the joint's position)
⑩ Gemelli	• Gemellus superior: ischial spine • Gemellus inferior: ischial tuberosity	Jointly with obturator internus tendon (medial surface, greater trochanter)		
⑪ Quadratus femoris	Lateral border of the ischial tuberosity	Intertrochanteric crest of the femur		External rotation and adduction of the hip joint

Fig. 31.18 Psoas and iliacus muscles
Right side, anterior view.

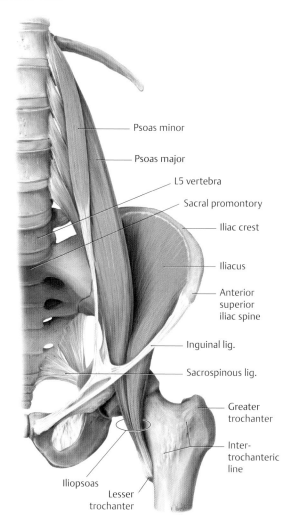

- Psoas minor
- Psoas major
- L5 vertebra
- Sacral promontory
- Iliac crest
- Iliacus
- Anterior superior iliac spine
- Inguinal lig.
- Sacrospinous lig.
- Greater trochanter
- Inter-trochanteric line
- Iliopsoas
- Lesser trochanter

Fig. 31.19 Superficial muscles of the gluteal region
Right side, posterior view.

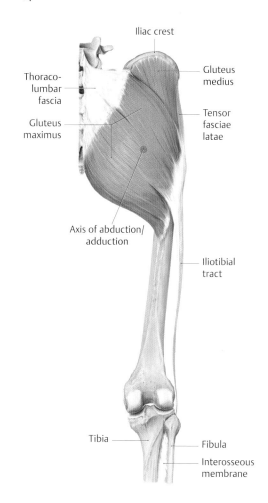

- Iliac crest
- Gluteus medius
- Thoraco-lumbar fascia
- Tensor fasciae latae
- Gluteus maximus
- Axis of abduction/adduction
- Iliotibial tract
- Tibia
- Fibula
- Interosseous membrane

Fig. 31.20 Deep muscles of the gluteal region

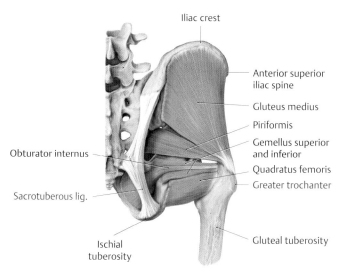

- Iliac crest
- Anterior superior iliac spine
- Gluteus medius
- Piriformis
- Gemellus superior and inferior
- Quadratus femoris
- Greater trochanter
- Obturator internus
- Sacrotuberous lig.
- Ischial tuberosity
- Gluteal tuberosity

A Deep layer with gluteus maximus removed.

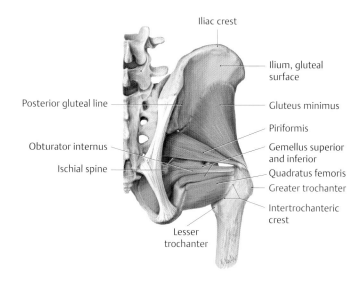

- Iliac crest
- Ilium, gluteal surface
- Gluteus minimus
- Posterior gluteal line
- Piriformis
- Obturator internus
- Gemellus superior and inferior
- Ischial spine
- Quadratus femoris
- Greater trochanter
- Intertrochanteric crest
- Lesser trochanter

B Deep layer with gluteus maximus and gluteus medius removed.

Muscle Facts (II)

Functionally, the medial thigh muscles are considered the adductors of the hip.

Fig. 31.21 Medial thigh muscles: Superficial layer
Right side, anterior view.

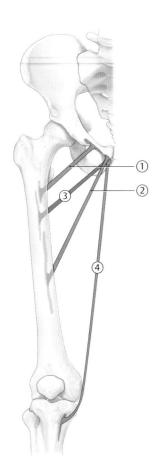

A Schematic.

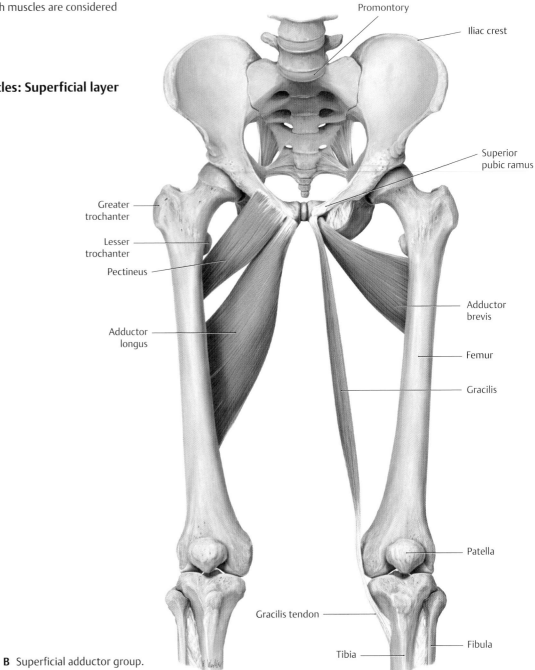

B Superficial adductor group.

Table 31.3	Medial thigh muscles: Superficial layer			
Muscle	**Origin**	**Insertion**	**Innervation**	**Action**
① Pectineus	Pecten pubis	Femur (pectineal line and the proximal linea aspera)	Femoral n., obturator n. (L2, L3)	• Hip joint: adduction, external rotation, and slight flexion • Stabilizes the pelvis in the coronal and sagittal planes
② Adductor longus	Superior pubic ramus and anterior side of the pubic symphysis	Femur (linea aspera, medial lip in the middle third of the femur)	Obturator n. (L2–L4)	• Hip joint: adduction and flexion (up to 70 degrees); extension (past 80 degrees of flexion) • Stabilizes the pelvis in the coronal and sagittal planes
③ Adductor brevis	Inferior pubic ramus			
④ Gracilis	Inferior pubic ramus below the pubic symphysis	Tibia (medial border of the tuberosity, along with the tendons of sartorius and semitendinosus)	Obturator n. (L2, L3)	• Hip joint: adduction and flexion • Knee joint: flexion and internal rotation

Fig. 31.22 Medial thigh muscles: Deep layer
Right side, anterior view.

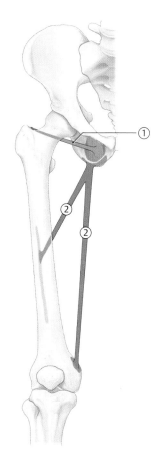

A Schematic.

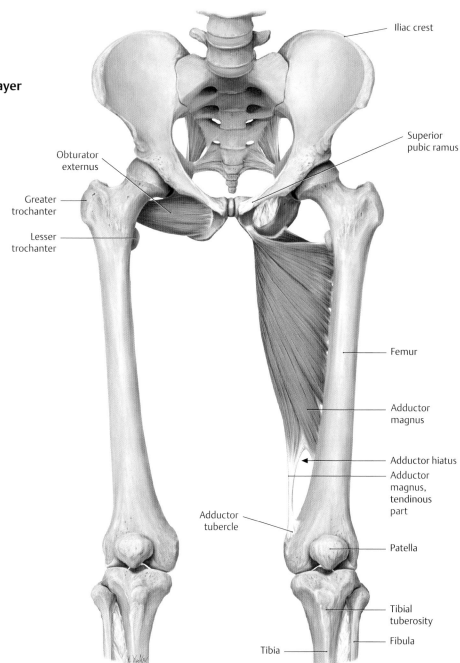

B Deep adductor group.

Table 31.4	**Medial thigh muscles: Deep layer**			
Muscle	**Origin**	**Insertion**	**Innervation**	**Action**
① Obturator externus	Outer surface of the obturator membrane and its bony boundaries	Trochanteric fossa of the femur	Obturator n. (L3, L4)	• Hip joint: adduction and external rotation • Stabilizes the pelvis in the sagittal plane
② Adductor magnus	Inferior pubic ramus, ischial ramus, and ischial tuberosity	• Deep part ("fleshy insertion"): medial lip of the linea aspera • Superficial part ("tendinous insertion"): adductor tubercle of the femur	• Deep part: obturator n. (L2–L4) • Superficial part: tibial n. (L4)	• Hip joint: adduction, extension, and slight flexion (the tendinous insertion is also active in internal rotation) • Stabilizes the pelvis in the coronal and sagittal planes

Muscle Facts (III)

The anterior and posterior muscles of the thigh can be classified as extensors and flexors, respectively, with regard to the knee joint.

Fig. 31.23 Anterior thigh muscles
Right side, anterior view.

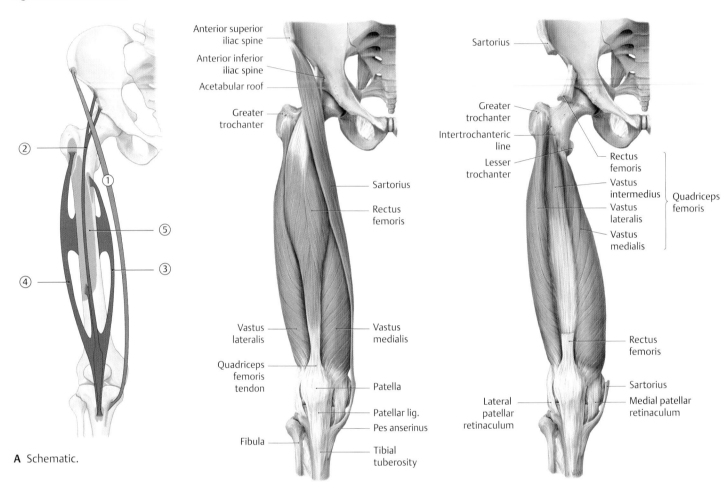

A Schematic.

B Superficial group.

C Deep group. *Removed:* Sartorius and rectus femoris.

Table 31.5	Anterior thigh muscles				
Muscle		**Origin**	**Insertion**	**Innervation**	**Action**
① Sartorius		Anterior superior iliac spine	Medial to the tibial tuberosity (together with gracilis and semitendinosus)	Femoral n. (L2, L3)	• Hip joint: flexion, abduction, and external rotation • Knee joint: flexion and internal rotation
Quadriceps femoris*	② Rectus femoris	Anterior inferior iliac spine, acetabular roof of hip joint	Tibial tuberosity (via patellar lig.)	Femoral n. (L2–L4)	• Hip joint: flexion • Knee joint: extension
	③ Vastus medialis	Linea aspera (medial lip), intertrochanteric line (distal part)	Both sides of tibial tuberosity on the medial and lateral condyles (via the medial and lateral patellar retinacula)		Knee joint: extension
	④ Vastus lateralis	Linea aspera (lateral lip), greater trochanter (lateral surface)			
	⑤ Vastus intermedius	Femoral shaft (anterior side)	Tibial tuberosity (via patellar lig.)		
	Articularis genus (distal fibers of vastus intermedius)	Anterior side of femoral shaft at level of the suprapatellar recess	Suprapatellar recess of knee joint capsule		Knee joint: extension; prevents entrapment of capsule

*The entire muscle inserts on the tibial tuberosity via the patellar lig.

Fig. 31.24 **Posterior thigh muscles**

Right side, posterior view.

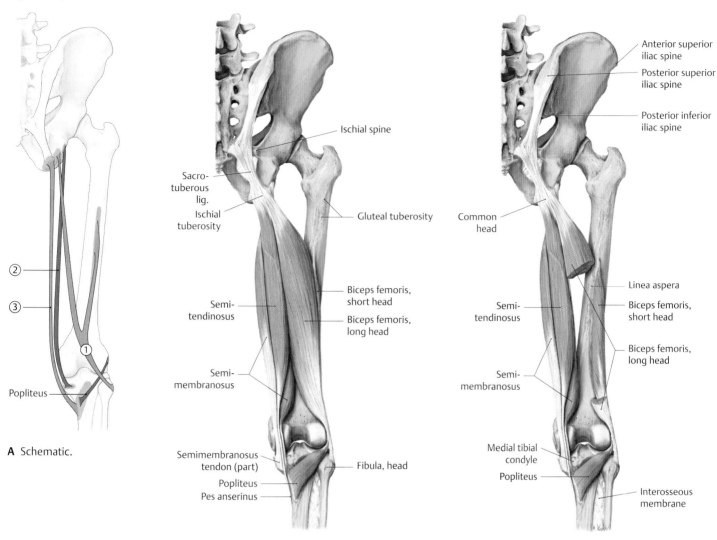

A Schematic.

B Superficial group.

C Deep group. *Removed:* Biceps femoris (long head) and semitendinosus.

Table 31.6	Posterior thigh muscles			
Muscle	**Origin**	**Insertion**	**Innervation**	**Action**
① Biceps femoris	Long head: ischial tuberosity, sacrotuberous lig. (common head with semitendinosus)	Head of fibula	Tibial n. (L5–S2)	• Hip joint (long head): extends the hip, stabilizes the pelvis in the sagittal plane • Knee joint: flexion and external rotation
	Short head: lateral lip of the linea aspera in the middle third of the femur		Common fibular n. (L5–S2)	Knee joint: flexion and external rotation
② Semimembranosus	Ischial tuberosity	Medial tibial condyle, oblique popliteal lig., popliteus fascia	Tibial n. (L5–S2)	• Hip joint: extends the hip, stabilizes the pelvis in the sagittal plane • Knee joint: flexion and internal rotation
③ Semitendinosus	Ischial tuberosity and sacrotuberous lig. (common head with long head of biceps femoris)	Medial to the tibial tuberosity in the pes anserinus (along with the tendons of gracilis and sartorius)		
See **p. 445** for the popliteus.				

Tibia & Fibula

 The tibia and fibula articulate at two joints, allowing limited motion (rotation). The crural interosseous membrane is a sheet of tough connective tissue that serves as an origin for several muscles in the leg. It also acts with the tibiofibular syndesmosis to stabilize the ankle joint.

Fig. 32.1 **Tibia and fibula**
Right leg.

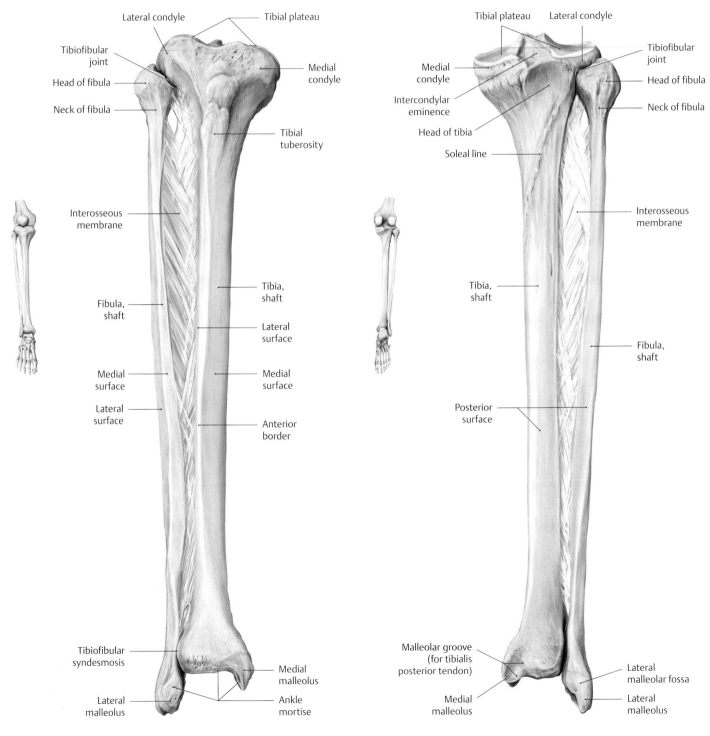

A Anterior view.

B Posterior view.

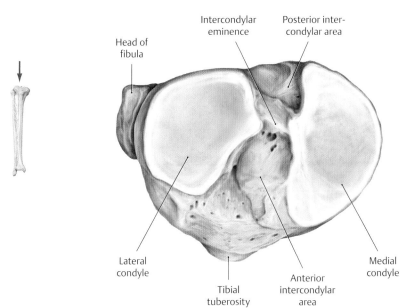

C Proximal view.

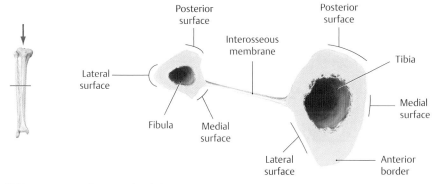

D Transverse section, proximal view.

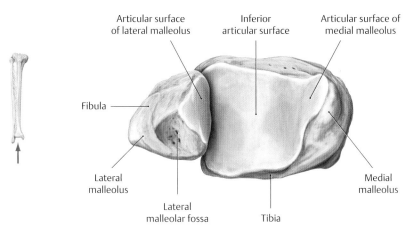

E Distal view.

Fibular fracture

When diagnosing a fibular fracture, it is important to determine whether the tibiofibular syndesmosis (see **p. 426**) is disrupted. Fibular fractures may occur distal to, level with, or proximal to the tibiofibular syndesmosis; the latter two frequently involve tearing of the syndesmosis.

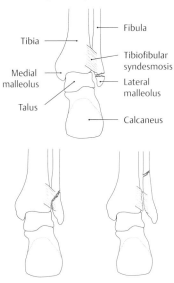

In this fracture located proximal to the syndesmosis (*arrow*), the syndesmosis is torn, as indicated by the widened medial joint space of the upper ankle joint (see **pp. 450–451**).

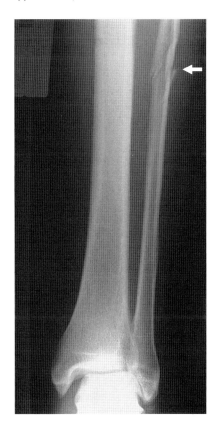

Knee Joint: Overview

In the knee joint, the femur articulates with the tibia and patella. Both joints are contained within a common capsule and have communicating articular cavities. *Note:* The fibula is not included in the knee joint (contrast to the humerus in the elbow; see **p. 322**). Instead, it forms a separate rigid articulation with the tibia.

***Fig. 32.2* Right knee joint**

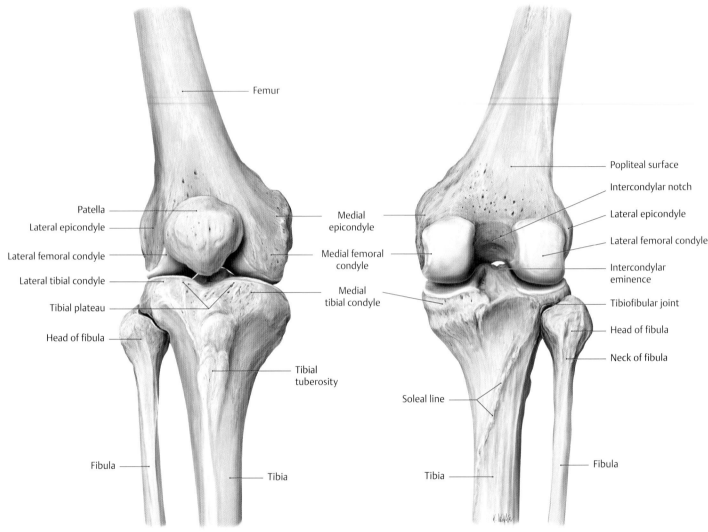

Femur

Patella
Lateral epicondyle
Lateral femoral condyle
Lateral tibial condyle
Tibial plateau
Head of fibula

Medial epicondyle
Medial femoral condyle
Medial tibial condyle

Tibial tuberosity

Fibula
Tibia

A Anterior view.

Popliteal surface
Intercondylar notch
Lateral epicondyle
Lateral femoral condyle
Intercondylar eminence
Tibiofibular joint
Head of fibula
Neck of fibula

Soleal line

Tibia
Fibula

B Posterior view.

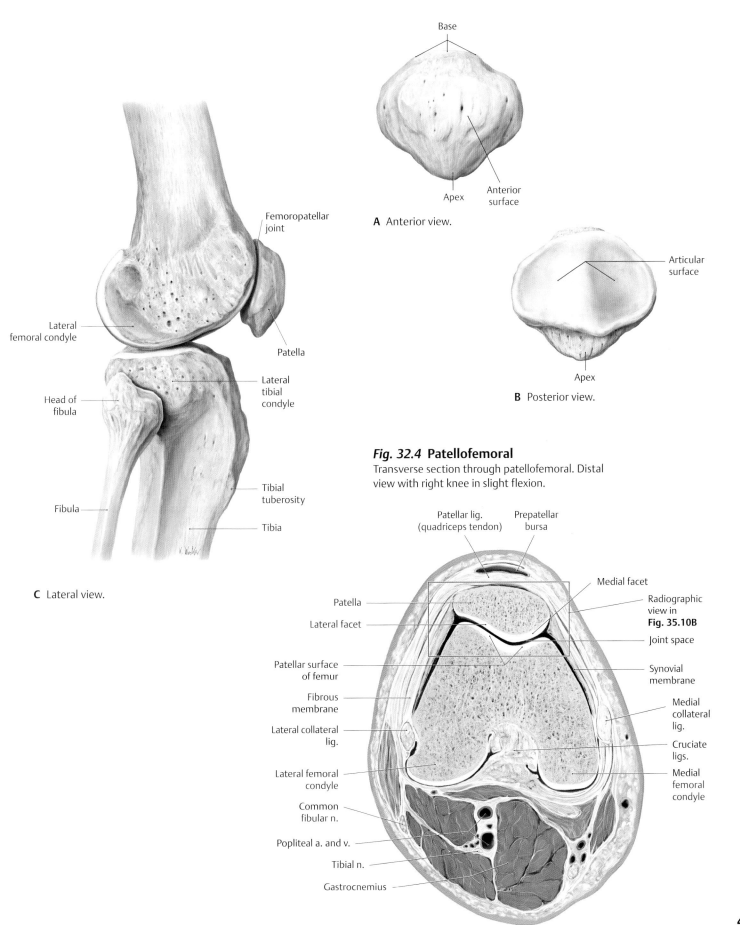

Fig. 32.3 Patella

Base

Apex

Anterior surface

A Anterior view.

Articular surface

Apex

B Posterior view.

Femoropatellar joint

Patella

Lateral femoral condyle

Lateral tibial condyle

Head of fibula

Fibula

Tibial tuberosity

Tibia

C Lateral view.

Fig. 32.4 Patellofemoral

Transverse section through patellofemoral. Distal view with right knee in slight flexion.

Patellar lig. (quadriceps tendon)

Prepatellar bursa

Patella

Lateral facet

Medial facet

Radiographic view in **Fig. 35.10B**

Joint space

Patellar surface of femur

Fibrous membrane

Lateral collateral lig.

Lateral femoral condyle

Common fibular n.

Popliteal a. and v.

Tibial n.

Gastrocnemius

Synovial membrane

Medial collateral lig.

Cruciate ligs.

Medial femoral condyle

Knee Joint: Capsule, Ligaments & Bursae

Table 32.1	Ligaments of the knee joint	
Extrinsic ligaments		
		Patellar lig.
	Anterior side	Medial longitudinal patellar retinaculum
		Lateral longitudinal patellar retinaculum
		Medial transverse patellar retinaculum
		Lateral transverse patellar retinaculum
	Medial and lateral sides	Medial (tibial) collateral lig.
		Lateral (fibular) collateral lig.
	Posterior side	Oblique popliteal lig.
		Arcuate popliteal lig.
Intrinsic ligaments		
	Anterior cruciate lig.	
	Posterior cruciate lig.	
	Transverse lig. of knee	
	Posterior meniscofemoral lig.	

Fig. 32.5 **Ligaments of the knee joint**
Anterior view of right knee.

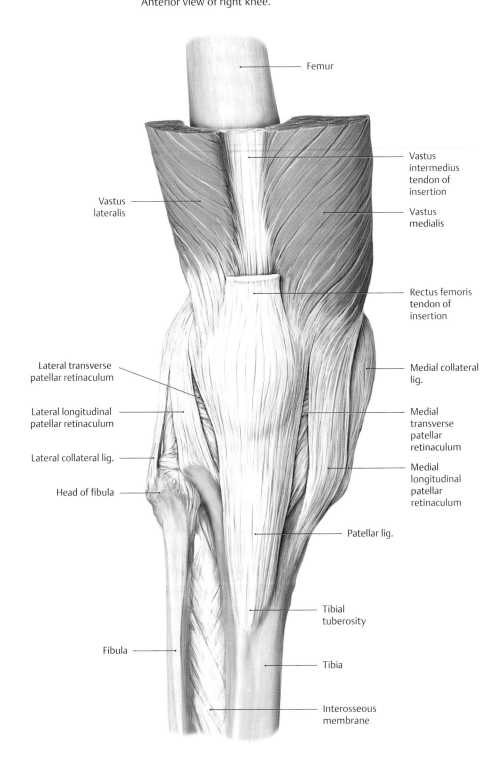

Femur

Vastus intermedius tendon of insertion

Vastus lateralis

Vastus medialis

Rectus femoris tendon of insertion

Lateral transverse patellar retinaculum

Medial collateral lig.

Lateral longitudinal patellar retinaculum

Medial transverse patellar retinaculum

Lateral collateral lig.

Medial longitudinal patellar retinaculum

Head of fibula

Patellar lig.

Tibial tuberosity

Fibula

Tibia

Interosseous membrane

Fig. 32.6 **Capsule, ligaments, and periarticular bursae**

Posterior view of right knee. The joint cavity communicates with peri-articular bursae at the subpopliteal recess, semimembranosus bursa, and medial subtendinous bursa of the gastrocnemius.

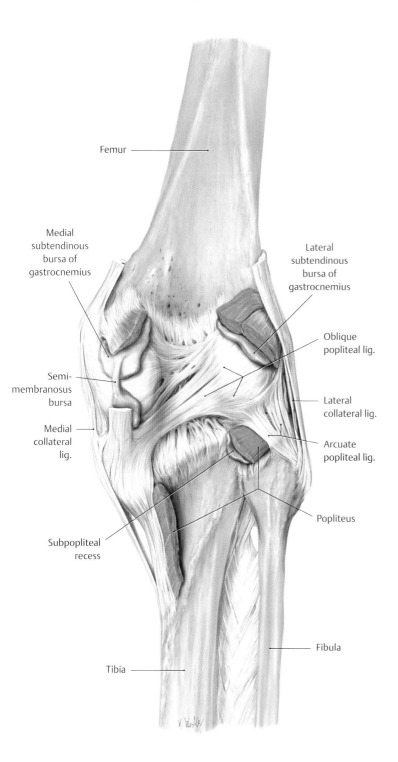

 Clinical box 32.2

Gastrocnemio-semimembranosus bursa (Baker's cyst)

Painful swelling behind the knee may be caused by a cystic outpouching of the joint capsule (synovial popliteal cyst). This frequently results from an increase in intra-articular pressure (e.g., in rheumatoid arthritis).

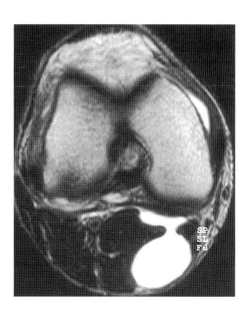

Axial MRI of a Baker's cyst in the popliteal fossa, inferior view. Baker's cyst in the right popliteal fossa. Baker's cysts often occur in the medial part of the popliteal fossa between the semimembranosus tendon and the medial head of the gastrocnemius at the level of the posteromedial femoral condyle.

431

Knee Joint: Ligaments & Menisci

Fig. 32.7 Collateral and patellar ligaments of the knee joint
Right knee joint. Each knee joint has medial and lateral collateral ligaments. The medial collateral ligament is attached to both the capsule
and the medial meniscus, whereas the lateral collateral ligament has no
direct contact with either the capsule or the lateral meniscus. Both
collateral ligaments are taut when the knee is in extension and stabilize
the joint in the coronal plane.

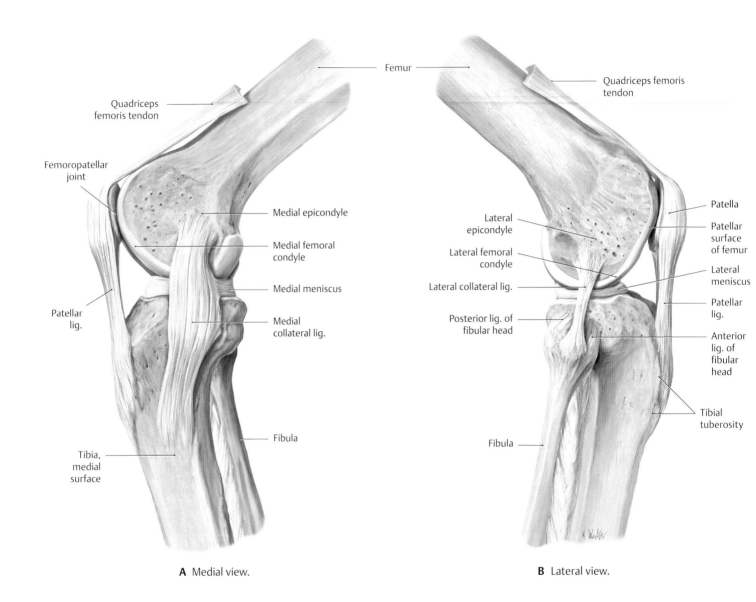

A Medial view.

B Lateral view.

Fig. 32.8 Menisci in the knee joint

Right tibial plateau, proximal view.

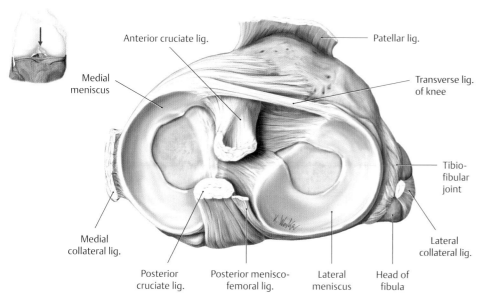

A Right tibial plateau with cruciate, patellar, and collateral ligaments divided.

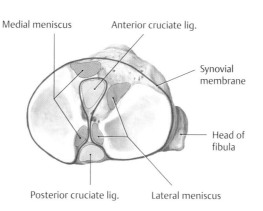

B Attachment sites of menisci and cruciate ligaments. Red line indicates the tibial attachment of the synovial membrane that covers the cruciate ligaments. The cruciate ligaments lie in the subsynovial connective tissue.

Fig. 32.9 Movements of the menisci

Right knee joint.

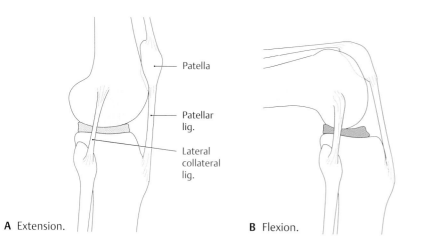

A Extension.　　**B** Flexion.　　**C** Tibial plateau, proximal view.

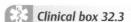 **Clinical box 32.3**

Injury to the menisci

The less mobile medial meniscus is more susceptible to injury than the lateral meniscus. Trauma generally results from sudden extension or rotation of the flexed knee while the leg is fixed.

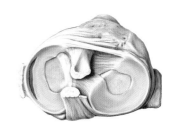

A Bucket-handle tear.

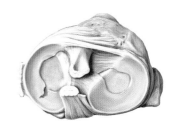

B Radial tear of posterior horn.

Cruciate Ligaments

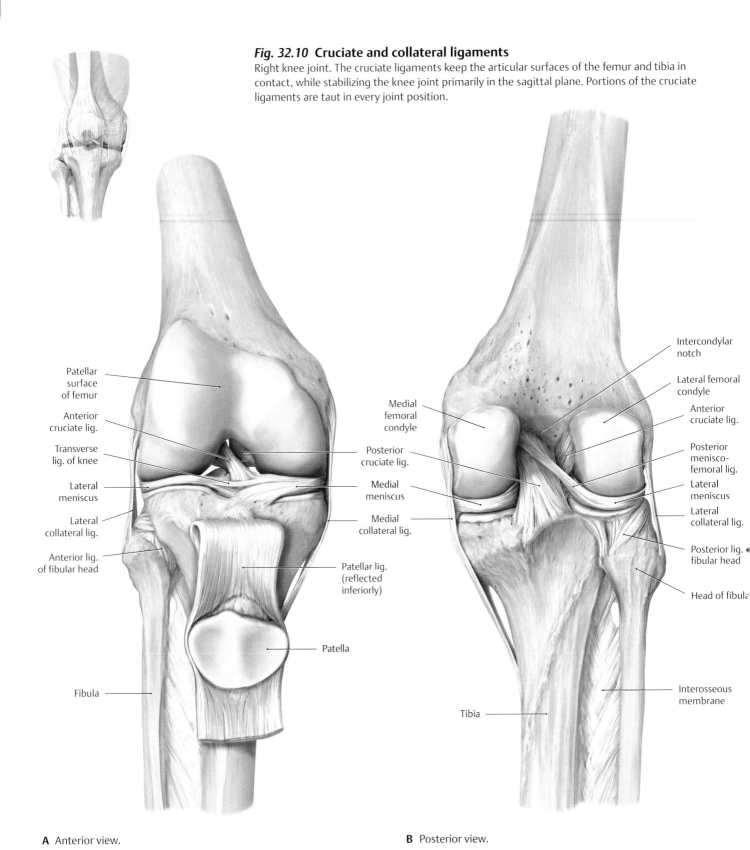

Fig. 32.10 Cruciate and collateral ligaments

Right knee joint. The cruciate ligaments keep the articular surfaces of the femur and tibia in contact, while stabilizing the knee joint primarily in the sagittal plane. Portions of the cruciate ligaments are taut in every joint position.

Patellar surface of femur

Anterior cruciate lig.

Transverse lig. of knee

Lateral meniscus

Lateral collateral lig.

Anterior lig. of fibular head

Fibula

Posterior cruciate lig.

Medial meniscus

Medial collateral lig.

Patellar lig. (reflected inferiorly)

Patella

A Anterior view.

Intercondylar notch

Lateral femoral condyle

Anterior cruciate lig.

Posterior menisco-femoral lig.

Lateral meniscus

Lateral collateral lig.

Posterior lig. fibular head

Head of fibula

Interosseous membrane

Medial femoral condyle

Tibia

B Posterior view.

Fig. 32.11 **Right knee joint in flexion**

Anterior view with joint capsule and patella removed.

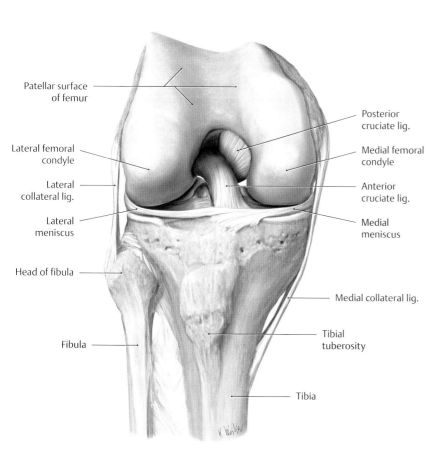

- Patellar surface of femur
- Lateral femoral condyle
- Lateral collateral lig.
- Lateral meniscus
- Head of fibula
- Fibula
- Posterior cruciate lig.
- Medial femoral condyle
- Anterior cruciate lig.
- Medial meniscus
- Medial collateral lig.
- Tibial tuberosity
- Tibia

Fig. 32.12 **Cruciate and collateral ligaments in flexion and extension**

Right knee, anterior view. Taut ligament fibers in red.

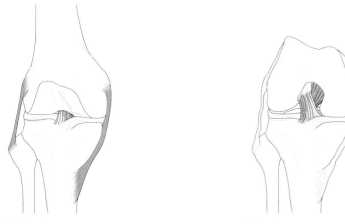

A Extension.

B Flexion.

C Flexion and internal rotation.

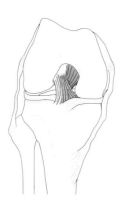

✴ Clinical box 32.4

Rupture of cruciate ligaments

Cruciate ligament rupture destabilizes the knee joint, allowing the tibia to move forward (anterior "drawer sign") or backward (posterior "drawer sign") relative to the femur. *Anterior* cruciate ligament ruptures are approximately 10 times more common than posterior ligament ruptures. The most common mechanism of injury is an internal rotation trauma with the leg fixed. A lateral blow to the fully extended knee with the foot planted tends to cause concomitant rupture of the anterior cruciate and medial collateral ligaments, as well as tearing of the attached medial meniscus.

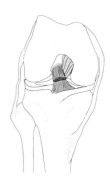

A Right knee in flexion, rupture of anterior cruciate ligament, anterior view.

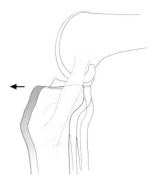

B Right knee in flexion, anterior "drawer sign," medial view. During examination of the flexed knee, the tibia can be pulled forward.

435

Knee Joint Cavity

Fig. 32.13 Joint cavity

Right knee, lateral view. The joint cavity was demonstrated by injecting liquid plastic into the knee joint and later removing the capsule.

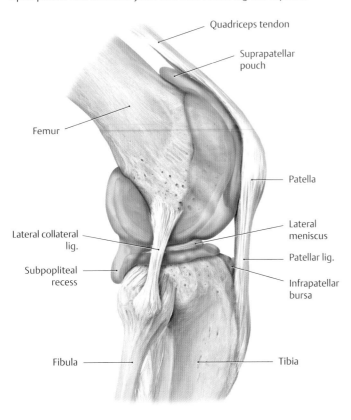

Fig. 32.15 Attachments of the joint capsule

Right knee joint, anterior view.

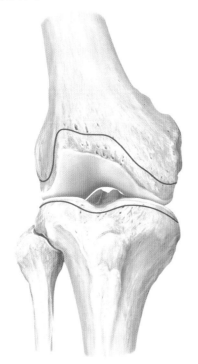

Fig. 32.14 Opened joint capsule

Right knee, anterior view with patella reflected downward.

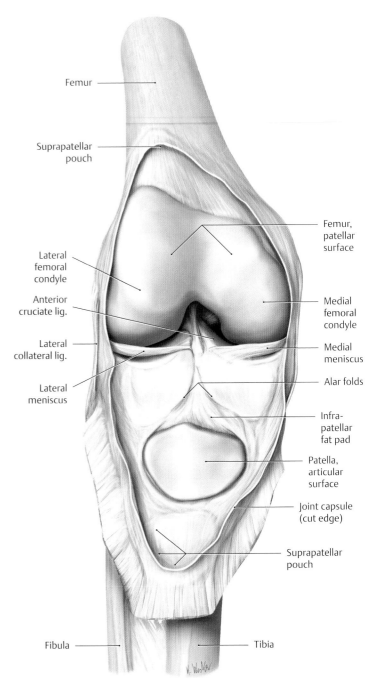

Fig. 32.16 Suprapatellar pouch during flexion

Right knee joint, medial view.

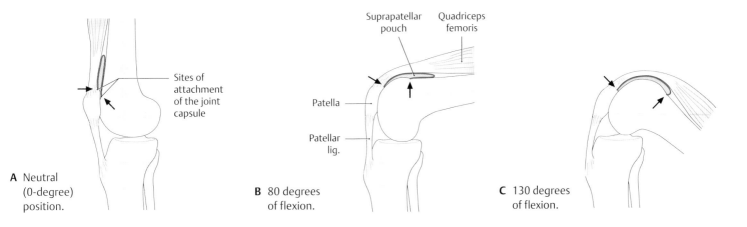

A Neutral (0-degree) position.

Sites of attachment of the joint capsule

Suprapatellar pouch

Quadriceps femoris

Patella

Patellar lig.

B 80 degrees of flexion.

C 130 degrees of flexion.

Fig. 32.17 Right knee joint: Midsagittal section

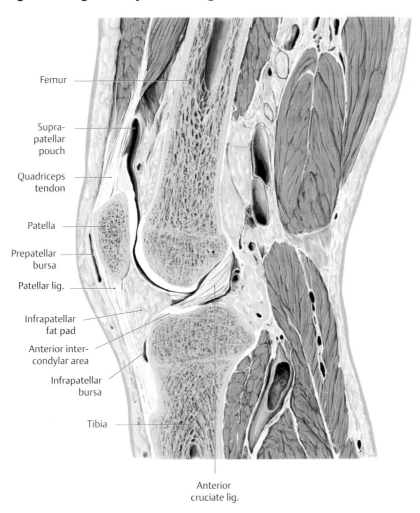

Femur

Supra-patellar pouch

Quadriceps tendon

Patella

Prepatellar bursa

Patellar lig.

Infrapatellar fat pad

Anterior inter-condylar area

Infrapatellar bursa

Tibia

Anterior cruciate lig.

Muscles of the Leg: Anterior & Lateral Compartments

***Fig. 32.18* Muscles of the anterior compartment of the leg**
Right leg. Muscle origins shown in red, insertions in blue.

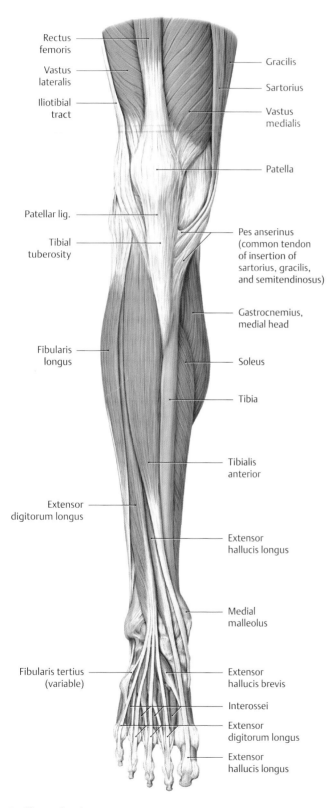

Rectus femoris
Vastus lateralis
Iliotibial tract
Patellar lig.
Tibial tuberosity
Fibularis longus
Extensor digitorum longus
Fibularis tertius (variable)

Gracilis
Sartorius
Vastus medialis
Patella
Pes anserinus (common tendon of insertion of sartorius, gracilis, and semitendinosus)
Gastrocnemius, medial head
Soleus
Tibia
Tibialis anterior
Extensor hallucis longus
Medial malleolus
Extensor hallucis brevis
Interossei
Extensor digitorum longus
Extensor hallucis longus

A All muscles shown.

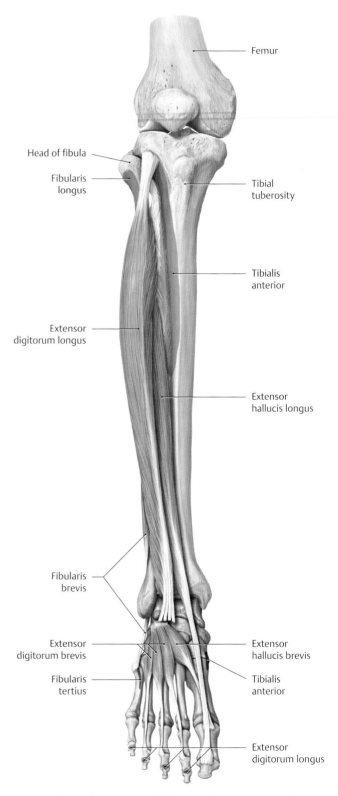

Femur
Head of fibula
Fibularis longus
Extensor digitorum longus
Fibularis brevis
Extensor digitorum brevis
Fibularis tertius

Tibial tuberosity
Tibialis anterior
Tibialis anterior
Extensor hallucis longus
Extensor hallucis brevis
Tibialis anterior
Extensor digitorum longus

B *Removed:* Tibialis anterior and fibularis longus; extensor digitorum longus tendons (distal portions). *Note:* The fibularis tertius is a division of the extensor digitorum longus.

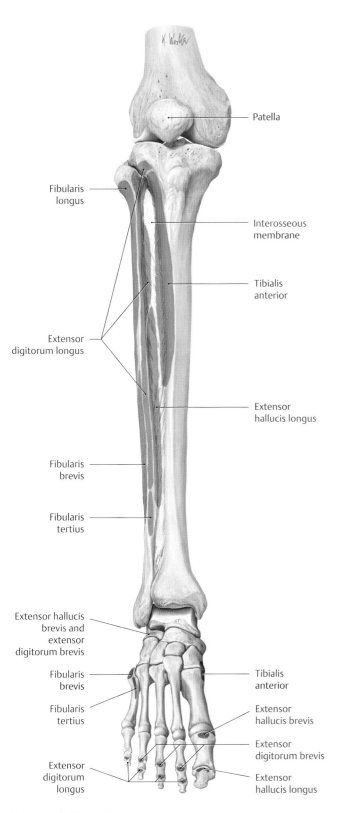

C *Removed:* All muscles.

Fibularis longus

Extensor digitorum longus

Fibularis brevis

Fibularis tertius

Extensor hallucis brevis and extensor digitorum brevis

Fibularis brevis

Fibularis tertius

Extensor digitorum longus

Patella

Interosseous membrane

Tibialis anterior

Extensor hallucis longus

Tibialis anterior

Extensor hallucis brevis

Extensor digitorum brevis

Extensor hallucis longus

Fig. 32.19 **Muscles of the lateral compartment of the leg**
Right leg. The triceps surae is comprised of the soleus and two heads of the gastrocnemius.

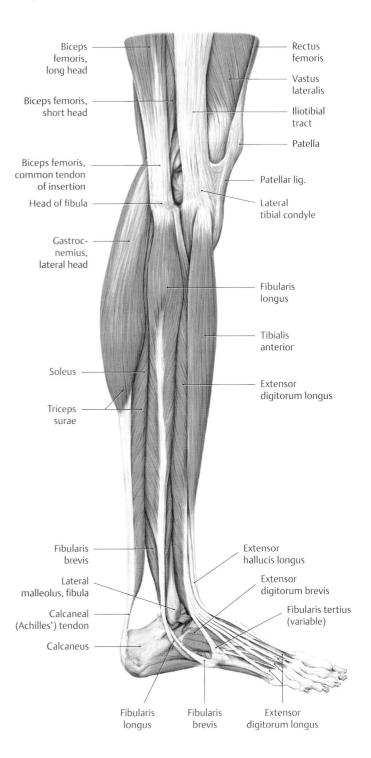

Biceps femoris, long head

Biceps femoris, short head

Biceps femoris, common tendon of insertion

Head of fibula

Gastroc-nemius, lateral head

Soleus

Triceps surae

Fibularis brevis

Lateral malleolus, fibula

Calcaneal (Achilles') tendon

Calcaneus

Fibularis longus

Fibularis brevis

Extensor digitorum longus

Rectus femoris

Vastus lateralis

Iliotibial tract

Patella

Patellar lig.

Lateral tibial condyle

Fibularis longus

Tibialis anterior

Extensor digitorum longus

Extensor hallucis longus

Extensor digitorum brevis

Fibularis tertius (variable)

439

Muscles of the Leg: Posterior Compartment

Fig. 32.20 Muscles of the posterior compartment of the leg
Right leg. Muscle origins shown in red, insertions in blue.

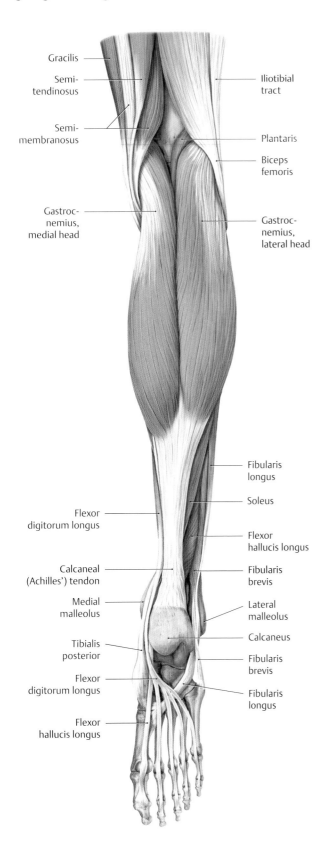

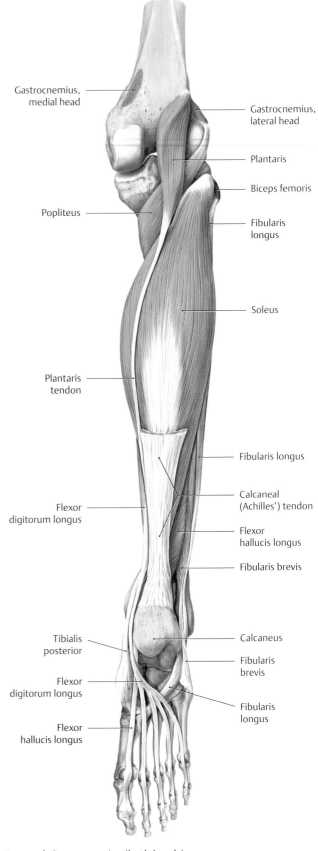

A *Note:* The bulge of the calf is produced mainly by the triceps surae (soleus and the two heads of the gastrocnemius).

B *Removed:* Gastrocnemius (both heads).

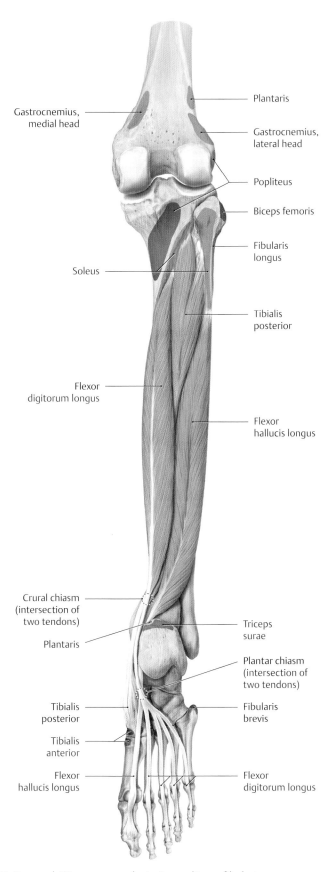

Gastrocnemius, medial head

Plantaris

Gastrocnemius, lateral head

Popliteus

Biceps femoris

Fibularis longus

Soleus

Tibialis posterior

Flexor digitorum longus

Flexor hallucis longus

Crural chiasm (intersection of two tendons)

Plantaris

Tibialis posterior

Tibialis anterior

Flexor hallucis longus

Triceps surae

Plantar chiasm (intersection of two tendons)

Fibularis brevis

Flexor digitorum longus

Gastrocnemius, medial head

Plantaris

Gastrocnemius, lateral head

Popliteus

Biceps femoris

Fibularis longus

Soleus

Tibialis posterior

Flexor digitorum longus

Flexor hallucis longus

Interosseous membrane

Fibularis brevis

Plantaris

Triceps surae

Tibialis posterior

Fibularis brevis

Tibialis anterior

Fibularis longus

Flexor hallucis longus

Flexor digitorum longus

C *Removed:* Triceps surae, plantaris, popliteus, fibularis longus, and fibularis brevis muscles.

D *Removed:* All muscles.

441

Muscle Facts (I)

The muscles of the leg control the flexion/extension and inversion/eversion of the foot, which provide stability to the lower limb during movements at the knee and hip joint.

Fig. 32.21 Muscles of the lateral compartment of the leg
Right leg and foot.

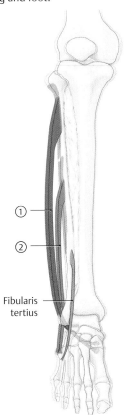

A Fibularis muscles, anterior view, schematic.

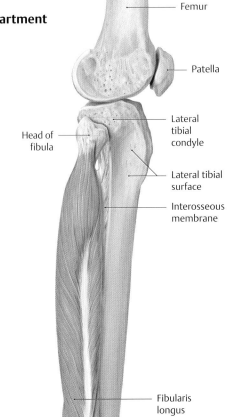

B Lateral compartment, right lateral view.

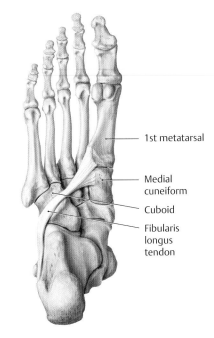

C Course of the fibularis longus tendon, plantar view.

Table 32.2	Lateral compartment			
Muscle	**Origin**	**Insertion**	**Innervation**	**Action**
① Fibularis longus	Fibula (head and proximal two thirds of the lateral surface, arising partly from the intermuscular septa)	Medial cuneiform (plantar side), 1st metatarsal (base)	Superficial fibular n. (L5, S1)	• Talocrural joint: plantar flexion • Subtalar joint: eversion (pronation) • Supports the transverse arch of the foot
② Fibularis brevis	Fibula (distal half of the lateral surface), intermuscular septa	5th metatarsal (tuberosity at the base, with an occasional division to the dorsal aponeurosis of the 5th toe)		• Talocrural joint: plantar flexion • Subtalar joint: eversion (pronation)

Fig. 32.22 **Muscles of the anterior compartment of the leg**

Right leg, anterior view.

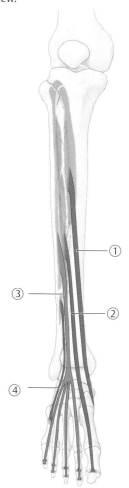

A Schematic.

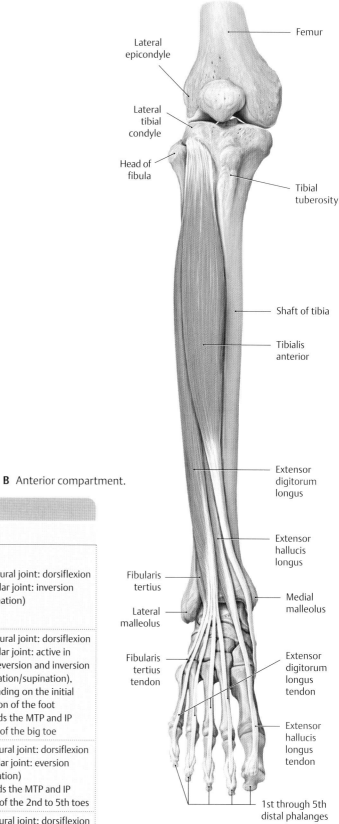

B Anterior compartment.

Table 32.3	**Anterior compartment**			
Muscle	**Origin**	**Insertion**	**Innervation**	**Action**
① Tibialis anterior	Tibia (upper two thirds of the lateral surface), interosseous membrane, and superficial crural fascia (highest part)	Medial cuneiform (medial and plantar surface), first metatarsal (medial base)	Deep fibular n. (L4, L5)	• Talocrural joint: dorsiflexion • Subtalar joint: inversion (supination)
② Extensor hallucis longus	Fibula (middle third of the medial surface), interosseous membrane	1st toe (at the dorsal aponeurosis at the base of its distal phalanx)	Deep fibular n. (L4, L5)	• Talocrural joint: dorsiflexion • Subtalar joint: active in both eversion and inversion (pronation/supination), depending on the initial position of the foot • Extends the MTP and IP joints of the big toe
③ Extensor digitorum longus	Fibula (head and medial surface), tibia (lateral condyle), and interosseous membrane	2nd to 5th toes (at the dorsal aponeuroses at the bases of the distal phalanges)	Deep fibular n. (L4, L5)	• Talocrural joint: dorsiflexion • Subtalar joint: eversion (pronation) • Extends the MTP and IP joints of the 2nd to 5th toes
④ Fibularis tertius	Distal fibula (anterior border)	5th metatarsal (base)	Deep fibular n. (L4, L5)	• Talocrural joint: dorsiflexion • Subtalar joint: eversion (pronation)

IP, interphalangeal; MTP, metatarsophalangeal.

Muscle Facts (II)

The muscles of the posterior compartment are divided into two groups: the superficial and deep flexors. These groups are separated by the transverse intermuscular septum.

Fig. 32.23 **Muscles of the posterior compartment of the leg: Superficial flexors**
Right leg, posterior view.

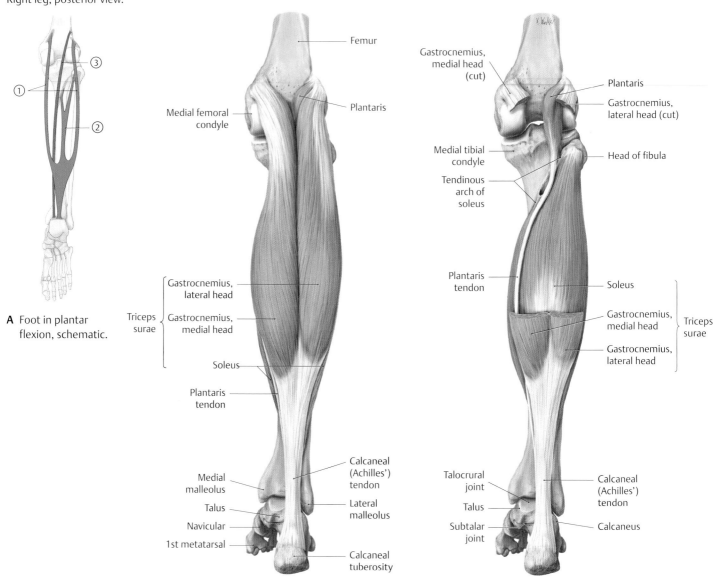

A Foot in plantar flexion, schematic.

B Superficial flexors.

C Superficial flexors with gastrocnemius removed (portions of medial and lateral heads).

Table 32.4		Superficial flexors of the posterior compartment			
Muscle		**Origin**	**Insertion**	**Innervation**	**Action**
Triceps surae	① Gastrocnemius	Femur (medial head: superior posterior part of the medial femoral condyle. lateral head: lateral surface of lateral femoral condyle)	Calcaneal tuberosity via the calcaneal (Achilles') tendon	Tibial n. (S1, S2)	• Talocrural joint: plantar flexion when knee is extended (gastrocnemius) • Knee joint: flexion (gastrocnemius) • Talocrural joint: plantar flexion (soleus)
	② Soleus	Fibula (head and neck, posterior surface), tibia (soleal line via a tendinous arch)			
③ Plantaris		Femur (lateral epicondyle, proximal to lateral head of gastrocnemius)	Calcaneal tuberosity		Negligible; may act with gastrocnemius in plantar flexion

Fig. 32.24 Posterior compartment of the leg: Deep flexors

Right leg with foot in plantar flexion, posterior view.

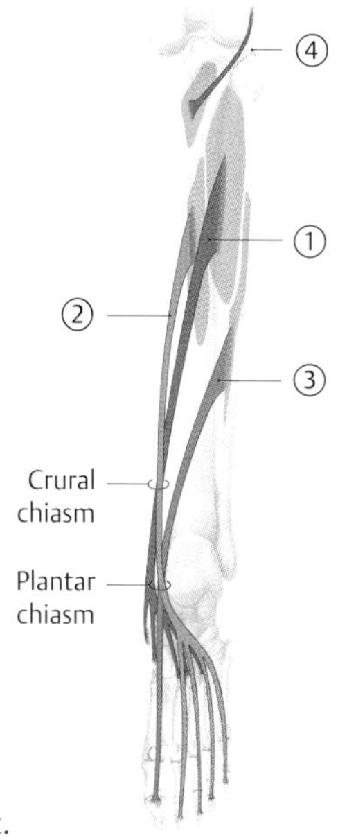

A Schematic.

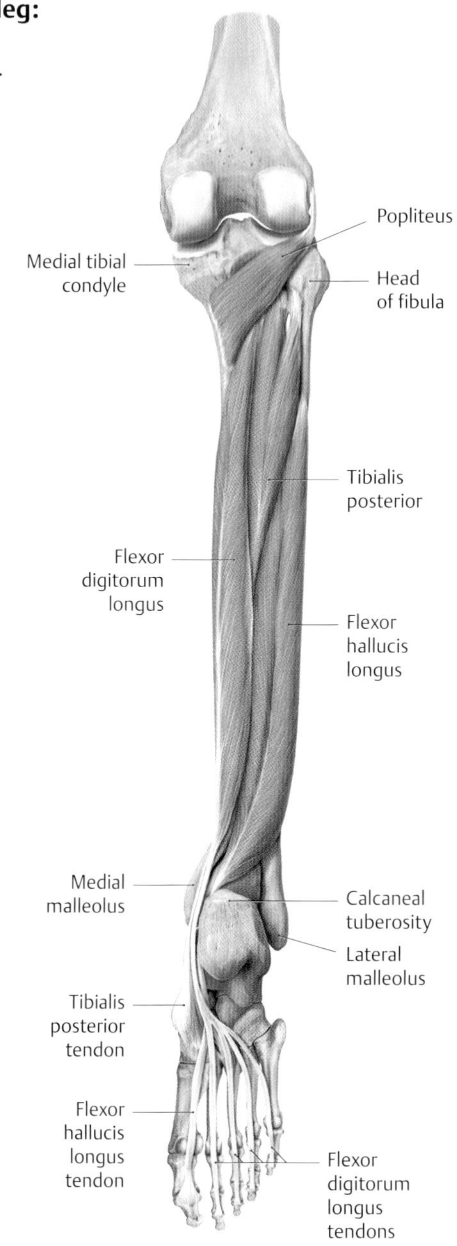

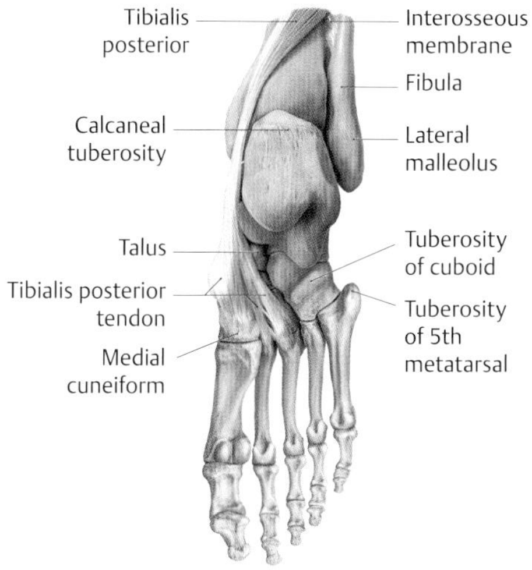

D Insertion of the tibialis posterior.

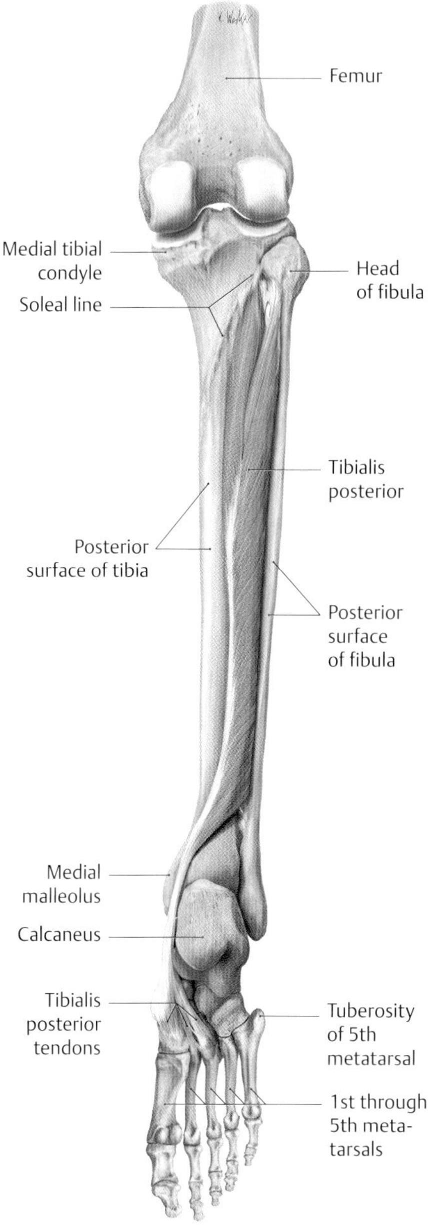

B Deep flexors.

C Tibialis posterior.

Table 32.5	Deep flexors of the posterior compartment			
Muscle	**Origin**	**Insertion**	**Innervation**	**Action**
① Tibialis posterior	Interosseous membrane, adjacent borders of tibia and fibula	Navicular tuberosity; cuneiforms (medial, intermediate, and lateral); 2nd to 4th metatarsals (bases)	Tibial n. (L4, L5)	• Talocrural joint: plantar flexion • Subtalar joint: inversion (supination) • Supports the longitudinal and transverse arches
② Flexor digitorum longus	Tibia (middle third of posterior surface)	2nd to 5th distal phalanges (bases)	Tibial n. (L5–S2)	• Talocrural joint: plantar flexion • Subtalar joint: inversion (supination) • MTP and IP joints of the 2nd to 5th toes: plantar flexion
③ Flexor hallucis longus	Fibula (distal two thirds of posterior surface), adjacent interosseous membrane	1st distal phalanx (base)		• Talocrural joint: plantar flexion • Subtalar joint: inversion (supination) • MTP and IP joints of the 1st toe: plantar flexion • Supports the medial longitudinal arch
④ Popliteus	Lateral femoral condyle, posterior horn of the lateral meniscus	Posterior tibial surface (above the origin at the soleus)	Tibial n. (L4–S1)	Knee joint: flexes and unlocks the knee by internally rotating the femur on the fixed tibia 5°

IP, interphalangeal; MTP, metatarsophalangeal.

445

Bones of the Foot

Fig. 33.1 Subdivisions of the pedal skeleton

Right foot, dorsal view. Descriptive anatomy divides the skeletal elements of the foot into the tarsus, metatarsus, and forefoot (antetarsus). Functional and clinical criteria divide the pedal skeleton into hindfoot, midfoot, and forefoot.

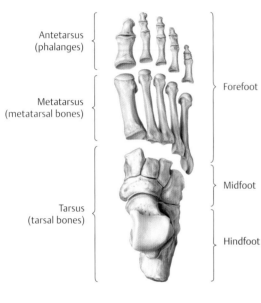

Antetarsus (phalanges)

Metatarsus (metatarsal bones)

Tarsus (tarsal bones)

Forefoot

Midfoot

Hindfoot

Fig. 33.2 Bones of the foot

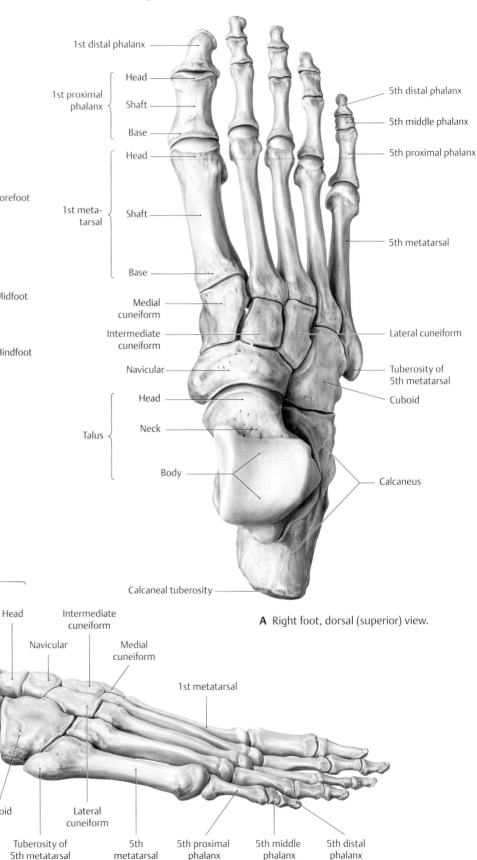

1st distal phalanx

1st proximal phalanx
- Head
- Shaft
- Base

1st metatarsal
- Head
- Shaft
- Base

Medial cuneiform

Intermediate cuneiform

Navicular

Talus
- Head
- Neck
- Body

5th distal phalanx

5th middle phalanx

5th proximal phalanx

5th metatarsal

Lateral cuneiform

Tuberosity of 5th metatarsal

Cuboid

Calcaneus

Calcaneal tuberosity

A Right foot, dorsal (superior) view.

Talus
- Neck
- Body
- Head

Posterior process

Calcaneus

Cal-caneal tuber-osity

Intermediate cuneiform

Navicular

Medial cuneiform

1st metatarsal

Lateral process of calcaneal tuberosity

Medial process of calcaneal tuberosity

Cuboid

Tuberosity of 5th metatarsal

Lateral cuneiform

5th metatarsal

5th proximal phalanx

5th middle phalanx

5th distal phalanx

B Right foot, lateral view.

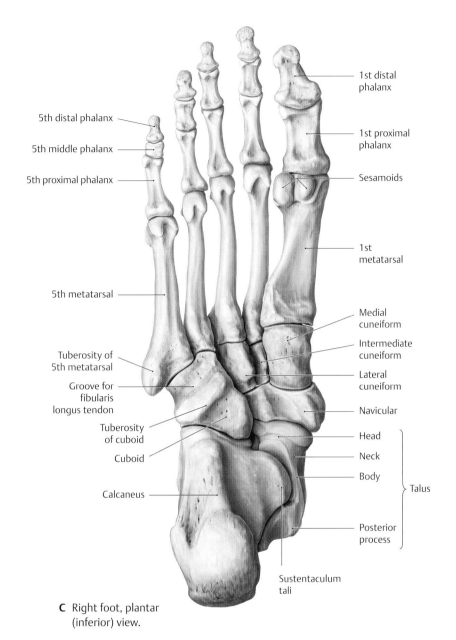

5th distal phalanx

5th middle phalanx

5th proximal phalanx

5th metatarsal

Tuberosity of
5th metatarsal

Groove for
fibularis
longus tendon

Tuberosity
of cuboid

Cuboid

Calcaneus

1st distal
phalanx

1st proximal
phalanx

Sesamoids

1st
metatarsal

Medial
cuneiform

Intermediate
cuneiform

Lateral
cuneiform

Navicular

Head
Neck
Body   } Talus

Posterior
process

Sustentaculum
tali

C Right foot, plantar
(inferior) view.

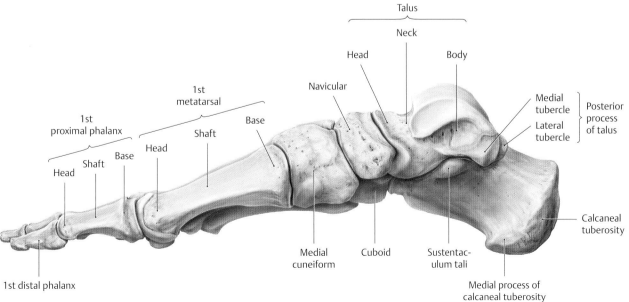

Talus

Neck

Head   Body

Navicular

1st
metatarsal

Base

Medial
tubercle

Lateral
tubercle

} Posterior
process
of talus

1st
proximal phalanx

Head

Shaft

Base

Head

Shaft

Head   Shaft   Base

1st distal phalanx

Medial
cuneiform

Cuboid

Sustentac-
ulum tali

Medial process of
calcaneal tuberosity

Calcaneal
tuberosity

D Right foot, medial view.

447

Joints of the Foot (I)

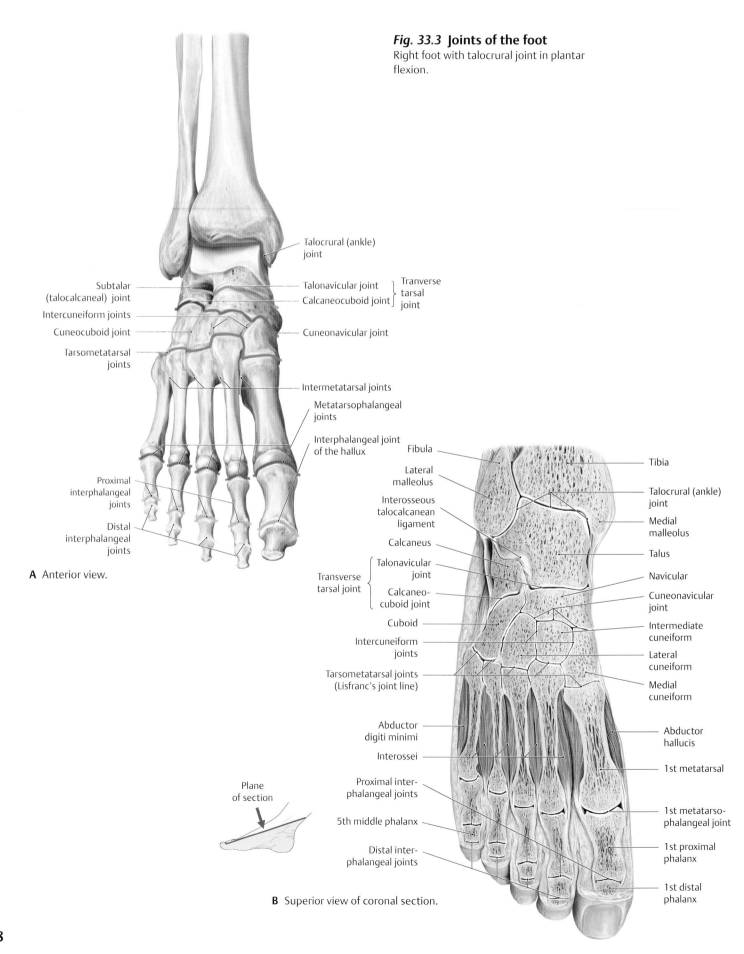

Fig. 33.3 Joints of the foot
Right foot with talocrural joint in plantar flexion.

Talocrural (ankle) joint

Subtalar (talocalcaneal) joint

Talonavicular joint
Calcaneocuboid joint
} Tranverse tarsal joint

Intercuneiform joints

Cuneocuboid joint

Cuneonavicular joint

Tarsometatarsal joints

Intermetatarsal joints

Metatarsophalangeal joints

Interphalangeal joint of the hallux

Proximal interphalangeal joints

Distal interphalangeal joints

A Anterior view.

Fibula

Lateral malleolus

Interosseous talocalcanean ligament

Calcaneus

Transverse tarsal joint {
Talonavicular joint
Calcaneo-cuboid joint
}

Cuboid

Intercuneiform joints

Tarsometatarsal joints (Lisfranc's joint line)

Abductor digiti minimi

Interossei

Proximal inter-phalangeal joints

5th middle phalanx

Distal inter-phalangeal joints

Tibia

Talocrural (ankle) joint

Medial malleolus

Talus

Navicular

Cuneonavicular joint

Intermediate cuneiform

Lateral cuneiform

Medial cuneiform

Abductor hallucis

1st metatarsal

1st metatarso-phalangeal joint

1st proximal phalanx

1st distal phalanx

Plane of section

B Superior view of coronal section.

Fig. 33.4 Proximal articular surfaces

Right foot, proximal view.

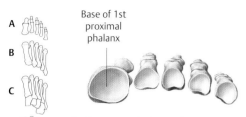

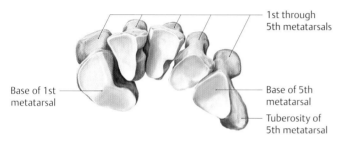

Base of 1st
proximal
phalanx

A Metatarsophalangeal joints.

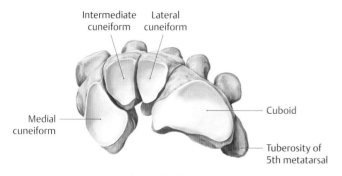

1st through
5th metatarsals

Base of 1st
metatarsal

Base of 5th
metatarsal

Tuberosity of
5th metatarsal

B Tarsometatarsal joints.

Intermediate
cuneiform · Lateral
cuneiform

Medial
cuneiform

Cuboid

Tuberosity of
5th metatarsal

C Cuneonavicular and calcaneocuboid joints.

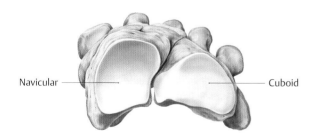

Navicular

Cuboid

D Talonavicular and calcaneocuboid joints.

Fig. 33.5 Distal articular surfaces

Right foot, distal view.

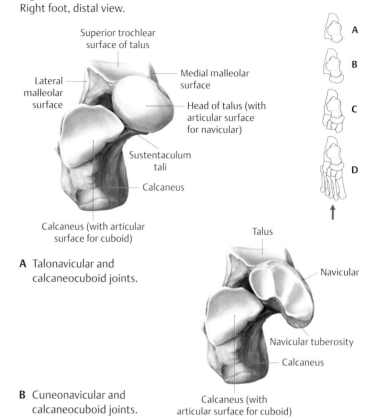

Superior trochlear
surface of talus

Lateral
malleolar
surface

Medial malleolar
surface

Head of talus (with
articular surface
for navicular)

Sustentaculum
tali

Calcaneus

Calcaneus (with articular
surface for cuboid)

A Talonavicular and
calcaneocuboid joints.

Talus

Navicular

Navicular tuberosity

Calcaneus

Calcaneus (with
articular surface for cuboid)

B Cuneonavicular and
calcaneocuboid joints.

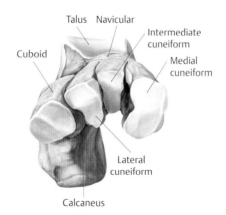

Talus   Navicular

Cuboid

Intermediate
cuneiform

Medial
cuneiform

Lateral
cuneiform

Calcaneus

C Tarsometatarsal joints.

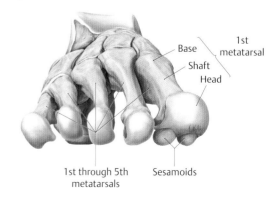

1st
metatarsal

Base

Shaft

Head

1st through 5th
metatarsals

Sesamoids

D Metatarsophalangeal joints.

Joints of the Foot (II)

Fig. 33.6 Talocrural and subtalar joints
Right foot. The talocrural (ankle) joint is formed by the distal ends of the tibia and fibula (ankle mortise) articulating with the trochlea of the talus. The subtalar joint consists of an anterior and a posterior compartment (the talocalcaneal and talocalcaneonavicular joints, respectively) divided by the interosseous talocalcaneal ligament (see **p. 452**).

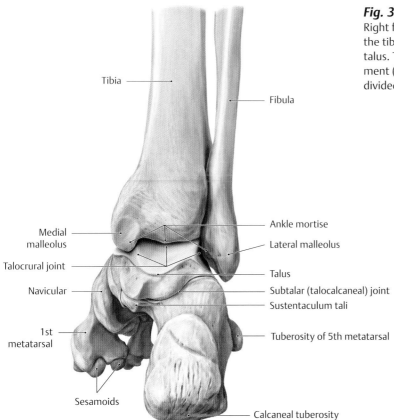

Tibia
Fibula
Medial malleolus
Ankle mortise
Lateral malleolus
Talocrural joint
Talus
Navicular
Subtalar (talocalcaneal) joint
Sustentaculum tali
1st metatarsal
Tuberosity of 5th metatarsal
Sesamoids
Calcaneal tuberosity

A Posterior view with foot in neutral (0-degree) position.

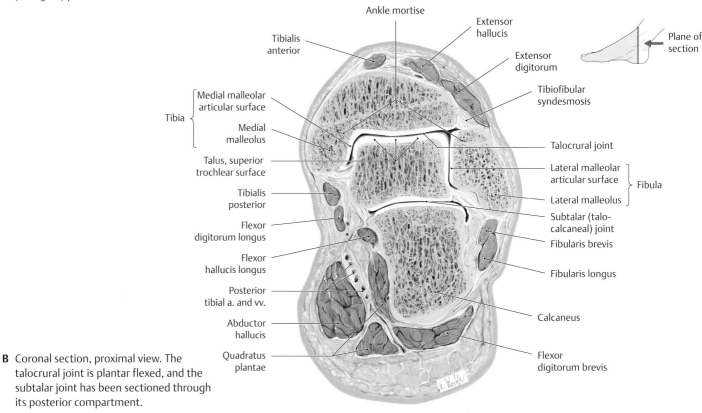

Ankle mortise
Extensor hallucis
Tibialis anterior
Extensor digitorum
Plane of section
Tibia — Medial malleolar articular surface
Tibiofibular syndesmosis
Medial malleolus
Talocrural joint
Talus, superior trochlear surface
Lateral malleolar articular surface — Fibula
Tibialis posterior
Lateral malleolus
Flexor digitorum longus
Subtalar (talocalcaneal) joint
Flexor hallucis longus
Fibularis brevis
Posterior tibial a. and vv.
Fibularis longus
Abductor hallucis
Calcaneus
Quadratus plantae
Flexor digitorum brevis

B Coronal section, proximal view. The talocrural joint is plantar flexed, and the subtalar joint has been sectioned through its posterior compartment.

Fig. 33.7 Talocrural and subtalar joints: Sagittal section
Right foot, medial view.

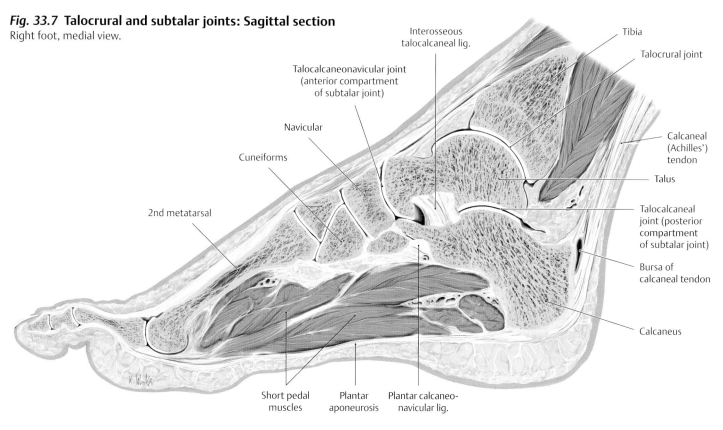

Interosseous talocalcaneal lig.
Talocalcaneonavicular joint (anterior compartment of subtalar joint)
Navicular
Cuneiforms
2nd metatarsal
Tibia
Talocrural joint
Calcaneal (Achilles') tendon
Talus
Talocalcaneal joint (posterior compartment of subtalar joint)
Bursa of calcaneal tendon
Calcaneus
Short pedal muscles
Plantar aponeurosis
Plantar calcaneo-navicular lig.

Fig. 33.8 Talocrural joint
Right foot.

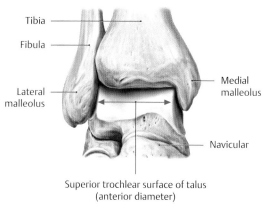

Tibia
Fibula
Lateral malleolus
Medial malleolus
Navicular
Superior trochlear surface of talus (anterior diameter)

A Anterior view.

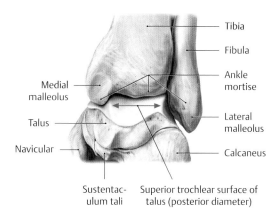

Tibia
Fibula
Ankle mortise
Medial malleolus
Talus
Navicular
Lateral malleolus
Calcaneus
Sustentaculum tali
Superior trochlear surface of talus (posterior diameter)

B Posterior view.

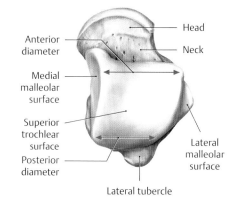

Head
Anterior diameter
Neck
Medial malleolar surface
Superior trochlear surface
Posterior diameter
Lateral malleolar surface
Lateral tubercle

C Proximal (superior) view of talus.

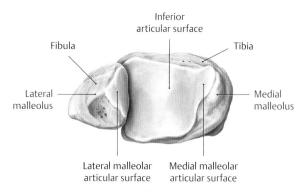

Inferior articular surface
Fibula
Tibia
Lateral malleolus
Medial malleolus
Lateral malleolar articular surface
Medial malleolar articular surface

D Distal (inferior) view of ankle mortise.

Joints of the Foot (III)

***Fig. 33.9* Subtalar joint and ligaments**

Right foot with opened subtalar joint. The subtalar joint consists of two distinct articulations separated by the interosseous talocalcaneal liga-

ment: the posterior compartment (talocalcaneal joint) and the anterior compartment (talocalcaneonavicular joint).

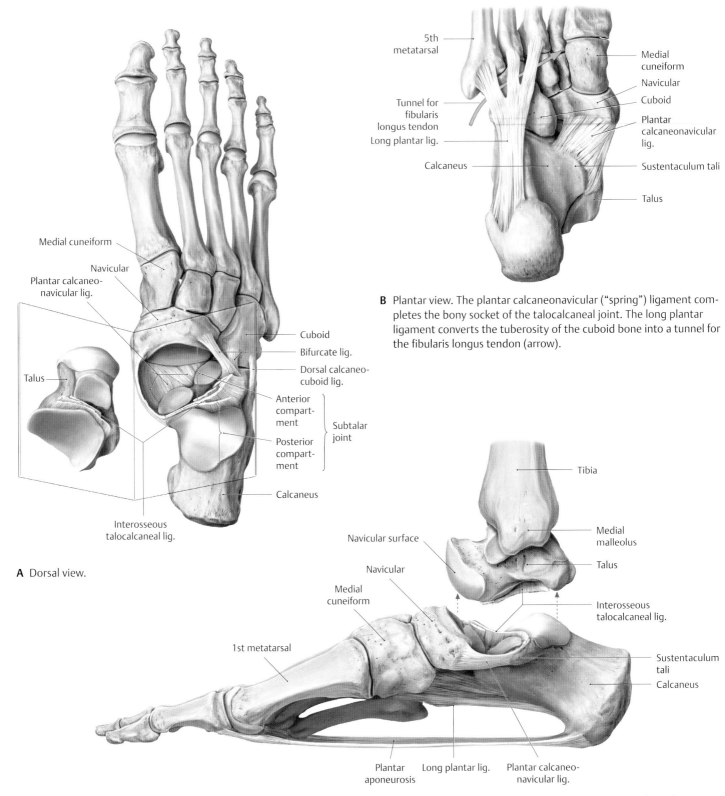

B Plantar view. The plantar calcaneonavicular ("spring") ligament completes the bony socket of the talocalcaneal joint. The long plantar ligament converts the tuberosity of the cuboid bone into a tunnel for the fibularis longus tendon (arrow).

A Dorsal view.

C Medial view. The interosseous talocalcaneal ligament has been divided and the talus displaced upward. Note the course of the plantar calca-

neonavicular ligament, which functions with the long plantar ligament and plantar aponeurosis to support the longitudinal arch of the foot.

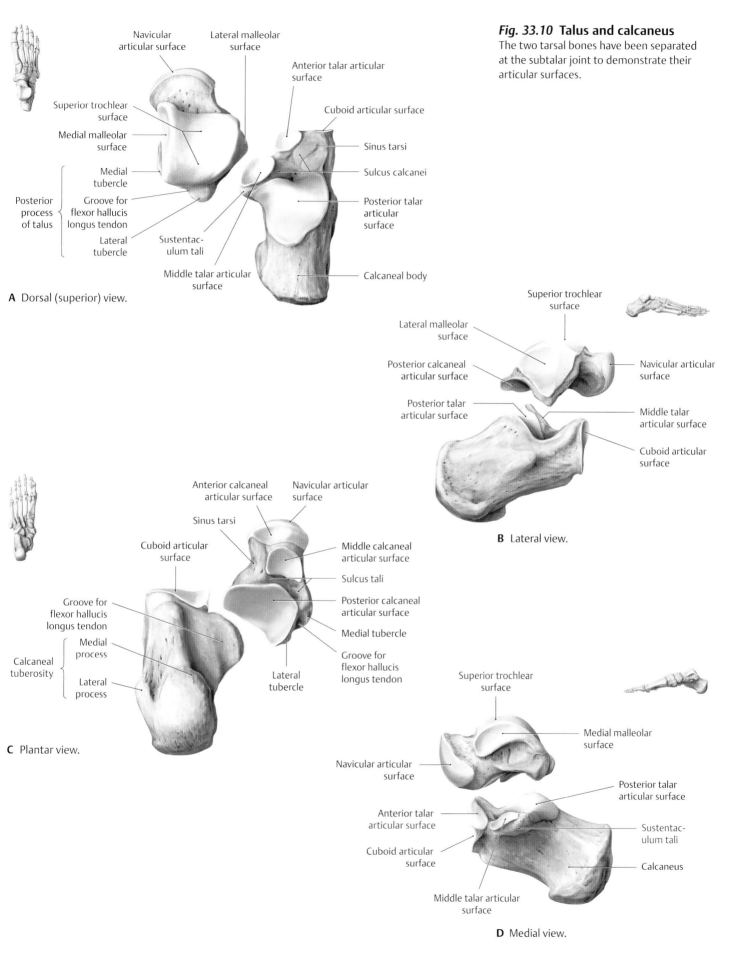

Fig. 33.10 Talus and calcaneus
The two tarsal bones have been separated at the subtalar joint to demonstrate their articular surfaces.

A Dorsal (superior) view.

Navicular articular surface

Lateral malleolar surface

Superior trochlear surface

Medial malleolar surface

Anterior talar articular surface

Cuboid articular surface

Sinus tarsi

Sulcus calcanei

Posterior talar articular surface

Posterior process of talus
- Medial tubercle
- Groove for flexor hallucis longus tendon
- Lateral tubercle

Sustentaculum tali

Middle talar articular surface

Calcaneal body

B Lateral view.

Superior trochlear surface

Lateral malleolar surface

Posterior calcaneal articular surface

Posterior talar articular surface

Navicular articular surface

Middle talar articular surface

Cuboid articular surface

C Plantar view.

Anterior calcaneal articular surface

Navicular articular surface

Sinus tarsi

Cuboid articular surface

Groove for flexor hallucis longus tendon

Middle calcaneal articular surface

Sulcus tali

Posterior calcaneal articular surface

Medial tubercle

Groove for flexor hallucis longus tendon

Calcaneal tuberosity
- Medial process
- Lateral process

Lateral tubercle

D Medial view.

Superior trochlear surface

Medial malleolar surface

Navicular articular surface

Posterior talar articular surface

Sustentaculum tali

Anterior talar articular surface

Cuboid articular surface

Calcaneus

Middle talar articular surface

Ligaments of the Ankle & Foot

The ligaments of the foot are classified as belonging to the talocrural joint, subtalar joint, metatarsus, forefoot, or sole of the foot. The medial and lateral collateral ligaments, along with the syndesmotic ligaments, are of major importance in the stabilization of the subtalar joint.

Fig. 33.11 Ligaments of the ankle and foot
Right foot. See **p. 452** for inferior view.

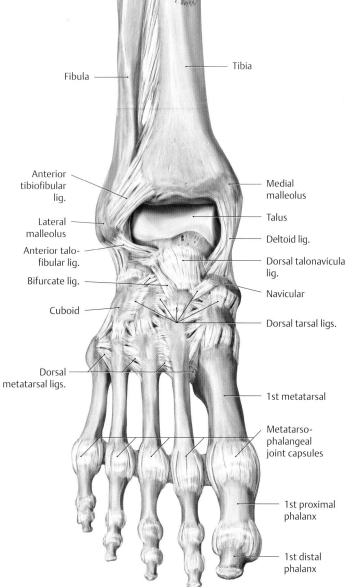

Table 33.1	Ligaments of the talocrural joint		
Lateral ligs.*	Anterior talofibular lig.		
	Posterior talofibular lig.		
	Calcaneofibular lig.		
Medial ligs.*	Deltoid lig.	Anterior tibiotalar part	
		Posterior tibiotalar part	
		Tibionavicular part	
		Tibiocalcaneal part	
Syndesmotic ligs. of the ankle mortise	Anterior tibiofibular lig.		
	Posterior tibiofibular lig.		

*The medial and lateral ligs. are also known as the medial and lateral collateral ligs.

Labels on image 1:
- Fibula
- Tibia
- Anterior tibiofibular lig.
- Medial malleolus
- Lateral malleolus
- Talus
- Anterior talo-fibular lig.
- Deltoid lig.
- Bifurcate lig.
- Dorsal talonavicular lig.
- Cuboid
- Navicular
- Dorsal tarsal ligs.
- Dorsal metatarsal ligs.
- 1st metatarsal
- Metatarsophalangeal joint capsules
- 1st proximal phalanx
- 1st distal phalanx

A Anterior view with talocrural joint in plantar flexion.

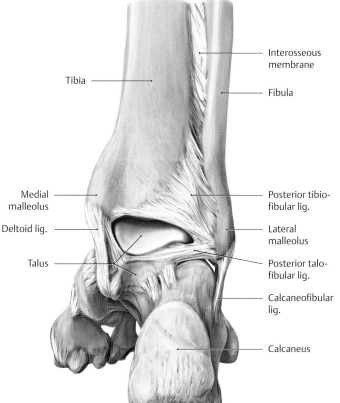

Labels on image 3:
- Interosseous membrane
- Tibia
- Fibula
- Medial malleolus
- Posterior tibiofibular lig.
- Deltoid lig.
- Lateral malleolus
- Talus
- Posterior talofibular lig.
- Calcaneofibular lig.
- Calcaneus

B Posterior view in plantigrade foot position.

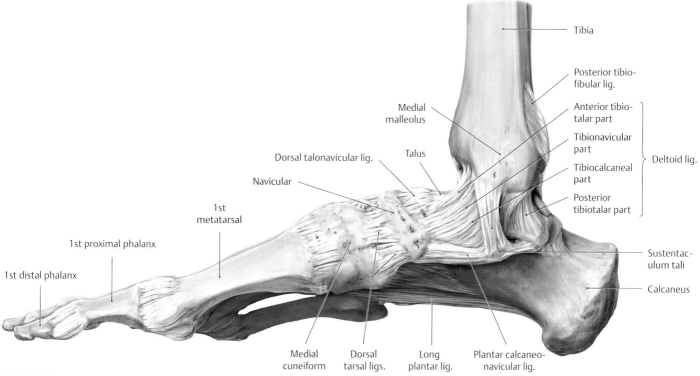

Tibia

Posterior tibio-fibular lig.

Medial malleolus

Anterior tibio-talar part

Tibionavicular part

Dorsal talonavicular lig.

Talus

Tibiocalcaneal part

Navicular

Posterior tibiotalar part

Deltoid lig.

1st metatarsal

1st proximal phalanx

Sustentaculum tali

1st distal phalanx

Calcaneus

Medial cuneiform

Dorsal tarsal ligs.

Long plantar lig.

Plantar calcaneo-navicular lig.

C Medial view.

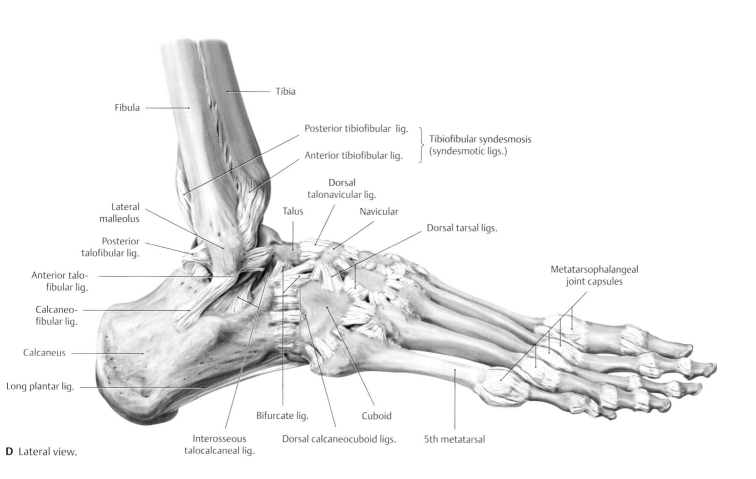

Tibia

Fibula

Posterior tibiofibular lig.

Anterior tibiofibular lig.

Tibiofibular syndesmosis (syndesmotic ligs.)

Dorsal talonavicular lig.

Lateral malleolus

Talus

Navicular

Posterior talofibular lig.

Dorsal tarsal ligs.

Anterior talo-fibular lig.

Metatarsophalangeal joint capsules

Calcaneo-fibular lig.

Calcaneus

Long plantar lig.

Bifurcate lig.

Cuboid

Interosseous talocalcaneal lig.

Dorsal calcaneocuboid ligs.

5th metatarsal

D Lateral view.

Plantar Vault & Arches of the Foot

Fig. 33.12 Plantar vault

Right foot. The forces of the foot are distributed among two lateral (fibular) and three medial (tibial) rays. The arrangement of these rays creates a longitudinal and a transverse arch in the sole of the foot, helping the foot absorb vertical loads.

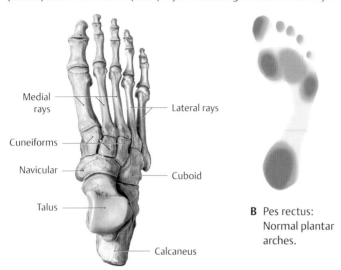

A Plantar vault, superior view. Lateral rays in green, medial rays in red.

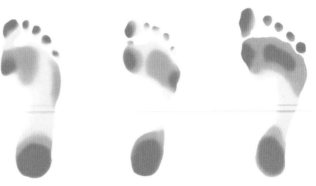

B Pes rectus: Normal plantar arches.

C Pes planus: Loss of longitudinal arch (flat foot).

D Pes cavus: Increased height of longitudinal arch.

E Pes transverso-planus: Loss of transverse arch (splayfoot).

Fig. 33.13 Stabilizers of the transverse arch

Right foot. The transverse pedal arch is supported by both active and passive stabilizing structures (muscles and ligaments, respectively).

Note: The arch of the forefoot has only passive stabilizers, whereas the arches of the metatarsus and tarsus have only active stabilizers.

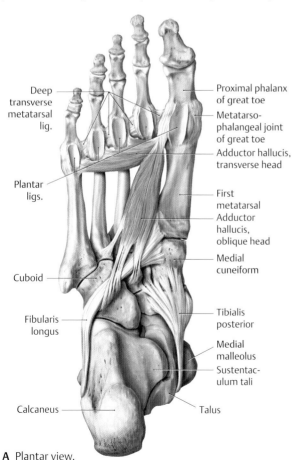

A Plantar view.

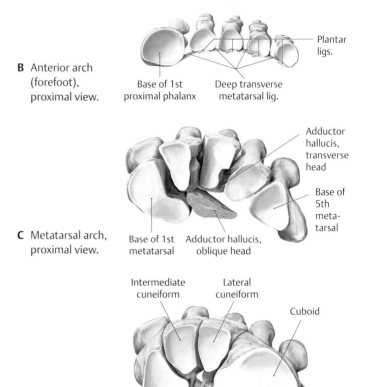

B Anterior arch (forefoot), proximal view.

C Metatarsal arch, proximal view.

D Tarsal region, proximal view.

Fig. 33.14 Stabilizers of the longitudinal arch

Right foot, medial view.

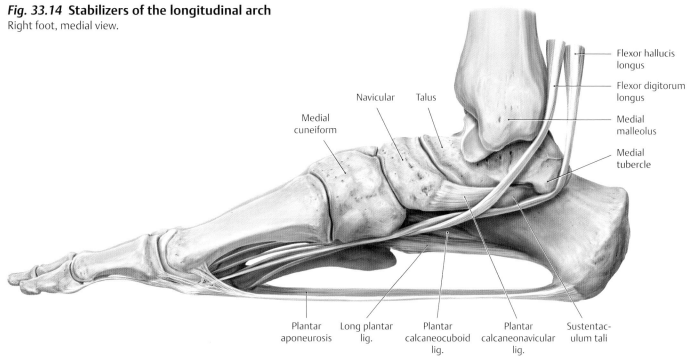

Flexor hallucis longus

Flexor digitorum longus

Medial malleolus

Medial tubercle

Navicular Talus

Medial cuneiform

Plantar aponeurosis Long plantar lig. Plantar calcaneocuboid lig. Plantar calcaneonavicular lig. Sustentaculum tali

A Passive stabilizers of the longitudinal arch. The main passive stabilizers of the longitudinal arch are the plantar aponeurosis (strongest component), the long plantar ligament, and the plantar calcaneonavicular ligament (weakest component).

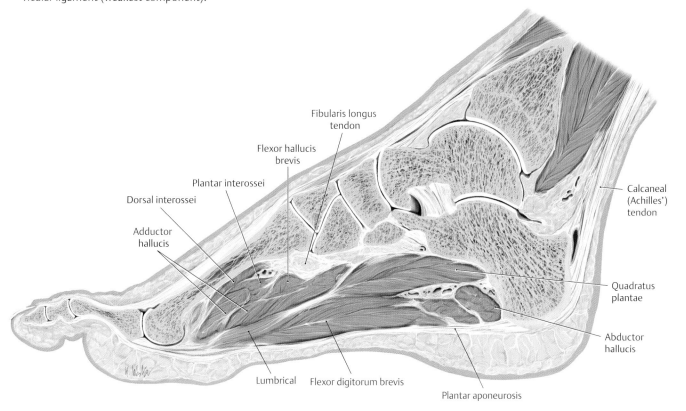

Fibularis longus tendon

Flexor hallucis brevis

Plantar interossei

Dorsal interossei

Adductor hallucis

Calcaneal (Achilles') tendon

Quadratus plantae

Abductor hallucis

Lumbrical Flexor digitorum brevis Plantar aponeurosis

B Active stabilizers of the longitudinal arch. Sagittal section at the level of the second ray. The major active stabilizers of the foot are the abductor hallucis, flexor hallucis brevis, flexor digitorum brevis, quadratus plantae, and abductor digiti minimi.

Muscles of the Sole of the Foot

Fig. 33.15 Plantar aponeurosis

Right foot, plantar view. The plantar aponeurosis is a tough aponeurotic sheet, thickest at the center, that blends with the dorsal fascia (not shown) at the borders of the foot.

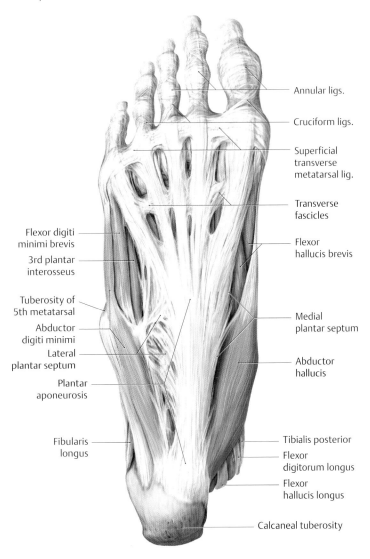

Fig. 33.16 Intrinsic muscles of the sole of the foot

Right foot, plantar view.

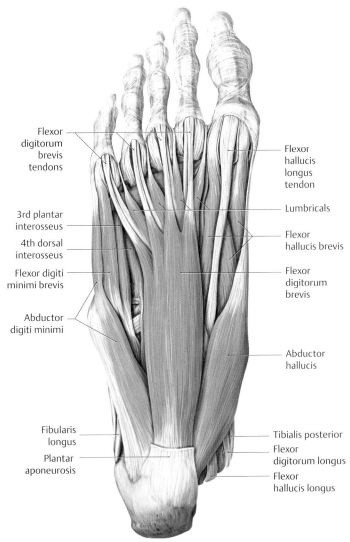

A Superficial (first) layer. *Removed:* Plantar aponeurosis, including the superficial transverse metacarpal ligament.

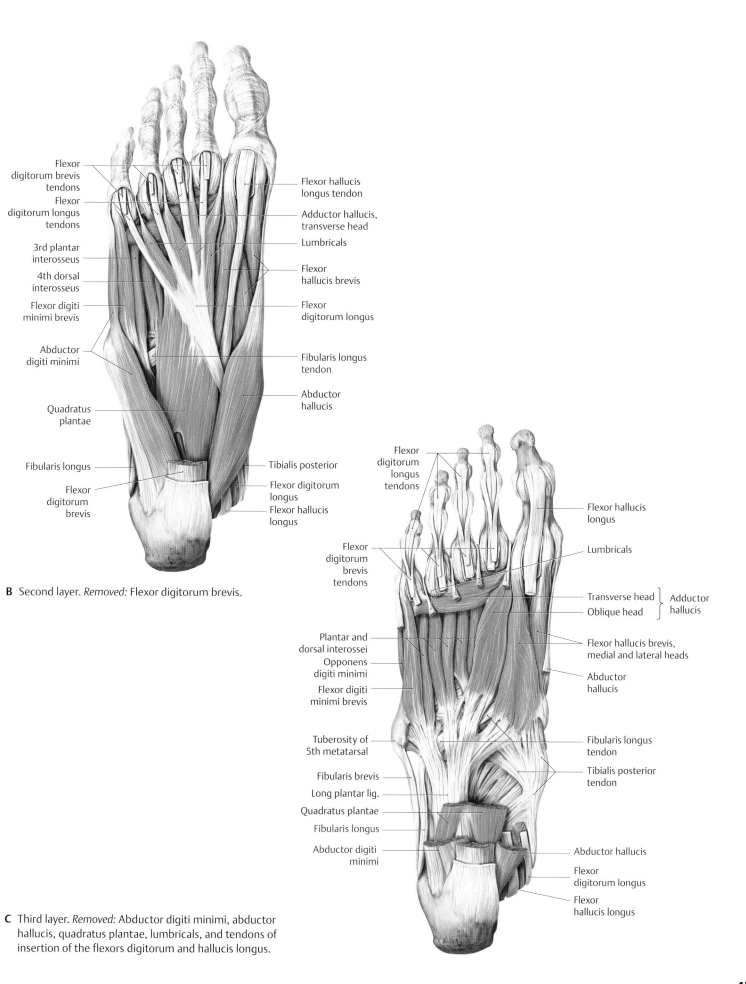

Flexor digitorum brevis tendons

Flexor digitorum longus tendons

3rd plantar interosseus

4th dorsal interosseus

Flexor digiti minimi brevis

Abductor digiti minimi

Quadratus plantae

Fibularis longus

Flexor digitorum brevis

Flexor hallucis longus tendon

Adductor hallucis, transverse head

Lumbricals

Flexor hallucis brevis

Flexor digitorum longus

Fibularis longus tendon

Abductor hallucis

Tibialis posterior

Flexor digitorum longus

Flexor hallucis longus

B Second layer. *Removed:* Flexor digitorum brevis.

Flexor digitorum longus tendons

Flexor digitorum brevis tendons

Plantar and dorsal interossei

Opponens digiti minimi

Flexor digiti minimi brevis

Tuberosity of 5th metatarsal

Fibularis brevis

Long plantar lig.

Quadratus plantae

Fibularis longus

Abductor digiti minimi

Flexor hallucis longus

Lumbricals

Transverse head — Adductor
Oblique head — hallucis

Flexor hallucis brevis, medial and lateral heads

Abductor hallucis

Fibularis longus tendon

Tibialis posterior tendon

Abductor hallucis

Flexor digitorum longus

Flexor hallucis longus

C Third layer. *Removed:* Abductor digiti minimi, abductor hallucis, quadratus plantae, lumbricals, and tendons of insertion of the flexors digitorum and hallucis longus.

Muscles & Tendon Sheaths of the Foot

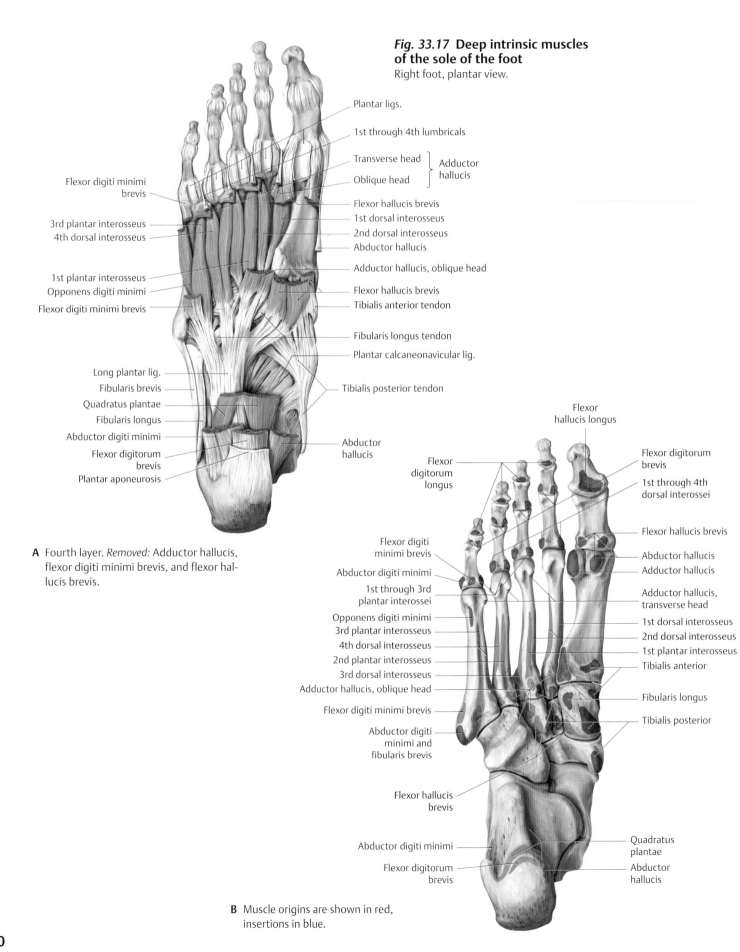

***Fig. 33.17* Deep intrinsic muscles of the sole of the foot**
Right foot, plantar view.

Plantar ligs.

1st through 4th lumbricals

Transverse head ⎤
Oblique head ⎦ Adductor hallucis

Flexor digiti minimi brevis

Flexor hallucis brevis

3rd plantar interosseus
4th dorsal interosseus

1st dorsal interosseus
2nd dorsal interosseus
Abductor hallucis
Adductor hallucis, oblique head

1st plantar interosseus
Opponens digiti minimi
Flexor digiti minimi brevis

Flexor hallucis brevis
Tibialis anterior tendon

Fibularis longus tendon
Plantar calcaneonavicular lig.

Long plantar lig.
Fibularis brevis
Quadratus plantae
Fibularis longus
Abductor digiti minimi
Flexor digitorum brevis
Plantar aponeurosis

Tibialis posterior tendon

Abductor hallucis

A Fourth layer. *Removed:* Adductor hallucis, flexor digiti minimi brevis, and flexor hallucis brevis.

Flexor hallucis longus

Flexor digitorum longus

Flexor digitorum brevis
1st through 4th dorsal interossei

Flexor digiti minimi brevis

Flexor hallucis brevis
Abductor hallucis
Adductor hallucis

Abductor digiti minimi
1st through 3rd plantar interossei

Adductor hallucis, transverse head

Opponens digiti minimi
3rd plantar interosseus
4th dorsal interosseus
2nd plantar interosseus
3rd dorsal interosseus
Adductor hallucis, oblique head
Flexor digiti minimi brevis

1st dorsal interosseus
2nd dorsal interosseus
1st plantar interosseus
Tibialis anterior

Fibularis longus

Tibialis posterior

Abductor digiti minimi and fibularis brevis

Flexor hallucis brevis

Abductor digiti minimi
Flexor digitorum brevis

Quadratus plantae
Abductor hallucis

B Muscle origins are shown in red, insertions in blue.

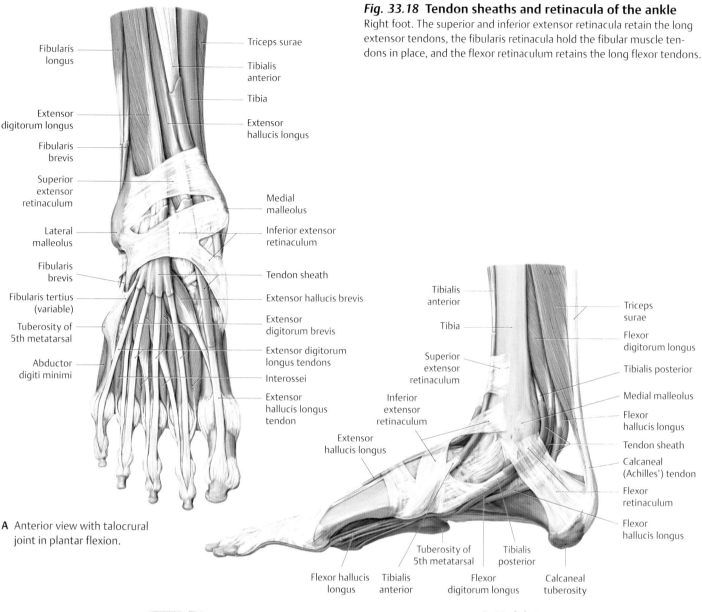

Fibularis longus

Triceps surae

Tibialis anterior

Tibia

Extensor digitorum longus

Extensor hallucis longus

Fibularis brevis

Superior extensor retinaculum

Medial malleolus

Lateral malleolus

Inferior extensor retinaculum

Fibularis brevis

Tendon sheath

Fibularis tertius (variable)

Extensor hallucis brevis

Tuberosity of 5th metatarsal

Extensor digitorum brevis

Abductor digiti minimi

Extensor digitorum longus tendons

Interossei

Extensor hallucis longus tendon

Fig. 33.18 Tendon sheaths and retinacula of the ankle
Right foot. The superior and inferior extensor retinacula retain the long extensor tendons, the fibularis retinacula hold the fibular muscle tendons in place, and the flexor retinaculum retains the long flexor tendons.

Tibialis anterior

Tibia

Triceps surae

Flexor digitorum longus

Tibialis posterior

Superior extensor retinaculum

Medial malleolus

Inferior extensor retinaculum

Flexor hallucis longus

Extensor hallucis longus

Tendon sheath

Calcaneal (Achilles') tendon

Flexor retinaculum

Tuberosity of 5th metatarsal

Tibialis posterior

Flexor hallucis longus

Flexor hallucis longus

Tibialis anterior

Flexor digitorum longus

Calcaneal tuberosity

A Anterior view with talocrural joint in plantar flexion.

B Medial view.

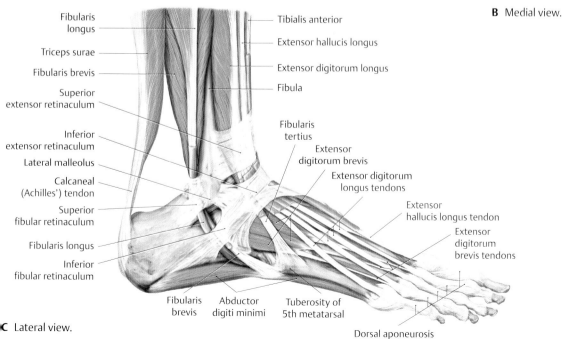

Fibularis longus

Tibialis anterior

Triceps surae

Extensor hallucis longus

Fibularis brevis

Extensor digitorum longus

Superior extensor retinaculum

Fibula

Inferior extensor retinaculum

Fibularis tertius

Lateral malleolus

Extensor digitorum brevis

Calcaneal (Achilles') tendon

Extensor digitorum longus tendons

Superior fibular retinaculum

Extensor hallucis longus tendon

Fibularis longus

Extensor digitorum brevis tendons

Inferior fibular retinaculum

Fibularis brevis

Abductor digiti minimi

Tuberosity of 5th metatarsal

Dorsal aponeurosis

C Lateral view.

Muscle Facts (I)

The dorsal surface (dorsum) of the foot contains only two muscles, the extensor digitorum brevis and the extensor hallucis brevis. The sole of the foot, however, is composed of four complex layers that maintain the arches of the foot.

Fig. 33.19 Intrinsic muscles of the dorsum of the foot
Right foot, dorsal view.

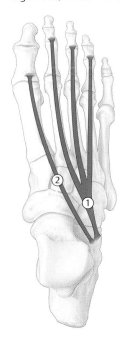

A Schematic.

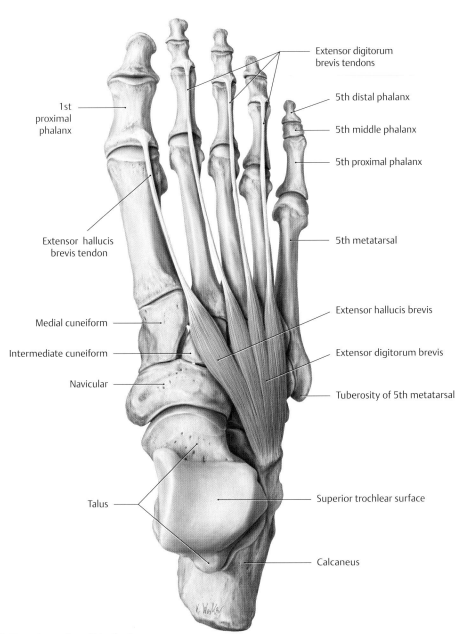

B Dorsal muscles of the foot.

Table 33.2	Intrinsic muscles of the dorsum of the foot				
Muscle	**Origin**	**Insertion**		**Innervation**	**Action**
① Extensor digitorum brevis	Calcaneus (dorsal surface)	2nd to 4th toes (at dorsal aponeuroses and bases of the middle phalanges)		Deep fibular n. (L5, S1)	Extension of the MTP and PIP joints of the 2nd to 4th toes
② Extensor hallucis brevis		1st toe (at dorsal aponeurosis and proximal phalanx)			Extension of the MTP joints of the 1st toe
MTP, metatarsophalangeal; PIP, proximal interphalangeal.					

Fig. 33.20 Superficial intrinsic muscles of the sole of the foot

Right foot, plantar view.

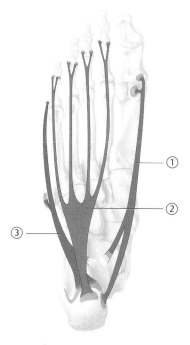

A First layer, schematic.

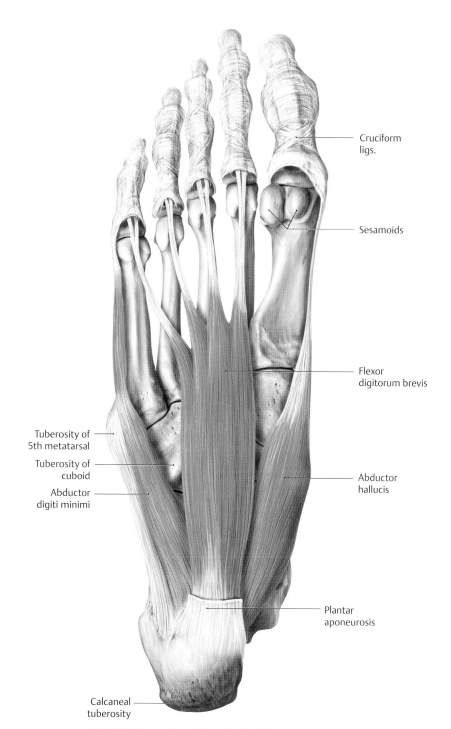

B Intrinsic muscles of the sole, first layer.

Table 33.3	Superficial intrinsic muscles of the sole of the foot			
Muscle	**Origin**	**Insertion**	**Innervation**	**Action**
① Abductor hallucis	Calcaneal tuberosity (medial process); flexor retinaculum, plantar aponeurosis	1st toe (base of proximal phalanx via the medial sesamoid)	Medial plantar n. (S1, S2)	• 1st MTP joint: flexion and abduction of the 1st toe • Supports the longitudinal arch
② Flexor digitorum brevis	Calcaneal tuberosity (medial tubercle), plantar aponeurosis	2nd to 5th toes (sides of middle phalanges)		• Flexes the MTP and PIP joints of the 2nd to 5th toes • Supports the longitudinal arch
③ Abductor digiti minimi		5th toe (base of proximal phalanx), 5th metatarsal (at tuberosity)	Lateral plantar n. (S1–S3)	• Flexes the MTP joint of the 5th toe • Abducts the 5th toe • Supports the longitudinal arch

MTP, metatarsophalangeal; PIP, proximal interphalangeal.

Muscle Facts (II)

Fig. 33.21 Deep intrinsic muscles of the sole of the foot

Right foot, plantar view, schematics.

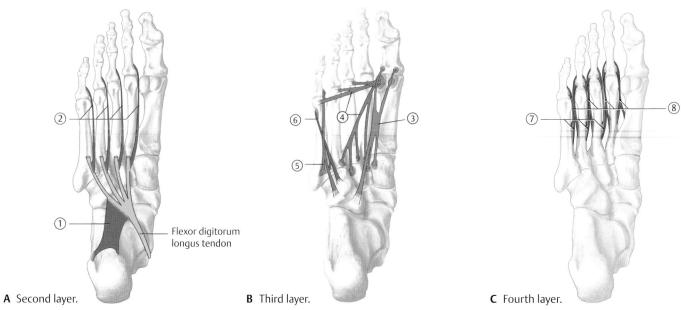

Flexor digitorum longus tendon

A Second layer.　　　**B** Third layer.　　　**C** Fourth layer.

Table 33.4	Deep intrinsic muscles of the sole of the foot			
Muscle	**Origin**	**Insertion**	**Innervation**	**Action**
① Quadratus plantae	Calcaneal tuberosity (medial and plantar borders on plantar side)	Flexor digitorum longus tendon (lateral border)	Lateral plantar n. (S1–S3)	Redirects and augments the pull of flexor digitorum longus
② Lumbricals (four muscles)	Flexor digitorum longus tendons (medial borders)	2nd to 5th toes (at dorsal aponeuroses)	1st lumbrical: medial plantar n. (S2, S3)	• Flexes the MTP joints of 2nd to 5th toes • Extension of IP joints of 2nd to 5th toes • Adducts 2nd to 5th toes toward the big toe
			2nd to 4th lumbrical: lateral plantar n. (S2, S3)	
③ Flexor hallucis brevis	Cuboid, lateral cuneiforms, and plantar calcaneocuboid lig.	1st toe (at base of proximal phalanx via medial and lateral sesamoids)	Medial head: medial plantar n. (S1, S2)	• Flexes the first MTP joint • Supports the longitudinal arch
			Lateral head: lateral plantar n. (S1, S2)	
④ Adductor hallucis	Oblique head: 2nd to 4th metatarsals (at bases) cuboid and lateral cuneiforms	1st proximal phalanx (at base, by a common tendon via the lateral sesamoid)	Lateral plantar n., deep branch (S2, S3)	• Flexes the first MTP joint • Adducts big toe • Transverse head: supports transverse arch • Oblique head: supports longitudinal arch
	Transverse head: MTP joints of 3rd to 5th toes, deep transverse metatarsal lig.			
⑤ Flexor digiti minimi brevis	5th metatarsal (base), long plantar lig.	5th toe (base of proximal phalanx)	Lateral plantar n., superficial branch (S2, S3)	Flexes the MTP joint of the little toe
⑥ Opponens digiti minimi*	Long plantar lig.; fibularis longus (at plantar tendon sheath)	5th metatarsal		Pulls 5th metatarsal in plantar and medial direction
⑦ Plantar interossei (three muscles)	3rd to 5th metatarsals (medial border)	3rd to 5th toes (medial base of proximal phalanx)	Lateral plantar n. (S2, S3)	• Flexes the MTP joints of 3rd to 5th toes • Extension of IP joints of 3rd to 5th toes • Adducts 3rd to 5th toes toward 2nd toe
⑧ Dorsal interossei (four muscles)	1st to 5th metatarsals (by two heads on opposing sides)	1st interosseus: 2nd proximal phalanx (medial base)		• Flexes the MTP joints of 2nd to 4th toes • Extension of IP joints of 2nd to 4th toes • Abducts 3rd and 4th toes from 2nd toe
		2nd to 4th interossei: 2nd to 4th proximal phalanges (lateral base), 2nd to 4th toes (at dorsal aponeuroses)		

IP, interphalangeal; MTP, metatarsophalangeal. *May be absent.

Fig. 33.22 Deep intrinsic muscles of the sole of the foot
Right foot, plantar view.

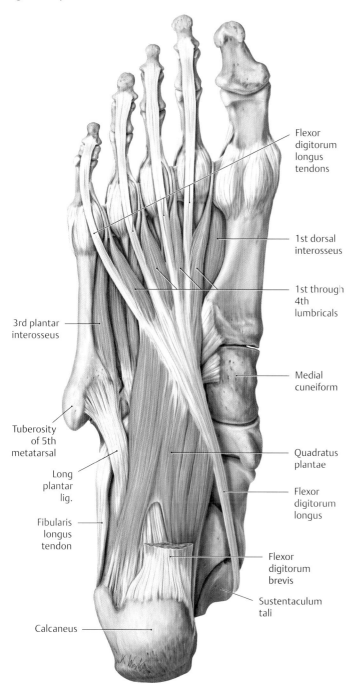

Flexor digitorum longus tendons

1st dorsal interosseus

1st through 4th lumbricals

3rd plantar interosseus

Medial cuneiform

Tuberosity of 5th metatarsal

Quadratus plantae

Long plantar lig.

Flexor digitorum longus

Fibularis longus tendon

Flexor digitorum brevis

Sustentaculum tali

Calcaneus

A Intrinsic muscles of the sole, second and fourth layers.

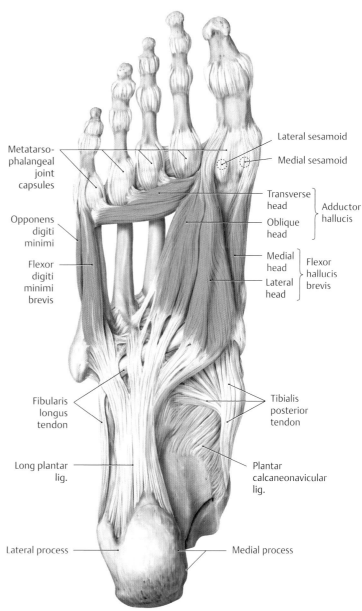

Lateral sesamoid

Medial sesamoid

Metatarso-phalangeal joint capsules

Transverse head | Adductor hallucis
Oblique head

Opponens digiti minimi

Medial head | Flexor hallucis brevis
Lateral head

Flexor digiti minimi brevis

Fibularis longus tendon

Tibialis posterior tendon

Long plantar lig.

Plantar calcaneonavicular lig.

Lateral process

Medial process

B Intrinsic muscles of the sole, third layer.

Arteries of the Lower Limb

Fig. 34.1 Arteries of the lower limb and the sole of the foot

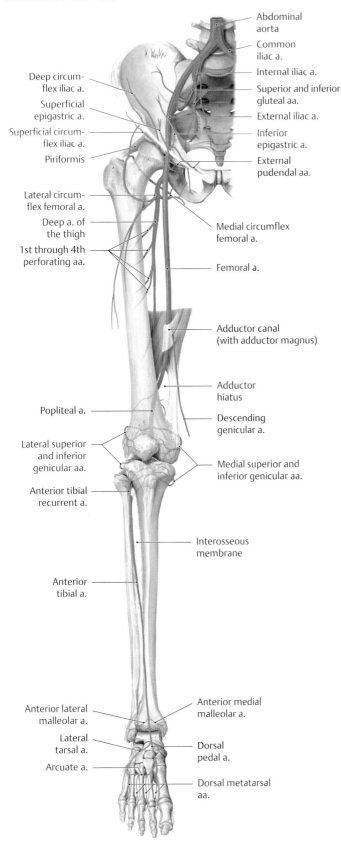

Abdominal aorta
Common iliac a.
Internal iliac a.
Superior and inferior gluteal aa.
External iliac a.
Inferior epigastric a.
External pudendal aa.
Medial circumflex femoral a.
Femoral a.
Adductor canal (with adductor magnus)
Adductor hiatus
Descending genicular a.
Medial superior and inferior genicular aa.

Deep circumflex iliac a.
Superficial epigastric a.
Superficial circumflex iliac a.
Piriformis
Lateral circumflex femoral a.
Deep a. of the thigh
1st through 4th perforating aa.
Popliteal a.
Lateral superior and inferior genicular aa.
Anterior tibial recurrent a.
Interosseous membrane
Anterior tibial a.
Anterior lateral malleolar a.
Lateral tarsal a.
Arcuate a.
Anterior medial malleolar a.
Dorsal pedal a.
Dorsal metatarsal aa.

A Right leg, anterior view.

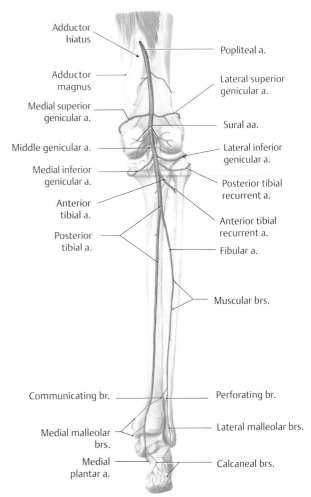

Adductor hiatus
Adductor magnus
Medial superior genicular a.
Middle genicular a.
Medial inferior genicular a.
Anterior tibial a.
Posterior tibial a.
Communicating br.
Medial malleolar brs.
Medial plantar a.

Popliteal a.
Lateral superior genicular a.
Sural aa.
Lateral inferior genicular a.
Posterior tibial recurrent a.
Anterior tibial recurrent a.
Fibular a.
Muscular brs.
Perforating br.
Lateral malleolar brs.
Calcaneal brs.

B Right leg, posterior view.

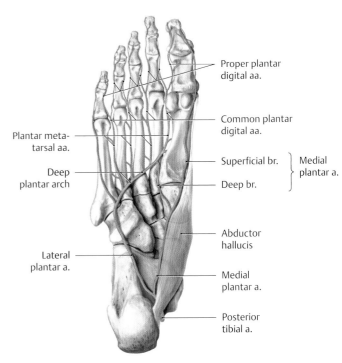

Proper plantar digital aa.
Common plantar digital aa.
Superficial br.
Deep br.
Medial plantar a.
Abductor hallucis
Medial plantar a.
Posterior tibial a.

Plantar metatarsal aa.
Deep plantar arch
Lateral plantar a.

C Sole of right foot, plantar view.

Fig. 34.2 Segments of the femoral artery

The blood supply to the lower limbs originates from the femoral artery. Color is used to identify the named distal segments of this vessel.

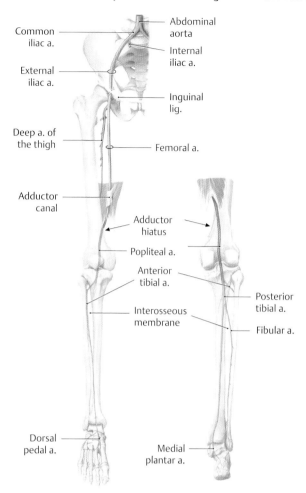

Fig. 34.3 Deep artery of the thigh

Right leg. The artery passes posteriorly through the adductor muscles of the medial thigh to supply the muscles of the posterior compartment via three to five perforating branches. Ligation of the femoral artery proximal to the origin of the deep artery of the thigh (*left*) is well tolerated owing to the collateral blood supply (*arrows*) from branches of the internal iliac artery that anastomose with the perforating branches.

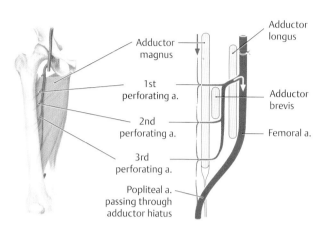

Clinical box 34.1

Femoral head necrosis

Dislocation or fracture of the femoral head (e.g., in patients with osteoporosis) may tear the femoral neck vessels, resulting in femoral head necrosis.

Fig. 34.4 Arteries of the femoral head

Anterior view.

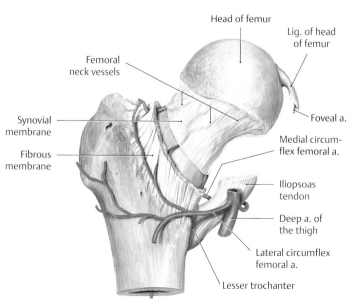

A Right femur.

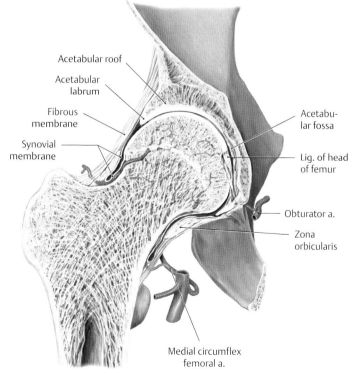

B Right femur, coronal section.

467

Veins & Lymphatics of the Lower Limb

Fig. 34.5 Superficial (epifascial) veins of the lower limb

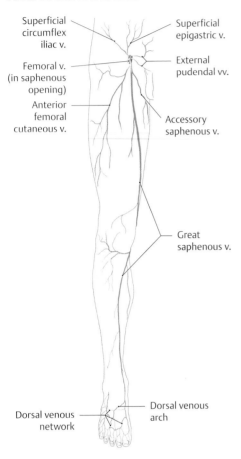

- Superficial circumflex iliac v.
- Femoral v. (in saphenous opening)
- Anterior femoral cutaneous v.
- Superficial epigastric v.
- External pudendal vv.
- Accessory saphenous v.
- Great saphenous v.
- Dorsal venous network
- Dorsal venous arch

A Right limb, anterior view.

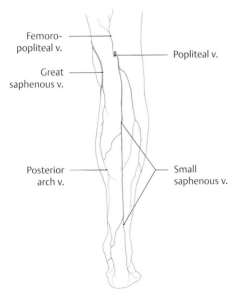

- Femoro-popliteal v.
- Great saphenous v.
- Posterior arch v.
- Popliteal v.
- Small saphenous v.

B Right limb, posterior view.

Fig. 34.6 Deep veins of the lower limb

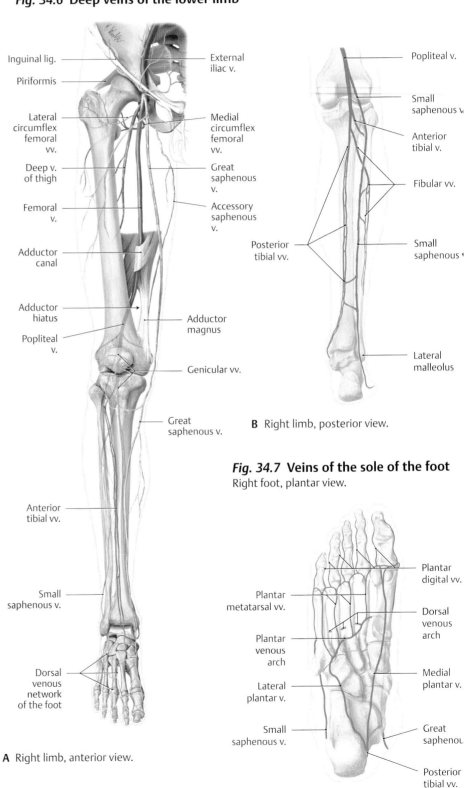

- Inguinal lig.
- Piriformis
- Lateral circumflex femoral vv.
- Deep v. of thigh
- Femoral v.
- Adductor canal
- Adductor hiatus
- Popliteal v.
- External iliac v.
- Medial circumflex femoral vv.
- Great saphenous v.
- Accessory saphenous v.
- Adductor magnus
- Genicular vv.
- Great saphenous v.
- Anterior tibial vv.
- Small saphenous v.
- Dorsal venous network of the foot

A Right limb, anterior view.

- Popliteal v.
- Small saphenous v.
- Anterior tibial v.
- Fibular vv.
- Posterior tibial vv.
- Small saphenous v.
- Lateral malleolus

B Right limb, posterior view.

Fig. 34.7 Veins of the sole of the foot
Right foot, plantar view.

- Plantar metatarsal vv.
- Plantar venous arch
- Lateral plantar v.
- Small saphenous v.
- Plantar digital vv.
- Dorsal venous arch
- Medial plantar v.
- Great saphenou
- Posterior tibial vv.

Fig. 34.8 Clinically important perforating veins

Right leg, medial view.

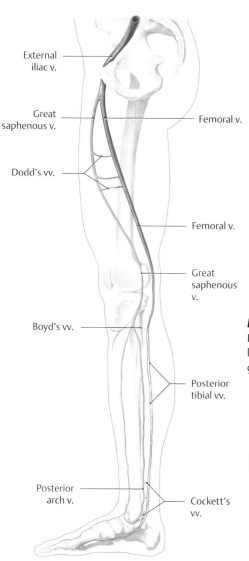

- External iliac v.
- Great saphenous v.
- Dodd's vv.
- Femoral v.
- Femoral v.
- Great saphenous v.
- Boyd's vv.
- Posterior tibial vv.
- Posterior arch v.
- Cockett's vv.

Fig. 34.9 Superficial lymph nodes

Right limb. Arrows indicate the main directions of lymphatic drainage.

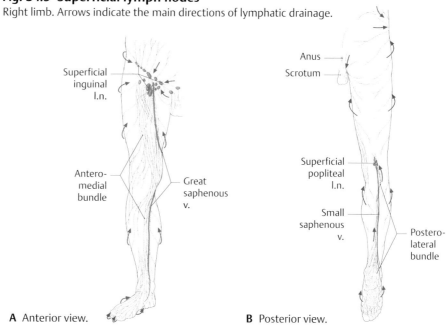

- Superficial inguinal l.n.
- Antero-medial bundle
- Great saphenous v.

A Anterior view.

- Anus
- Scrotum
- Superficial popliteal l.n.
- Small saphenous v.
- Postero-lateral bundle

B Posterior view.

Fig. 34.10 Lymph nodes and drainage

Right limb, anterior view. Arrows indicate direction of lymphatic drainage. Yellow: superficial nodes; green: deep nodes.

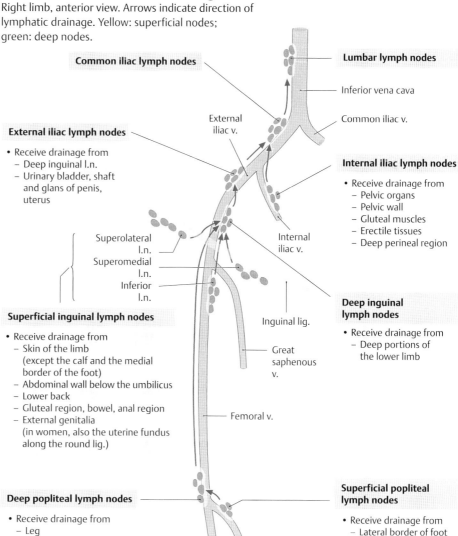

Common iliac lymph nodes

External iliac lymph nodes

- Receive drainage from
  - Deep inguinal l.n.
  - Urinary bladder, shaft and glans of penis, uterus

Lumbar lymph nodes

- Inferior vena cava
- Common iliac v.
- External iliac v.
- Internal iliac v.

Internal iliac lymph nodes

- Receive drainage from
  - Pelvic organs
  - Pelvic wall
  - Gluteal muscles
  - Erectile tissues
  - Deep perineal region

- Superolateral l.n.
- Superomedial l.n.
- Inferior l.n.

Superficial inguinal lymph nodes

- Receive drainage from
  - Skin of the limb (except the calf and the medial border of the foot)
  - Abdominal wall below the umbilicus
  - Lower back
  - Gluteal region, bowel, anal region
  - External genitalia (in women, also the uterine fundus along the round lig.)

- Inguinal lig.
- Great saphenous v.
- Femoral v.

Deep inguinal lymph nodes

- Receive drainage from
  - Deep portions of the lower limb

Deep popliteal lymph nodes

- Receive drainage from
  - Leg
  - Foot

- Popliteal v.
- Small saphenous v.

Superficial popliteal lymph nodes

- Receive drainage from
  - Lateral border of foot
  - Calf

Lumbosacral Plexus

 The lumbosacral plexus supplies sensory and motor innervation to the lower limb. It is formed by the anterior (ventral) rami of the lumbar and sacral spinal nerves, with contributions from the sub-costal nerve (T12) and coccygeal nerve (Co1).

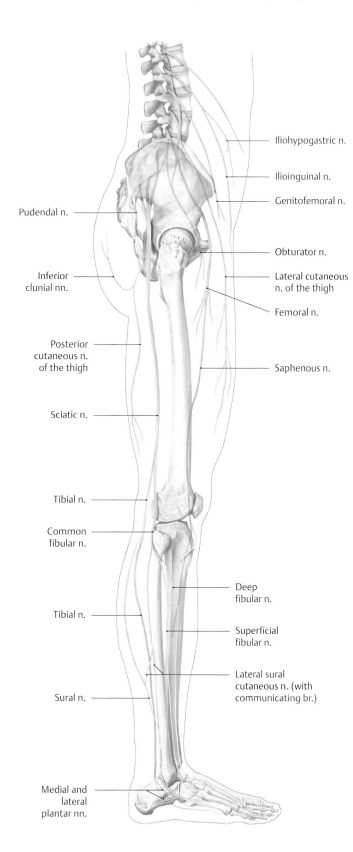

Iliohypogastric n.

Ilioinguinal n.

Genitofemoral n.

Pudendal n.

Obturator n.

Inferior clunial nn.

Lateral cutaneous n. of the thigh

Femoral n.

Posterior cutaneous n. of the thigh

Saphenous n.

Sciatic n.

Tibial n.

Common fibular n.

Tibial n.

Deep fibular n.

Superficial fibular n.

Lateral sural cutaneous n. (with communicating br.)

Sural n.

Medial and lateral plantar nn.

Table 34.1	Nerves of the lumbosacral plexus	
Lumbar plexus		
Iliohypogastric n.	L1	
Ilioinguinal n.	L1	
Genitofemoral n.	L1–L2	p. 473
Lateral cutaneous n. of the thigh	L2–L3	
Obturator n.	L2–L4	**p. 474**
Femoral n.		**p. 475**
Sacral plexus		
Superior gluteal n.	L4–S1	p. 477
Inferior gluteal n.	L5–S2	
Posterior cutaneous n. of the thigh	S1–S3	**p. 476**
Sciatic n. Common fibular n.	L4–S2	**p. 478**
Sciatic n. Tibial n.	L4–S3	**p. 479**
Pudendal n.	S2–S4	**pp. 278, 281**

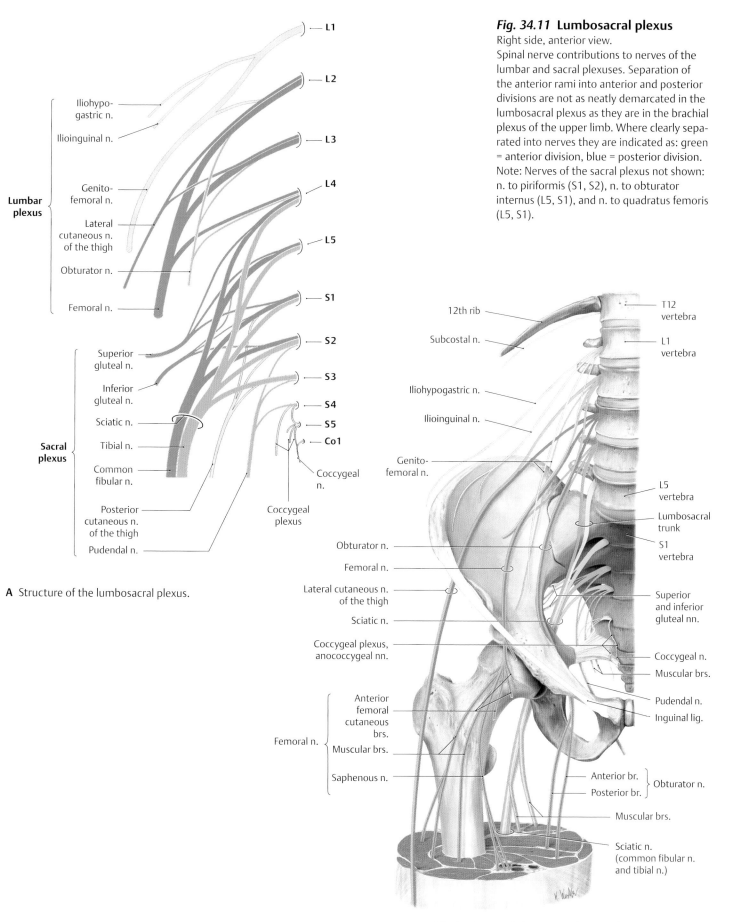

Fig. 34.11 Lumbosacral plexus

Right side, anterior view.

Spinal nerve contributions to nerves of the lumbar and sacral plexuses. Separation of the anterior rami into anterior and posterior divisions are not as neatly demarcated in the lumbosacral plexus as they are in the brachial plexus of the upper limb. Where clearly separated into nerves they are indicated as: green = anterior division, blue = posterior division. Note: Nerves of the sacral plexus not shown: n. to piriformis (S1, S2), n. to obturator internus (L5, S1), and n. to quadratus femoris (L5, S1).

A Structure of the lumbosacral plexus.

B Course of the lumbosacral plexus. Distribution of anterior rami of lumbar (yellow/orange) and sacral (blue/green) spinal nerves to the gluteal region and lower limb.

Nerves of the Lumbar Plexus

Table 34.2	Nerves of the lumbar plexus		
Nerve	**Level**	**Innervated muscle**	**Cutaneous branches**
Iliohypogastric n.	L1	Transversus abdominis and internal oblique (inferior portions)	Anterior and lateral cutaneous brs.
Ilioinguinal n.	L1		♂: Anterior scrotal nn. ♀: Anterior labial nn.
Genitofemoral n.	L1–L2	♂: Cremaster (genital br.)	Genital br. Femoral br.
Lateral cutaneous n. of the thigh	L2–L3	—	lateral cutaneous n. of the thigh
Obturator n.	L2–L4	See **p. 474**	
Femoral n.	L2–L4	See **p. 475**	
Short, direct muscular brs.	T12–L4	Psoas major Quadratus lumborum Iliacus Intertransversarii lumborum	—

Fig. 34.12 Cutaneous innervation of the inguinal region

Right male inguinal region, anterior view.

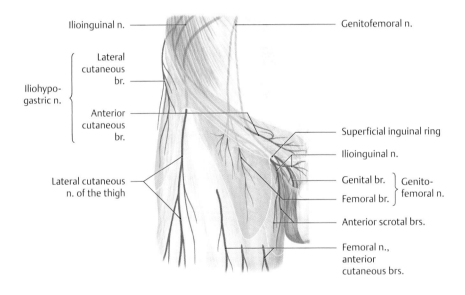

Clinical box 34.2

Entrapment of the lateral femoral cutaneous nerve (meralgia paresthetica)

Ischemia (diminished blood flow) of the lateral cutaneous nerve of the thigh can result when the nerve is stretched or entrapped by the inguinal ligament (see **Fig. 34.11B**) during hyperextension of the hip or with increased lordosis (curvature) of the lumbar spine, as often occurs during pregnancy.

This results in pain, numbness, or paresthesia (tingling or burning) on the outer aspect of the thigh. It is most commonly found in obese or diabetic individuals and in pregnant women.

Fig. 34.13 Nerves of the lumbar plexus

Right side, anterior view with the anterior abdominal wall removed.

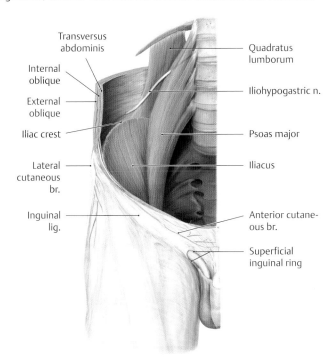

Transversus abdominis

Internal oblique

External oblique

Iliac crest

Lateral cutaneous br.

Inguinal lig.

Quadratus lumborum

Iliohypogastric n.

Psoas major

Iliacus

Anterior cutaneous br.

Superficial inguinal ring

A Iliohypogastric nerve.

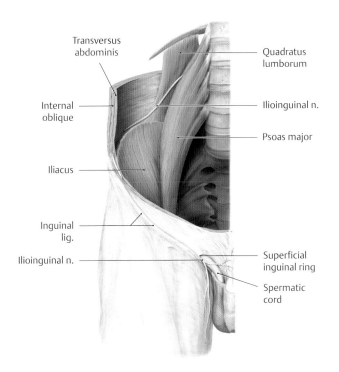

Transversus abdominis

Internal oblique

Iliacus

Inguinal lig.

Ilioinguinal n.

Quadratus lumborum

Ilioinguinal n.

Psoas major

Superficial inguinal ring

Spermatic cord

B Ilioinguinal nerve.

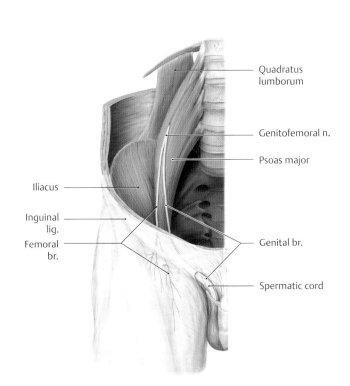

Iliacus

Inguinal lig.

Femoral br.

Quadratus lumborum

Genitofemoral n.

Psoas major

Genital br.

Spermatic cord

C Genitofemoral nerve.

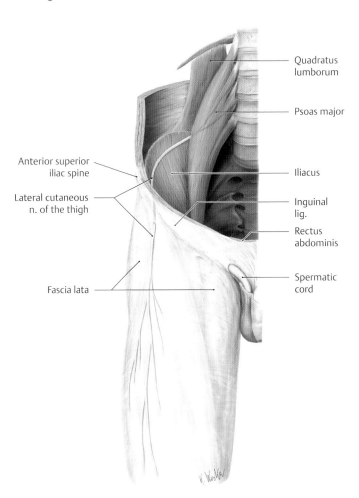

Anterior superior iliac spine

Lateral cutaneous n. of the thigh

Fascia lata

Quadratus lumborum

Psoas major

Iliacus

Inguinal lig.

Rectus abdominis

Spermatic cord

D Lateral cutaneous nerve of the thigh.

Nerves of the Lumbar Plexus: Obturator & Femoral Nerves

Fig. 34.14 **Obturator nerve: Cutaneous distribution**
Right leg, medial view.

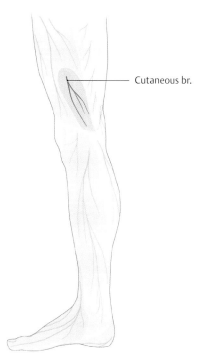

Cutaneous br.

Fig. 34.15 **Obturator nerve**
Right side, anterior view.

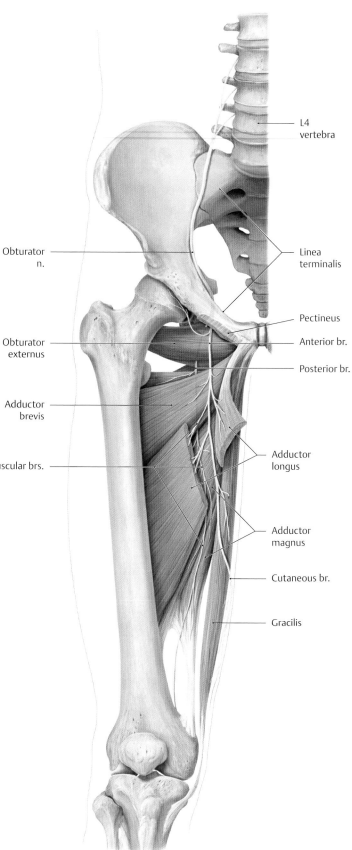

L4 vertebra

Obturator n.

Linea terminalis

Pectineus

Obturator externus

Anterior br.

Posterior br.

Adductor brevis

Muscular brs.

Adductor longus

Adductor magnus

Cutaneous br.

Gracilis

Table 34.3	Obturator nerve (L2–L4)
Motor branches	**Innervated muscles**
Direct br.	Obturator externus
Anterior br.	Adductor longus
	Adductor brevis
	Gracilis
	Pectineus
Posterior br.	Adductor magnus
Sensory branches	
Cutaneous br.	

Fig. 34.16 Femoral nerve
Right side, anterior view.

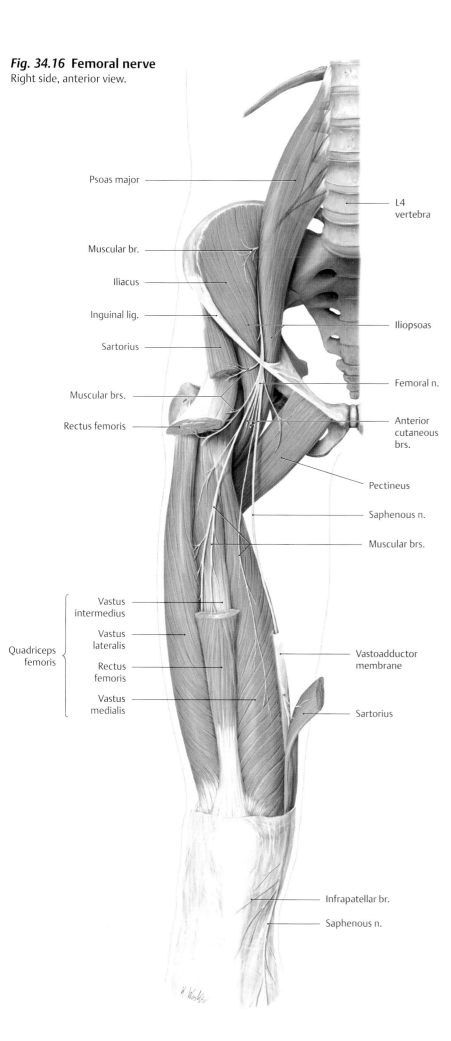

Psoas major

Muscular br.

Iliacus

Inguinal lig.

Sartorius

Muscular brs.

Rectus femoris

L4 vertebra

Iliopsoas

Femoral n.

Anterior cutaneous brs.

Pectineus

Saphenous n.

Muscular brs.

Quadriceps femoris

Vastus intermedius

Vastus lateralis

Rectus femoris

Vastus medialis

Vastoadductor membrane

Sartorius

Infrapatellar br.

Saphenous n.

Fig. 34.17 Femoral nerve: Cutaneous distribution
Right limb, anterior view.

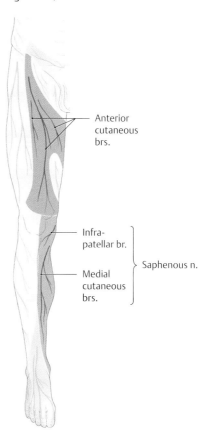

Anterior cutaneous brs.

Infrapatellar br.

Medial cutaneous brs.

Saphenous n.

Table 34.4	Femoral nerve (L2–L4)
Motor branches	**Innervated muscles**
Muscular brs.	Iliopsoas
	Pectineus
	Sartorius
	Quadriceps femoris
Sensory branches	
Anterior cutaneous br.	
Saphenous n.	

Nerves of the Sacral Plexus

Table 34.5   **Nerves of the sacral plexus**

Nerve		Level	Innervated muscle	Cutaneous branches	
Superior gluteal n.		L4–S1	Gluteus medius Gluteus minimus Tensor fasciae latae	—	
Inferior gluteal n.		L5–S2	Gluteus maximus	—	
Posterior cutaneous n. of the thigh		S1–S3	—	Posterior cutaneous n. of the thigh	Inferior clunial nn.
					Perineal brs.
Direct branches	N. of piriformis	S1–S2	Piriformis	—	
	N. of obturator internus	L5–S1	Obturator internus Gemelli	—	
	N. of quadratus femoris		Quadratus femoris	—	
Sciatic n.	Common fibular n.	L4–S2	See **p. 478**		
	Tibial n.	L4–S3	See **p. 479**		
Pudenal n.		S2–S4	See **pp. 278, 281**		

Fig. 34.18 Cutaneous innervation of the gluteal region
Right limb, posterior view.

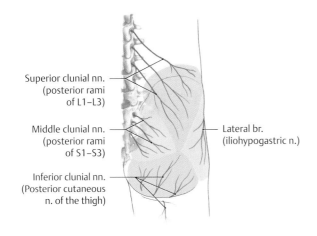

Fig. 34.19 Posterior cutaneous nerve of the thigh: Cutaneous distribution
Right limb, posterior view.

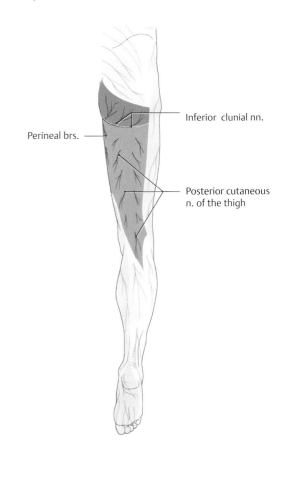

Fig. 34.20 Emerging spinal nerve
Horizontal section, superior view.

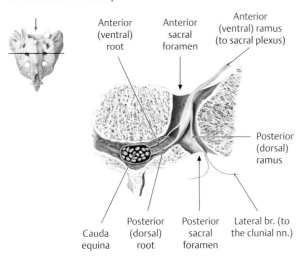

Fig. 34.21 **Nerves of the sacral plexus**
Right limb.

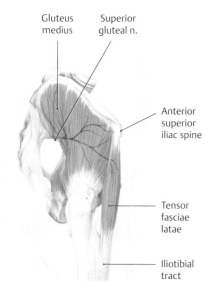

A Superior gluteal nerve. Lateral view.

Gluteus medius — Superior gluteal n. — Anterior superior iliac spine — Tensor fasciae latae — Iliotibial tract

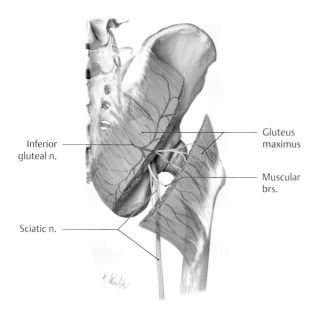

B Inferior gluteal nerve. Posterior view.

Inferior gluteal n. — Sciatic n. — Gluteus maximus — Muscular brs.

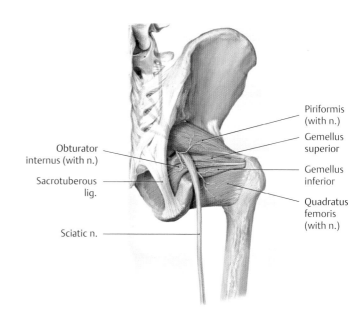

C Direct branches. Posterior view.

Obturator internus (with n.) — Sacrotuberous lig. — Sciatic n. — Piriformis (with n.) — Gemellus superior — Gemellus inferior — Quadratus femoris (with n.)

❖❖ Clinical box 34.3

Small gluteal muscle weakness
The small gluteal muscles on the stance side stabilize the pelvis in the coronal plane (**A**). Weakness or paralysis of the small gluteal muscles from damage to the superior gluteal nerve (e.g., due to a faulty intramuscular injection) is manifested by weak abduction of the affected hip joint. In a positive Trendelenburg's test, the pelvis sags toward the normal, unsupported side (**B**). Tilting the upper body toward the affected side shifts the center of gravity onto the stance side, thereby elevating the pelvis on the swing side (Duchenne's limp) (**C**). With bilateral loss of the small gluteals, the patient exhibits a typical waddling gait.

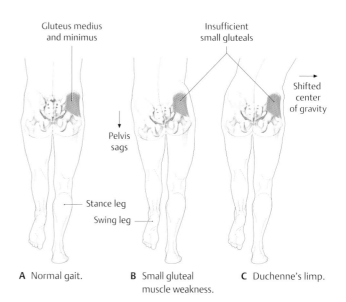

Gluteus medius and minimus — Insufficient small gluteals — Shifted center of gravity — Pelvis sags — Stance leg — Swing leg

A Normal gait. **B** Small gluteal muscle weakness. **C** Duchenne's limp.

Nerves of the Sacral Plexus: Sciatic Nerve

 The sciatic nerve gives off several direct muscular branches before dividing into the tibial and common fibular nerves proximal to the popliteal fossa.

Fig. 34.22 **Common fibular nerve: Cutaneous distribution**

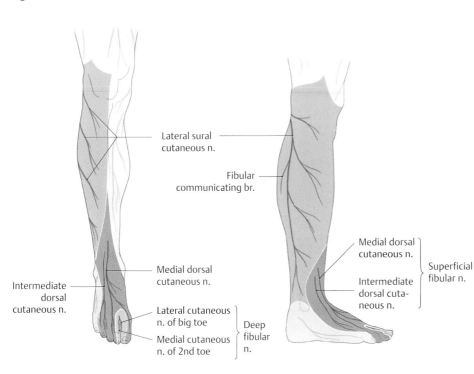

A Right leg, anterior view.   **B** Right leg, lateral view.

Fig. 34.23 **Common fibular nerve**
Right limb, lateral view.

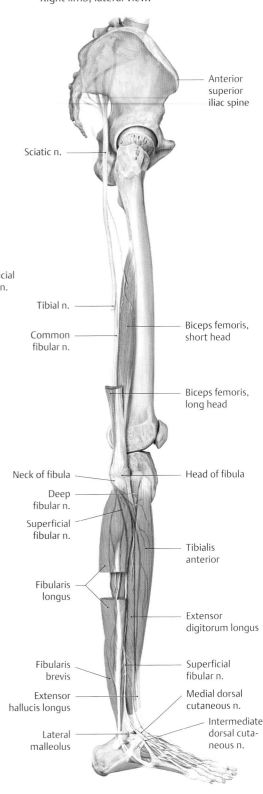

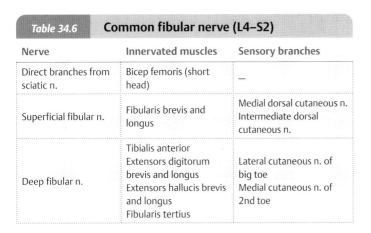

Table 34.6	Common fibular nerve (L4–S2)	
Nerve	**Innervated muscles**	**Sensory branches**
Direct branches from sciatic n.	Bicep femoris (short head)	—
Superficial fibular n.	Fibularis brevis and longus	Medial dorsal cutaneous n. Intermediate dorsal cutaneous n.
Deep fibular n.	Tibialis anterior Extensors digitorum brevis and longus Extensors hallucis brevis and longus Fibularis tertius	Lateral cutaneous n. of big toe Medial cutaneous n. of 2nd toe

***Fig. 34.24* Tibial nerve**
Right limb.

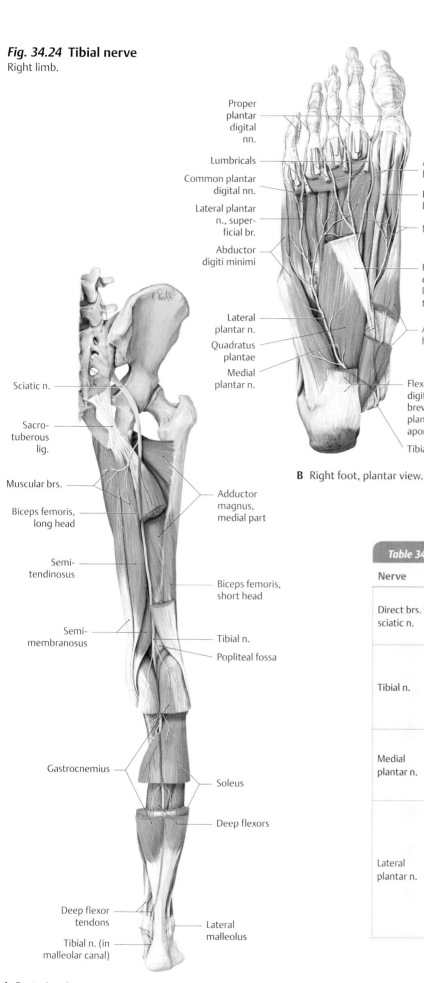

A Posterior view.

***Fig. 34.25* Tibial nerve: Cutaneous distribution**
Right lower limb, posterior view.

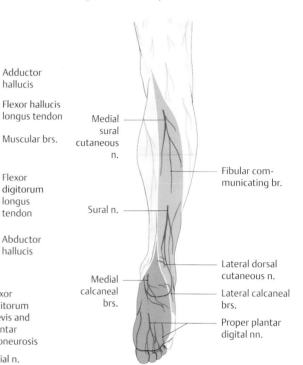

B Right foot, plantar view.

Table 34.7	Tibial nerve (L4–S3)	
Nerve	**Innervated muscles**	**Sensory branches**
Direct brs. from sciatic n.	Semitendinosus Semimembranosus Biceps femoris (long head) Adductor magnus (medial part)	–
Tibial n.	Triceps surae Plantaris Popliteus Tibialis posterior Flexor digitorum longus Flexor hallucis longus	Medial sural cutaneous n. Medial and lateral calcaneal brs. Lateral dorsal cutaneous n.
Medial plantar n.	Adductor hallucis Flexor digitorum brevis Flexor hallucis brevis (medial head) 1st lumbricals	Proper plantar digital nn.
Lateral plantar n.	Flexor hallucis brevis (lateral head) Quadratus plantae Abductor digiti minimi Flexor digiti minimi brevis Opponens digiti minimi 2nd to 4th lumbricals 1st to 3rd plantar interossei 1st to 4th dorsal interossei Adductor hallucis	Proper plantar digital nn.

Superficial Nerves & Vessels of the Lower Limb

Fig. 34.26 **Superficial cutaneous veins and nerves of right lower limb**

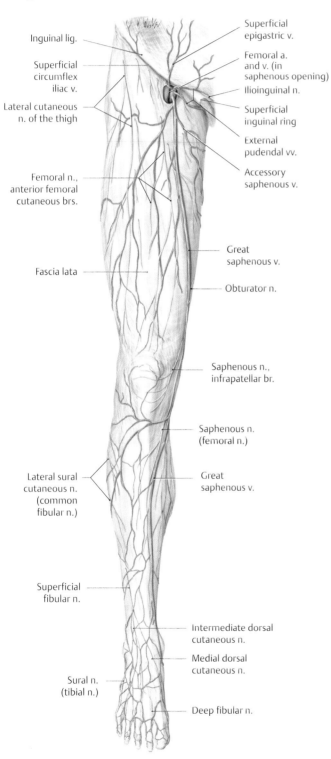

Inguinal lig.

Superficial circumflex iliac v.

Lateral cutaneous n. of the thigh

Femoral n., anterior femoral cutaneous brs.

Fascia lata

Lateral sural cutaneous n. (common fibular n.)

Superficial fibular n.

Sural n. (tibial n.)

Superficial epigastric v.

Femoral a. and v. (in saphenous opening)

Ilioinguinal n.

Superficial inguinal ring

External pudendal vv.

Accessory saphenous v.

Great saphenous v.

Obturator n.

Saphenous n., infrapatellar br.

Saphenous n. (femoral n.)

Great saphenous v.

Intermediate dorsal cutaneous n.

Medial dorsal cutaneous n.

Deep fibular n.

A Anterior view.

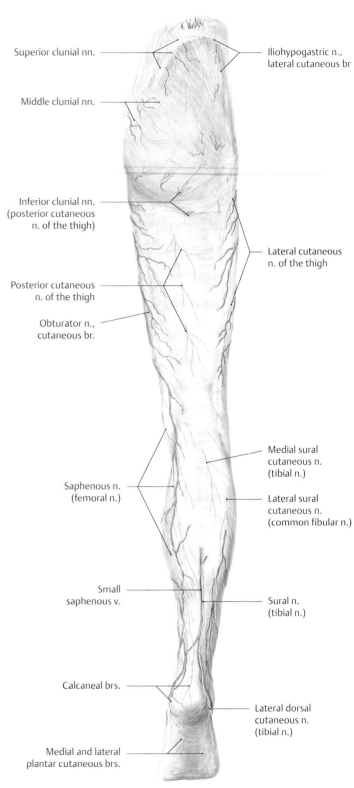

Superior clunial nn.

Middle clunial nn.

Inferior clunial nn. (posterior cutaneous n. of the thigh)

Posterior cutaneous n. of the thigh

Obturator n., cutaneous br.

Saphenous n. (femoral n.)

Small saphenous v.

Calcaneal brs.

Medial and lateral plantar cutaneous brs.

Iliohypogastric n., lateral cutaneous br

Lateral cutaneous n. of the thigh

Medial sural cutaneous n. (tibial n.)

Lateral sural cutaneous n. (common fibular n.)

Sural n. (tibial n.)

Lateral dorsal cutaneous n. (tibial n.)

B Posterior view.

Fig. 34.27 Cutaneous innervation of the lower limb
Right lower limb.

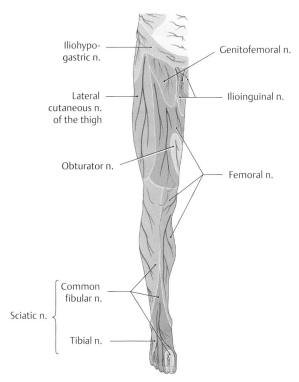

Iliohypo-gastric n.

Lateral cutaneous n. of the thigh

Obturator n.

Common fibular n.

Sciatic n.

Tibial n.

Genitofemoral n.

Ilioinguinal n.

Femoral n.

A Anterior view.

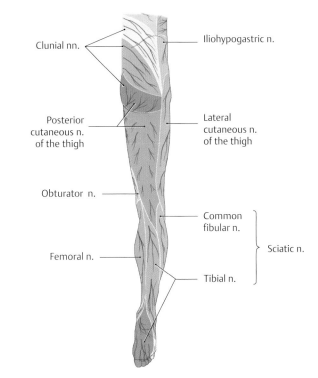

Clunial nn.

Posterior cutaneous n. of the thigh

Obturator n.

Femoral n.

Iliohypogastric n.

Lateral cutaneous n. of the thigh

Common fibular n.

Sciatic n.

Tibial n.

B Posterior view.

Fig. 34.28 Dermatomes of the lower limb
Right lower limb.

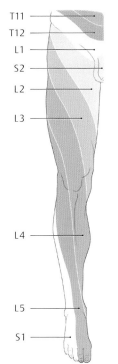

T11
T12
L1
S2
L2
L3

L4

L5

S1

A Anterior view.

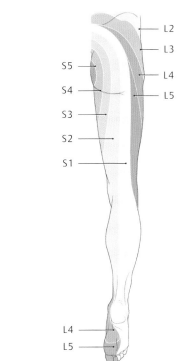

S5
S4
S3
S2
S1

L2
L3
L4
L5

L4
L5

B Posterior view.

Topography of the Inguinal Region

Fig. 34.29 Superficial veins and lymph nodes

Right male inguinal region, anterior view. *Removed:* Cribriform fascia over the saphenous opening (see **pp. 150–151**).

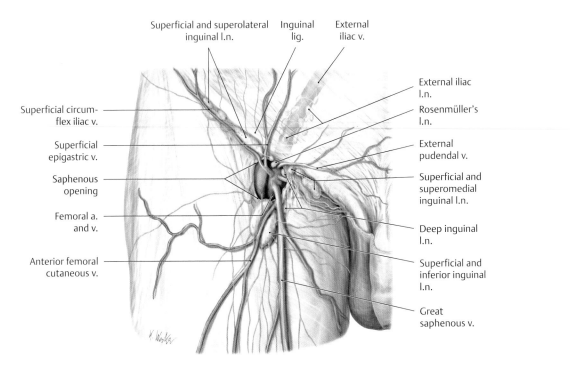

Fig. 34.30 Inguinal region

Right male inguinal region, anterior view.

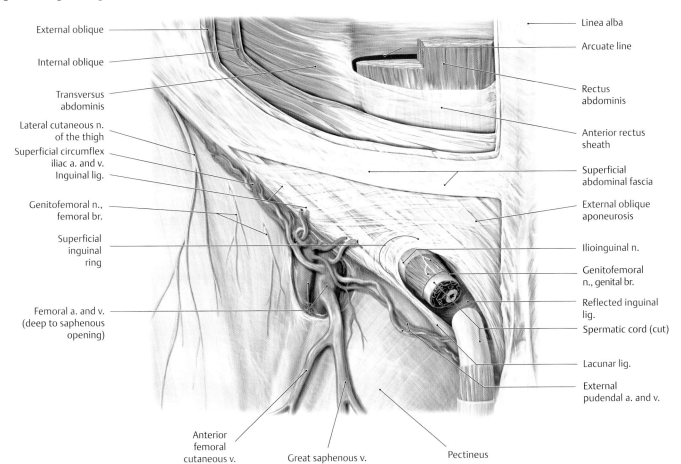

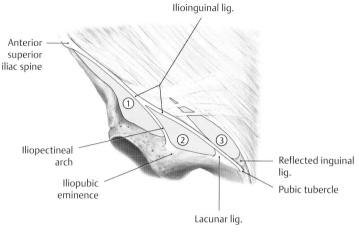

Anterior superior iliac spine

Ilioinguinal lig.

Iliopectineal arch

Iliopubic eminence

Lacunar lig.

Reflected inguinal lig.

Pubic tubercle

Table 34.8	Structures in the inguinal region	
Region	**Boundaries**	**Contents**
Retro-inguinal space		
① Muscular compartment	Anterior superior iliac spine Inguinal lig. Iliopectineal arch	Femoral n. Lateral cutaneous n. of the thigh Iliacus Psoas major
② Vascular compartment	Inguinal lig. Iliopectineal arch Lacunar lig.	Femoral a. and v. Genitofemoral n., femoral br. Rosenmüller's lymph node
Inguinal canal		
③ Superficial inguinal ring	Medial crus Lateral crus Reflected inguinal lig.	Ilioinguinal n. Genitofemoral n., genital br. Spermatic cord

Fig. 34.31 Retro-inguinal space: Muscular and vascular compartments

Right inguinal region, anterior view.

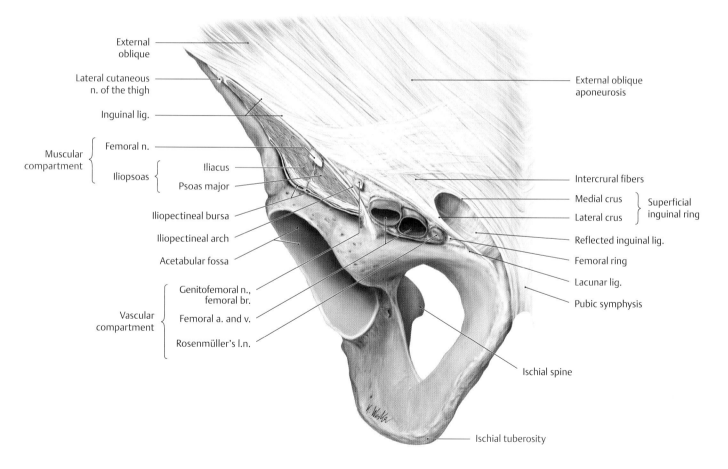

External oblique

Lateral cutaneous n. of the thigh

Inguinal lig.

Muscular compartment

Femoral n.

Iliopsoas — Iliacus

Psoas major

Iliopectineal bursa

Iliopectineal arch

Acetabular fossa

Genitofemoral n., femoral br.

Vascular compartment — Femoral a. and v.

Rosenmüller's l.n.

External oblique aponeurosis

Intercrural fibers

Medial crus

Lateral crus

Superficial inguinal ring

Reflected inguinal lig.

Femoral ring

Lacunar lig.

Pubic symphysis

Ischial spine

Ischial tuberosity

Topography of the Gluteal Region

Fig. 34.32 **Gluteal region**
Right gluteal region, posterior view.

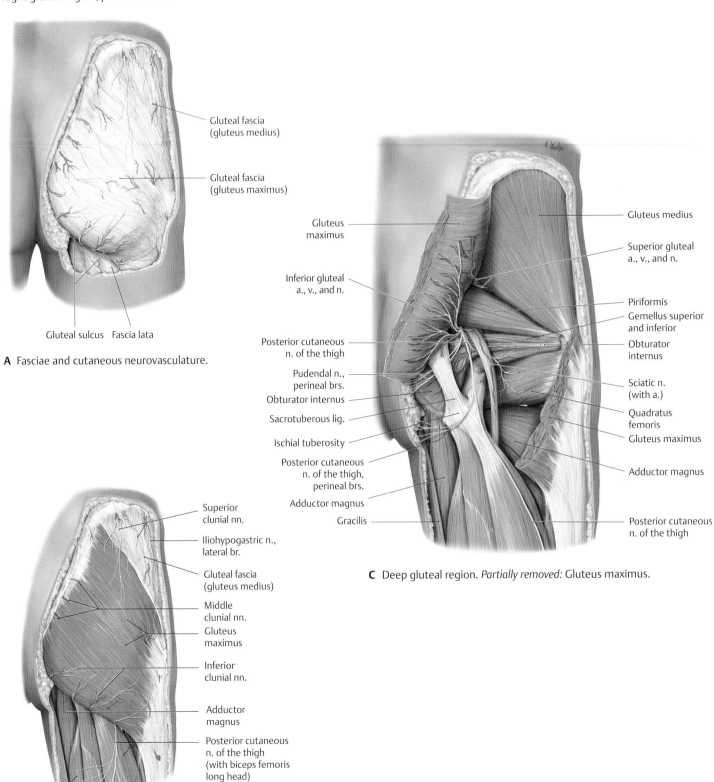

A Fasciae and cutaneous neurovasculature.

Gluteal fascia
(gluteus medius)

Gluteal fascia
(gluteus maximus)

Gluteal sulcus   Fascia lata

Gluteus
maximus

Inferior gluteal
a., v., and n.

Posterior cutaneous
n. of the thigh

Pudendal n.,
perineal brs.

Obturator internus

Sacrotuberous lig.

Ischial tuberosity

Posterior cutaneous
n. of the thigh,
perineal brs.

Adductor magnus

Gracilis

Gluteus medius

Superior gluteal
a., v., and n.

Piriformis

Gemellus superior
and inferior

Obturator
internus

Sciatic n.
(with a.)

Quadratus
femoris

Gluteus maximus

Adductor magnus

Posterior cutaneous
n. of the thigh

C Deep gluteal region. *Partially removed:* Gluteus maximus.

Superior
clunial nn.

Iliohypogastric n.,
lateral br.

Gluteal fascia
(gluteus medius)

Middle
clunial nn.

Gluteus
maximus

Inferior
clunial nn.

Adductor
magnus

Posterior cutaneous
n. of the thigh
(with biceps femoris
long head)

Semi-
membranosus   Semitendinosus

B Gluteal region. *Removed:* Fascia lata.

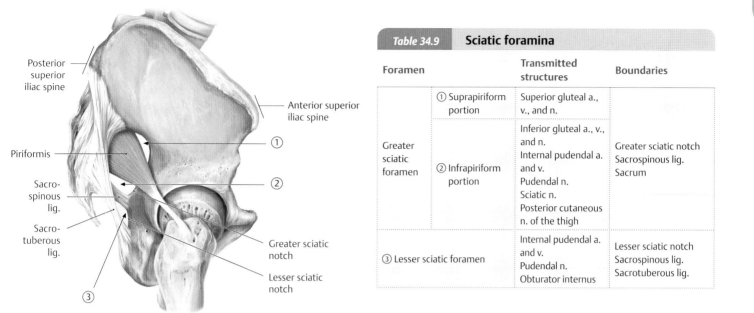

Posterior superior iliac spine

Anterior superior iliac spine

Piriformis

Sacro-spinous lig.

Sacro-tuberous lig.

①

②

③

Greater sciatic notch

Lesser sciatic notch

Table 34.9		Sciatic foramina	
Foramen		**Transmitted structures**	**Boundaries**
Greater sciatic foramen	① Suprapiriform portion	Superior gluteal a., v., and n.	Greater sciatic notch Sacrospinous lig. Sacrum
	② Infrapiriform portion	Inferior gluteal a., v., and n. Internal pudendal a. and v. Pudendal n. Sciatic n. Posterior cutaneous n. of the thigh	
③ Lesser sciatic foramen		Internal pudendal a. and v. Pudendal n. Obturator internus	Lesser sciatic notch Sacrospinous lig. Sacrotuberous lig.

***Fig. 34.33* Gluteal region and ischioanal fossa**

Right gluteal region, posterior view.
Removed: Gluteus maximus and medius.

Posterior superior iliac spine

Superior gluteal a. and n.

Inferior gluteal n.

Inferior gluteal aa. and vv.

Pudendal n.

Internal pudendal a. and v.

Obturator internus

Pudendal canal (Alcock's canal)

Sacrotuberous lig.

Adductor magnus

Gracilis

Semitendinosus

Anterior superior iliac spine

Gluteus minimus

Tensor fasciae latae

Piriformis

Gemellus superior

Obturator internus

Gemellus inferior

Br. of medial circumflex femoral a.

Trochanteric bursa

Quadratus femoris

Sciatic n.

Adductor magnus

1st perforating a.

Semi-membranosus

Biceps femoris, long head

Posterior cutaneous n. of the thigh

Topography of the Anterior, Medial & Posterior Thigh

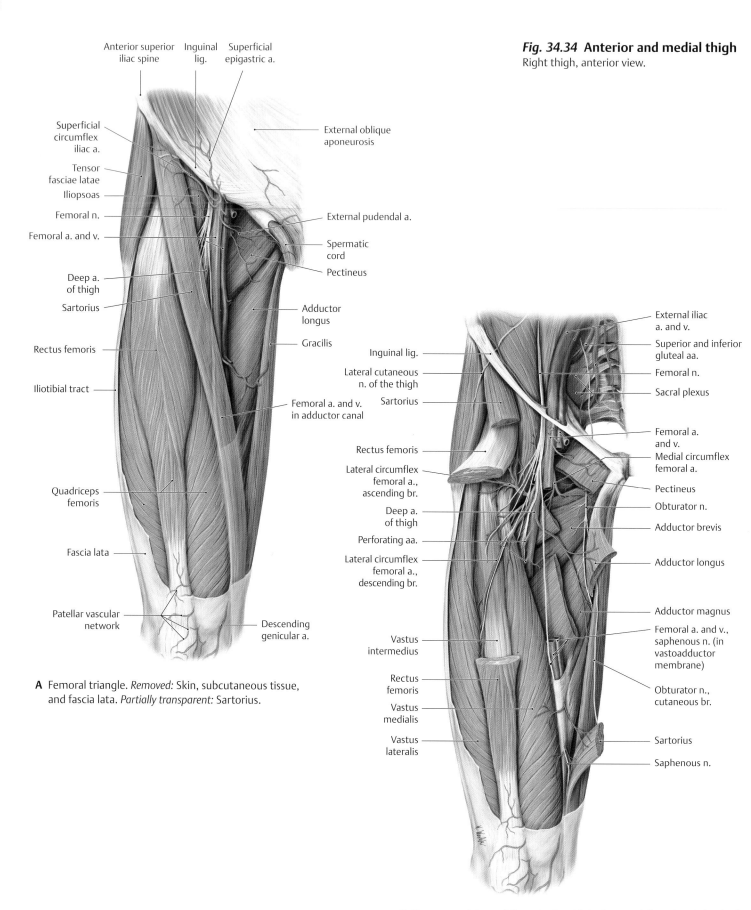

Lower Limb

Fig. 34.34 Anterior and medial thigh
Right thigh, anterior view.

A Femoral triangle. *Removed:* Skin, subcutaneous tissue, and fascia lata. *Partially transparent:* Sartorius.

B Neurovasculature of the anterior thigh. *Removed:* Anterior abdominal wall. *Partially removed:* Sartorius, rectus femoris, adductor longus, and pectineus.

486

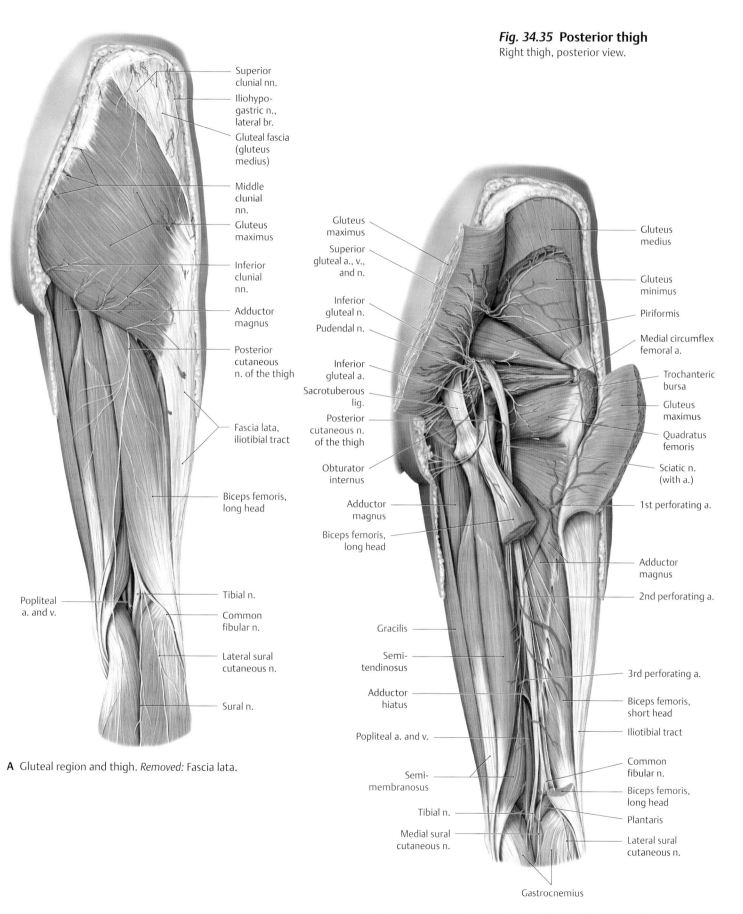

Fig. 34.35 Posterior thigh
Right thigh, posterior view.

Superior
clunial nn.

Iliohypo-
gastric n.,
lateral br.

Gluteal fascia
(gluteus
medius)

Middle
clunial
nn.

Gluteus
maximus

Inferior
clunial
nn.

Adductor
magnus

Posterior
cutaneous
n. of the thigh

Fascia lata,
iliotibial tract

Biceps femoris,
long head

Popliteal
a. and v.

Tibial n.

Common
fibular n.

Lateral sural
cutaneous n.

Sural n.

A Gluteal region and thigh. *Removed:* Fascia lata.

Gluteus
maximus

Superior
gluteal a., v.,
and n.

Inferior
gluteal n.

Pudendal n.

Inferior
gluteal a.

Sacrotuberous
lig.

Posterior
cutaneous n.
of the thigh

Obturator
internus

Adductor
magnus

Biceps femoris,
long head

Gracilis

Semi-
tendinosus

Adductor
hiatus

Popliteal a. and v.

Semi-
membranosus

Tibial n.

Medial sural
cutaneous n.

Gastrocnemius

Gluteus
medius

Gluteus
minimus

Piriformis

Medial circumflex
femoral a.

Trochanteric
bursa

Gluteus
maximus

Quadratus
femoris

Sciatic n.
(with a.)

1st perforating a.

Adductor
magnus

2nd perforating a.

3rd perforating a.

Biceps femoris,
short head

Iliotibial tract

Common
fibular n.

Biceps femoris,
long head

Plantaris

Lateral sural
cutaneous n.

B Neurovasculature of the posterior thigh. *Partially removed:* Gluteus maximus, gluteus medius, and biceps femoris. *Retracted:* Semimembranosus.

Topography of the Posterior Compartment of the Leg & Foot

Lower Limb

***Fig. 34.36* Posterior compartment of leg**
Right leg, posterior view.

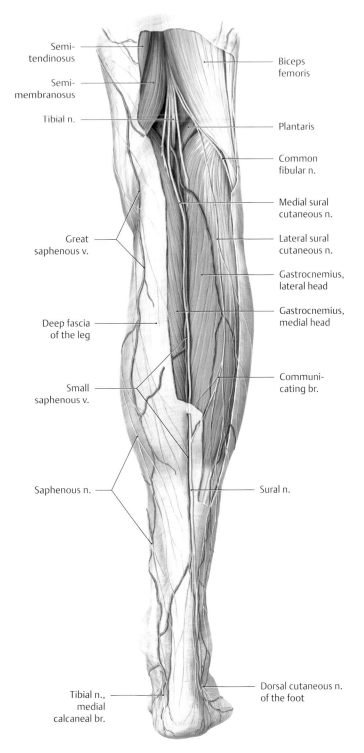

Semi-tendinosus

Semi-membranosus

Tibial n.

Great saphenous v.

Deep fascia of the leg

Small saphenous v.

Saphenous n.

Tibial n., medial calcaneal br.

Biceps femoris

Plantaris

Common fibular n.

Medial sural cutaneous n.

Lateral sural cutaneous n.

Gastrocnemius, lateral head

Gastrocnemius, medial head

Communicating br.

Sural n.

Dorsal cutaneous n. of the foot

A Superficial neurovascular structures.

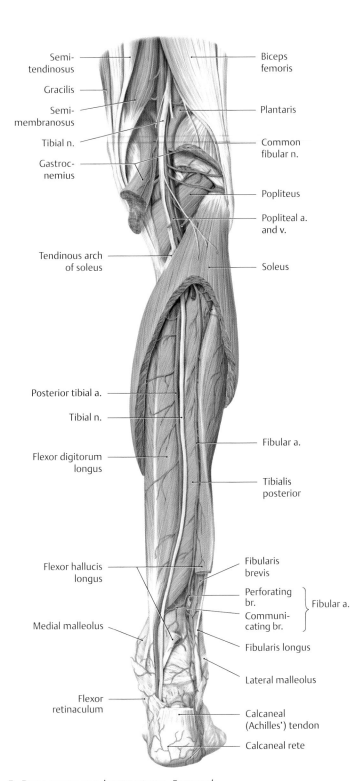

Semi-tendinosus

Gracilis

Semi-membranosus

Tibial n.

Gastrocnemius

Tendinous arch of soleus

Posterior tibial a.

Tibial n.

Flexor digitorum longus

Flexor hallucis longus

Medial malleolus

Flexor retinaculum

Biceps femoris

Plantaris

Common fibular n.

Popliteus

Popliteal a. and v.

Soleus

Fibular a.

Tibialis posterior

Fibularis brevis

Perforating br.

Communicating br.

Fibular a.

Fibularis longus

Lateral malleolus

Calcaneal (Achilles') tendon

Calcaneal rete

B Deep neurovascular structures. *Removed:* Gastrocnemius. *Windowed:* Soleus.

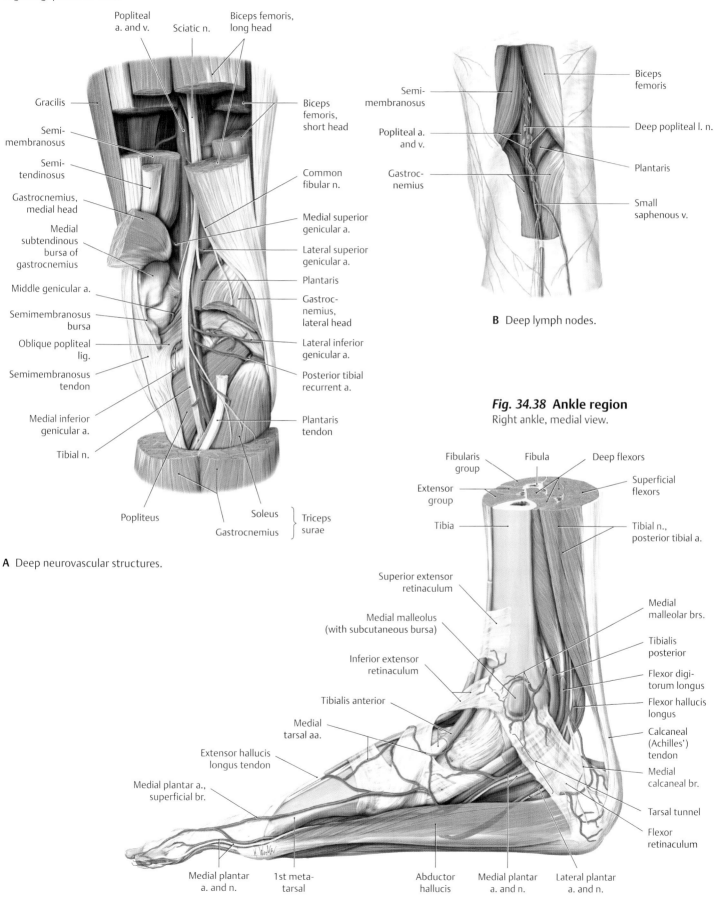

Fig. 34.37 Popliteal region
Right leg, posterior view.

Popliteal a. and v.

Sciatic n.

Biceps femoris, long head

Gracilis

Semi-membranosus

Semi-tendinosus

Gastrocnemius, medial head

Medial subtendinous bursa of gastrocnemius

Middle genicular a.

Semimembranosus bursa

Oblique popliteal lig.

Semimembranosus tendon

Medial inferior genicular a.

Tibial n.

Biceps femoris, short head

Common fibular n.

Medial superior genicular a.

Lateral superior genicular a.

Plantaris

Gastroc-nemius, lateral head

Lateral inferior genicular a.

Posterior tibial recurrent a.

Plantaris tendon

Popliteus

Soleus

Gastrocnemius

} Triceps surae

A Deep neurovascular structures.

Semi-membranosus

Popliteal a. and v.

Gastroc-nemius

Biceps femoris

Deep popliteal l. n.

Plantaris

Small saphenous v.

B Deep lymph nodes.

Fig. 34.38 Ankle region
Right ankle, medial view.

Fibularis group

Fibula

Deep flexors

Extensor group

Tibia

Superficial flexors

Tibial n., posterior tibial a.

Superior extensor retinaculum

Medial malleolus (with subcutaneous bursa)

Inferior extensor retinaculum

Tibialis anterior

Medial tarsal aa.

Extensor hallucis longus tendon

Medial plantar a., superficial br.

Medial plantar a. and n.

1st meta-tarsal

Abductor hallucis

Medial plantar a. and n.

Lateral plantar a. and n.

Medial malleolar brs.

Tibialis posterior

Flexor digi-torum longus

Flexor hallucis longus

Calcaneal (Achilles') tendon

Medial calcaneal br.

Tarsal tunnel

Flexor retinaculum

Topography of the Lateral & Anterior Compartments of the Leg and Dorsum of the Foot

Fig. 34.39 Neurovasculature of the lateral compartment of the leg

Right limb. *Removed:* Origins of the fibularis longus and extensor digitorum longus.

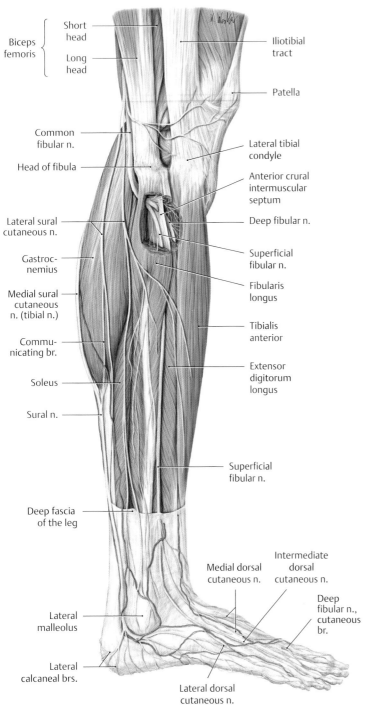

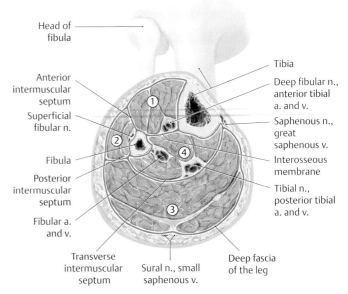

Table 34.10	**Compartments of the leg**		
Compartment		**Muscular contents**	**Neurovascular contents**
① Anterior compartment		Tibialis anterior	Deep fibular n. Anterior tibial a. and v.
		Extensor digitorum longus	
		Extensor hallucis longus	
		Fibularis tertius	
② Lateral compartment		Fibularis longus	Superficial fibular n.
		Fibularis brevis	
Posterior compartment	③ Superficial part	Triceps surae (gastrocnemius and soleus)	—
		Plantaris	
	④ Deep part	Tibialis posterior	Tibial n. Posterior tibial a. and v. Fibular a. and v.
		Flexor digitorum longus	
		Flexor hallucis longus	

Fig. 34.40 Neurovasculature of the anterior compartment of the leg and foot

Right limb with foot in plantar flexion.

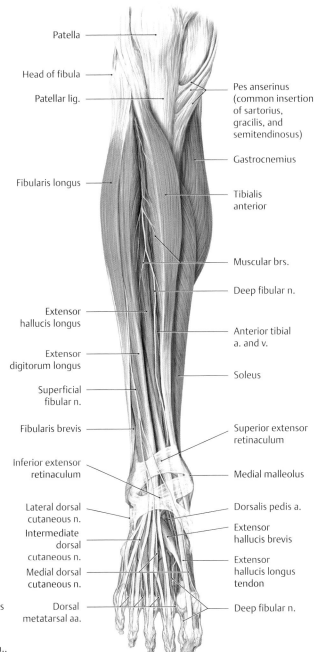

B Neurovasculature of the leg. *Removed:* Skin, subcutaneous tissue, and fasciae. *Retracted:* Tibialis anterior and extensor hallucis longus.

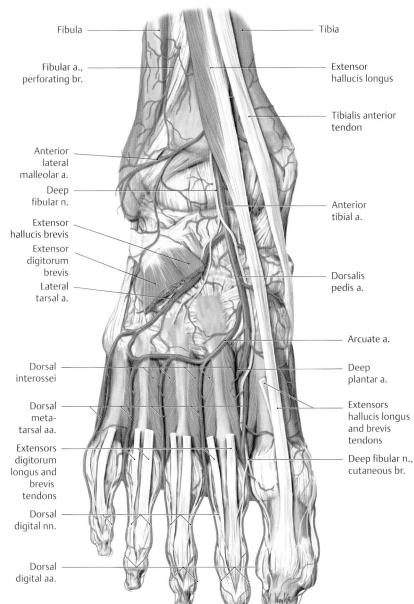

A Neurovasculature of the dorsum of the foot.

491

Topography of the Sole of the Foot

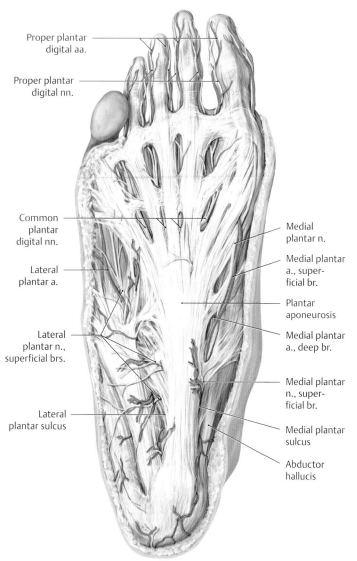

Proper plantar digital aa.

Proper plantar digital nn.

Common plantar digital nn.

Lateral plantar a.

Lateral plantar n., superficial brs.

Lateral plantar sulcus

Medial plantar n.

Medial plantar a., superficial br.

Plantar aponeurosis

Medial plantar a., deep br.

Medial plantar n., superficial br.

Medial plantar sulcus

Abductor hallucis

A Superficial layer. *Removed:* Skin, subcutaneous tissue, and fascia.

Fig. 34.41 Neurovasculature of the sole of the foot
Right foot, plantar view.

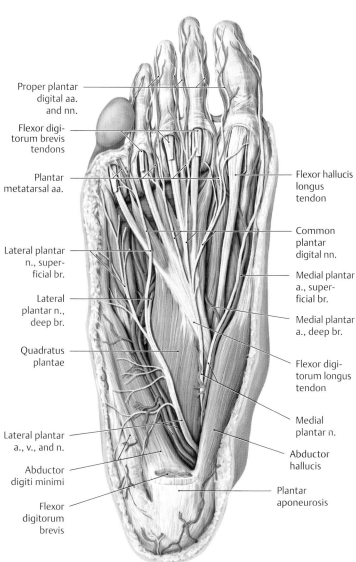

Proper plantar digital aa. and nn.

Flexor digitorum brevis tendons

Plantar metatarsal aa.

Lateral plantar n., superficial br.

Lateral plantar n., deep br.

Quadratus plantae

Lateral plantar a., v., and n.

Abductor digiti minimi

Flexor digitorum brevis

Flexor hallucis longus tendon

Common plantar digital nn.

Medial plantar a., superficial br.

Medial plantar a., deep br.

Flexor digitorum longus tendon

Medial plantar n.

Abductor hallucis

Plantar aponeurosis

B Middle layer. *Removed:* Plantar aponeurosis and flexor digitorum brevis.

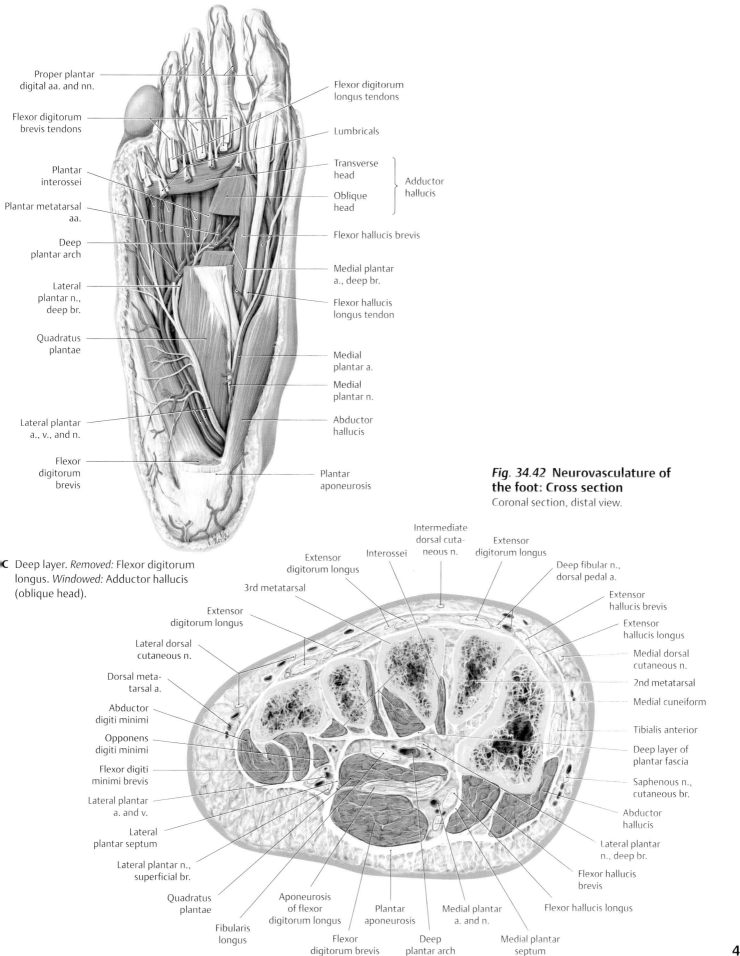

Proper plantar digital aa. and nn.

Flexor digitorum brevis tendons

Plantar interossei

Plantar metatarsal aa.

Deep plantar arch

Lateral plantar n., deep br.

Quadratus plantae

Lateral plantar a., v., and n.

Flexor digitorum brevis

Flexor digitorum longus tendons

Lumbricals

Transverse head

Oblique head

} Adductor hallucis

Flexor hallucis brevis

Medial plantar a., deep br.

Flexor hallucis longus tendon

Medial plantar a.

Medial plantar n.

Abductor hallucis

Plantar aponeurosis

Fig. 34.42 Neurovasculature of the foot: Cross section
Coronal section, distal view.

C Deep layer. *Removed:* Flexor digitorum longus. *Windowed:* Adductor hallucis (oblique head).

Extensor digitorum longus

3rd metatarsal

Extensor digitorum longus

Lateral dorsal cutaneous n.

Dorsal metatarsal a.

Abductor digiti minimi

Opponens digiti minimi

Flexor digiti minimi brevis

Lateral plantar a. and v.

Lateral plantar septum

Lateral plantar n., superficial br.

Quadratus plantae

Fibularis longus

Aponeurosis of flexor digitorum longus

Flexor digitorum brevis

Plantar aponeurosis

Deep plantar arch

Medial plantar a. and n.

Medial plantar septum

Interossei

Intermediate dorsal cutaneous n.

Extensor digitorum longus

Deep fibular n., dorsal pedal a.

Extensor hallucis brevis

Extensor hallucis longus

Medial dorsal cutaneous n.

2nd metatarsal

Medial cuneiform

Tibialis anterior

Deep layer of plantar fascia

Saphenous n., cutaneous br.

Abductor hallucis

Lateral plantar n., deep br.

Flexor hallucis brevis

Flexor hallucis longus

Sectional Anatomy of the Lower Limb

Fig. 35.1 **Compartments of the lower limb**
Right limb, transverse section, distal (inferior) view.

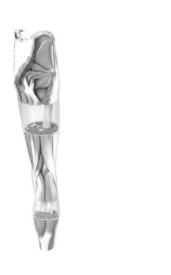

Anterior ↑

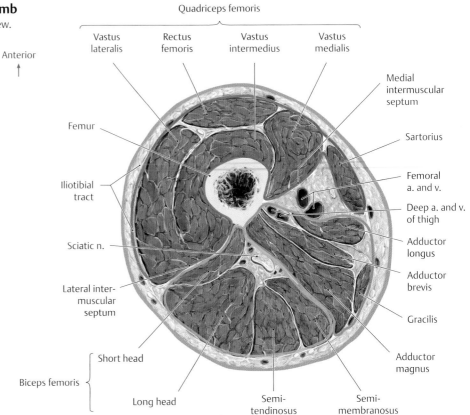

Quadriceps femoris

- Vastus lateralis
- Rectus femoris
- Vastus intermedius
- Vastus medialis

Medial intermuscular septum

Sartorius

Femoral a. and v.

Deep a. and v. of thigh

Adductor longus

Adductor brevis

Gracilis

Adductor magnus

Femur

Iliotibial tract

Sciatic n.

Lateral inter- muscular septum

Biceps femoris
- Short head
- Long head

Semi- tendinosus

Semi- membranosus

A Thigh. Anterior compartment–red; posterior compartment–green, medial compartment–orange.

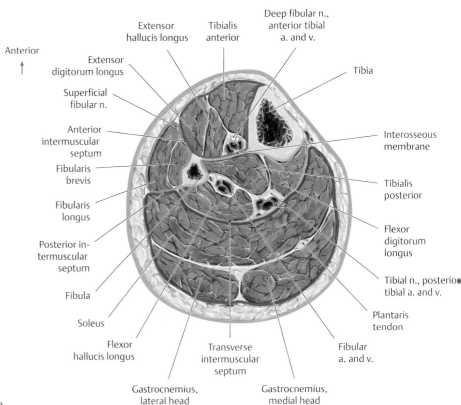

Anterior ↑

Extensor hallucis longus

Tibialis anterior

Deep fibular n., anterior tibial a. and v.

Extensor digitorum longus

Superficial fibular n.

Anterior intermuscular septum

Fibularis brevis

Fibularis longus

Posterior in- termuscular septum

Fibula

Soleus

Flexor hallucis longus

Transverse intermuscular septum

Gastrocnemius, lateral head

Gastrocnemius, medial head

Tibia

Interosseous membrane

Tibialis posterior

Flexor digitorum longus

Tibial n., posterior tibial a. and v.

Plantaris tendon

Fibular a. and v.

B Leg. Anterior compartment–red; deep posterior compartment–green, superficial posterior compartment–blue, lateral compartment–orange.

Fig. 35.2 MRI of right thigh

Transverse section, distal (inferior) view.

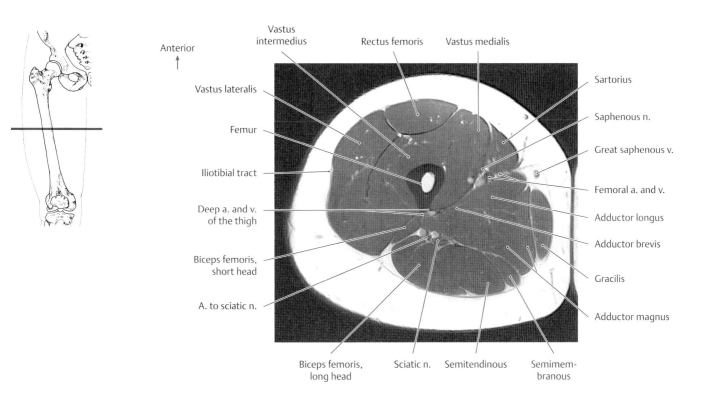

Anterior

Vastus intermedius — Rectus femoris — Vastus medialis

Vastus lateralis

Femur

Iliotibial tract

Deep a. and v. of the thigh

Biceps femoris, short head

A. to sciatic n.

Sartorius

Saphenous n.

Great saphenous v.

Femoral a. and v.

Adductor longus

Adductor brevis

Gracilis

Adductor magnus

Biceps femoris, long head — Sciatic n. — Semitendinous — Semimembranous

Fig. 35.3 MRI of right leg

Transverse section, distal (inferior) view.

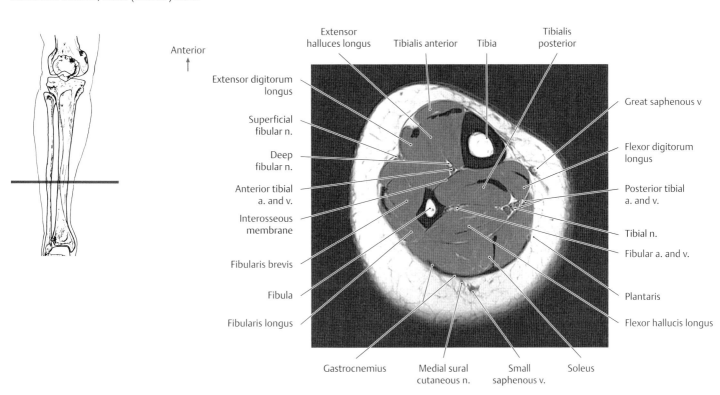

Anterior

Extensor halluces longus — Tibialis anterior — Tibia — Tibialis posterior

Extensor digitorum longus

Superficial fibular n.

Deep fibular n.

Anterior tibial a. and v.

Interosseous membrane

Fibularis brevis

Fibula

Fibularis longus

Great saphenous v

Flexor digitorum longus

Posterior tibial a. and v.

Tibial n.

Fibular a. and v.

Plantaris

Flexor hallucis longus

Gastrocnemius — Medial sural cutaneous n. — Small saphenous v. — Soleus

Radiographic Anatomy of the Lower Limb (I)

Fig. 35.4 **Radiograph of the right hip joint**
Anteroposterior view.

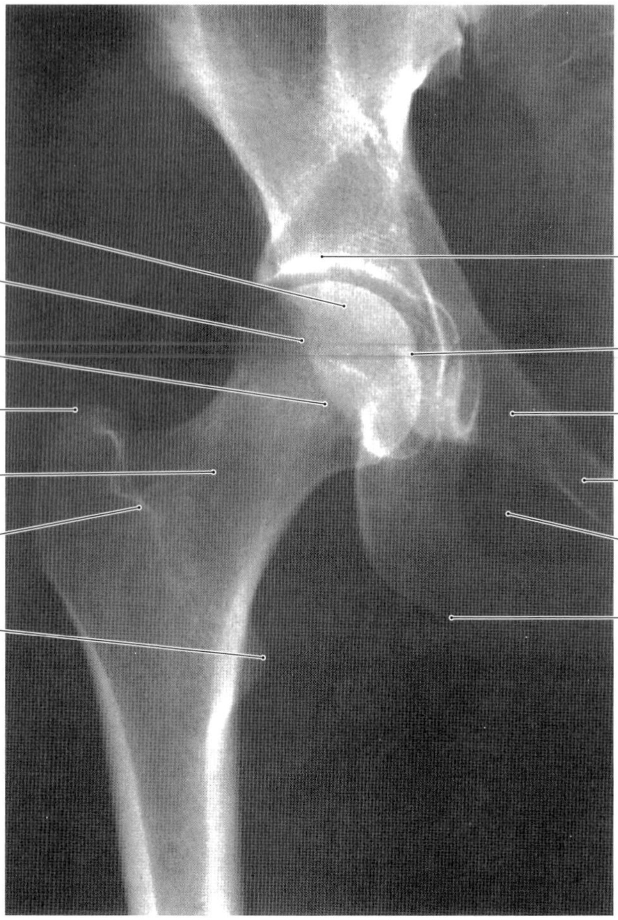

Anterior acetabular rim

Posterior acetabular rim

Femoral head

Greater trochanter

Femoral neck

Intertrochanteric crest

Lesser trochanter

Roof of the acetabulum

Fovea of the femoral head

Köhler's teardrop figure

Superior pubic ramus

Obturator foramen

Ischial tuberosity

Fig. 35.5 **Radiograph of right hip joint with limb abducted laterally (Lauenstein view)**

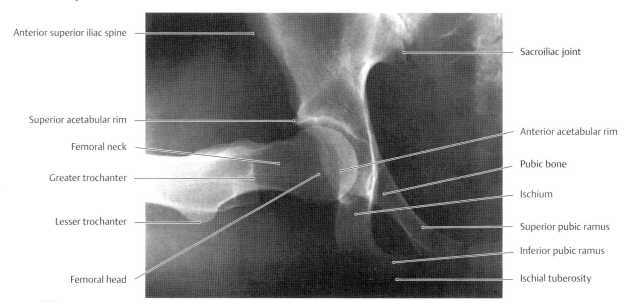

Anterior superior iliac spine

Superior acetabular rim

Femoral neck

Greater trochanter

Lesser trochanter

Femoral head

Sacroiliac joint

Anterior acetabular rim

Pubic bone

Ischium

Superior pubic ramus

Inferior pubic ramus

Ischial tuberosity

Fig. 35.6 MRI of the right hip joint
Transverse section, inferior view.

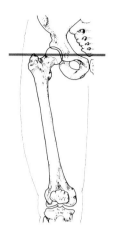

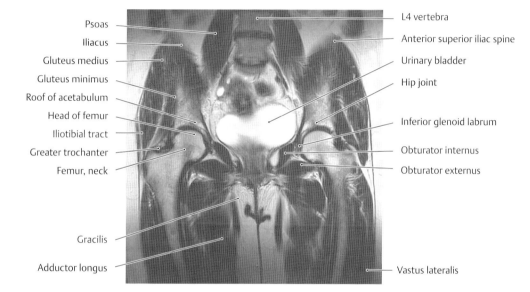

Sartorius
Iliopsoas
Tensor fascia lata
Head of femur
Gluteus medius
Iliotibial tract
Gemellus inferior
Sciatic n.

Femoral a., v., and n.
Urinary bladder
Pubis, superior ramus
Obturator a., v., and n.
Rectum
Levator ani
Obturator internus
Ischium
Gluteus maximus

Fig. 35.7 MRI of the hip joints
Coronal section, anterior view.

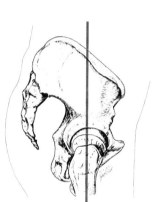

Psoas
Iliacus
Gluteus medius
Gluteus minimus
Roof of acetabulum
Head of femur
Iliotibial tract
Greater trochanter
Femur, neck
Gracilis
Adductor longus

L4 vertebra
Anterior superior iliac spine
Urinary bladder
Hip joint
Inferior glenoid labrum
Obturator internus
Obturator externus
Vastus lateralis

Fig. 35.8 MRI of the right hip joint
Sagittal section, medial view.

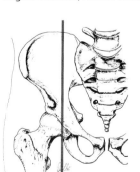

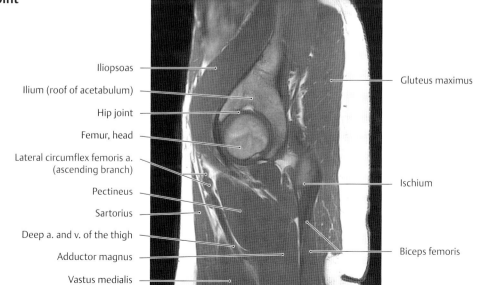

Iliopsoas
Ilium (roof of acetabulum)
Hip joint
Femur, head
Lateral circumflex femoris a.
(ascending branch)
Pectineus
Sartorius
Deep a. and v. of the thigh
Adductor magnus
Vastus medialis

Gluteus maximus
Ischium
Biceps femoris

Radiographic Anatomy of the Lower Limb (II)

Fig. 35.9 **Radiograph of the right knee joint**
Anteroposterior view.

Femur

Patella

Lateral femoral epicondyle

Medial femoral epicondyle

Growth plate

Lateral femoral condyle

Medial femoral condyle

Medial tibial condyle

Lateral tibial condyle

Medial and lateral tubercles of intercondylar eminence

Epiphyseal plate

Fibular head

Tibia

Fibula

Cortex

Fig. 35.10 **Radiograph of the knee in flexion**

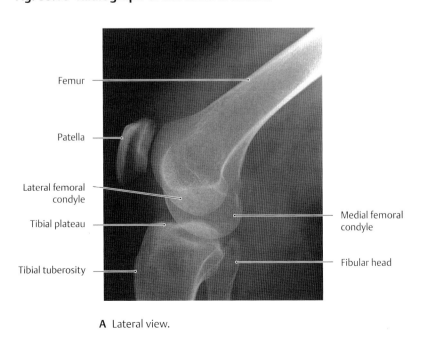

Femur

Patella

Lateral femoral condyle

Medial femoral condyle

Tibial plateau

Fibular head

Tibial tuberosity

A Lateral view.

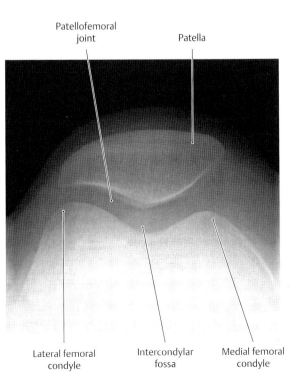

Patellofemoral joint

Patella

Lateral femoral condyle

Intercondylar fossa

Medial femoral condyle

B Sunrise view.

Fig. 35.11 MRI of the knee joint

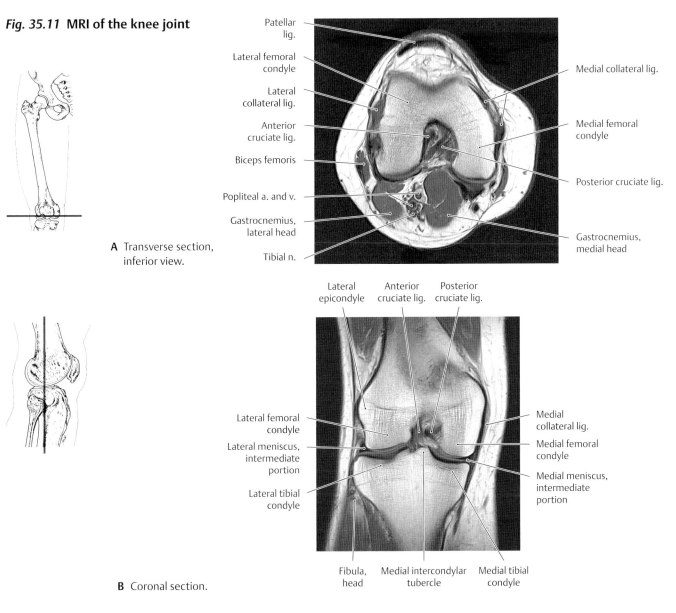

Patellar lig.

Lateral femoral condyle

Lateral collateral lig.

Anterior cruciate lig.

Biceps femoris

Popliteal a. and v.

Gastrocnemius, lateral head

Tibial n.

Medial collateral lig.

Medial femoral condyle

Posterior cruciate lig.

Gastrocnemius, medial head

A Transverse section, inferior view.

Lateral epicondyle

Anterior cruciate lig.

Posterior cruciate lig.

Lateral femoral condyle

Lateral meniscus, intermediate portion

Lateral tibial condyle

Medial collateral lig.

Medial femoral condyle

Medial meniscus, intermediate portion

Fibula, head

Medial intercondylar tubercle

Medial tibial condyle

B Coronal section.

Fig. 35.12 MRI of the knee joint

Sagittal section.

Vastus lateralis

Biceps femoris

Gastrocnemius, lateral head

Femur, lateral condyle

Lateral meniscus, posterior horn

Tibiofibular joint

Fibula, head

A

Lateral meniscus, anterior horn

Lateral tibial condyle

Quadriceps tendon

Popliteal a.

Popliteal v.

Patella

Anterior cruciate lig.

Patellar lig.

B

Infrapatellar fat pad

Posterior cruciate lig.

Radiographic Anatomy of the Lower Limb (III)

Lower Limb

Fig. 35.13 Radiograph of the ankle

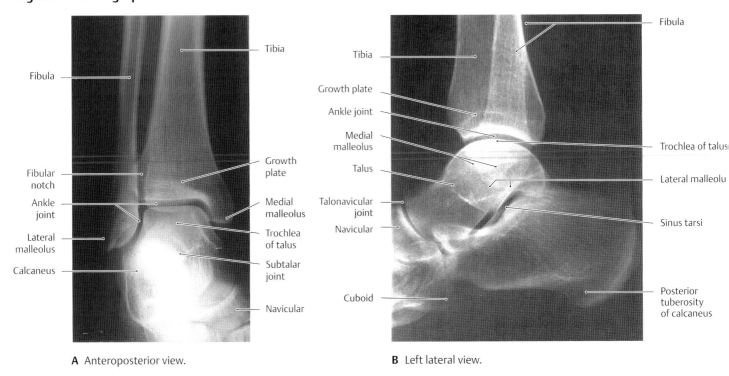

A Anteroposterior view.

B Left lateral view.

Fig. 35.14 Anterior-posterior view of the forefoot

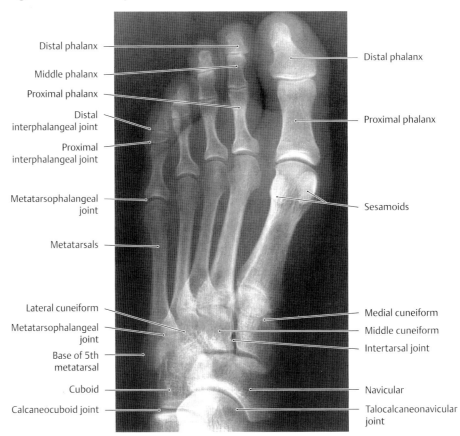

500

Fig. 35.15 MRI of the right ankle
Coronal section, anterior view.

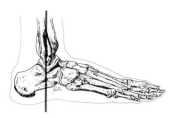

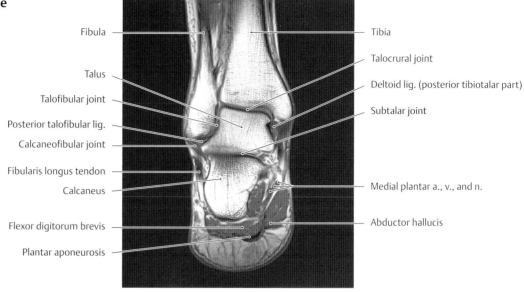

Fibula — Tibia

Talus — Talocrural joint

Talofibular joint — Deltoid lig. (posterior tibiotalar part)

Posterior talofibular lig. — Subtalar joint

Calcaneofibular joint

Fibularis longus tendon

Calcaneus — Medial plantar a., v., and n.

Flexor digitorum brevis — Abductor hallucis

Plantar aponeurosis

Fig. 35.16 MRI of the right foot
Coronal section, anterior (distal) view.

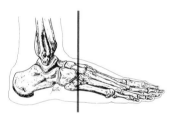

Dorsal ↑

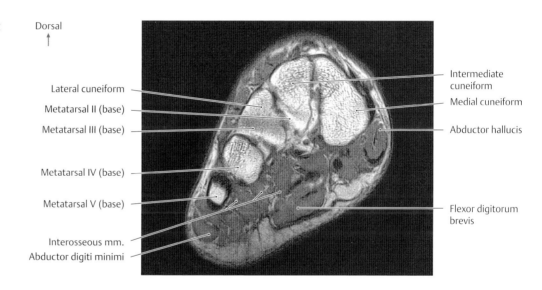

Lateral cuneiform — Intermediate cuneiform

Metatarsal II (base) — Medial cuneiform

Metatarsal III (base) — Abductor hallucis

Metatarsal IV (base)

Metatarsal V (base)

Interosseous mm. — Flexor digitorum brevis

Abductor digiti minimi

Fig. 35.17 MRI of the right foot and ankle
Sagittal section.

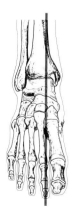

Talonavicular joint — Talocalcaneal interosseous lig. — Talus — Tibia — Talocrural joint

Calcaneal (Achilles) tendon)

Navicular — Subtalar joint

Medial cuneiform — Calcaneous

2 Proximal, middle, and distal phalanx of second toe — Plantar calcaneonavicular lig.

Plantar aponeurosis

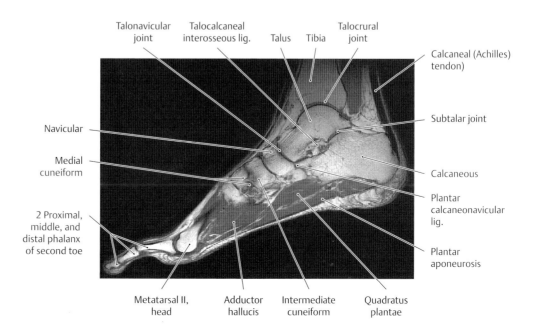

Metatarsal II, head — Adductor hallucis — Intermediate cuneiform — Quadratus plantae

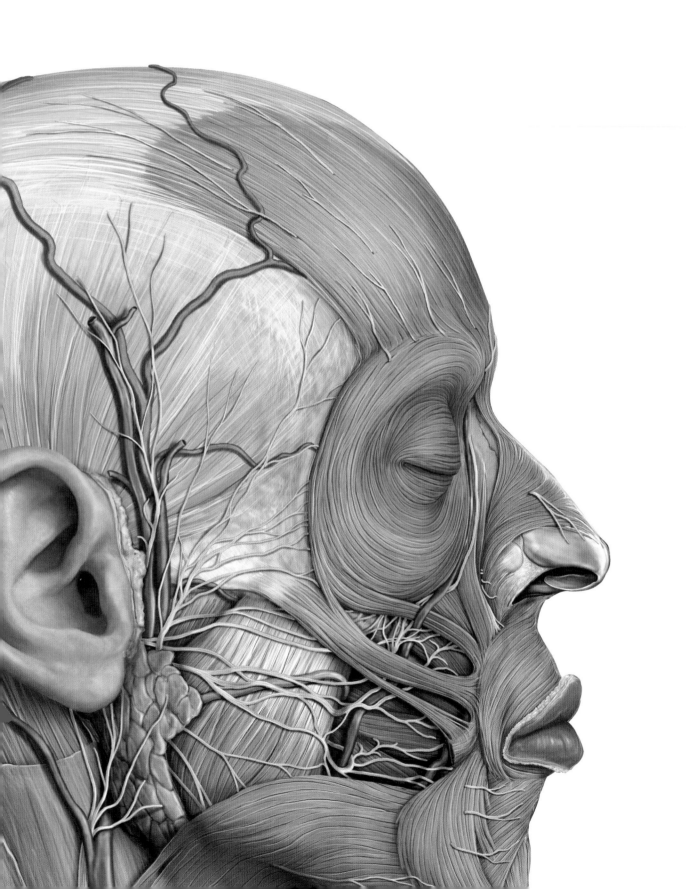

Head & Neck

Surface Anatomy

Fig. 36.1 Regions of the head and neck

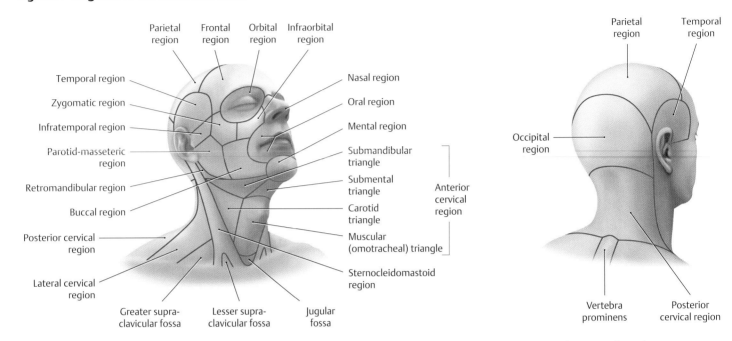

Parietal region — Frontal region — Orbital region — Infraorbital region

Temporal region
Zygomatic region
Infratemporal region
Parotid-masseteric region
Retromandibular region
Buccal region
Posterior cervical region
Lateral cervical region

Nasal region
Oral region
Mental region
Submandibular triangle
Submental triangle
Carotid triangle
Muscular (omotracheal) triangle

Anterior cervical region

Sternocleidomastoid region

Greater supra-clavicular fossa — Lesser supra-clavicular fossa — Jugular fossa

A Right anterolateral view.

Parietal region — Temporal region

Occipital region

Vertebra prominens — Posterior cervical region

B Right posterolateral view.

Fig. 36.2 Surface anatomy of the head and neck

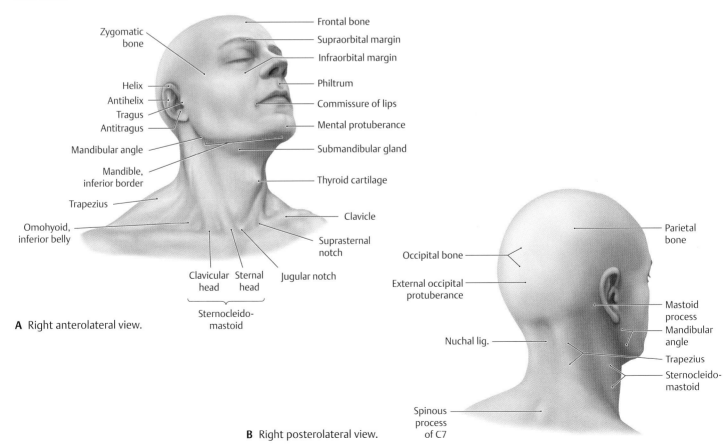

Zygomatic bone

Helix
Antihelix
Tragus
Antitragus
Mandibular angle
Mandible, inferior border
Trapezius
Omohyoid, inferior belly

Frontal bone
Supraorbital margin
Infraorbital margin
Philtrum
Commissure of lips
Mental protuberance
Submandibular gland
Thyroid cartilage
Clavicle
Suprasternal notch

Clavicular head — Sternal head — Jugular notch

Sternocleido-mastoid

A Right anterolateral view.

Occipital bone
External occipital protuberance
Nuchal lig.

Parietal bone

Mastoid process
Mandibular angle
Trapezius
Sternocleido-mastoid

Spinous process of C7

B Right posterolateral view.

Fig. 36.3 **Palpable bony prominences of the head and neck**

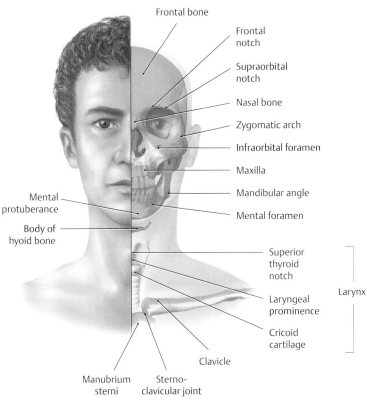

Frontal bone

Frontal notch

Supraorbital notch

Nasal bone

Zygomatic arch

Infraorbital foramen

Maxilla

Mandibular angle

Mental foramen

Mental protuberance

Body of hyoid bone

Superior thyroid notch

Laryngeal prominence

Cricoid cartilage

Larynx

Clavicle

Manubrium sterni

Sterno-clavicular joint

A Anterior view.

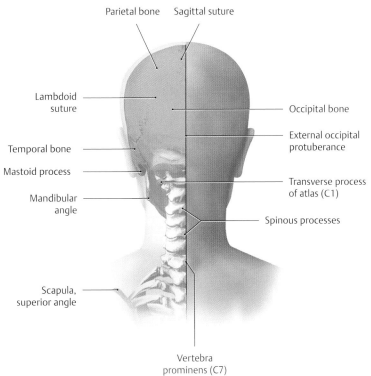

Parietal bone   Sagittal suture

Lambdoid suture

Temporal bone

Mastoid process

Mandibular angle

Scapula, superior angle

Occipital bone

External occipital protuberance

Transverse process of atlas (C1)

Spinous processes

Vertebra prominens (C7)

B Posterior view.

Anterior & Lateral Skull

Fig. 37.1 Lateral skull
Left lateral view.

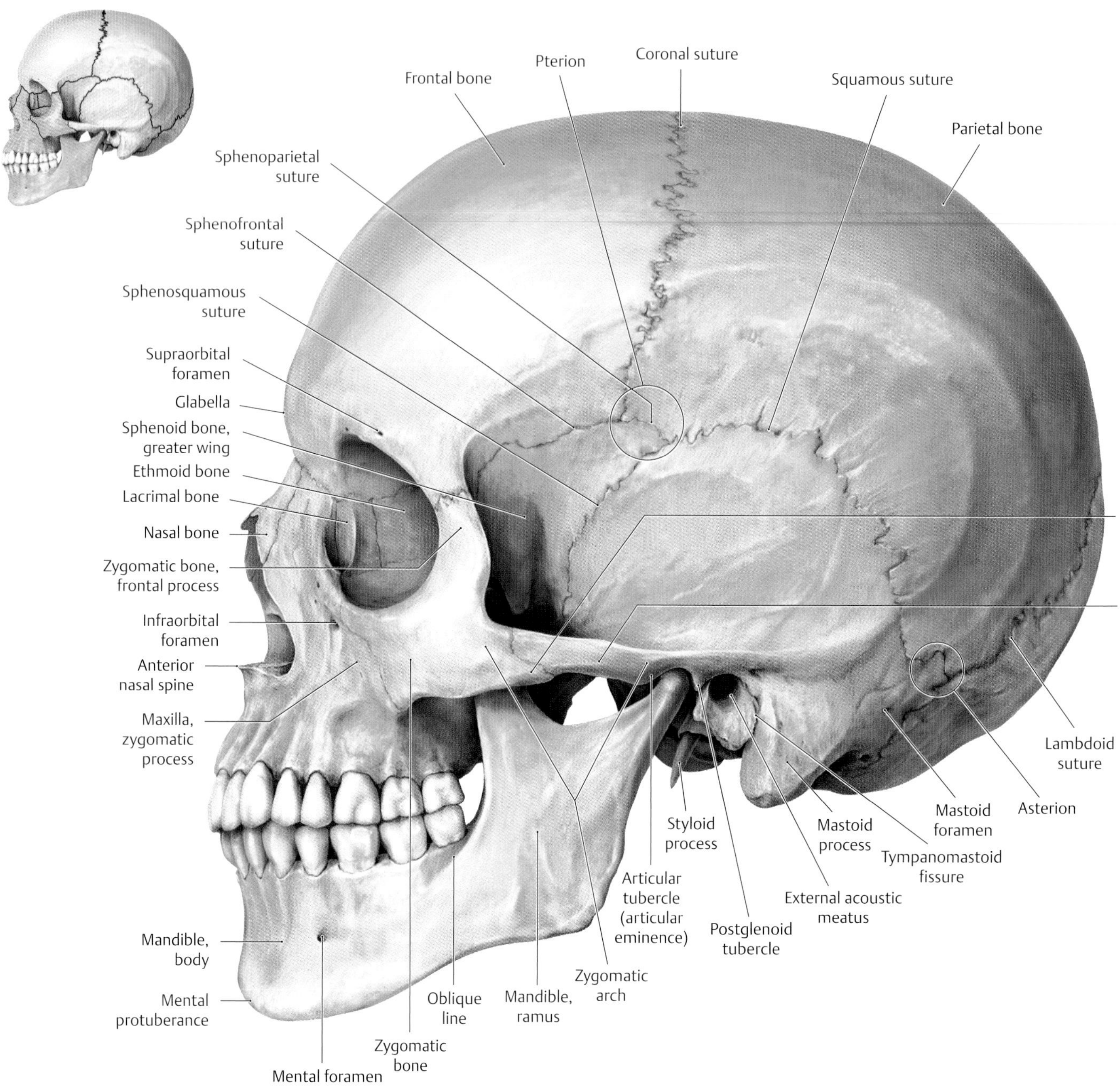
Frontal bone
Pterion
Coronal suture
Squamous suture
Parietal bone
Sphenoparietal suture
Sphenofrontal suture
Sphenosquamous suture
Supraorbital foramen
Glabella
Sphenoid bone, greater wing
Ethmoid bone
Lacrimal bone
Nasal bone
Zygomatic bone, frontal process
Infraorbital foramen
Anterior nasal spine
Maxilla, zygomatic process
Mandible, body
Mental protuberance
Mental foramen
Zygomatic bone
Oblique line
Mandible, ramus
Zygomatic arch
Articular tubercle (articular eminence)
Styloid process
Postglenoid tubercle
External acoustic meatus
Mastoid process
Tympanomastoid fissure
Mastoid foramen
Asterion
Lambdoid suture
Zygomatic bone, temporal process
Temporal bone, zygomatic process

Table 37.1 Bones of the skull

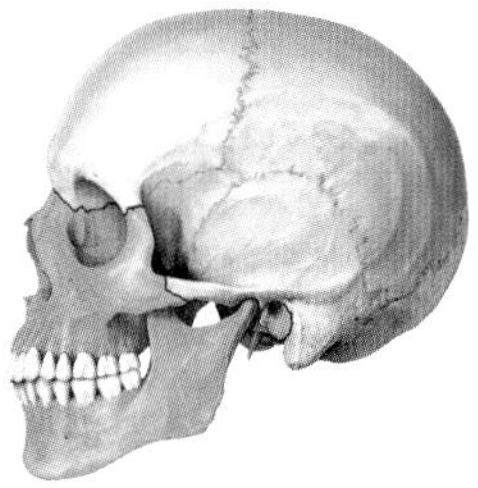

The skull is subdivided into the neurocranium (gray) and viscerocranium (orange). The neurocranium protects the brain, while the viscerocranium houses and protects the facial regions.

Neurocranium	Viscerocranium	
• Ethmoid bone (cribriform plate)*	• Ethmoid bone	• Mandible
• Frontal bone	• Hyoid bone	• Maxilla
• Occipital bone	• Inferior nasal concha	• Nasal bone
• Parietal bone	• Lacrimal bone	• Palatine bone
• Sphenoid bone	• Sphenoid bone (pterygoid process)	
• Temporal bone (petrous and squamous parts)	• Temporal bone	
	• Vomer	

*Most of the ethmoid bone is in the viscerocranium; most of the sphenoid bone is in the neurocranium. The temporal bone is divided between the two.

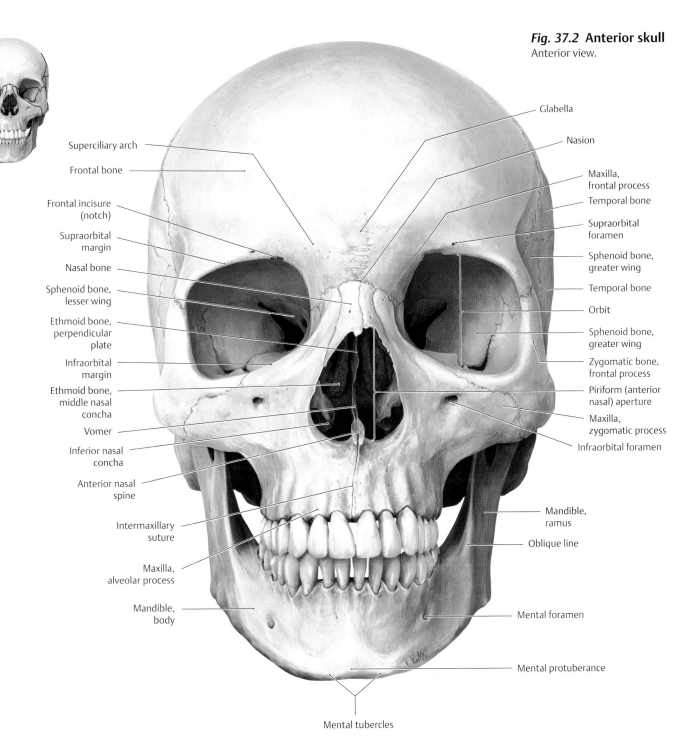

Fig. 37.2 **Anterior skull**
Anterior view.

Glabella

Nasion

Superciliary arch

Frontal bone

Maxilla, frontal process

Temporal bone

Frontal incisure (notch)

Supraorbital foramen

Supraorbital margin

Sphenoid bone, greater wing

Nasal bone

Temporal bone

Sphenoid bone, lesser wing

Orbit

Ethmoid bone, perpendicular plate

Sphenoid bone, greater wing

Infraorbital margin

Zygomatic bone, frontal process

Ethmoid bone, middle nasal concha

Piriform (anterior nasal) aperture

Vomer

Maxilla, zygomatic process

Inferior nasal concha

Infraorbital foramen

Anterior nasal spine

Intermaxillary suture

Mandible, ramus

Oblique line

Maxilla, alveolar process

Mandible, body

Mental foramen

Mental protuberance

Mental tubercles

Fractures of the face

The framelike construction of the facial skeleton leads to characteristic patterns for fracture lines (classified as Le Fort I, II, and III fractures).

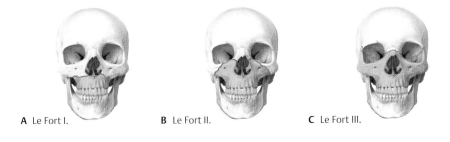

A Le Fort I.   **B** Le Fort II.   **C** Le Fort III.

Posterior Skull & Calvaria

Fig. 37.3 **Posterior skull**
Posterior view.

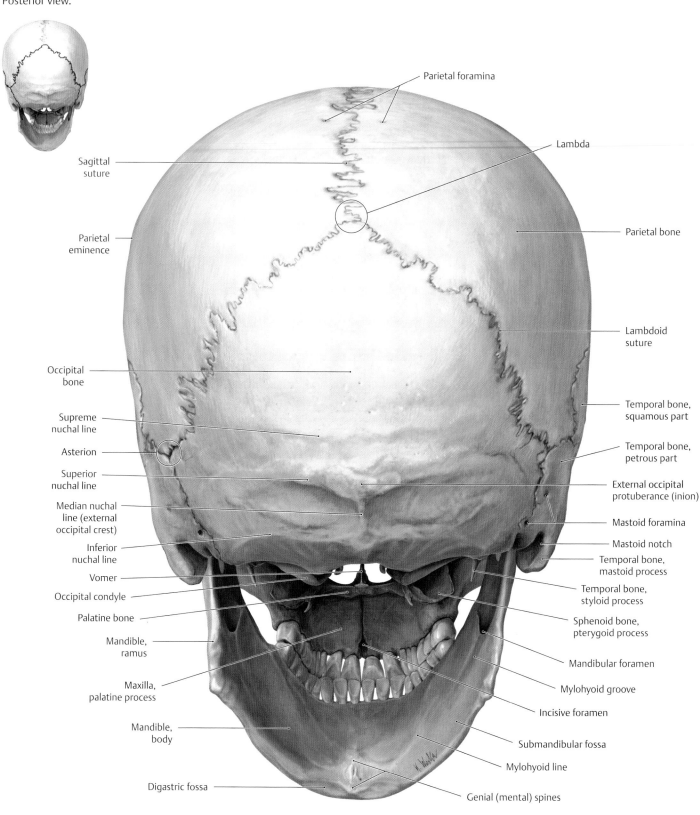

Parietal foramina

Lambda

Sagittal suture

Parietal bone

Parietal eminence

Lambdoid suture

Occipital bone

Temporal bone, squamous part

Supreme nuchal line

Temporal bone, petrous part

Asterion

External occipital protuberance (inion)

Superior nuchal line

Mastoid foramina

Median nuchal line (external occipital crest)

Mastoid notch

Inferior nuchal line

Temporal bone, mastoid process

Vomer

Temporal bone, styloid process

Occipital condyle

Sphenoid bone, pterygoid process

Palatine bone

Mandibular foramen

Mandible, ramus

Mylohyoid groove

Maxilla, palatine process

Incisive foramen

Mandible, body

Submandibular fossa

Mylohyoid line

Digastric fossa

Genial (mental) spines

Fig. 37.4 **Calvaria**

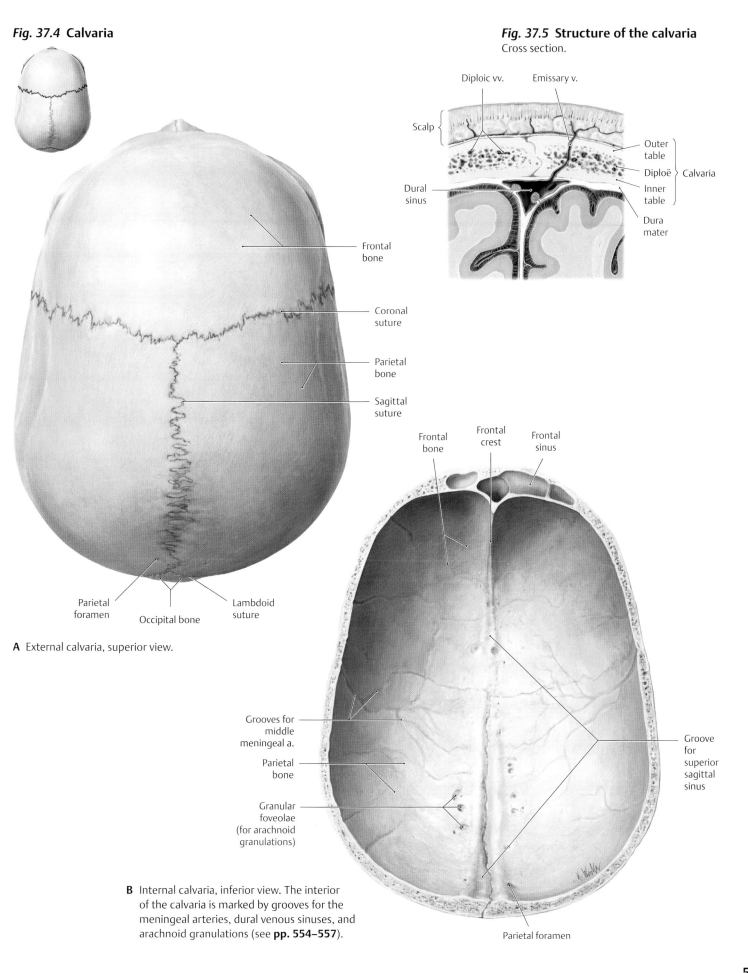

Fig. 37.5 **Structure of the calvaria**
Cross section.

Diploic vv.   Emissary v.

Scalp

Outer table
Diploë ⟩ Calvaria
Inner table

Dural sinus

Dura mater

Frontal bone

Coronal suture

Parietal bone

Sagittal suture

Parietal foramen   Lambdoid suture
Occipital bone

A External calvaria, superior view.

Frontal bone   Frontal crest   Frontal sinus

Grooves for middle meningeal a.

Parietal bone

Granular foveolae (for arachnoid granulations)

Groove for superior sagittal sinus

Parietal foramen

B Internal calvaria, inferior view. The interior of the calvaria is marked by grooves for the meningeal arteries, dural venous sinuses, and arachnoid granulations (see **pp. 554–557**).

509

Base of the Skull

Fig. 37.6 Base of the skull: Exterior
Inferior view. *Revealed:* Foramina and canals for blood vessels
(see **p. 546**) and cranial nerves. *Note:* This view allows visual
access into the posterior region of the nasal cavity.

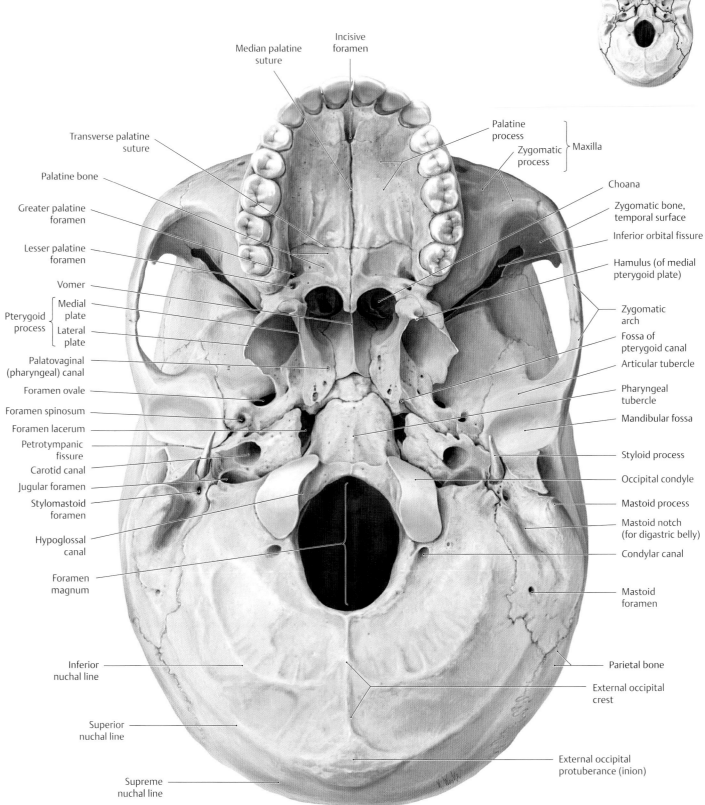

Incisive
foramen

Median palatine
suture

Transverse palatine
suture

Palatine bone

Greater palatine
foramen

Lesser palatine
foramen

Vomer

Pterygoid
process { Medial
plate

Lateral
plate

Palatovaginal
(pharyngeal) canal

Foramen ovale

Foramen spinosum

Foramen lacerum

Petrotympanic
fissure

Carotid canal

Jugular foramen

Stylomastoid
foramen

Hypoglossal
canal

Foramen
magnum

Inferior
nuchal line

Superior
nuchal line

Supreme
nuchal line

Palatine
process

Zygomatic
process } Maxilla

Choana

Zygomatic bone,
temporal surface

Inferior orbital fissure

Hamulus (of medial
pterygoid plate)

Zygomatic
arch

Fossa of
pterygoid canal

Articular tubercle

Pharyngeal
tubercle

Mandibular fossa

Styloid process

Occipital condyle

Mastoid process

Mastoid notch
(for digastric belly)

Condylar canal

Mastoid
foramen

Parietal bone

External occipital
crest

External occipital
protuberance (inion)

Fig. 37.7 Cranial fossae

The interior of the skull base consists of three successive fossae that become progressively deeper in the frontal-to-occipital direction.

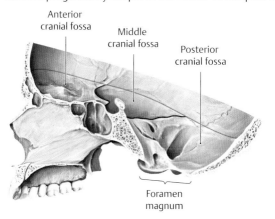

A Midsagittal section, left lateral view.

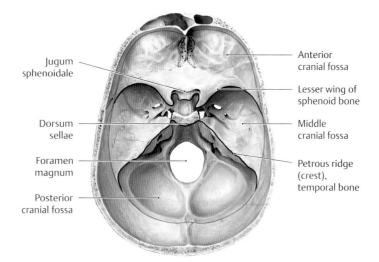

B Superior view of opened skull.

Fig. 37.8 Base of the skull: Interior

Superior view.

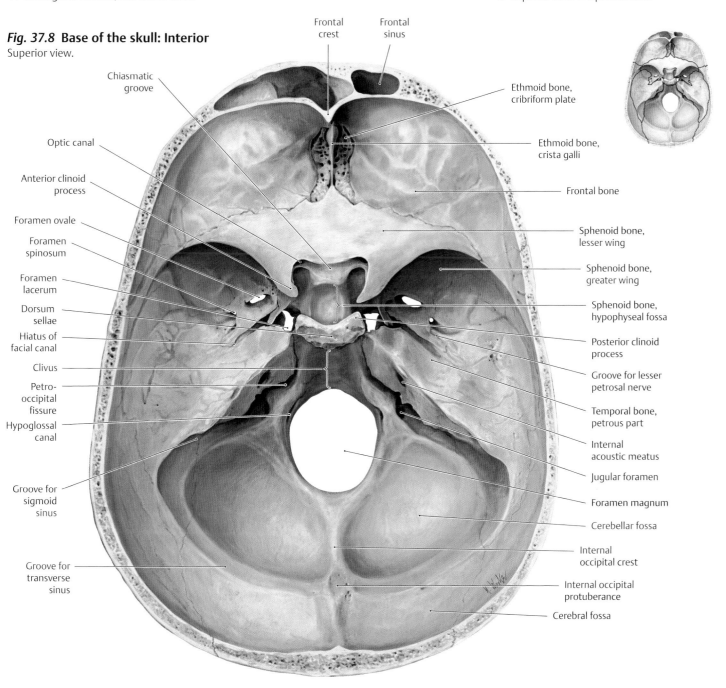

Neurovascular Pathways Exiting or Entering the Cranial Cavity

Fig. 37.9 **Summary of the neurovascular structures exiting or entering the cranial cavity**

Cribriform plate

Olfactory n., anterior and posterior ethmoidal aa.

Optic canal

Optic n., ophthalmic a.

Superior orbital fissure

① Superior oph-thalmic v.
② Lacrimal n.
③ Frontal n.
④ Trochlear n.
⑤ Abducent n.
⑥ Oculomotor n.
⑦ Nasociliary n.

Foramen rotundum

Maxillary n. (CN V₂)

Foramen ovale

Mandibular n. (CN V₃), lesser petrosal n. accessory meningeal a.

Carotid canal

Internal carotid a., internal carotid sympathetic plexus

Foramen spinosum

Middle meningeal a., meningeal br. of mandibular n. (CN V₃)

Hiatus of canal for lesser petrosal n.

Lesser petrosal n., superior tympanic a.

Hiatus of canal for greater petrosal n.

Greater petrosal n.

Internal acoustic meatus

Labyrinthine a. and v.
① Vestibulocochlear n.
② Facial n.

Incisive canal

Nasopalatine n., nasopalatine a.

Greater palatine foramen

Greater palatine n. and a.

Lesser palatine foramina

Lesser palatine n. and a.

Foramen lacerum

Deep petrosal n., greater petrosal n.

Foramen spinosum

Middle meningeal a., meningeal br. of mandibular n. (CN V₃)

Carotid canal

Internal carotid a., internal carotid sympathetic plexus

Petrotympanic fissure

Anterior tympanic a., chorda tympani

Stylomastoid foramen

Facial n., stylomastoid a.

Jugular foramen

① Internal jugular v.
② Glossopharyngeal n.
③ Vagus n.
④ Accessory n.
⑤ Inferior petrosal sinus
⑥ Posterior meningeal a.

Mastoid foramen

Emissary v.

Hypoglossal canal

Hypoglossal n., venous plexus of hypoglossal canal

Condylar canal

Condylar emissary v.

Jugular foramen

① Sigmoid sinus
② Glossopharyngeal n.
③ Vagus n.
④ Accessory n.
⑤ Inferior petrosal sinus
⑥ Posterior meningeal a.

Foramen magnum

① Spinal v.
② Anterior spinal a.
③ Posterior spinal a.
④ Medulla oblongata
⑤ Accessory n.
⑥ Vertebral a.

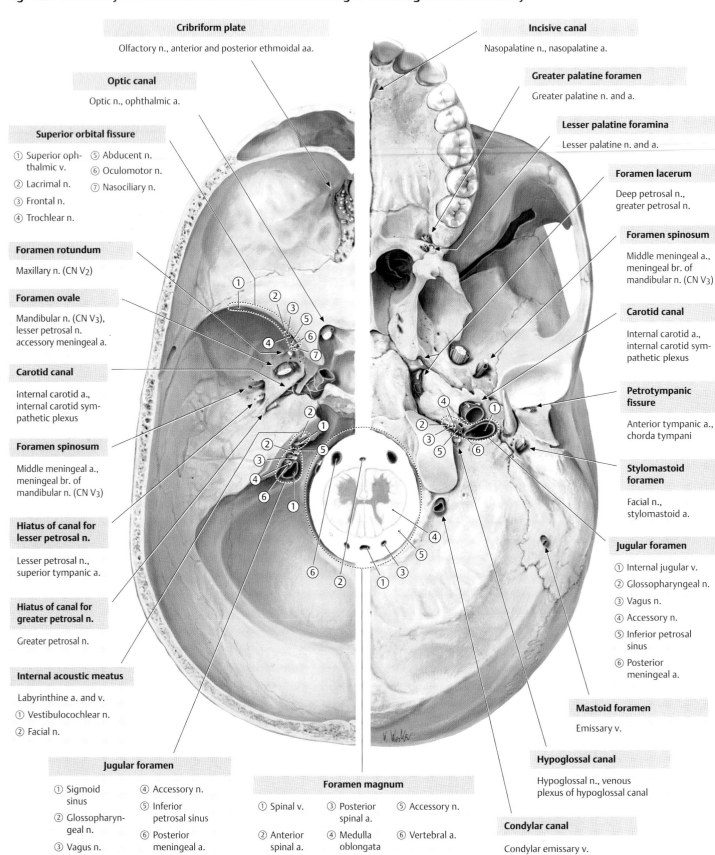

A Cranial cavity (interior of skull base), left side, superior view.

B Exterior of skull base, left side, inferior view

Fig. 37.10 Cranial nerves exiting the cranial cavity

Cranial cavity (interior of skull base), left side, superior view. *Removed:* Brain and tentorium cerebelli. The ends of the cranial nerves have been cut to reveal the fissures, fossa, or dural cave where they pass through the cranial fossa.

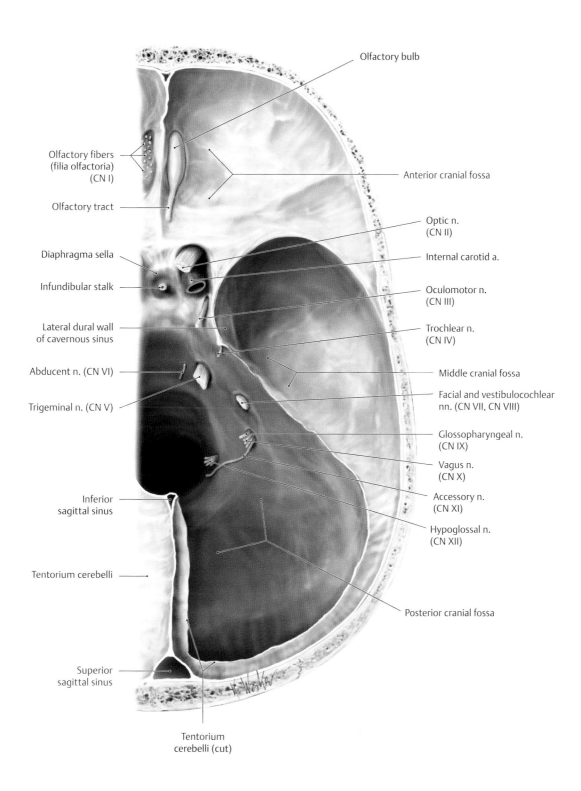

Olfactory bulb

Olfactory fibers (filia olfactoria) (CN I)

Olfactory tract

Anterior cranial fossa

Diaphragma sella

Infundibular stalk

Lateral dural wall of cavernous sinus

Abducent n. (CN VI)

Trigeminal n. (CN V)

Optic n. (CN II)

Internal carotid a.

Oculomotor n. (CN III)

Trochlear n. (CN IV)

Middle cranial fossa

Facial and vestibulocochlear nn. (CN VII, CN VIII)

Glossopharyngeal n. (CN IX)

Vagus n. (CN X)

Accessory n. (CN XI)

Hypoglossal n. (CN XII)

Inferior sagittal sinus

Tentorium cerebelli

Posterior cranial fossa

Superior sagittal sinus

Tentorium cerebelli (cut)

Ethmoid & Sphenoid Bones

 The structurally complex ethmoid and sphenoid bones are shown here in isolation. The other bones of the skull are shown in their respective regions: orbit (see **pp. 556–557**), nasal cavity (see **pp. 580–581**), oral cavity (see **pp. 598–599**), and ear (see **pp. 586–587**).

Fig. 37.11 **Ethmoid bone**

The ethmoid bone is the central bone of the nose and paranasal air sinuses (see **pp. 580–583**).

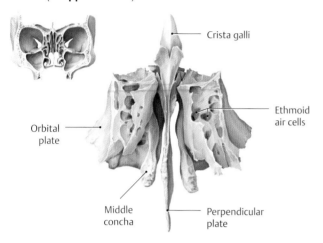

Crista galli

Ethmoid air cells

Orbital plate

Middle concha

Perpendicular plate

A Anterior view.

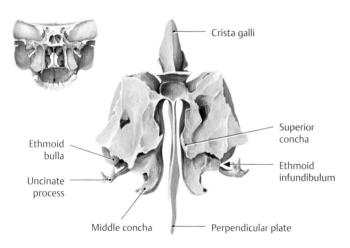

Crista galli

Superior concha

Ethmoid bulla

Uncinate process

Ethmoid infundibulum

Middle concha

Perpendicular plate

C Posterior view.

Perpendicular plate

Crista galli

Ethmoid air cells

Cribriform plate

Orbital plate

B Superior view.

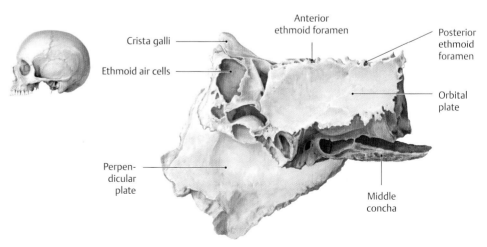

Anterior ethmoid foramen

Posterior ethmoid foramen

Crista galli

Ethmoid air cells

Orbital plate

Perpendicular plate

Middle concha

D Left lateral view.

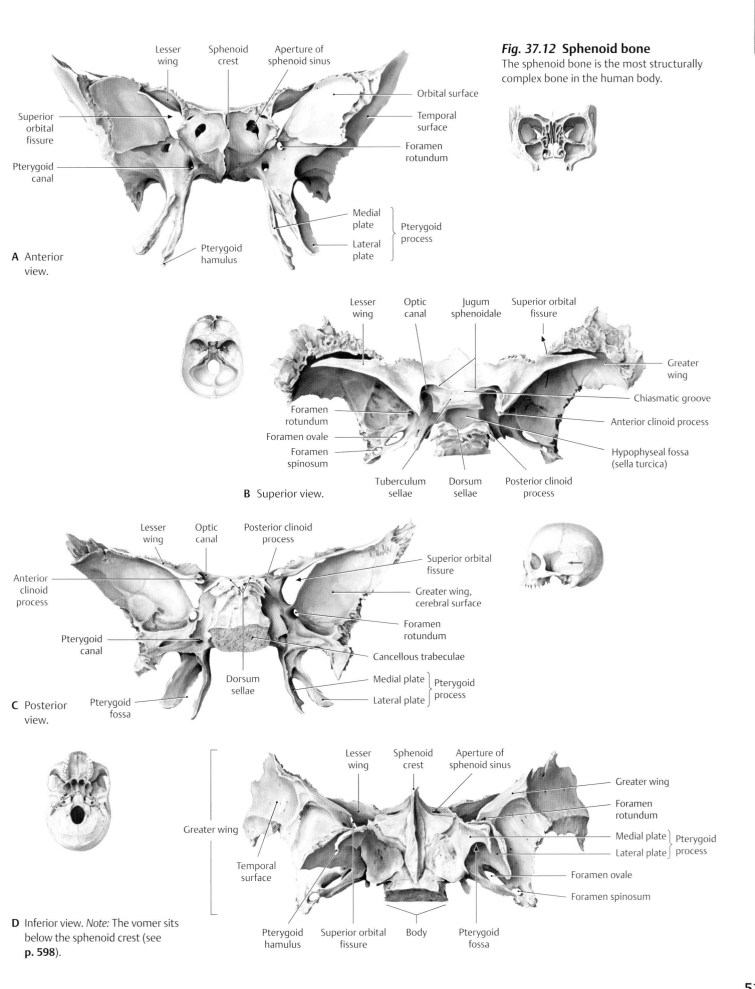

Lesser wing
Sphenoid crest
Aperture of sphenoid sinus
Orbital surface
Temporal surface
Foramen rotundum
Superior orbital fissure
Pterygoid canal
Medial plate
Lateral plate
Pterygoid process
Pterygoid hamulus

A Anterior view.

Lesser wing
Optic canal
Jugum sphenoidale
Superior orbital fissure
Greater wing
Chiasmatic groove
Foramen rotundum
Anterior clinoid process
Foramen ovale
Foramen spinosum
Tuberculum sellae
Dorsum sellae
Posterior clinoid process
Hypophyseal fossa (sella turcica)

B Superior view.

Lesser wing
Optic canal
Posterior clinoid process
Superior orbital fissure
Anterior clinoid process
Greater wing, cerebral surface
Foramen rotundum
Pterygoid canal
Cancellous trabeculae
Dorsum sellae
Medial plate
Lateral plate
Pterygoid process
Pterygoid fossa

C Posterior view.

Lesser wing
Sphenoid crest
Aperture of sphenoid sinus
Greater wing
Foramen rotundum
Medial plate
Lateral plate
Pterygoid process
Foramen ovale
Foramen spinosum
Greater wing
Temporal surface
Pterygoid hamulus
Superior orbital fissure
Body
Pterygoid fossa

D Inferior view. *Note:* The vomer sits below the sphenoid crest (see **p. 598**).

Fig. 37.12 **Sphenoid bone**

The sphenoid bone is the most structurally complex bone in the human body.

Muscles of Facial Expression & of Mastication

 The muscles of the skull and face are divided into two groups. The muscles of facial expression make up the superficial muscle layer in the face. The muscles of mastication are responsible for the movement of the mandible during mastication (chewing).

***Fig. 38.1* Muscles of facial expression**

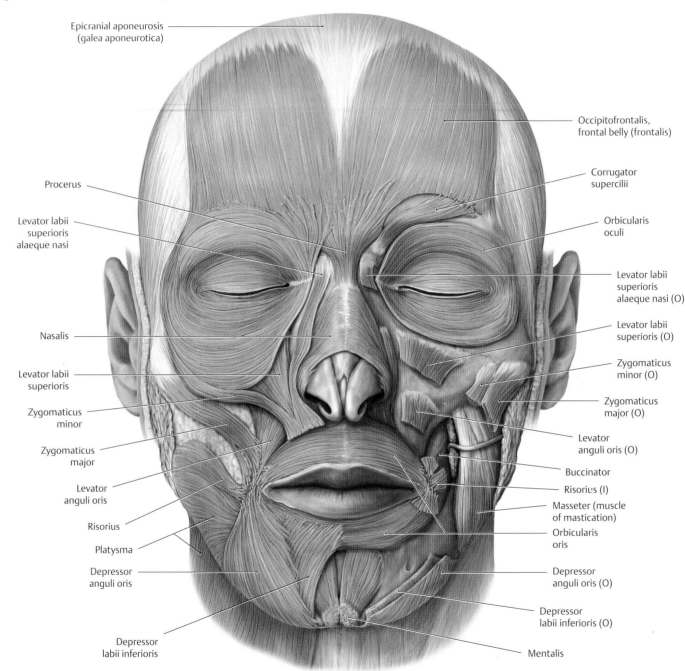

Epicranial aponeurosis
(galea aponeurotica)

Procerus

Levator labii
superioris
alaeque nasi

Nasalis

Levator labii
superioris

Zygomaticus
minor

Zygomaticus
major

Levator
anguli oris

Risorius

Platysma

Depressor
anguli oris

Depressor
labii inferioris

Occipitofrontalis,
frontal belly (frontalis)

Corrugator
supercilii

Orbicularis
oculi

Levator labii
superioris
alaeque nasi (O)

Levator labii
superioris (O)

Zygomaticus
minor (O)

Zygomaticus
major (O)

Levator
anguli oris (O)

Buccinator

Risorius (I)

Masseter (muscle
of mastication)

Orbicularis
oris

Depressor
anguli oris (O)

Depressor
labii inferioris (O)

Mentalis

A Anterior view. Muscle origins (O) and insertions (I) indicated on left side of face.

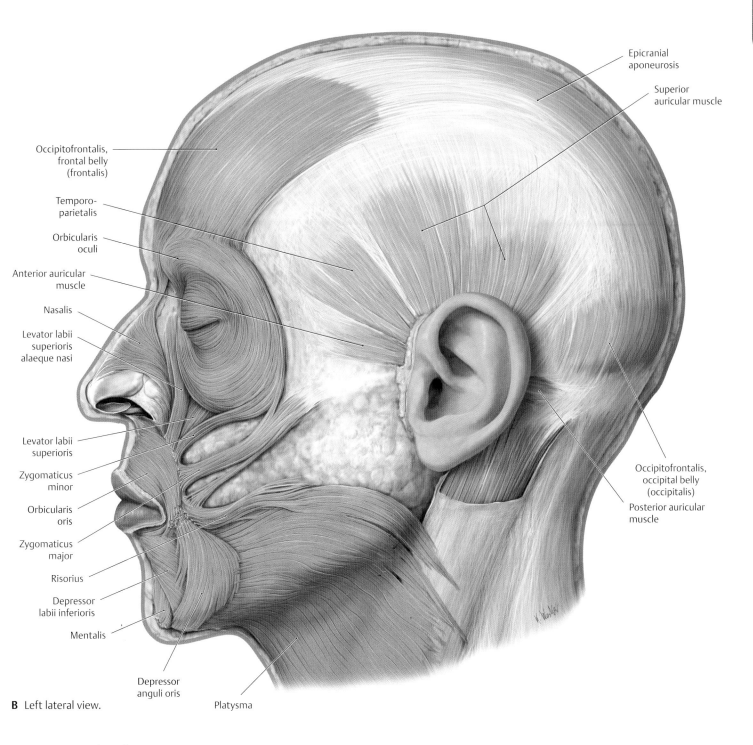

Epicranial
aponeurosis

Superior
auricular muscle

Occipitofrontalis,
frontal belly
(frontalis)

Temporo-
parietalis

Orbicularis
oculi

Anterior auricular
muscle

Nasalis

Levator labii
superioris
alaeque nasi

Levator labii
superioris

Zygomaticus
minor

Orbicularis
oris

Zygomaticus
major

Risorius

Depressor
labii inferioris

Mentalis

Occipitofrontalis,
occipital belly
(occipitalis)

Posterior auricular
muscle

Depressor
anguli oris

Platysma

B Left lateral view.

Fig. 38.2 **Muscles of mastication**
Left lateral view.

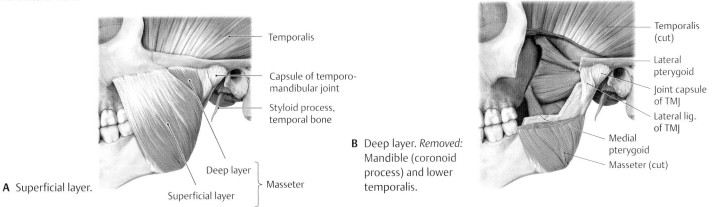

Temporalis

Capsule of temporo-
mandibular joint

Styloid process,
temporal bone

Deep layer

Superficial layer

Masseter

A Superficial layer.

B Deep layer. *Removed:*
Mandible (coronoid
process) and lower
temporalis.

Temporalis
(cut)

Lateral
pterygoid

Joint capsule
of TMJ

Lateral lig.
of TMJ

Medial
pterygoid

Masseter (cut)

Muscle Origins & Insertions on the Skull

Fig. 38.3 Lateral skull: Origins and insertions

Left lateral view. Muscle origins are shown in red, insertions in blue. *Note*: There are generally no bony insertions for the muscles of facial expression. These muscles insert into skin and other muscles of facial expression.

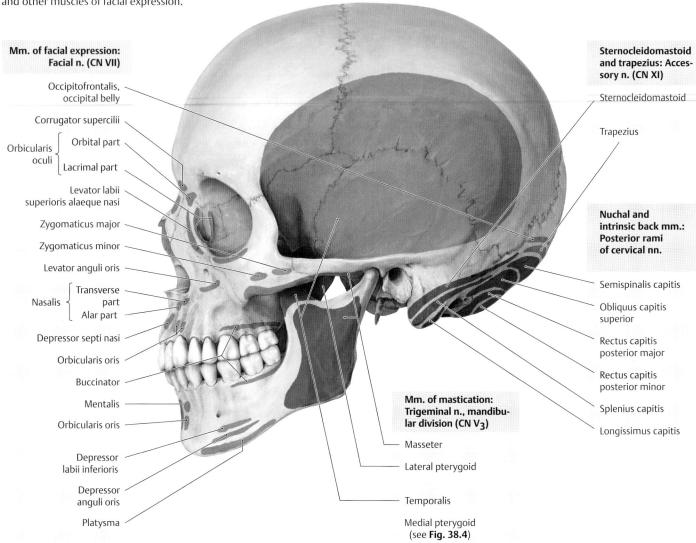

Mm. of facial expression: Facial n. (CN VII)

Occipitofrontalis, occipital belly

Corrugator supercilii

Orbicularis oculi — Orbital part / Lacrimal part

Levator labii superioris alaeque nasi

Zygomaticus major

Zygomaticus minor

Levator anguli oris

Nasalis — Transverse part / Alar part

Depressor septi nasi

Orbicularis oris

Buccinator

Mentalis

Orbicularis oris

Depressor labii inferioris

Depressor anguli oris

Platysma

Sternocleidomastoid and trapezius: Accessory n. (CN XI)

Sternocleidomastoid

Trapezius

Nuchal and intrinsic back mm.: Posterior rami of cervical nn.

Semispinalis capitis

Obliquus capitis superior

Rectus capitis posterior major

Rectus capitis posterior minor

Splenius capitis

Longissimus capitis

Mm. of mastication: Trigeminal n., mandibular division (CN V₃)

Masseter

Lateral pterygoid

Temporalis

Medial pterygoid (see **Fig. 38.4**)

Fig. 38.4 Mandible: Origins and insertions

Medial view of right hemimandible (inner surface). Muscle origins are shown in red, insertions in blue.

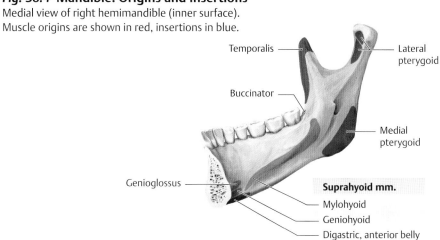

Temporalis

Lateral pterygoid

Buccinator

Medial pterygoid

Genioglossus

Suprahyoid mm.

Mylohyoid

Geniohyoid

Digastric, anterior belly

Fig. 38.5 Skull base: Origins and insertions

Inferior view of external skull.
Muscle origins are shown in red, insertions in blue.

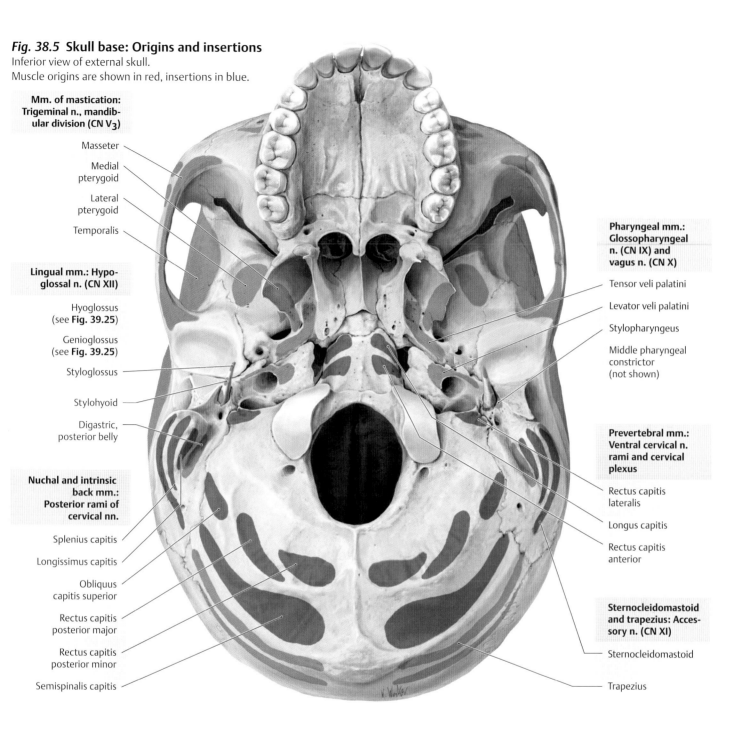

Mm. of mastication: Trigeminal n., mandibular division (CN V₃)

Masseter

Medial pterygoid

Lateral pterygoid

Temporalis

Lingual mm.: Hypoglossal n. (CN XII)

Hyoglossus (see Fig. 39.25)

Genioglossus (see Fig. 39.25)

Styloglossus

Stylohyoid

Digastric, posterior belly

Nuchal and intrinsic back mm.: Posterior rami of cervical nn.

Splenius capitis

Longissimus capitis

Obliquus capitis superior

Rectus capitis posterior major

Rectus capitis posterior minor

Semispinalis capitis

Pharyngeal mm.: Glossopharyngeal n. (CN IX) and vagus n. (CN X)

Tensor veli palatini

Levator veli palatini

Stylopharyngeus

Middle pharyngeal constrictor (not shown)

Prevertebral mm.: Ventral cervical n. rami and cervical plexus

Rectus capitis lateralis

Longus capitis

Rectus capitis anterior

Sternocleidomastoid and trapezius: Accessory n. (CN XI)

Sternocleidomastoid

Trapezius

Fig. 38.6 Hyoid bone: Origins and insertions

The larynx is suspended from the hyoid bone, primarily by the thyrohyoid membrane. The hyoid bone is the site for attachment for the suprahyoid and infrahyoid muscles. Muscle insertions are shown in blue.

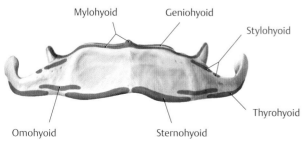

Mylohyoid

Geniohyoid

Stylohyoid

Thyrohyoid

Omohyoid

Sternohyoid

A Anterior view.

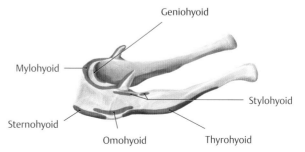

Geniohyoid

Mylohyoid

Sternohyoid

Stylohyoid

Omohyoid

Thyrohyoid

B Oblique left lateral view.

Muscle Facts (I)

 The muscles of facial expression originate on bone and/or fascia and insert into the subcutaneous tissue of the face. This allows them to produce their effects by pulling on the skin.

Fig. 38.7 Occipitofrontalis
Anterior view.

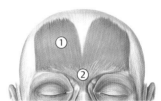

Fig. 38.8 Muscles of the palpebral fissure and nose
Anterior view.

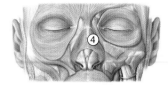

A Orbicularis oculi.

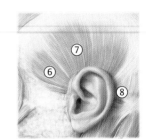

B Nasalis.

Fig. 38.9 Muscles of the ear
Left lateral view.

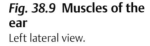

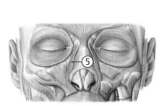

C Levator labii superioris alaeque nasi.

Table 38.1	Muscles of facial expression: Forehead, nose, and ear		
Muscle	**Origin**	**Insertion***	**Main action(s)****
Calvaria			
① Occipitofrontalis (frontal belly)	Epicranial aponeurosis	Skin and subcutaneous tissue of eyebrows and forehead	Elevates eyebrows, wrinkles skin of forehead
Palpebral fissure and nose			
② Procerus	Nasal bone, lateral nasal cartilage (upper part)	Skin of lower forehead between eyebrows	Pulls medial angle of eyebrows inferiorly, producing transverse wrinkles over bridge of nose
③ Orbicularis oculi	Medial orbital margin, medial palpebral ligament, lacrimal bone	Skin around margin of orbit, superior and inferior tarsal plates	Acts as orbital sphincter (closes eyelids) • Palpebral portion gently closes • Orbital portion tightly closes (as in winking)
④ Nasalis	Maxilla (superior region of canine ridge)	Nasal cartilages	Flares nostrils by drawing ala (side) of nose toward nasal septum
⑤ Levator labii superioris alaeque nasi	Maxilla (frontal process)	Alar cartilage of nose and upper lip	Elevates upper lip, opens nostril
Ear			
⑥ Anterior auricular muscle	Temporal fascia (anterior portion)	Helix of the ear	Pulls ear superiorly and anteriorly
⑦ Superior auricular muscle	Epicranial aponeurosis on side of head	Upper portion of auricle	Elevates ear
⑧ Posterior auricular muscle	Mastoid process	Convexity of concha of ear	Pulls ear superiorly and posteriorly

*There are no bony insertions for the muscles of facial expression.
All muscles of facial expression are innervated by the facial nerve (CN VII) via temporal, zygomatic, buccal, mandibular, or cervical branches arising from the parotid plexus (see **pp. 532–533).

Fig. 38.10 Muscles of the mouth

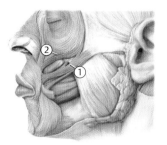

A Zygomaticus major and minor, left lateral view.

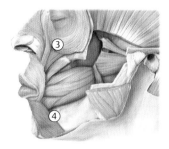

B Levator labii superioris and depressor labii inferioris, left lateral view.

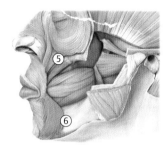

C Levator and depressor anguli oris, left lateral view.

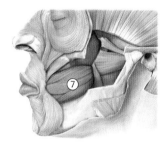

D Buccinator, left lateral view.

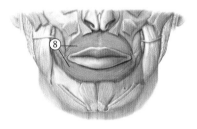

E Orbicularis oris, anterior view.

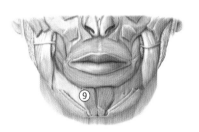

F Mentalis, anterior view.

Table 38.2	Muscles of facial expression: Mouth and neck		
Muscle	**Origin**	**Insertion***	**Main action(s)****
Mouth			
① Zygomaticus major	Zygomatic bone (lateral surface, posterior part)	Skin at corner of the mouth	Pulls corner of mouth superiorly and laterally
② Zygomaticus minor		Upper lip just medial to corner of the mouth	Pulls upper lip superiorly
Levator labii superioris alaeque nasi (see **Fig. 38.8C**)	Maxilla (frontal process)	Alar cartilage of nose and upper lip	Elevates upper lip, opens nostril
③ Levator labii superioris	Maxilla (frontal process) and infraorbital region	Skin of upper lip, alar cartilages of nose	Elevates upper lip, dilates nostril, raises angle of the mouth
④ Depressor labii inferioris	Mandible (anterior portion of oblique line)	Lower lip at midline; blends with muscle from opposite side	Pulls lower lip inferiorly and laterally
⑤ Levator anguli oris	Maxilla (below infraorbital foramen)	Skin at corner of the mouth	Raises angle of mouth, helps form nasolabial furrow
⑥ Depressor anguli oris	Mandible (oblique line below canine, premolar, and first molar teeth)	Skin at corner of the mouth; blends with orbicularis oris	Pulls angle of mouth inferiorly and laterally
⑦ Buccinator	Mandible, alveolar processes of maxilla and mandible, pterygo-mandibular raphe	Angle of mouth, orbicularis oris	Presses cheek against molar teeth, working with tongue to keep food between occlusal surfaces and out of oral vestibule; expels air from oral cavity/resists distension when blowing *Unilateral:* Draws mouth to one side
⑧ Orbicularis oris	Deep surface of skin Superiorly: maxilla (median plane) Inferiorly: mandible	Mucous membrane of lips	Acts as oral sphincter • Compresses and protrudes lips (e.g., when whistling, sucking, and kissing) • Resists distension (when blowing)
Risorius (see **pp. 519–517**)	Fascia over masseter	Skin of corner of the mouth	Retracts corner of mouth as in grimacing
⑨ Mentalis	Mandible (incisive fossa)	Skin of chin	Elevates and protrudes lower lip
Neck			
Platysma (see **pp. 516–517**)	Skin over lower neck and upper lateral thorax	Mandible (inferior border), skin over lower face, angle of mouth	Depresses and wrinkles skin of lower face and mouth; tenses skin of neck; aids in forced depression of the mandible

*There are no bony insertions for the muscles of facial expression.
**All muscles of facial expression are innervated by the facial nerve (CN VII) via temporal, zygomatic, buccal, mandibular, or cervical branches arising from its parotid plexus.

Muscle Facts (II)

 The muscles of mastication are located at various depths in the parotid and infratemporal regions of the face. They attach to the mandible and receive their motor innervation from the mandibu-lar division of the trigeminal nerve (CN V₃). The muscles of the oral floor that aid in opening the mouth are found on **p. 620**.

Table 38.3 | **Muscles of mastication: Masseter and temporalis**

Muscle	Origin	Insertion	Innervation	Action
① Masseter	Superficial layer: zygomatic arch (anterior two thirds)	Mandibular angle (masseteric tuberosity)	Mandibular n. (CN V₃) via masseteric n.	Elevates (adducts) and protrudes mandible
	Deep layer: zygomatic arch (posterior one third)			
② Temporalis	Temporal fossa (inferior temporal line)	Coronoid process of mandible (apex and medial surface)	Mandibular n. (CN V₃) via deep temporal nn.	*Vertical fibers:* Elevate (adduct) mandible *Horizontal fibers:* Retract (retrude) mandible *Unilateral:* Lateral movement of mandible (chewing)

Fig. 38.11 Masseter muscle
Left lateral view.

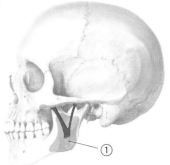

A Schematic.

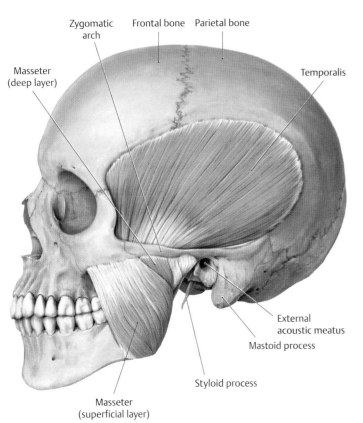

B Masseter with temporalis muscle.

Fig. 38.12 Temporalis muscle
Left lateral view.

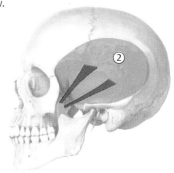

A Schematic.

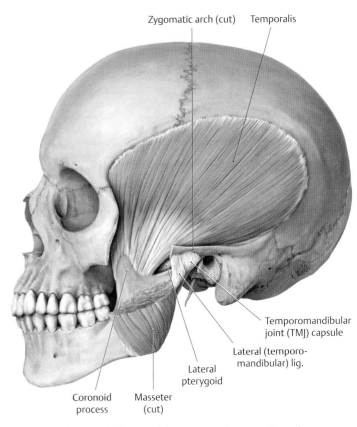

B Temporalis muscle. *Removed:* Masseter and zygomatic arch.

Table 38.4	Muscles of mastication: Pterygoid muscles				
Muscle		**Origin**	**Insertion**	**Innervation**	**Action**
Lateral pterygoid	③ Superior head	Greater wing of sphenoid bone (infratemporal crest)	Temporomandibular joint (articular disk)	Mandibular n. (CN V₃) via lateral pterygoid n.	*Bilateral:* Protrudes mandible (pulls articular disk forward) *Unilateral:* Lateral movements of mandible (chewing)
	④ Inferior head	Lateral pterygoid plate (lateral surface)	Mandible (condylar process)		
Medial pterygoid	⑤ Superficial head	Maxilla (tuberosity)	Pterygoid tuberosity on medial surface of the mandibular angle	Mandibular n. (CN V₃) via medial pterygoid n.	*Bilateral:* Elevates (adducts) mandible with masseter; contributes to protrusion. *Unilateral:* small grinding movements.
	⑥ Deep head	Medial surface of lateral pterygoid plate and pterygoid fossa			

Fig. 38.13 Lateral pterygoid muscle
Left lateral view.

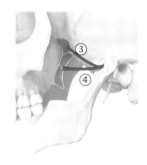

A Schematic.

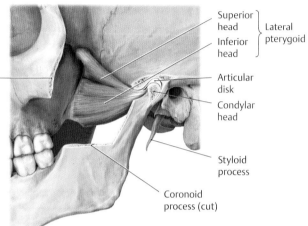

B Left lateral pterygoid muscle. *Removed:* Coronoid process and part of ramus of mandible.

Fig. 38.14 Medial pterygoid muscle
Left lateral view.

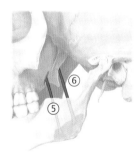

A Schematic.

B Left medial pterygoid muscle. *Removed:* Coronoid process of mandible.

Fig. 38.15 Masticatory muscle sling
Oblique posterior view.

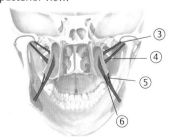

A Schematic.

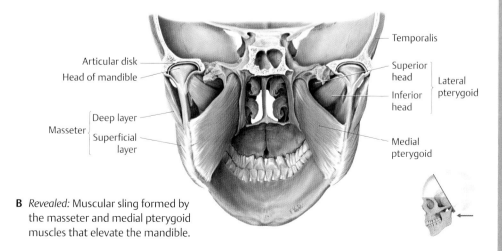

B *Revealed:* Muscular sling formed by the masseter and medial pterygoid muscles that elevate the mandible.

Cranial Nerves: Overview

Fig. 39.1 **Cranial nerves**

Inferior (basal) view. The 12 pairs of cranial nerves (CN) are numbered according to the order of their emergence from the brainstem. *Note:* The sensory and motor fibers of the cranial nerves enter and exit the brainstem at the same sites (in contrast to spinal nerves, whose sensory and motor fibers enter and leave through posterior and anterior roots, respectively).

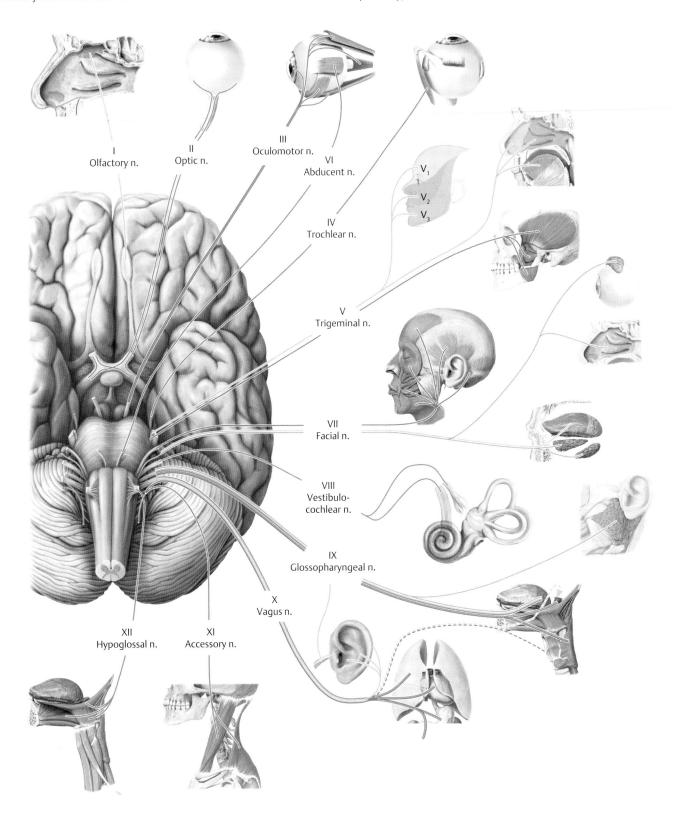

I
Olfactory n.

II
Optic n.

III
Oculomotor n.

VI
Abducent n.

IV
Trochlear n.

V₁
V₂
V₃

V
Trigeminal n.

VII
Facial n.

VIII
Vestibulo-
cochlear n.

IX
Glossopharyngeal n.

X
Vagus n.

XII
Hypoglossal n.

XI
Accessory n.

The cranial nerves contain both afferent (sensory) and efferent (motor) axons that belong to either the somatic or the autonomic (visceral) nervous system (see **pp. 682–683**). The somatic fibers allow interaction with the environment, whereas the visceral fibers regulate the autonomic activity of internal organs.

In addition to the general fiber types, the cranial nerves may contain special fiber types associated with particular structures (e.g., auditory apparatus and taste buds). The cranial nerve fibers originate or terminate at specific nuclei, which are similarly classified as either general or special, somatic or visceral, and afferent or efferent.

Table 39.1 Classification of cranial nerve fibers and nuclei

This color coding is used in subsequent chapters to indicate fiber and nuclei classifications.

Fiber type	Example	Fiber type	Example
General somatic efferent (somatomotor function)	Innervate skeletal muscles	General somatic afferent (somatic sensation)	Conduct impulses from skin, skeletal muscle spindles
General visceral efferent (visceromotor function)	Innervate smooth muscle of the viscera, intraocular muscles, heart, salivary glands, etc.	Special somatic afferent	Conduct impulses from retina, auditory and vestibular apparatuses
Special visceral efferent	Innervate skeletal muscles derived from branchial arches	General visceral afferent (visceral sensation)	Conduct impulses from viscera, blood vessels
		Special visceral afferent	Conduct impulses from taste buds, olfactory mucosa

Fig. 39.2 Cranial nerve nuclei

The sensory and motor fibers of cranial nerves III to XII originate and terminate in the brainstem at specific nuclei.

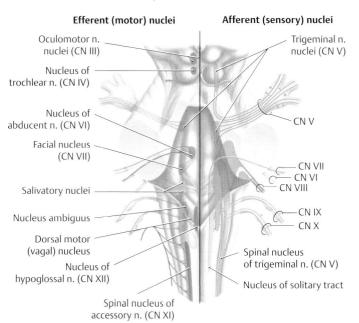

Efferent (motor) nuclei

- Oculomotor n. nuclei (CN III)
- Nucleus of trochlear n. (CN IV)
- Nucleus of abducent n. (CN VI)
- Facial nucleus (CN VII)
- Salivatory nuclei
- Nucleus ambiguus
- Dorsal motor (vagal) nucleus
- Nucleus of hypoglossal n. (CN XII)
- Spinal nucleus of accessory n. (CN XI)

Afferent (sensory) nuclei

- Trigeminal n. nuclei (CN V)
- CN V
- CN VII
- CN VI
- CN VIII
- CN IX
- CN X
- Spinal nucleus of trigeminal n. (CN V)
- Nucleus of solitary tract

A Posterior view with the cerebellum removed.

Table 39.2 Cranial nerves

Cranial nerve	Origin	Functional fiber types
CN I: Olfactory n.	Telencephalon*	●
CN II: Optic n.	Diencephalon*	●
CN III: Oculomotor n.	Mesencephalon	● ●
CN IV: Trochlear n.		●
CN V: Trigeminal n.	Pons	● ●
CN VI: Abducent n.		●
CN VII: Facial n.		● ● ● ●
CN VIII: Vestibulocochlear n.		●
CN IX: Glossopharyngeal n.	Medulla oblongata	● ● ● ● ●
CN X: Vagus n.		● ● ● ● ●
CN XI: Accessory n.		● ●
CN XII: Hypoglossal n.		●

* The olfactory and optic nerves are extensions of the brain rather than true nerves; they are therefore not associated with nuclei in the brainstem.

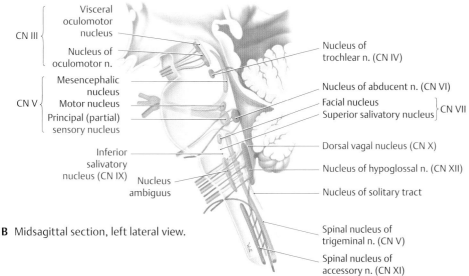

- CN III
  - Visceral oculomotor nucleus
  - Nucleus of oculomotor n.
- CN V
  - Mesencephalic nucleus
  - Motor nucleus
  - Principal (partial) sensory nucleus
- Inferior salivatory nucleus (CN IX)
- Nucleus ambiguus
- Nucleus of trochlear n. (CN IV)
- Nucleus of abducent n. (CN VI)
- Facial nucleus
- Superior salivatory nucleus } CN VII
- Dorsal vagal nucleus (CN X)
- Nucleus of hypoglossal n. (CN XII)
- Nucleus of solitary tract
- Spinal nucleus of trigeminal n. (CN V)
- Spinal nucleus of accessory n. (CN XI)

B Midsagittal section, left lateral view.

CN I & II: Olfactory & Optic Nerves

 The olfactory and optic nerves are not true peripheral nerves but extensions (tracts) of the telencephalon and diencephalon, respectively. They are therefore not associated with cranial nerve nuclei in the brainstem.

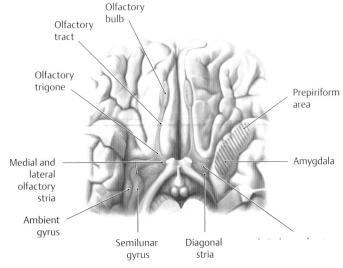

A Olfactory bulb and tract, inferior view. *Note*: The amygdala and prepiriform area are deep to the basal surface of the brain.

Fig. 39.3 Olfactory nerve (CN I)

Fiber bundles in the olfactory mucosa pass from the nasal cavity through the cribriform plate of the ethmoid bone into the anterior cranial fossa, where they synapse in the olfactory bulb. Axons from second-order afferent neurons in the olfactory bulb pass through the olfactory tract and medial or lateral olfactory stria, terminating in the cerebral cortex of the prepiriform area, in the amygdala, or in neighboring areas.

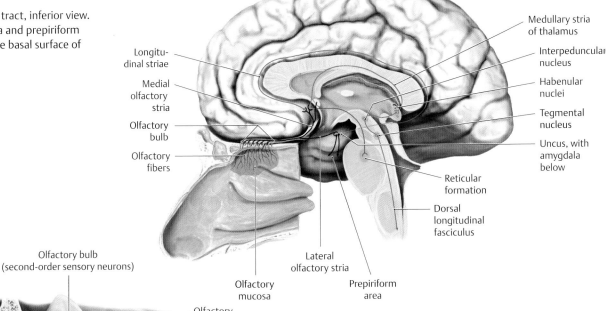

B Course of the olfactory nerve. Parasagittal section, viewed from left side.

C Olfactory fibers. Portion of left nasal septum and lateral wall of right nasal cavity, left lateral view.

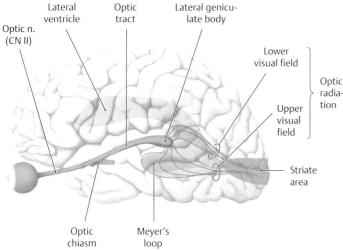

A Optic nerve in the geniculate visual pathway, left lateral view.

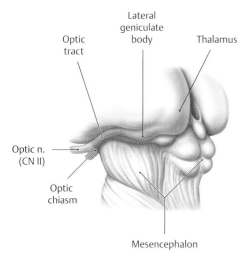

B Termination of the optic tract, left posterolateral view of the brainstem. The optic nerve contains the axons of retinal ganglion cells, which terminate mainly in the lateral geniculate body of the diencephalon and in the mesencephalon (superior colliculus).

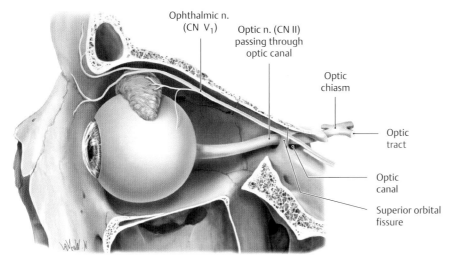

Fig. 39.4 Optic nerve (CN II)

The optic nerve passes from the eyeball through the optic canal into the middle cranial fossa. The two optic nerves join below the base of the diencephalon to form the optic chiasm, before dividing into the two optic tracts. Each of these tracts divides into a lateral and medial root. Many retinal cell ganglion axons cross the midline to the contralateral side of the brain in the optic chiasm.

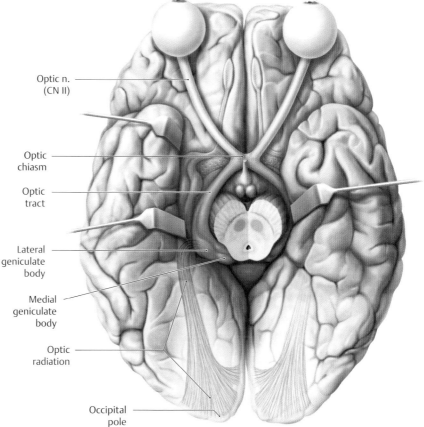

C Course of the optic nerve, inferior (basal) view.

D Optic nerve in the left orbit, lateral view. The optic nerve exits the orbit via the optic canal. *Note*: The other cranial nerves entering the orbit do so via the superior orbital fissure.

CN III, IV & VI: Oculomotor, Trochlear & Abducent Nerves

Cranial nerves III, IV, and VI innervate the extraocular muscles (see **p. 569**). Of the three, only the oculomotor nerve (CN III) contains both somatic and visceral efferent fibers; it is also the only cranial nerve of the extraocular muscles to innervate multiple extra- and intraocular muscles.

Fig. 39.5 Nuclei of the oculomotor, trochlear, and abducent nerves

The trochlear nerve (CN IV) is the only cranial nerve in which all the fibers cross to the opposite side. It is also the only cranial nerve to emerge from the dorsal side of the brainstem and, consequently, has the longest intradural (intracranial) course of any cranial nerve.

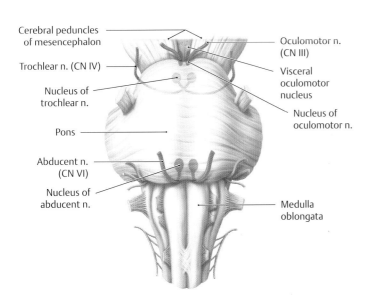

A Emergence of the cranial nerves of the extraocular muscles. Anterior view of the brainstem.

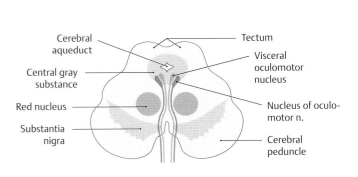

B Oculomotor nerve nuclei. Transverse section, superior view.

Table 39.3	Cranial nerves of the extraocular muscles

Course*	Fibers	Nuclei	Function	Effects of nerve injury
Oculomotor nerve (CN III)				
Runs anteriorly from mesencephalon	Somatic efferent	Oculomotor nucleus	Innervates: • Levator palpebrae superioris • Superior, medial, and inferior rectus • Inferior oblique	Complete oculomotor palsy (paralysis of extra- and intraocular muscles): • Ptosis (drooping of eyelid) • Downward and lateral gaze deviation • Diplopia (double vision) • Mydriasis (pupil dilation) • Accommodation difficulties (ciliary paralysis)
	Visceral efferent	Visceral oculomotor (Edinger-Westphal) nucleus	Synapse with neurons in ciliary ganglia. Innervates: • Pupillary sphincter • Ciliary muscle	
Trochlear nerve (CN IV)				
Emerges from posterior surface of brainstem near midline, courses anteriorly around the cerebral peduncle	Somatic efferent	Nucleus of the trochlear n.	Innervates: • Superior oblique	• Diplopia • Affected eye is higher and deviated medially (dominance of inferior oblique)
Abducent nerve (CN VI)				
Follows a long extradural path**	Somatic efferent	Nucleus of the abducent n.	Innervates: • Lateral rectus	• Diplopia • Medial strabismas (due to unopposed action of medial rectus)

* All three nerves enter the orbit through the superior orbital fissure; CN III and CN VI pass through the common tendinous ring of the extraocular muscles.
** The abducent nerve follows an extradural course; abducent nerve palsy may therefore develop in association with meningitis and subarachnoid hemorrhage.

Note: The oculomotor nerve supplies parasympathetic innervation to the intraocular muscles and somatic motor innervation to most of the extraocular muscles (also the levator palpebrae superioris). Its parasympathetic fibers synapse in the ciliary ganglion. Oculomotor nerve palsy may affect exclusively the parasympathetic or somatic fibers, or both concurrently.

Fig. 39.6 **Course of the nerves innervating the extraocular muscles**
Right orbit.

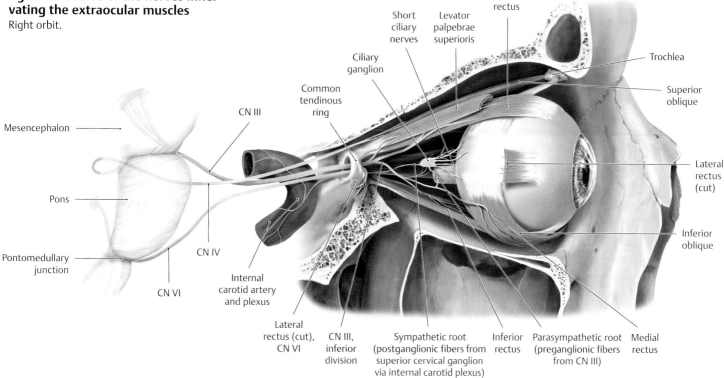

A Lateral view.

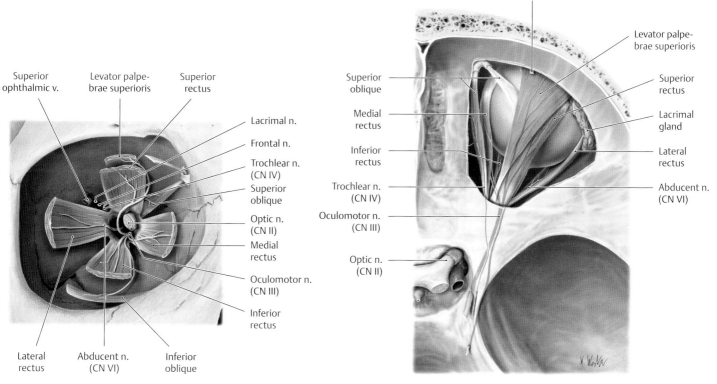

B Anterior view. CN II exits the orbit via the optic canal, which lies medial to the superior orbital fissure (site of emergence of CN III, IV, and VI).

C Superior view of the opened orbit. Note the relationship between the optic canal and the superior orbital fissure.

CN V: Trigeminal Nerve

 The trigeminal nerve, the sensory nerve of the head, has three somatic afferent nuclei: the mesencephalic nucleus, which receives proprioceptive fibers from the muscles of mastication; the principal (pontine) sensory nucleus, which chiefly mediates touch; and the spinal nucleus, which mediates pain and temperature sensation. The motor nucleus supplies motor innervation to the muscles of mastication.

Fig. 39.7 Trigeminal nerve nuclei

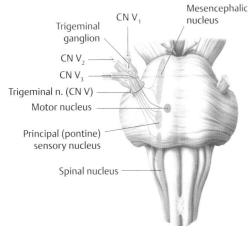

A Anterior view of the brainstem.

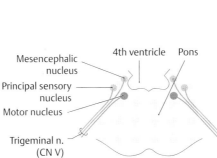

B Cross section through the pons, superior view.

Fig. 39.8 Divisions of the trigeminal nerve (CN V)
Right lateral view.

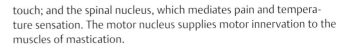
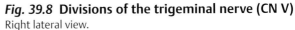

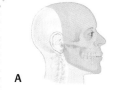 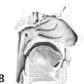 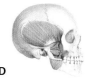

A   B   C   D

Table 39.4		Trigeminal nerve (CN V)			
Course	**Fibers**	**Nuclei**	**Function**		**Effects of nerve injury**
Exits from the middle cranial fossa. **Ophthalmic division (CN V₁):** Enters orbit through superior orbital fissure **Maxillary division (CN V₂):** Enters pterygopalatine fossa through foramen rotundum **Mandibular division (CN V₃):** Passes through foramen ovale into infratemporal fossa	Somatic afferent	• Principal (pontine) sensory nucleus of the trigeminal n. • Mesencephalic nucleus of the trigeminal n. • Spinal nucleus of the trigeminal n.	Innervates: • Facial skin (**A**) • Nasopharyngeal mucosa (**B**) • Tongue (anterior two thirds) (**C**) Involved in the corneal reflex (reflex closure of eyelid)		• Sensory loss (traumatic nerve lesions) • Herpes zoster ophthalmicus (varicella-zoster virus); herpes zoster of the face
	Special visceral efferent	Motor nucleus of the trigeminal n.	Innervates (via CN V₃): • Muscles of mastication (temporalis, masseter, medial and lateral pterygoids (**D**)) • Oral floor muscles (mylohyoid, anterior digastric) • Tensor tympani • Tensor veli palatini		
	Visceral efferent pathway*	• Lacrimal n. (CN V₁) conveys parasympathetic fibers from CN VII along the zygomatic n. (CN V₂) to the lacrimal gland • Lingual n. (CN V₃) conveys parasympathetic fibers from CN VII (via the chorda tympani) to the submandibular and sublingual glands • Auriculotemporal n. (CN V₃) conveys parasympathetic fibers from CN IX to the parotid gland			
	Visceral afferent pathway*	Gustatory (taste) fibers from CN VII (via chorda tympani) travel with the lingual n. (CN V₃) to the anterior two thirds of the tongue			

* Fibers of certain cranial nerves adhere to divisions or branches of the trigeminal nerve, by which they travel to their destination.

Fig. 39.9 Course of the trigeminal nerve divisions
Right lateral view.

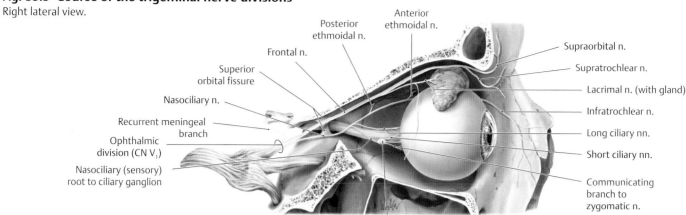

Posterior ethmoidal n.
Anterior ethmoidal n.
Frontal n.
Superior orbital fissure
Nasociliary n.
Recurrent meningeal branch
Ophthalmic division (CN V₁)
Nasociliary (sensory) root to ciliary ganglion
Supraorbital n.
Supratrochlear n.
Lacrimal n. (with gland)
Infratrochlear n.
Long ciliary nn.
Short ciliary nn.
Communicating branch to zygomatic n.
Ciliary ganglion

A Ophthalmic division (CN V₁). Partially opened right orbit.

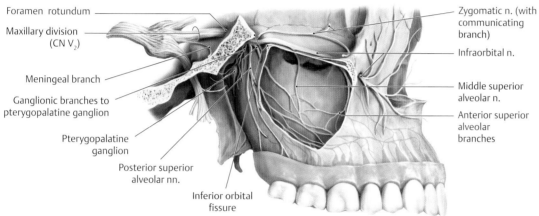

Foramen rotundum
Maxillary division (CN V₂)
Meningeal branch
Ganglionic branches to pterygopalatine ganglion
Pterygopalatine ganglion
Posterior superior alveolar nn.
Inferior orbital fissure
Zygomatic n. (with communicating branch)
Infraorbital n.
Middle superior alveolar n.
Anterior superior alveolar branches

B Maxillary division (CN V₂). Partially opened right maxillary sinus with the zygomatic arch removed.

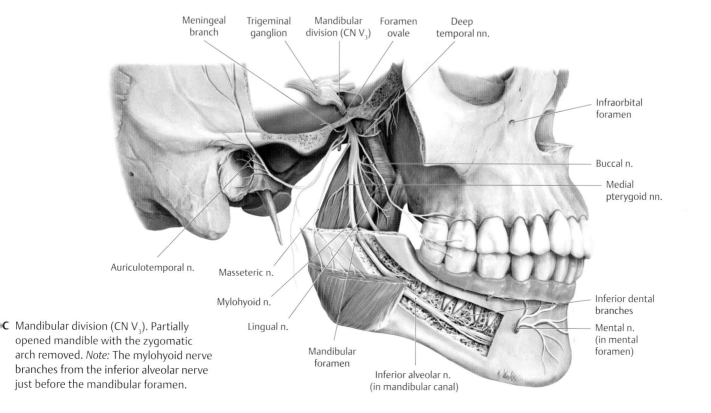

Meningeal branch
Trigeminal ganglion
Mandibular division (CN V₃)
Foramen ovale
Deep temporal nn.
Infraorbital foramen
Buccal n.
Medial pterygoid nn.
Auriculotemporal n.
Masseteric n.
Mylohyoid n.
Lingual n.
Mandibular foramen
Inferior alveolar n. (in mandibular canal)
Inferior dental branches
Mental n. (in mental foramen)

C Mandibular division (CN V₃). Partially opened mandible with the zygomatic arch removed. *Note:* The mylohyoid nerve branches from the inferior alveolar nerve just before the mandibular foramen.

CN VII: Facial Nerve

 The facial nerve mainly conveys special visceral efferent (branchiogenic) fibers from the facial nerve nucleus to the muscles of facial expression. The other visceral efferent (para-sympathetic) fibers from the superior salivatory nucleus are grouped with the visceral afferent (gustatory) fibers to form the nervus intermedius.

Fig. 39.10 Facial nerve nuclei

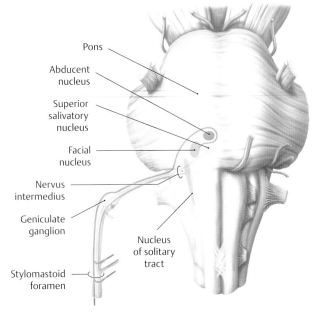

A Anterior view of the brainstem.

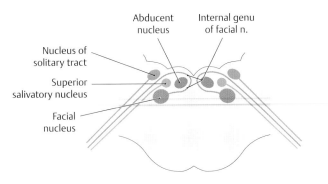

B Cross section through the pons, superior view.

Fig. 39.11 Branches of the facial nerve
Right lateral view.

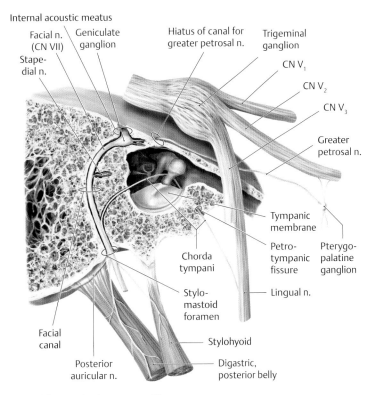

A Facial nerve in the temporal bone.

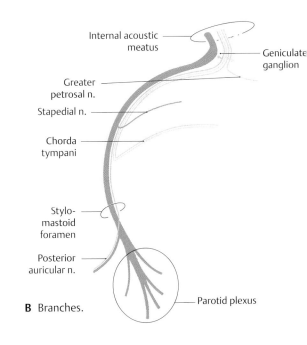

B Branches.

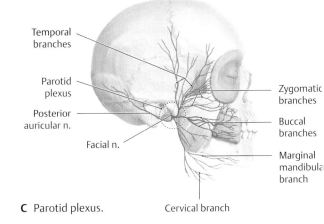

C Parotid plexus.

Table 39.5 **Facial nerve (CN VII)**

Course	Fibers	Nuclei	Function	Effects of nerve injury
Emerges in the cerebellopontine angle between the pons and olive; passes through the internal acoustic meatus into the temporal bone (petrous part), where it divides into: • Greater petrosal n. • Stapedial n. • Chorda tympani Certain special visceral efferent fibers pass through the stylomastoid foramen to the skull base, forming the intraparotid plexus	Special visceral afferent	Facial nucleus	Innervate: • Muscles of facial expression • Stylohyoid • Digastric (posterior belly) • Stapedius	Peripheral facial nerve injury: paralysis of muscles of facial expression on affected side Associated disturbances of taste, lacrimation, salivation, hyperacusis, etc.
	Visceral efferent (para-sympathetic)*	Superior salivatory nucleus	Synapse with neurons in the pterygopalatine or submandibular ganglion. Innervate: • Lacrimal gland • Small glands of nasal mucosa, hard and soft palate • Submandibular gland • Sublingual gland • Small salivary glands of tongue (dorsum)	
	Special visceral afferent*	Nucleus of the solitary tract	Peripheral processes of fibers from geniculate ganglion form the chorda tympani (gustatory fibers from tongue)	
	Somatic afferent		Sensory fibers from the auricle, skin of the auditory canal, and outer surface of the tympanic membrane travel via CN VII to the principal sensory nucleus of the trigeminal n.	

* Grouped to form nervus intermedius, which aggregates with the visceral efferent fibers from the facial n. nucleus.

Fig. 39.12 Course of the facial nerve

Right lateral view. Visceral efferent (parasympathetic) and special visceral afferent (taste) fibers shown in black.

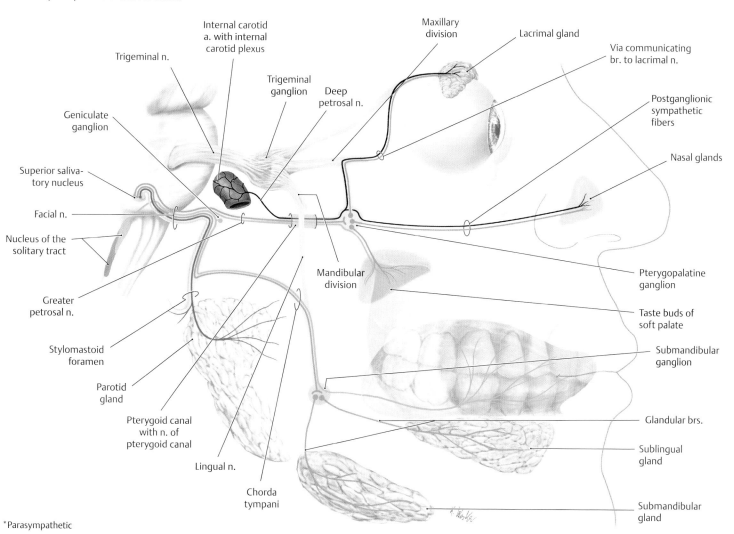

*Parasympathetic

CN VIII: Vestibulocochlear Nerve

 The vestibulochochlear nerve is a special somatic afferent nerve that consists of two roots. The vestibular root transmits impulses from the vestibular apparatus; the cochlear root transmits impulses from the auditory apparatus.

Fig. 39.13 **Vestibulocochlear nerve: Vestibular part**

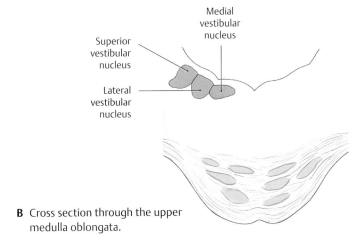

Flocculus of cerebellum
Direct fibers to cerebellum
Vestibulo-cochlear n. (CN VIII)
Vestibular root
Vestibular ganglion
Semi-circular canals
Superior vestibular nucleus
Medial vestibular nucleus
Lateral vestibular nucleus
Inferior vestibular nucleus

A Anterior view of the medulla oblon-gata and pons with cerebellum.

Superior vestibular nucleus
Medial vestibular nucleus
Lateral vestibular nucleus

B Cross section through the upper medulla oblongata.

Fig. 39.14 **Vestibulocochlear nerve: Cochlear part**

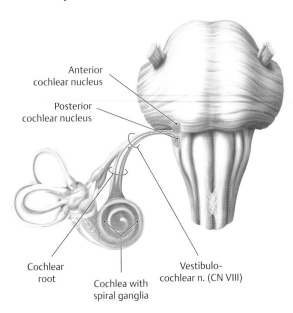

Anterior cochlear nucleus
Posterior cochlear nucleus
Cochlear root
Cochlea with spiral ganglia
Vestibulo-cochlear n. (CN VIII)

A Anterior view of the medulla oblon-gata and pons.

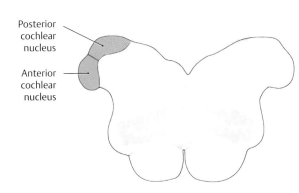

Posterior cochlear nucleus
Anterior cochlear nucleus

B Cross section through the upper medulla oblongata.

Table 39.6	Vestibulocochlear nerve (CN VIII)				
Part	**Course**	**Fibers**	**Nuclei**	**Function**	**Effects of nerve injury**
Vestibular part	Pass from the inner ear through the internal acoustic meatus to the cerebellopontine angle, where they enter the brain	Special somatic afferent	Superior, lateral, medial, and inferior vestibular nuclei	Peripheral processes from the semicircular canals, saccule, and utricle pass to the vestibular ganglion and then to the four vestibular nuclei	Dizziness
Cochlear part			Anterior and posterior cochlear nuclei	Peripheral processes beginning at the hair cells of the organ of Corti pass to the spiral ganglion and then to the two cochlear nuclei	Hearing loss

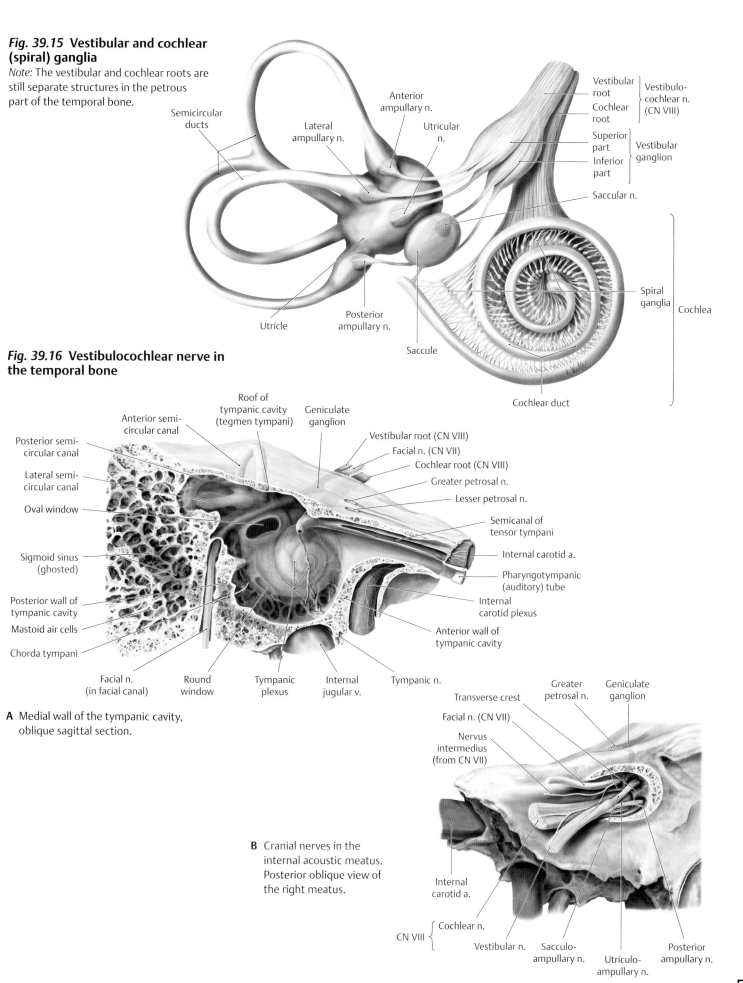

Fig. 39.15 Vestibular and cochlear (spiral) ganglia

Note: The vestibular and cochlear roots are still separate structures in the petrous part of the temporal bone.

Semicircular ducts

Anterior ampullary n.

Lateral ampullary n.

Utricular n.

Vestibular root

Cochlear root

Vestibulo-cochlear n. (CN VIII)

Superior part

Inferior part

Vestibular ganglion

Saccular n.

Spiral ganglia

Cochlea

Utricle

Posterior ampullary n.

Saccule

Cochlear duct

Fig. 39.16 Vestibulocochlear nerve in the temporal bone

Posterior semi-circular canal

Anterior semi-circular canal

Roof of tympanic cavity (tegmen tympani)

Geniculate ganglion

Vestibular root (CN VIII)

Facial n. (CN VII)

Lateral semi-circular canal

Oval window

Cochlear root (CN VIII)

Greater petrosal n.

Lesser petrosal n.

Semicanal of tensor tympani

Sigmoid sinus (ghosted)

Internal carotid a.

Pharyngotympanic (auditory) tube

Posterior wall of tympanic cavity

Mastoid air cells

Chorda tympani

Internal carotid plexus

Anterior wall of tympanic cavity

Facial n. (in facial canal)

Round window

Tympanic plexus

Internal jugular v.

Tympanic n.

A Medial wall of the tympanic cavity, oblique sagittal section.

Transverse crest

Greater petrosal n.

Geniculate ganglion

Facial n. (CN VII)

Nervus intermedius (from CN VII)

Internal carotid a.

B Cranial nerves in the internal acoustic meatus. Posterior oblique view of the right meatus.

CN VIII { Cochlear n.

Vestibular n.

Sacculo-ampullary n.

Utriculo-ampullary n.

Posterior ampullary n.

CN IX: Glossopharyngeal Nerve

Fig. 39.17 Glossopharyngeal nerve nuclei

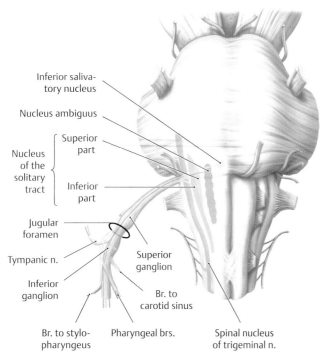

A Anterior view of the medulla oblongata.

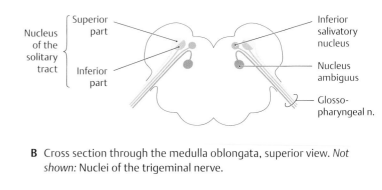

B Cross section through the medulla oblongata, superior view. *Not shown:* Nuclei of the trigeminal nerve.

Fig. 39.18 Course of the glossopharyngeal nerve

Left lateral view. *Note:* Fibers from the vagus nerve (CN X) combine with fibers from the glossopharyngeal nerve (CN IX) to form the pharyngeal plexus and supply the carotid sinus.

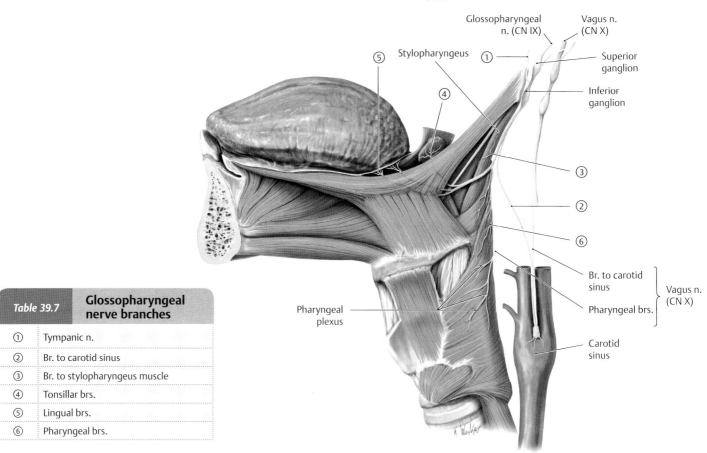

Table 39.7	Glossopharyngeal nerve branches
①	Tympanic n.
②	Br. to carotid sinus
③	Br. to stylopharyngeus muscle
④	Tonsillar brs.
⑤	Lingual brs.
⑥	Pharyngeal brs.

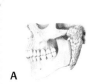
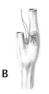

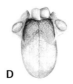

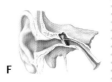

A B C D E F

Table 39.8   **Glossopharyngeal nerve (CN IX)**

Course	Fibers	Nuclei	Function	Effects of nerve injury
Emerges from the medulla oblongata; leaves cranial cavity through the jugular foramen	Visceral efferent (parasympathetic)	Inferior salivatory nucleus	Parasympathetic presynaptic fibers are sent to the otic ganglion; postsynaptic fibers are distributed to • Parotid gland (**A**) • Buccal gland • Labial gland	Isolated lesions of CN IX are rare. Lesions are generally accompanied by lesions of CN X and CN XI (cranial part), as all three emerge jointly from the jugular foramen and are susceptible to injury in basal skull fractures.
	Special visceral efferent (branchiogenic)	Nucleus ambiguus	Innervate: • Constrictor muscles of the pharynx (pharyngeal branches join with the vagus nerve to form the pharyngeal plexus) • Stylopharyngeus	
	Visceral afferent	Nucleus of the solitary tract (inferior part)	Receive sensory information from • Chemoreceptors in the carotid body (**B**) • Pressure receptors in the carotid sinus	
	Special visceral afferent	Nucleus of the solitary tract (superior part)	Receives sensory information from the posterior third of the tongue (via the inferior ganglion) (**C**)	
	Somatic afferent	Spinal nucleus of trigeminal nerve	Peripheral processes of the intracranial superior ganglion or the extracranial inferior ganglion arise from • Tongue, soft palate, pharyngeal mucosa, and tonsils (**D, E**) • Mucosa of the tympanic cavity, internal surface of the tympanic membrane, pharyngotympanic tube (tympanic plexus) (**F**) • Skin of the external ear and auditory canal (blends with the vagus n.)	

Fig. 39.19 **Glossopharyngeal nerve in the tympanic cavity**

Left anterolateral view. The tympanic nerve contains visceral efferent (presynaptic parasympathetic) fibers for the otic ganglion, as well as somatic afferent fibers for the tympanic cavity and pharyngotympanic tube. It joins with sympathetic fibers from the internal carotid plexus (via the caroticotympanic nerve) to form the tympanic plexus.

Fig. 39.20 **Visceral efferent (parasympathetic) fibers of CN IX**

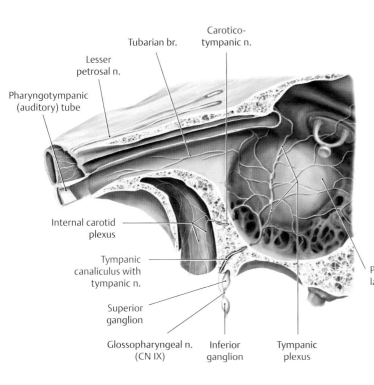

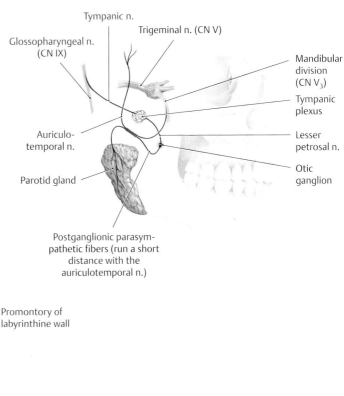

CN X: Vagus Nerve

Fig. 39.21 Vagus nerve nuclei

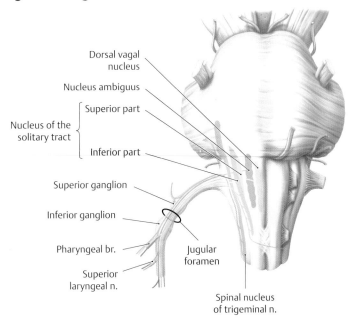

A Anterior view of the medulla oblongata.

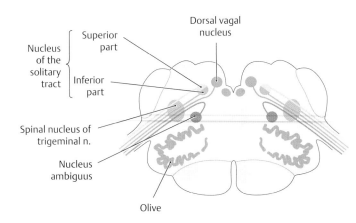

B Cross section through the medulla oblongata, superior view.

Table 39.9	Vagus nerve (CN X)			
Course	Fibers	Nuclei	Function	Effects of nerve injury
Emerges from the medulla oblongata; leaves the cranial cavity through the jugular foramen. CN X has the most extensive distribution of all the cranial nerves (vagus = "vagabond"), consisting of cranial, cervical, thoracic (see **p. 87**), and abdominal (see **p. 211**) parts.	Special visceral efferent (branchiogenic)	Nucleus ambiguus	Innervate: • Pharyngeal muscles (via pharyngeal plexus with CN IX) • Muscles of the soft palate • Laryngeal muscles (superior laryngeal n. supplies the cricothyroid; inferior laryngeal n. supplies all other laryngeal muscles)	The recurrent laryngeal n. supplies visceromotor innervation to the only muscle abducting the vocal cords, the posterior cricoarytenoid. Unilateral destruction of this nerve leads to hoarseness; bilateral destruction leads to respiratory distress (dyspnea).
	Visceral efferent (parasympathetic)	Dorsal vagal nucleus	Synapse in prevertebral or intramural ganglia. Innervate smooth muscle and glands of • Thoracic viscera (**A**) • Abdominal viscera (**A**)	
	Somatic afferent	Spinal nucleus of trigeminal nerve	Superior (jugular) ganglion receives peripheral fibers from • Dura in posterior cranial fossa (**C**) • Skin of ear (**D**), external auditory canal (**E**)	
	Special visceral afferent	Nucleus of solitary tract (superior part)	Inferior nodose ganglion receives peripheral processes from • Taste buds on the epiglottis and root of the tongue (**F**)	
	Visceral afferent	Nucleus of solitary tract (inferior part)	Inferior ganglion receives peripheral processes from • Mucosa of lower pharynx at its esophageal junction (**G**) • Laryngeal mucosa above (superior laryngeal n.) and below (inferior laryngeal n.) the vocal fold (**G**) • Pressure receptors in the aortic arch (**B**) • Chemoreceptors in the para-aortic body (**B**) • Thoracic and abdominal viscera (**A**)	

Fig. 39.22 **Course of the vagus nerve**

The vagus nerve gives off four major branches in the neck. The inferior laryngeal nerves are the terminal branches of the recurrent laryngeal nerves. *Note:* The left recurrent laryngeal nerve hooks around the aortic arch, while the right nerve hooks around the subclavian artery.

Table 39.10	Vagus nerve branches in the neck
①	Pharyngeal brs.
②	Superior laryngeal n.
③R	Right recurrent laryngeal n.
③L	Left recurrent laryngeal n.
④	Cervical cardiac brs.

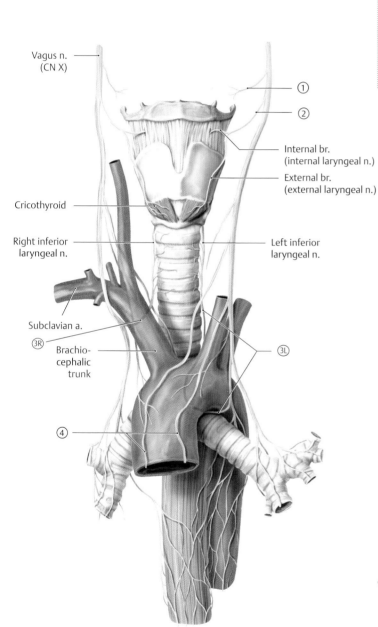

Vagus n. (CN X)
①
②
Internal br. (internal laryngeal n.)
External br. (external laryngeal n.)
Cricothyroid
Right inferior laryngeal n.
Left inferior laryngeal n.
Subclavian a.
③R
Brachio-cephalic trunk
③L
④

A Branches of the vagus nerve in the neck. Anterior view.

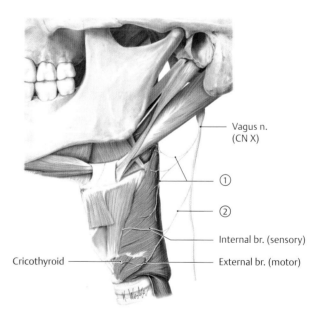

Vagus n. (CN X)
①
②
Internal br. (sensory)
External br. (motor)
Cricothyroid

B Innervation of the pharyngeal and laryngeal muscles. Left lateral view.

CN XI & XII: Accessory & Hypoglossal Nerves

 The traditional "cranial root" of the accessory nerve (CN XI) is now considered a part of the vagus nerve (CN X) that travels with the spinal root for a short distance before splitting. The cranial fibers are distributed via the vagus nerve while the spinal root fibers continue on as the accessory nerve (CN XI).

Fig. 39.23 Accessory nerve
Posterior view of the brainstem with the cerebellum removed. *Note:* For didactic reasons, the muscles are displayed from the right side.

Fig. 39.24 Accessory nerve lesions
Lesion of the right accessory nerve.

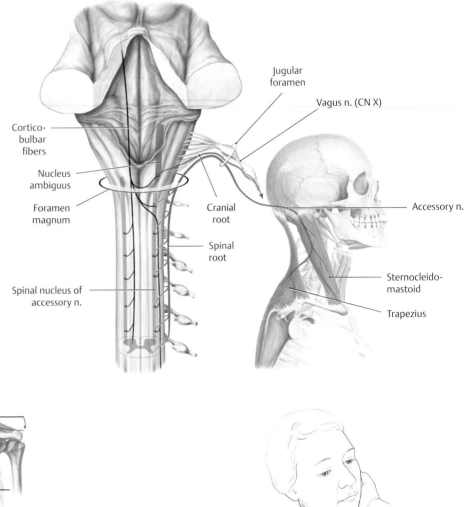

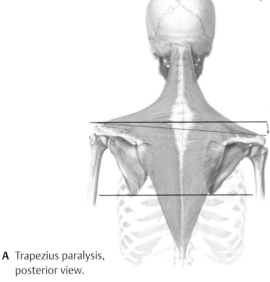

A Trapezius paralysis, posterior view.

B Sternocleidomastoid paralysis, right anterolateral view.

| Table 39.11 | Accessory nerve (CN XI) |

Course	Fibers	Nuclei	Function	Effects of nerve injury
The spinal root emerges from the spinal cord (at the level of C1–C5/6), passes superiorly, and enters the skull through the foramen magnum, where it joins with the cranial root from the medulla oblongata. Both roots leave the skull through the jugular foramen. Within the jugular foramen, fibers from the cranial root pass to the vagus n. (internal branch). The spinal portion descends to the nuchal region as the external branch.	Special visceral efferent	Nucleus ambiguus (caudal part)	Join CN X and are distributed with the recurrent laryngeal n. Innervate: • All laryngeal muscles (except cricothyroid)	*Trapezius paralysis:* drooping of shoulder on affected side and difficulty raising arm above horizontal plane. This paralysis is a concern during neck operations (e.g., lymph node biopsies). An injury of the accessory n. will not result in complete trapezius paralysis (the muscle is also innervated by segments C3 and C4/5). *Sternocleidomastoid paralysis:* torticollis (wry neck, i.e., difficulty turning head). Unilateral lesions cause flaccid paralysis (the muscle is supplied exclusively by the accessory n.). Bilateral lesions make it difficult to hold the head upright.
	Somatic efferent	Spinal nucleus of accessory n.	Form the external branch of the accessory n. Innervate: • Trapezius • Sternocleidomastoid	

Fig. 39.25 Hypoglossal nerve

Posterior view of the brainstem with the cerebellum removed.
Note: C1, which innervates the thyrohyoid and geniohyoid, runs briefly with the hypoglossal nerve.

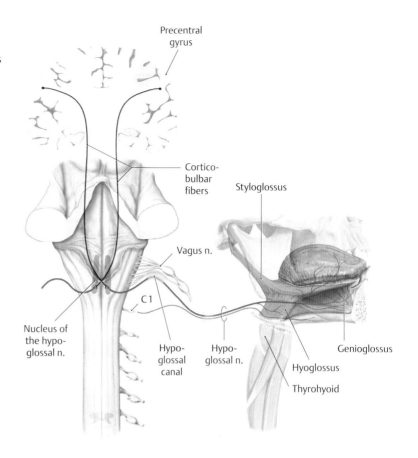

Fig. 39.26 Hypoglossal nerve nuclei

Note: The nucleus of the hypoglossal nerve is innervated by cortical neurons from the contralateral side.

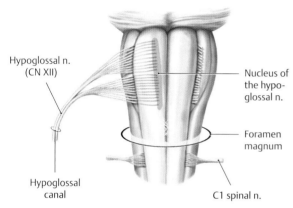

A Anterior view.

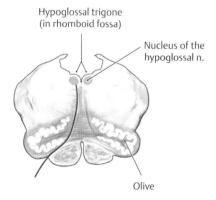

B Cross section through the medulla oblongata.

Fig. 39.27 Hypoglossal nerve lesions

Superior view.

A Normal genioglossus muscles.

B Unilateral nuclear or peripheral lesion.

Table 39.12	Hypoglossal nerve (CN XII)				

Course	Fibers	Nuclei	Function	Effects of nerve injury
Emerges from the medulla oblongata, leaves the cranial cavity through the hypoglossal canal, and descends laterally to the vagus nerve. CN XII enters the root of the tongue above the hyoid bone.	Somatic efferent	Nucleus of the hypoglossal n.	Innervates: • Intrinsic and extrinsic muscles of the tongue (except the palatoglossus, supplied by CN X)	Central hypoglossal paralysis (supranuclear): tongue deviates *away* from the side of the lesion. Nuclear or peripheral paralysis: tongue deviates *toward* the affected side (due to preponderance of muscle on healthy side) Flaccid paralysis: both nuclei injured; tongue cannot be protruded.

Autonomic Innervation

Fig. 39.28 Parasympathetic nervous system (cranial part): Overview

There are four parasympathetic nuclei in the brainstem. The visceral efferent fibers of these nuclei travel along particular cranial nn., listed below.

- Visceral oculomotor (Edinger–Westphal) nucleus: oculomotor n. (CN III)
- Superior salivatory nucleus: facial n. (CN VII)
- Inferior salivatory nucleus: glossopharyngeal n. (CN IX)
- Dorsal vagal nucleus: vagus n. (CN X)

The presynaptic parasympathetic fibers often travel with multiple cranial nn. to reach their target organs. The vagus n. supplies all of the thoracic and abdominal organs as far as a point near the left colic flexure.
Note: The sympathetic fibers to the head travel along the arteries to their target organs.

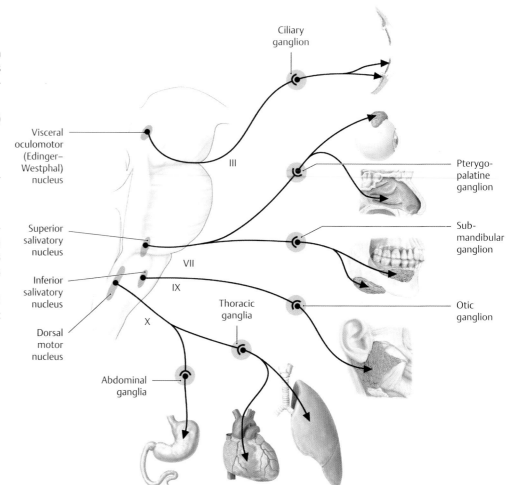

Table 39.13   Parasympathetic ganglia in the head

Nucleus	Path of presynaptic fibers	Ganglion	Postsynaptic fibers	Target organs
Edinger-Westphal nucleus	Oculomotor n. (CN III)	Ciliary ganglion	Short ciliary nn. (CN V$_1$)	Ciliary muscle (accommodation) Pupillary sphincter (miosis)
Superior salivary nucleus	Nervus intermedius (CN VII root) → greater petrosal n. → n. of pterygoid canal	Pterygopalatine ganglion	• Maxillary n. (CN V$_2$) → zygomatic n. → anastomosis → lacrimal n. (CN V$_1$) • Orbital branches • Posterior superior nasal brs. • Nasopalatine nn. • Greater and lesser palatine nn.	• Lacrimal gland • Glands of nasal cavity and paranasal sinuses • Glands of gingiva • Glands of hard and soft palate • Glands of pharynx
	Nervus intermedius (CN VII root) → chorda tympani → lingual n. (CN V$_3$)	Submandibular ganglion	Glandular branches	Submandibular gland Sublingual gland
Inferior salivary nucleus	Glossopharyngeal n. (CN IX) → tympanic n. → lesser petrosal n.	Otic ganglion	Auriculotemporal n. (CN V$_3$)	Parotid gland
Dorsal motor (vagal) nucleus	Vagus n. (X)	Ganglia near organs	Fine fibers in organs, not individually named	Thoracic and abdominal viscera
→ = is continuous with				

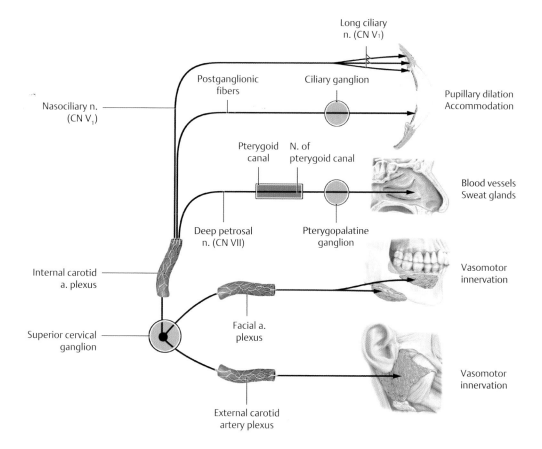

Fig. 39.29 Sympathetic innervation of the head

Sympathetic preganglionic neurons of the head originate in the lateral horn of the spinal cord (TI–L2). They exit into the sympathetic trunk and ascend to synapse in the superior cervical ganglion. Postganglionic neurons then travel with arterial plexuses. Postganglionic fibers that travel with the carotid plexus (on the internal carotid artery) join with the nasociliary nerves (of CN V₁) and then the long ciliary nerves to reach the dilator pupillae muscle (pupillary dilation); other postganglionic fibers travel through the ciliary ganglion (without synapsing) to reach the ciliary muscle (accommodation). Still other postganglionic fibers from the carotid plexus leave with the deep petrosal nerve, which joins with the greater petrosal nerve (CN VII), to form the nerve of the pterygoid canal (vidian nerve). This nerve travels to the pterygopalatine ganglion where it distributes fibers via branches of the maxillary nerve to the glands of the nasal cavity, maxillary sinus, hard and soft palate, gingiva, and pharynx, and to sweat glands and blood vessels in the head.

Postganglionic fibers from the superior cervical ganglion that travel with the facial artery plexus pass through the submandibular ganglion (without synapsing) to the submandibular and sublingual glands. Other postganglionic fibers travel with the middle meningeal plexus, through the otic ganglion (without synapsing), to the parotid gland.

Table 39.14 Sympathetic fibers in the head

Nucleus	Path of presynaptic fibers	Ganglion	Postsynaptic fibers	Target organs
Lateral horn of spinal cord (TI–L2)	Enter sympathetic trunk and ascend to superior cervical ganglion	Superior cervical ganglion	ICA plexus → nasociliary nn. (CN V₁) → long ciliary nn. (CN V₁)	Dilator pupillae muscle (mydriasis)
			Postganglionic fibers → ciliary ganglion* → short ciliary nn.	Ciliary muscle (accommodation)
			ICA plexus → deep petrosal n. → n. of pterygoid canal → pterygopalatine ganglion* → branches of maxillary n. (CN V₂)	Glands of nasal cavity / Sweat glands / Blood vessels
			Facial a. plexus → submandibular ganglion*	Submandibular gland / Sublingual gland
			External carotid a. plexus	Parotid gland

*passes through without synapsing; → = is continuous with
ICA, internal carotid a.

Innervation of the Face

Fig. 40.1 Motor innervation of the face

Left lateral view. Five branches of the facial nerve (CN VII) provide
motor innervation to the muscles of facial expression. The mandibular
division of the trigeminal nerve (CN V₃) supplies motor innervation to
the muscles of mastication.

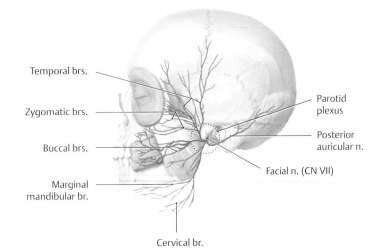

A Motor innervation of the muscles of facial expression.

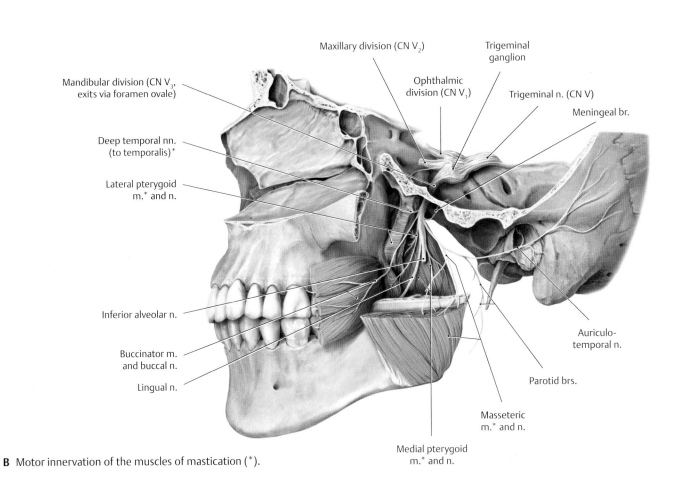

B Motor innervation of the muscles of mastication (*).

Fig. 40.2 Sensory innervation of the face

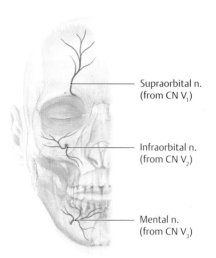

Supraorbital n.
(from CN V₁)

Infraorbital n.
(from CN V₂)

Mental n.
(from CN V₃)

A Sensory branches of the trigeminal nerve, anterior view. The sensory branches of the three divisions emerge from the supraorbital, infraorbital, and mental foramina, respectively.

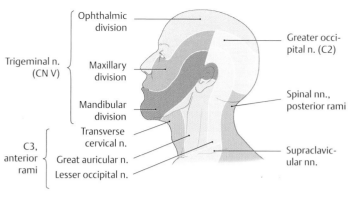

Ophthalmic division

Greater occipital n. (C2)

Trigeminal n. (CN V)

Maxillary division

Spinal nn., posterior rami

Mandibular division

C3, anterior rami

Transverse cervical n.

Great auricular n.

Lesser occipital n.

Supraclavicular nn.

B Cutaneous innervation of the head and neck, left lateral view. The occiput and nuchal regions are supplied by the posterior rami (blue) of the spinal nerves (the greater occipital nerve is the posterior ramus of C2).

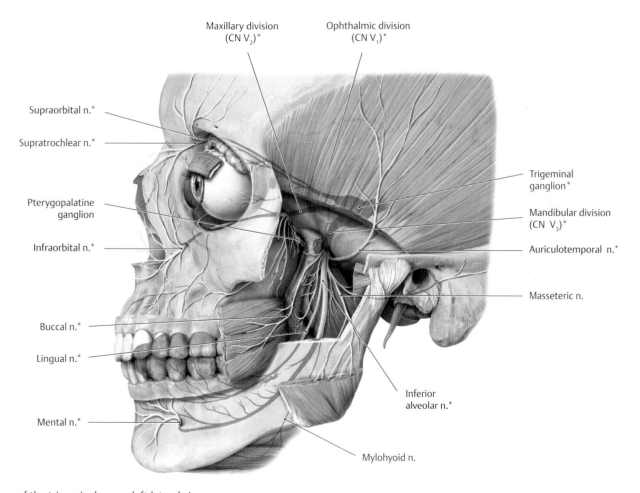

Maxillary division (CN V₂)*

Ophthalmic division (CN V₁)*

Supraorbital n.*

Supratrochlear n.*

Pterygopalatine ganglion

Infraorbital n.*

Buccal n.*

Lingual n.*

Mental n.*

Trigeminal ganglion*

Mandibular division (CN V₃)*

Auriculotemporal n.*

Masseteric n.

Inferior alveolar n.*

Mylohyoid n.

C Divisions of the trigeminal nerve, left lateral view.

*Indicate sensory nn.

Arteries of the Head & Neck

The head and neck are supplied by branches of the common carotid artery. The common carotid splits at the carotid bifurcation into two branches: the internal and external carotid arteries. The internal carotid chiefly supplies the brain (**p. 674**), although its branches anastomose with the external carotid in the orbit and nasal septum. The external carotid is the major supplier of structures of the head and neck.

Fig. 40.3 Internal carotid artery

Left lateral view. The most important extra-cerebral branch of the internal carotid artery is the ophthalmic artery, which supplies the upper nasal septum (**p. 584**) and the orbit (**p. 572**). See **pp. 676–677** for the arteries of the brain.

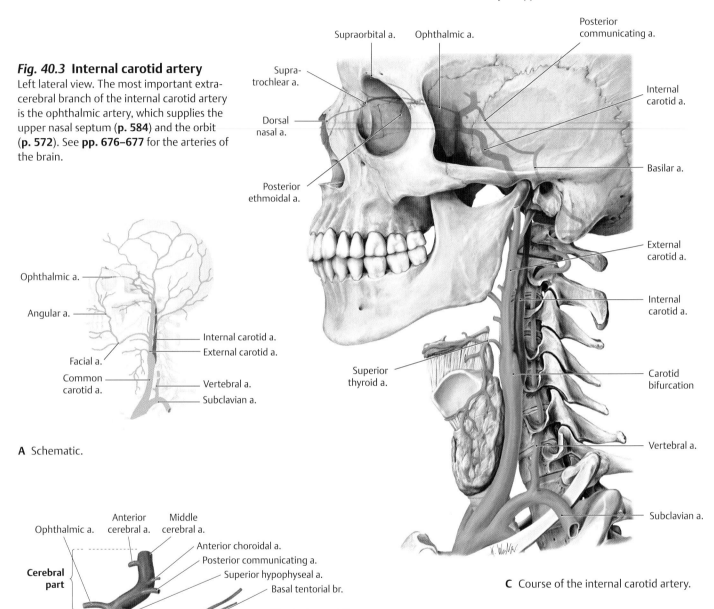

A Schematic.

C Course of the internal carotid artery.

B Parts and branches of the internal carotid artery.

Carotid artery atherosclerosis

The carotid artery is often affected by atherosclerosis, a hardening of arterial walls due to plaque formation. The examiner can determine the status of the arteries using ultrasound. *Note:* The absence of atherosclerosis in the carotid artery does not preclude coronary heart disease or atherosclerotic changes in other locations.

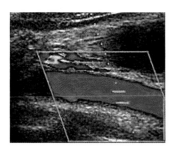

A Common carotid artery with "normal" flow.

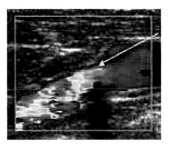

B Calcified plaque in the carotid bulb.

Fig. 40.4 **External carotid artery: Overview**
Left lateral view.

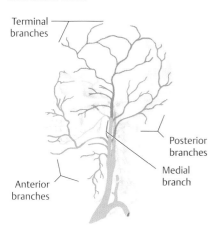

A Schematic of the external carotid artery.

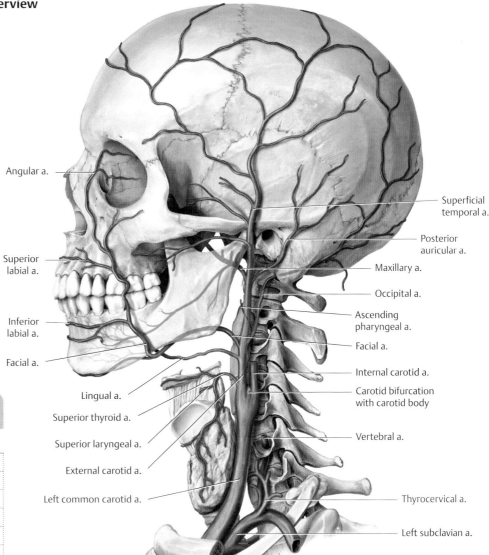

B Course of the external carotid artery.

Table 40.1	Branches of the external carotid artery
Group	**Artery**
Anterior (**p. 548**)	Superior thyroid a.
	Lingual a.
	Facial a.
Medial (**p. 548**)	Ascending pharyngeal a.
Posterior (**p. 549**)	Occipital a.
	Posterior auricular a.
Terminal (**p. 550**)	Maxillary a.
	Superficial temporal a.

External Carotid Artery: Anterior, Medial & Posterior Branches

Fig. 40.5 Anterior and medial branches

Left lateral view. The arteries of the anterior aspect supply the anterior structures of the head and neck, including the orbit (**p. 570**), ear (**p. 594**), larynx (**p. 635**), pharynx (**p. 616**), and oral cavity. *Note:* The angular artery anastomoses with the dorsal nasal artery of the internal carotid (via the ophthalmic artery).

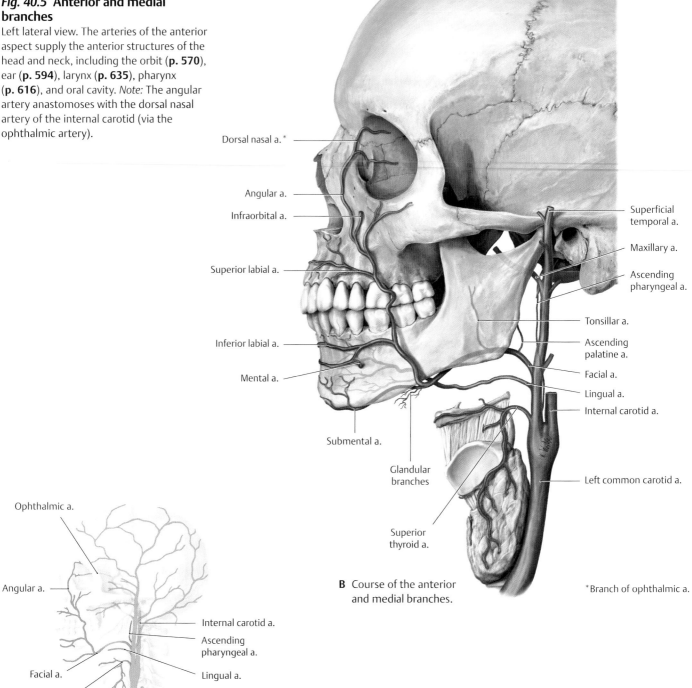

Dorsal nasal a.*

Angular a.

Infraorbital a.

Superior labial a.

Inferior labial a.

Mental a.

Submental a.

Glandular branches

Superior thyroid a.

Superficial temporal a.

Maxillary a.

Ascending pharyngeal a.

Tonsillar a.

Ascending palatine a.

Facial a.

Lingual a.

Internal carotid a.

Left common carotid a.

B Course of the anterior and medial branches.

*Branch of ophthalmic a.

Ophthalmic a.

Angular a.

Internal carotid a.

Ascending pharyngeal a.

Facial a.

Lingual a.

Superior thyroid a.

A Arteries of the anterior and medial branches. The copious blood supply to the face makes facial injuries bleed profusely but heal quickly. There are extensive anastomoses between branches of the external carotid artery and between the external carotid artery and branches of the ophthalmic artery.

Fig. 40.6 Posterior branches

Left lateral view. The posterior branches of the external carotid artery supply the ear (**p. 594**), posterior skull (**p. 559**), and posterior neck muscles (**p. 645**).

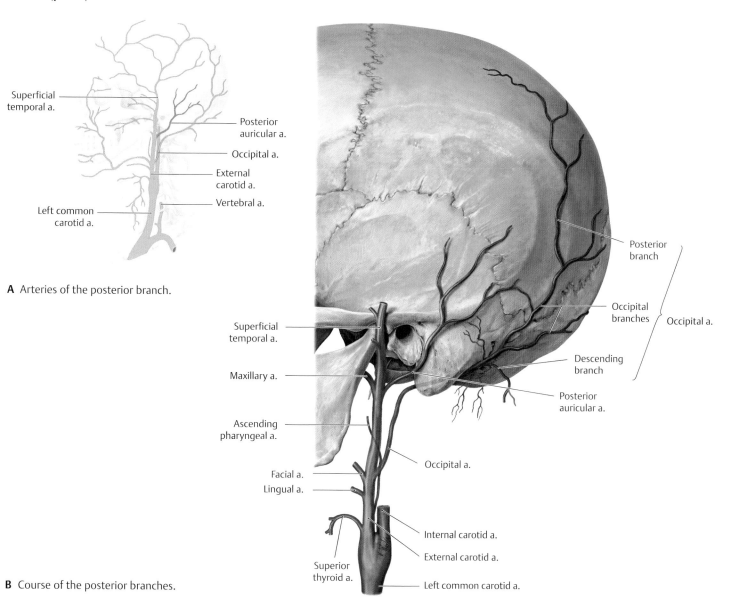

A Arteries of the posterior branch.

B Course of the posterior branches.

Table 40.2	Anterior, medial, and posterior branches of the external carotid artery	
Branch	**Artery**	**Divisions and distribution**
Anterior brs.	Superior thyroid a.	Glandular br. (to thyroid gland); superior laryngeal a.; sternocleidomastoid br.
	Lingual a.	Dorsal lingual brs. (to base of tongue, epiglottis); sublingual a. (to sublingual gland, tongue, oral floor, oral cavity)
	Facial a.	Ascending palatine a. (to pharyngeal wall, soft palate, pharyngotympanic tube); tonsillar branch (to palatine tonsils); submental a. (to oral floor, submandibular gland); labial aa.; angular a. (to nasal root)
Medial br.	Ascending pharyngeal a.	Pharyngeal brs.; interior tympanic a. (to mucosa of inner ear); posterior meningeal a.
Posterior brs.	Occipital a.	Occipital brs.; descending br. (to posterior neck muscles)
	Posterior auricular a.	Stylomastoid a. (to facial n. in facial canal); posterior tympanic a.; auricular br.; occipital br.; parotid br.
For terminal brs., see **Table 40.3 (p. 550).**		

External Carotid Artery: Terminal Branches

 The terminal branches of the external carotid artery consist of two major arteries: superficial temporal and maxillary. The superficial temporal artery supplies the lateral skull. The maxillary artery is a major artery for internal structures of the face.

Fig. 40.7 **Superficial temporal artery**

Left lateral view. Inflammation of the superficial temporal artery due to temporal arteritis can cause severe headaches. The course of the frontal branch of the artery can often be seen superficially under the skin of elderly patients.

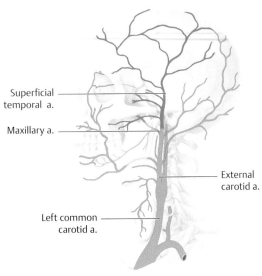

A Arteries of the terminal branch.

B Course of the superficial temporal artery.

Table 40.3	Terminal branches of the external carotid artery		
Branch	**Artery**		**Divisions and distribution**
Terminal brs.	Superficial temporal a.		Transverse facial a. (to soft tissues below the zygomatic arch); frontal brs.; parietal brs.; zygomatico-orbital a. (to lateral orbital wall)
	Maxillary a.	Mandibular part	Inferior alveolar a. (to mandible, teeth, gingiva); middle meningeal a.; deep auricular a. (to temporomandibular joint, external auditory canal); anterior tympanic a.
		Pterygoid part	Masseteric a.; deep temporal brs.; pterygoid brs.; buccal a.
		Pterygopalatine part	Posterosuperior alveolar a. (to maxillary molars, maxillary sinus, gingiva); infraorbital a. (to maxillary alveoli)
			Descending palatine a. — Greater palatine a. (to hard palate)
			Descending palatine a. — Lesser palatine a. (to soft palate, palatine tonsil, pharyngeal wall)
			Sphenopalatine a. — Lateral posterior nasal aa. (to lateral wall of nasal cavity, conchae)
			Sphenopalatine a. — Posterior septal brs. (to nasal septum)

* Parts not shown here. See **Fig 40.27 (p. 563)** and **Table 40.8 (p. 564).**

Fig. 40.8 Maxillary artery

Left lateral view. The maxillary artery consists of three parts: mandibular (blue), pterygoid (green), and pterygopalatine (yellow).

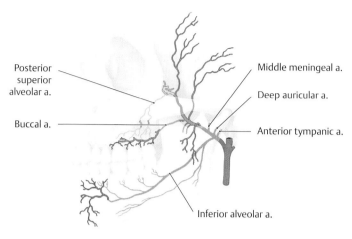

A Divisions of the maxillary artery.

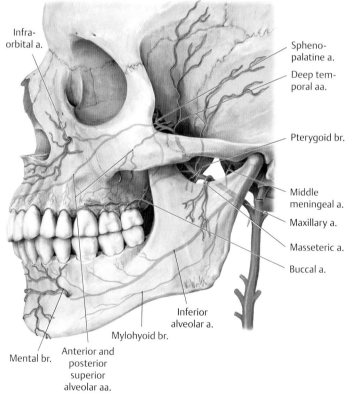

B Course of the maxillary artery.

Middle meningeal artery

The middle meningeal artery supplies the meninges and overlying calvaria. Rupture of the artery (generally due to head trauma) results in an epidural hematoma.

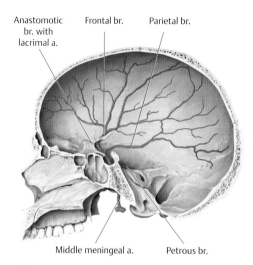

A Right middle meningeal artery, medial view of opened skull.

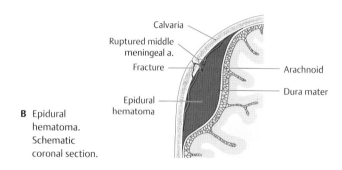

B Epidural hematoma. Schematic coronal section.

Sphenopalatine artery

The sphenopalatine artery supplies the wall of the nasal cavity. Excessive nasopharyngeal bleeding from the branches of the sphenopalatine artery may necessitate ligation of the maxillary artery in the pterygopalatine fossa.

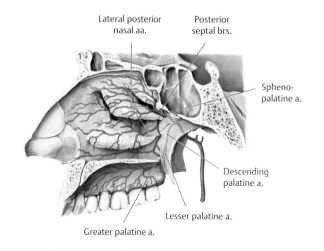

C Lateral wall of right nasal cavity, medial view.

Veins of the Head & Neck

Fig. 40.9 Veins of the head and neck

Left lateral view. The veins of the head and neck drain into the brachio-cephalic vein. *Note:* The left and right brachiocephalic veins are not symmetrical.

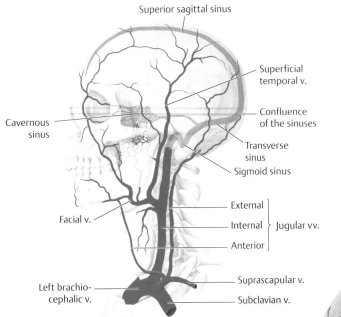

A Principal veins of the head and neck.

Table 40.4	**Principal superficial veins**	
Vein	**Region drained**	**Location**
Internal jugular v.	Interior of skull (including brain)	Within carotid sheath
External jugular v.	Superficial head	Within superficial cervical fascia
Anterior jugular v.	Neck, portions of head	

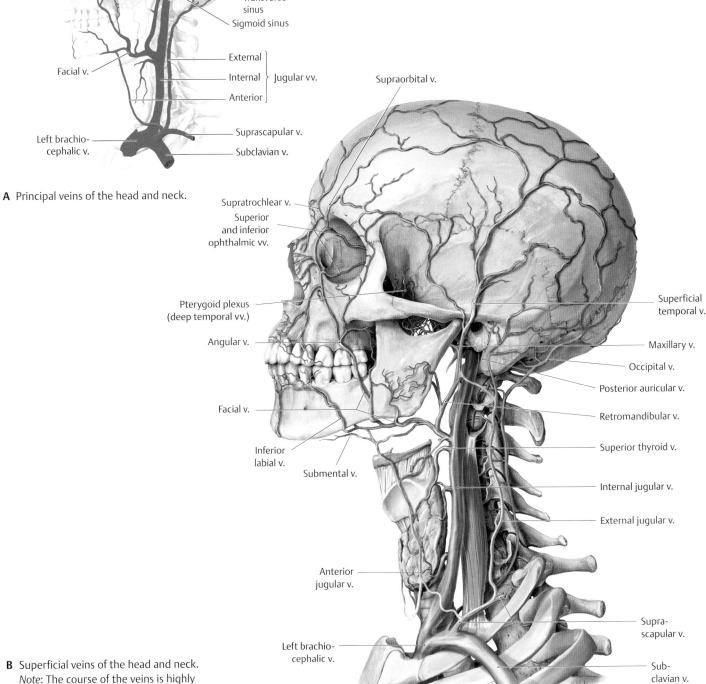

B Superficial veins of the head and neck.
Note: The course of the veins is highly variable.

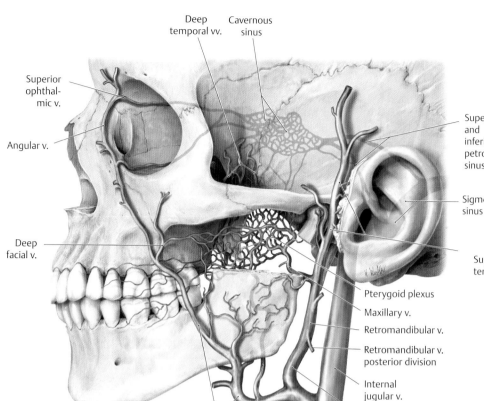

Fig. 40.10 Deep veins of the head

Left lateral view. *Removed:* Upper ramus, condylar and coronoid processes of mandible. The pterygoid plexus is a venous network situated between the mandibular ramus and the muscles of mastication. The cavernous sinus connects branches of the facial vein to the sigmoid sinuses.

Fig. 40.11 Veins of the occiput

Posterior view. The superficial veins of the occiput communicate with the dural venous sinuses via emissary veins that drain to diploic veins (calvaria, **p. 509**). *Note:* The external vertebral venous plexus traverses the entire length of the spine (**p. 45**).

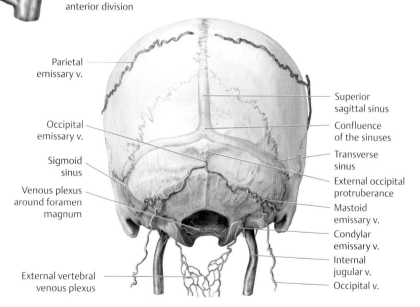

Table 40.5	**Venous anastomoses**

The extensive venous anastomoses in this region provide routes for the spread of infections.

Extracranial vein	Connecting vein	Venous sinus
Angular v.	Superior and inferior ophthalmic vv.	Cavernous sinus*
Vv. of palatine tonsil	Pterygoid plexus; inferior ophthalmic v.	
Superficial temporal v.	Parietal emissary vv.	Superior sagittal sinus
Occipital v.	Occipital emissary v.	Transverse sinus, confluence of the sinuses
Posterior auricular v.	Mastoid emissary v.	Sigmoid sinus
External vertebral venous plexus	Condylar emissary v.	

*Deep spread of bacterial infection from the facial region may result in cavernous sinus thrombosis.

Meninges

The brain and spinal cord are covered by membranes called meninges. The meninges are composed of three layers: dura mater (dura), arachnoid mater (arachnoid membrane), and pia mater.

The subarachnoid space, located between the arachnoid mater and pia mater, contains cerebrospinal fluid (CSF, see **p. 672**). See **p. 40** for the coverings of the spinal cord.

Fig. 40.12 Layers of the meninges

See **pp. 676–677** for the veins of the brain.

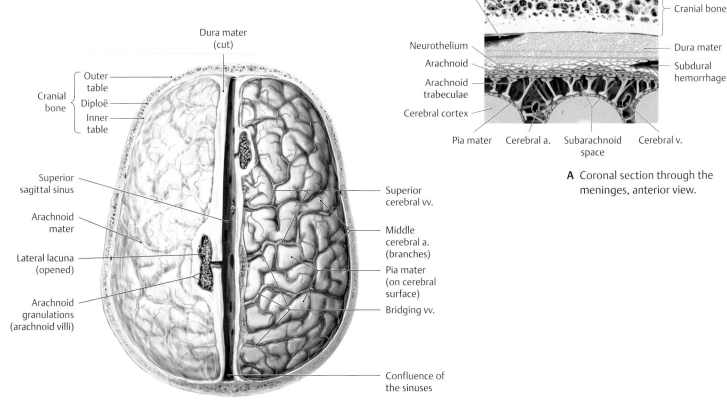

Dura mater (cut)

Cranial bone
{ Outer table
  Diploë
  Inner table }

Superior sagittal sinus

Arachnoid mater

Lateral lacuna (opened)

Arachnoid granulations (arachnoid villi)

Superior cerebral vv.

Middle cerebral a. (branches)

Pia mater (on cerebral surface)

Bridging vv.

Confluence of the sinuses

Diploic vv.

Epidural hematoma

Cranial bone

Neurothelium

Arachnoid

Arachnoid trabeculae

Cerebral cortex

Dura mater

Subdural hemorrhage

Pia mater   Cerebral a.   Subarachnoid space   Cerebral v.

A Coronal section through the meninges, anterior view.

B Superior view of opened cranium. *Left side:* Dura mater (outer layer) cut to reveal arachnoid (middle layer). *Right side:* Dura mater and arachnoid removed to reveal pia mater (inner layer) lining the surface of the brain. *Note:* Arachnoid granulations, sites for loss of cerebrospinal fluid into the venous blood, are protrusions of the arachnoid layer of the meninges into the venous sinus system.

Fig. 40.13 Dural septa (folds)

Left anterior oblique view. Two layers of meningeal dura come together, after separating from the periosteal dura during formation of a dural (venous) sinus, to form a dural fold or septum. These include the falx cerebri (separating right and left cerebral hemispheres); the tentorium cerebelli (supporting the cerebrum to keep it from crushing the underlying cerebellum); the falx cerebelli (not shown, separating right and left cerebellar lobes under the tentorium); and the diaphragma sellae (forming the roof over the hypophyseal fossa and invaginated by the hypophysis).

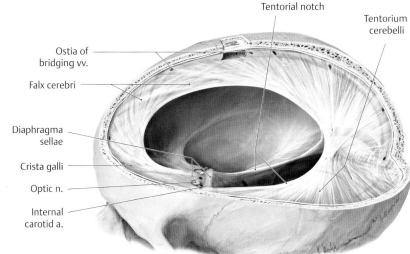

Ostia of bridging vv.

Falx cerebri

Diaphragma sellae

Crista galli

Optic n.

Internal carotid a.

Tentorial notch

Tentorium cerebelli

Extracerebral hemorrhages

Bleeding between the bony calvarium and the soft tissue of the brain (extracerebral hemorrhage) exerts pressure on the brain. A rise of intracranial pressure may damage brain tissue both at the bleeding site and in more remote brain areas. Three types of intracranial hemorrhage are distinguished based on the relationship to the dura mater. See **pp. 674–675** for the arteries of the brain.

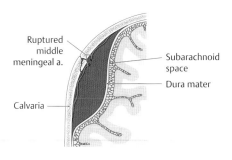
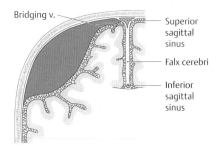
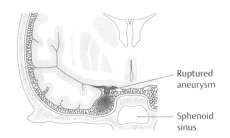

A Epidural hematoma (above the dura).

B Subdural hematoma (below the dura).

C Subarachnoid hemorrhage.

Fig. 40.14 **Arteries of the dura mater**
Midsagittal section, left lateral view. See **pp. 674–675** for the arteries of the brain.

Fig. 40.15 **Innervation of the dura mater**
Superior view. *Removed:* Tentorium cerebelli (right side).

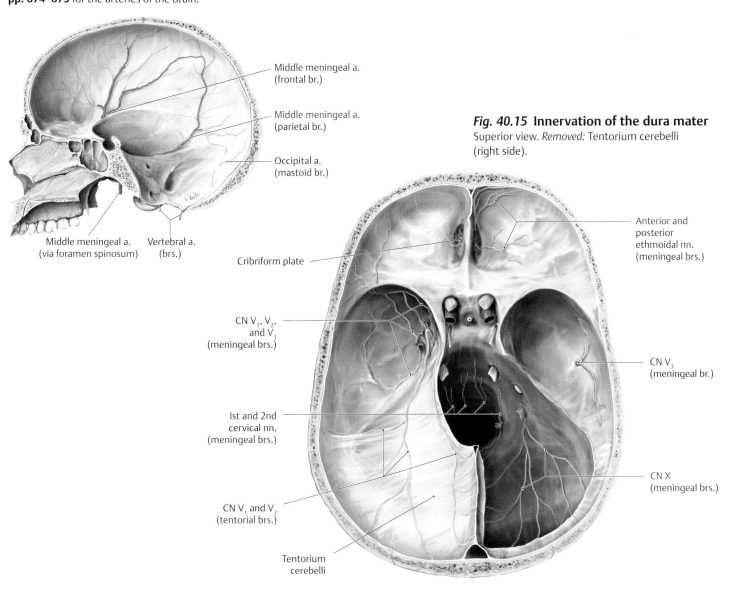

Dural Sinuses

The dura mater is composed of two layers that separate in the region of a venous sinus into an outer periosteal layer, which lines the calvaria and an inner meningeal layer, which forms the unattached boundaries of the sinus. In the region of a sinus, the two meningeal dural layers come together after forming the sinus to create a dural fold, or septa (see **Fig. 40.13, p. 554**). The network of venous sinuses collect blood from the scalp, the calvaria, and the brain and eventually drain into the internal jugular vein at the jugular foramen.

Fig. 40.16 Dural sinus

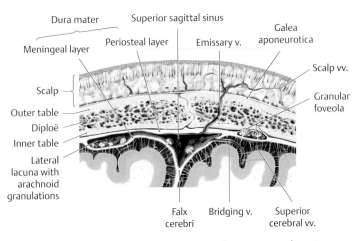

A Structure of a dural sinus. Superior sagittal sinus, coronal section, anterior view.

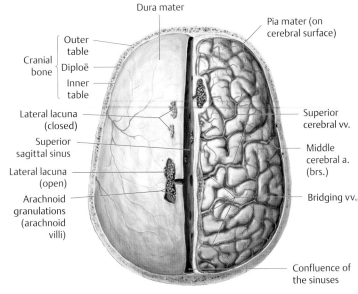

B Superior sagittal sinus in situ. Superior view of opened cranial cavity. The roof of the sinus (the periosteal layer of the dura attached to the calvaria) is removed. *Left side:* Areas of dura mater removed to show arachnoid granulations (protrusions of the arachnoid layer of the meninges) in the sinus. *Right side:* Dura mater and arachnoid layers removed to reveal pia mater adhering to the cerebral cortex.

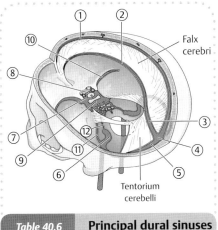

Fig. 40.17 Dural sinuses in the cranial cavity

Superior view of opened cranial cavity. Dural sinus system ghosted in blue. *Removed:* Tentorium cerebelli (right side).

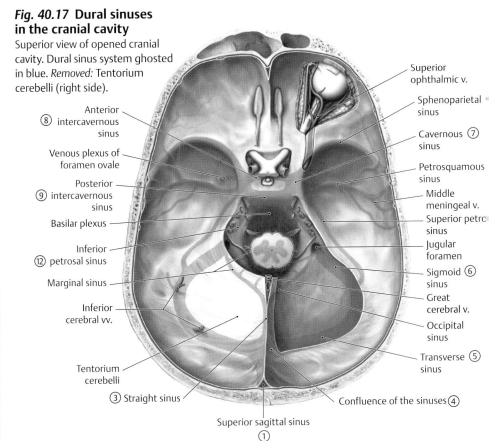

Table 40.6	Principal dural sinuses		
Upper group		**Lower group**	
①	Superior sagittal sinus	⑦	Cavernous sinus
②	Inferior sagittal sinus	⑧	Anterior inter-cavernous sinus
③	Straight sinus	⑨	Posterior inter-cavernous sinus
④	Confluence of the sinuses	⑩	Sphenoparietal sinus
⑤	Transverse sinus	⑪	Superior petrosal sinus
⑥	Sigmoid sinus	⑫	Inferior petrosal sinus

The occipital sinus is also included in the upper group (see **Fig. 48.1, p. 674**).

Fig. 40.18 Cavernous sinus and cranial nerves

Superior view of the right anterior and middle cranial fossae. *Removed:* Lateral dural wall and roof of the cavernous sinus. The trigeminal ganglion is cut and retracted laterally following removal of its dural covering

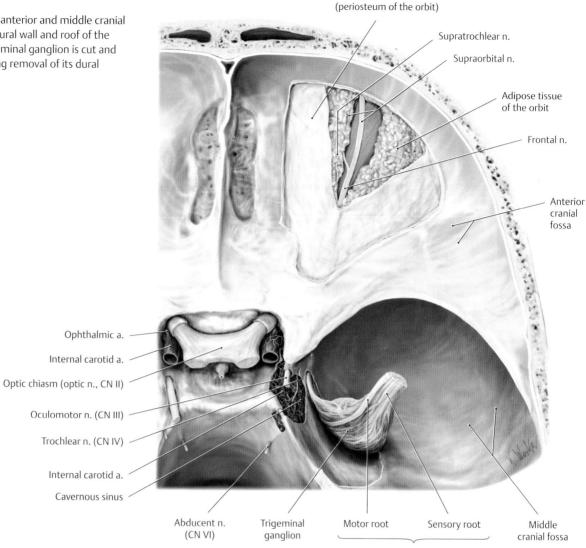

Periorbita (periosteum of the orbit)
Supratrochlear n.
Supraorbital n.
Adipose tissue of the orbit
Frontal n.
Anterior cranial fossa

Ophthalmic a.
Internal carotid a.
Optic chiasm (optic n., CN II)
Oculomotor n. (CN III)
Trochlear n. (CN IV)
Internal carotid a.
Cavernous sinus

Abducent n. (CN VI)
Trigeminal ganglion
Motor root
Sensory root
Middle cranial fossa

Trigeminal nerve (CN V)

Fig. 40.19 Cavernous sinus, coronal section through middle cranial fossa

Anterior view. The right and left cavernous sinuses connect via the intercavernous sinuses that pass around the hypophysis, which sits in the hypophysial fossa after invaginating the diaphragma sellae. On each side, this coronal section cuts through the internal carotid artery twice due to the presence of the carotid siphon, a 180 degree bend in the cavernous part of the artery. Of the five cranial nerves, or their divisions, associated with the sinus only the abducent nerve (CN VI) is not embedded in the lateral dural wall.

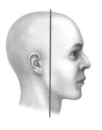
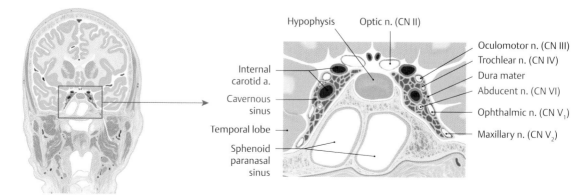

Hypophysis
Optic n. (CN II)
Oculomotor n. (CN III)
Trochlear n. (CN IV)
Dura mater
Abducent n. (CN VI)
Ophthalmic n. (CN V₁)
Maxillary n. (CN V₂)

Internal carotid a.
Cavernous sinus
Temporal lobe
Sphenoid paranasal sinus

Topography of the Superficial Face

Fig. 40.20 Superficial neurovasculature of the face
Anterior view. *Removed:* Skin and fatty subcutaneous tissue; muscles of facial expression (left side).

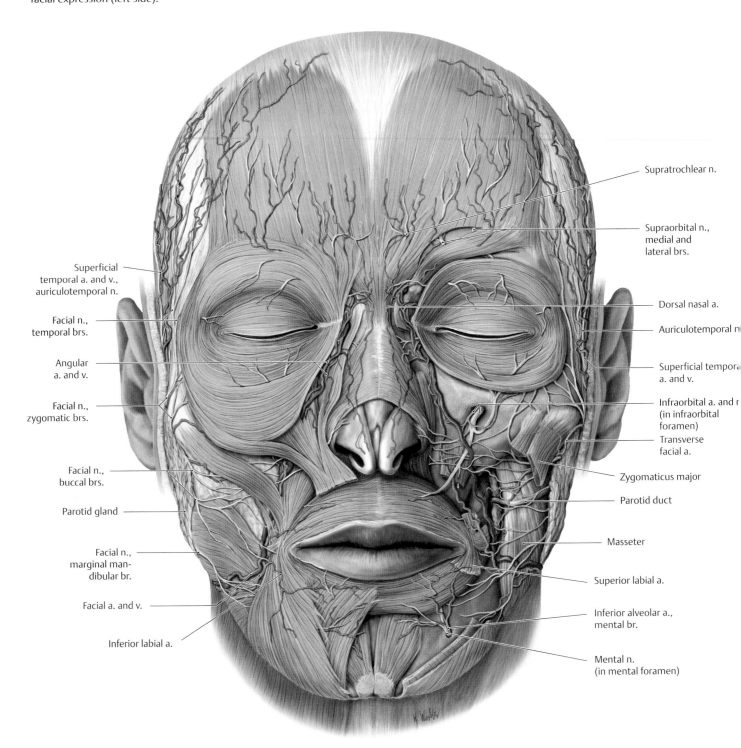

Supratrochlear n.

Supraorbital n., medial and lateral brs.

Superficial temporal a. and v., auriculotemporal n.

Facial n., temporal brs.

Angular a. and v.

Facial n., zygomatic brs.

Facial n., buccal brs.

Parotid gland

Facial n., marginal mandibular br.

Facial a. and v.

Inferior labial a.

Dorsal nasal a.

Auriculotemporal n.

Superficial temporal a. and v.

Infraorbital a. and n. (in infraorbital foramen)

Transverse facial a.

Zygomaticus major

Parotid duct

Masseter

Superior labial a.

Inferior alveolar a., mental br.

Mental n. (in mental foramen)

Fig. 40.21 **Superficial neurovasculature of the head**
Left lateral view.

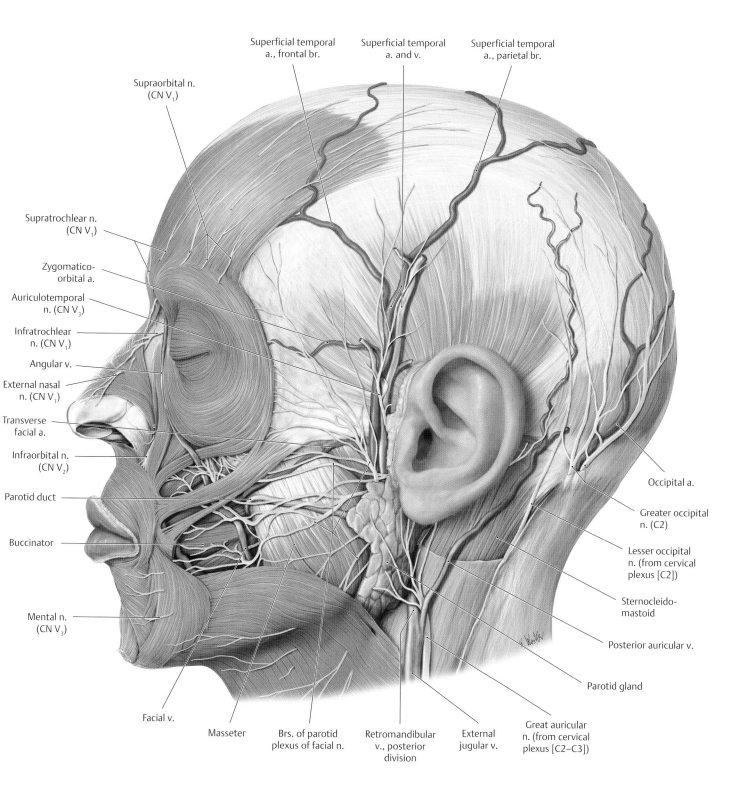

Supraorbital n. (CN V₁)

Superficial temporal a., frontal br.

Superficial temporal a. and v.

Superficial temporal a., parietal br.

Supratrochlear n. (CN V₁)

Zygomatico- orbital a.

Auriculotemporal n. (CN V₃)

Infratrochlear n. (CN V₁)

Angular v.

External nasal n. (CN V₁)

Transverse facial a.

Infraorbital n. (CN V₂)

Parotid duct

Buccinator

Mental n. (CN V₃)

Occipital a.

Greater occipital n. (C2)

Lesser occipital n. (from cervical plexus [C2])

Sternocleido- mastoid

Posterior auricular v.

Parotid gland

Facial v.

Masseter

Brs. of parotid plexus of facial n.

Retromandibular v., posterior division

External jugular v.

Great auricular n. (from cervical plexus [C2–C3])

Topography of the Parotid Region & Temporal Fossa

Fig. 40.22 Parotid region

Left lateral view. *Removed:* Parotid gland, sternocleidomastoid, and veins of the head. *Revealed:* Parotid bed and carotid triangle.

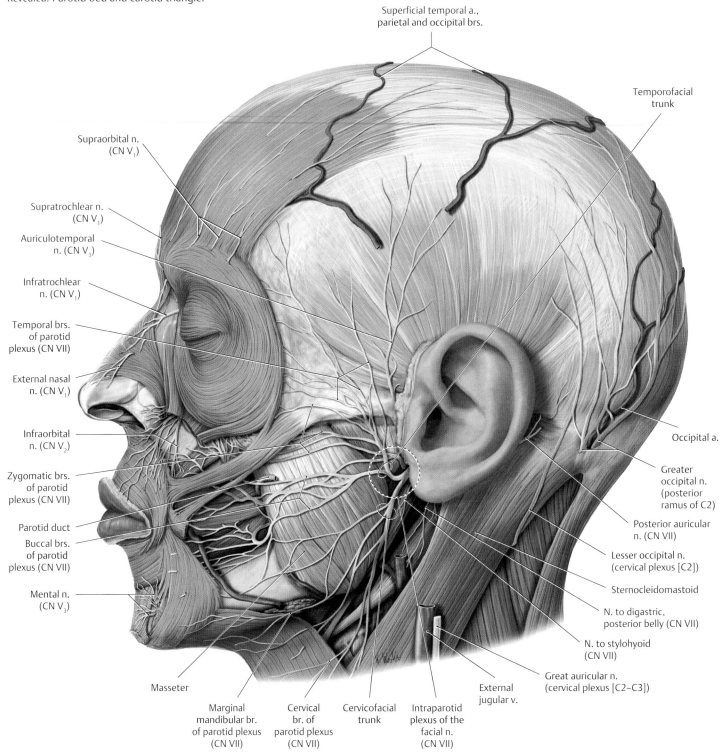

Superficial temporal a., parietal and occipital brs.

Temporofacial trunk

Supraorbital n. (CN V₁)

Supratrochlear n. (CN V₁)

Auriculotemporal n. (CN V₃)

Infratrochlear n. (CN V₁)

Temporal brs. of parotid plexus (CN VII)

External nasal n. (CN V₁)

Infraorbital n. (CN V₂)

Zygomatic brs. of parotid plexus (CN VII)

Parotid duct

Buccal brs. of parotid plexus (CN VII)

Mental n. (CN V₃)

Occipital a.

Greater occipital n. (posterior ramus of C2)

Posterior auricular n. (CN VII)

Lesser occipital n. (cervical plexus [C2])

Sternocleidomastoid

N. to digastric, posterior belly (CN VII)

N. to stylohyoid (CN VII)

Great auricular n. (cervical plexus [C2–C3])

Masseter

Marginal mandibular br. of parotid plexus (CN VII)

Cervical br. of parotid plexus (CN VII)

Cervicofacial trunk

Intraparotid plexus of the facial n. (CN VII)

External jugular v.

Fig. 40.23 Temporal fossa

Left lateral view. The temporal fossa is located on the lateral aspect of the skull. It communicates with the infratemporal fossa inferiorly (medial to the zygomatic arch). The pterygopalatine fossa can also be seen here medial to the infratemporal fossa due to the removal of the zygomatic arch and some of the zygomatic bone.

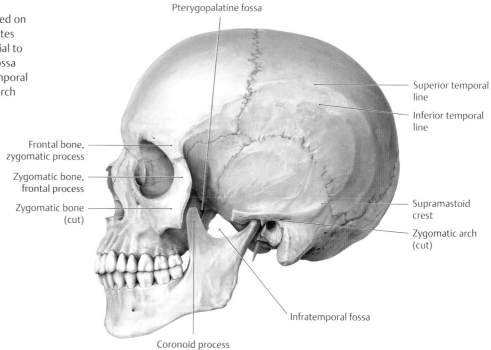

Pterygopalatine fossa

Superior temporal line

Inferior temporal line

Frontal bone, zygomatic process

Zygomatic bone, frontal process

Zygomatic bone (cut)

Supramastoid crest

Zygomatic arch (cut)

Infratemporal fossa

Coronoid process

Fig. 40.24 Temporal fossa

Left lateral view. *Removed:* Sternocleidomastoid and masseter. *Revealed:* Temporal fossa and temporomandibular joint (**p. 600**).

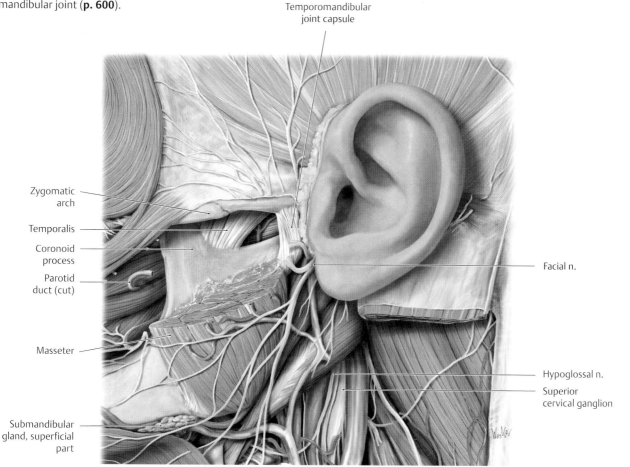

Temporomandibular joint capsule

Zygomatic arch

Temporalis

Coronoid process

Parotid duct (cut)

Masseter

Facial n.

Hypoglossal n.

Superior cervical ganglion

Submandibular gland, superficial part

Topography of the Infratemporal Fossa

Fig. 40.25 **Infratemporal fossa: Superficial layer**

Left lateral view. *Removed:* Ramus of mandible. *Note:* The mylohyoid
nerve (see **Fig. 44.15 and 44.17A**) branches from the inferior alveolar
nerve just before the mandibular foramen.

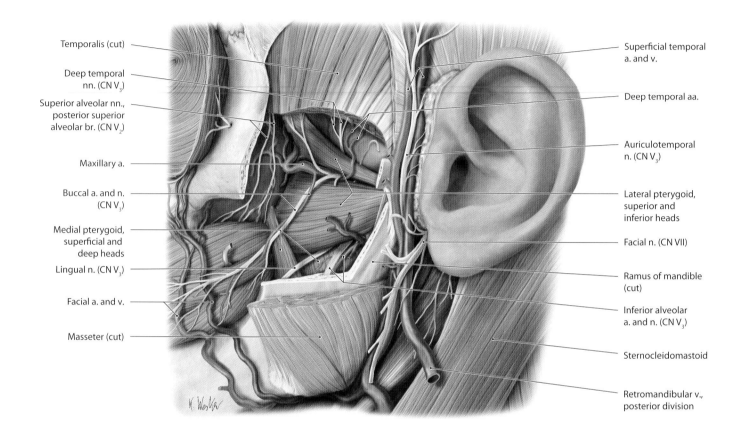

Temporalis (cut)

Deep temporal
nn. (CN V₃)

Superior alveolar nn.,
posterior superior
alveolar br. (CN V₂)

Maxillary a.

Buccal a. and n.
(CN V₃)

Medial pterygoid,
superficial and
deep heads

Lingual n. (CN V₃)

Facial a. and v.

Masseter (cut)

Superficial temporal
a. and v.

Deep temporal aa.

Auriculotemporal
n. (CN V₃)

Lateral pterygoid,
superior and
inferior heads

Facial n. (CN VII)

Ramus of mandible
(cut)

Inferior alveolar
a. and n. (CN V₃)

Sternocleidomastoid

Retromandibular v.,
posterior division

Fig. 40.26 Infratemporal fossa: Deep layer

Left lateral view. *Removed:* Lateral pterygoid muscle (both heads).
Revealed: Deep infratemporal fossa and mandibular nerve as it enters the
mandibular canal via the foramen ovale in the roof of the fossa.

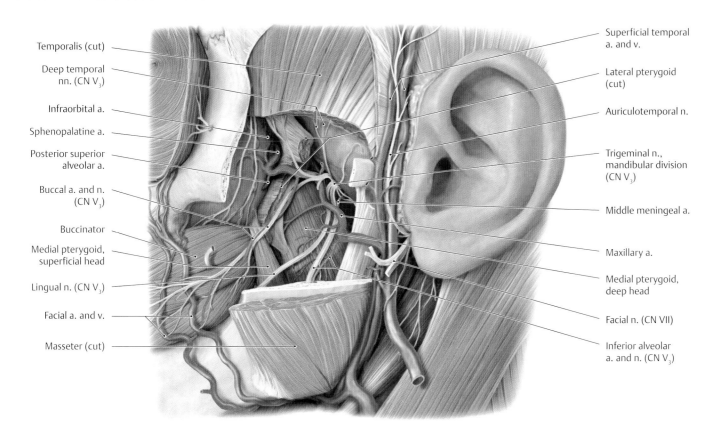

Temporalis (cut)

Deep temporal nn. (CN V₃)

Infraorbital a.

Sphenopalatine a.

Posterior superior alveolar a.

Buccal a. and n. (CN V₃)

Buccinator

Medial pterygoid, superficial head

Lingual n. (CN V₃)

Facial a. and v.

Masseter (cut)

Superficial temporal a. and v.

Lateral pterygoid (cut)

Auriculotemporal n.

Trigeminal n., mandibular division (CN V₃)

Middle meningeal a.

Maxillary a.

Medial pterygoid, deep head

Facial n. (CN VII)

Inferior alveolar a. and n. (CN V₃)

Fig. 40.27 Mandibular nerve (CN V₃) in the infratemporal fossa

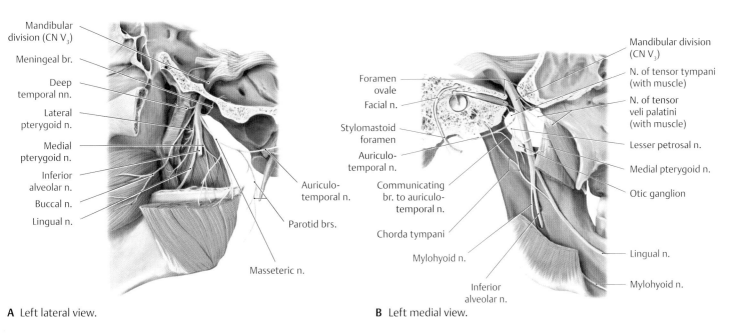

Mandibular division (CN V₃)

Meningeal br.

Deep temporal nn.

Lateral pterygoid n.

Medial pterygoid n.

Inferior alveolar n.

Buccal n.

Lingual n.

Auriculotemporal n.

Parotid brs.

Masseteric n.

A Left lateral view.

Mandibular division (CN V₃)

N. of tensor tympani (with muscle)

N. of tensor veli palatini (with muscle)

Lesser petrosal n.

Medial pterygoid n.

Otic ganglion

Lingual n.

Mylohyoid n.

Foramen ovale

Facial n.

Stylomastoid foramen

Auriculotemporal n.

Communicating br. to auriculotemporal n.

Chorda tympani

Mylohyoid n.

Inferior alveolar n.

B Left medial view.

Topography of the Pterygopalatine Fossa

The pterygopalatine fossa is a small pyramidal space just inferior to the apex of the orbit. It is continuous with the infratemporal fossa laterally through the pterygomaxillary fissure.

The pterygopalatine fossa is a crossroads for neurovascular structures traveling between the middle cranial fossa, orbit, nasal cavity, and oral cavity.

Table 40.7	Borders of the pterygopalatine fossa			
Direction	**Boundaries**		**Direction**	**Boundaries**
Superior	Sphenoid bone (greater wing), junction with inferior orbital fissure		Posterior	Pterygoid process (lateral plate)
Anterior	Maxillary tuberosity		Lateral	Communicates with the infratemporal fossa via the pterygomaxillary fissure
Medial	Palatine bone (perpendicular plate)		Inferior	None; opens into the retropharyngeal space

Fig. 40.28 Arteries in the pterygopalatine fossa

Left lateral view into area. The maxillary artery passes either superficial or deep to the lateral pterygoid in the infratemporal fossa (see **Fig. 40.24, p. 561**) and enters the pterygopalatine fossa through the pterygomaxillary fissure.

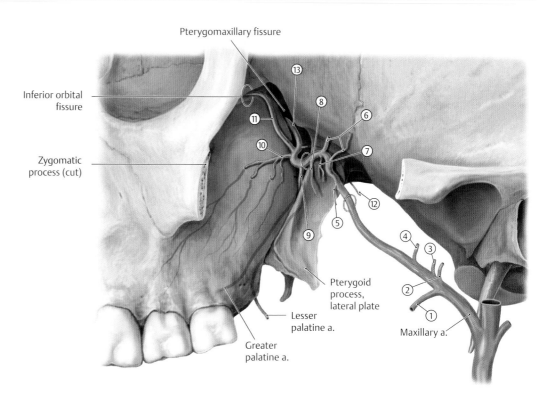

Table 40.8	Branches of the maxillary artery		
Part	**Artery**		**Distribution**
Mandibular part (between the origin and the first circle around artery in **Fig. 40.28**)	① Inferior alveolar a.		Mandible, teeth, gingiva
	② Anterior tympanic a.		Tympanic cavity
	③ Deep auricular a.		Temporomandibular joint, external auditory canal
	④ Middle meningeal a.		Calvaria, dura, anterior and middle cranial fossae
Pterygoid part (between the first and second circles around the artery)	⑤ Masseteric a.		Masseter m.
	⑥ Deep temporal aa.		Temporalis m.
	⑦ Pterygoid brs.		Pterygoid mm.
	⑧ Buccal a.		Buccal mucosa
Pterygopalatine part (between the second and third circles around the artery)	⑨ Descending palatine a.	Greater palatine a.	Hard palate
		Lesser palatine a.	Soft palate, palatine tonsil, pharyngeal wall
	⑩ Posterior superior alveolar a.		Maxillary molars, maxillary sinus, gingiva
	⑪ Infraorbital a.		Maxillary alveoli
	⑫ A. of pterygoid canal		
	⑬ Sphenopalatine a.	Lateral posterior nasal aa.	Lateral wall of nasal cavity, choanae
		Posterior septal brs.	Nasal septum

The maxillary division of the trigeminal nerve (CN V₂, see **p. 531**) passes from the middle cranial fossa through the foramen rotundum into the pterygopalatine fossa. The parasympathetic pterygopalatine ganglion receives presynaptic fibers from the greater petrosal nerve (the parasympathetic root of the nervus intermedius branch of the facial nerve). The preganglionic fibers of the pterygopalatine ganglion synapse with ganglion cells that innervate the lacrimal, small palatal, and small nasal glands. The sympathetic fibers of the deep petrosal nerve (sympathetic root) and sensory fibers of the maxillary nerve (sensory root) pass through the pterygopalatine ganglion without synapsing. The pterygopalatine structures can be seen from the medial view in **Fig. 42.8, p. 585.**

Fig. 40.29 Nerves in the pterygopalatine fossa
Left lateral view.

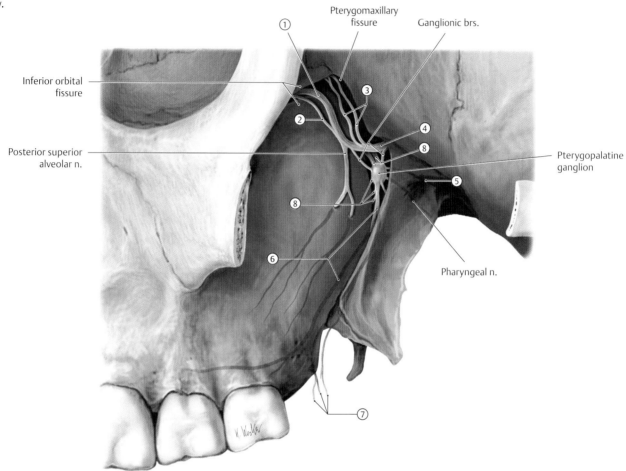

Table 40.9 Passage of neurovascular structures into pterygopalatine fossa

Origin of structures	Passageway	Transmitted nerves	Transmitted vessels
Orbit	Inferior orbital fissure	① Infraorbital n.	Infraorbital a. (and accompanying vv.)
		② Zygomatic n.	Inferior ophthalmic v.
		③ Orbital brs. (from CN V₂)	
Middle cranial fossa	Foramen rotundum	④ Maxillary n. (CN V₂)	
Base of skull	Pterygoid canal	⑤ N. of pterygoid canal (greater and deep petrosal nn.)	A. of pterygoid canal (with accompanying vv.)
Palate	Greater palatine canal	⑥ Greater palatine n.	Descending palatine a.
			Greater palatine a.
	Lesser palatine canals	⑦ Lesser palatine nn.	Lesser palatine aa. (terminal branches of descending palatine a.)
Nasal cavity	Sphenopalatine foramen	⑧ Medial and lateral posterior superior and posterior inferior nasal brs. (from nasopalatine n., CN V₂)	Sphenopalatine a. (with accompanying vv.)

Bones of the Orbit

Fig. 41.1 Bones of the orbit

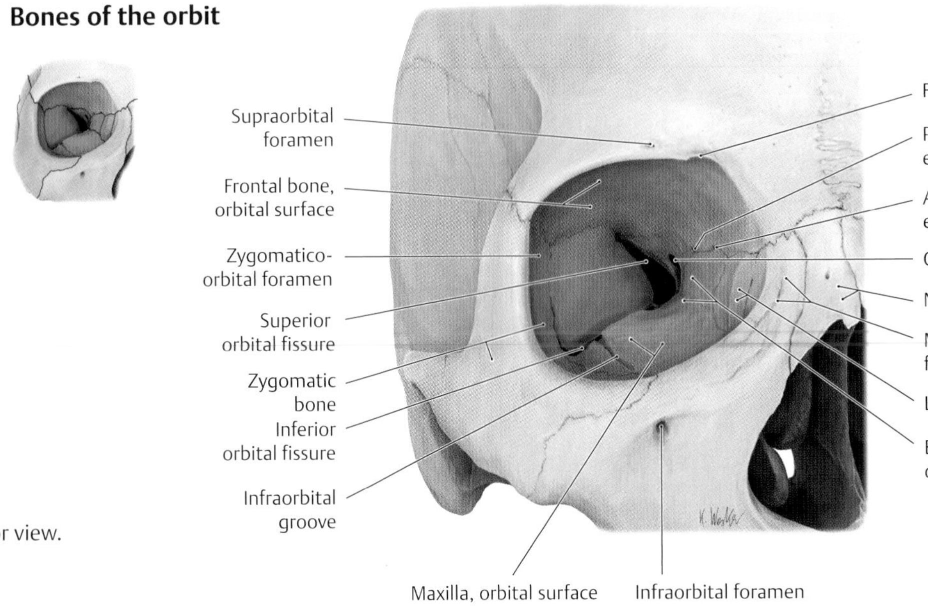

Supraorbital foramen
Frontal bone, orbital surface
Zygomatico-orbital foramen
Superior orbital fissure
Zygomatic bone
Inferior orbital fissure
Infraorbital groove

Frontal incisure
Posterior ethmoidal foramen
Anterior ethmoidal foramen
Optic canal (sphenoid bone)
Nasal bone
Maxilla, frontal process
Lacrimal bone
Ethmoid bone, orbital plate

Maxilla, orbital surface   Infraorbital foramen

A Anterior view.

Frontal bone, orbital surface   Lacrimal bone

Anterior and posterior ethmoidal foramina
Ethmoid bone
Sphenoid, optic canal
Superior orbital fissure
Foramen rotundum
Inferior orbital fissure

Maxilla, frontal process
Lacrimal bone, posterior lacrimal crest
Maxilla, anterior lacrimal crest
Fossa of lacrimal sac (with opening for nasolacrimal duct)
Maxilla, orbital surface
Infraorbital canal

Pterygopalatine fossa   Maxillary hiatus   Maxillary sinus   Infraorbital foramen

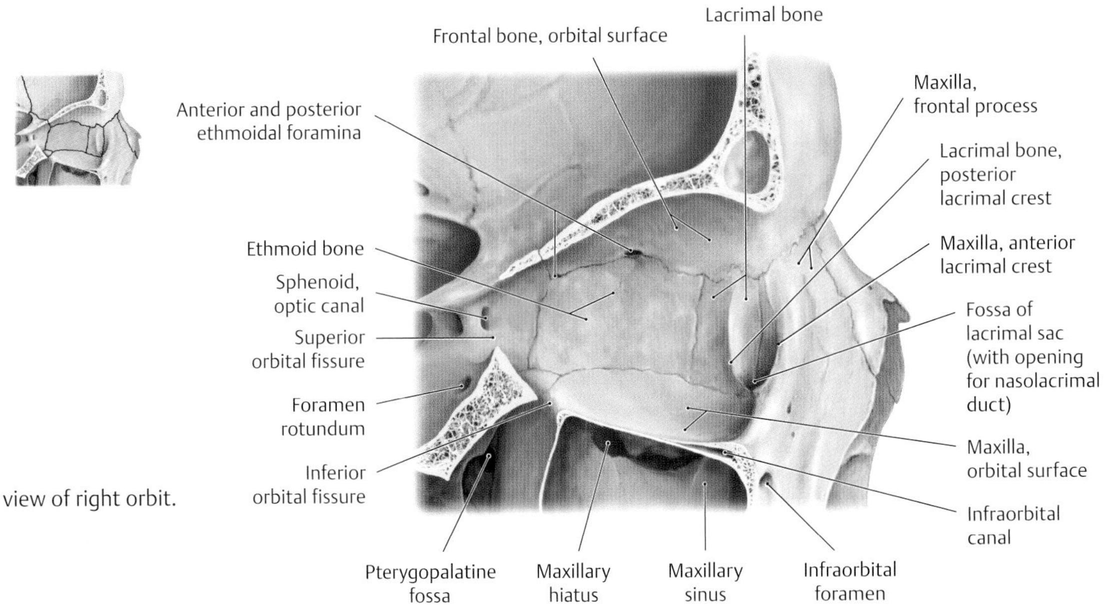

B Lateral view of right orbit.

Table 41.1	Openings in the orbit for neurovascular structures		
Opening*	**Nerves**		**Vessels**
Optic canal	Optic n. (CN II)		Ophthalmic a.
Superior orbital fissure	Oculomotor n. (CN III) Trochlear n. (CN IV) Abducent n. (CN VI)	Trigeminal n., ophthalmic division (CN V₁) • Lacrimal n. • Frontal n. • Nasociliary n.	Superior ophthalmic v.
Inferior orbital fissure	Infraorbital n. (CN V₂) Zygomatic n. (CN V₂)		Infraorbital a. and v., inferior ophthalmic v.
Infraorbital canal	Infraorbital n. (CN V₂), a., and v.		
Supraorbital foramen	Supraorbital n. (lateral br.)		Supraorbital a.
Frontal incisure	Supraorbital n. (medial br.)		Supratrochlear a.
Anterior ethmoidal foramen	Anterior ethmoidal n., a., and v.		
Posterior ethmoidal foramen	Posterior ethmoidal n., a., and v.		

* The nasolacrimal canal transmits the nasolacrimal duct.

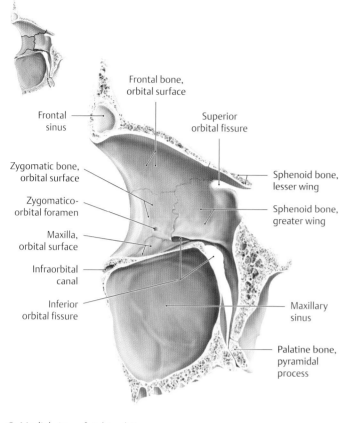

Frontal bone,
orbital surface

Frontal
sinus

Superior
orbital fissure

Zygomatic bone,
orbital surface

Sphenoid bone,
lesser wing

Zygomatico-
orbital foramen

Sphenoid bone,
greater wing

Maxilla,
orbital surface

Infraorbital
canal

Inferior
orbital fissure

Maxillary
sinus

Palatine bone,
pyramidal
process

C Medial view of right orbit.

Table 41.2	Structures surrounding the orbit
Direction	**Bordering structure**
Superior	Frontal sinus
	Anterior cranial fossa
Medial	Ethmoid sinus
Inferior	Maxillary sinus
Certain deeper structures also have a clinically important relationship to the orbit:	
Sphenoid sinus	Hypophysis (pituitary)
Middle cranial fossa	Cavernous sinus
Optic chiasm	Pterygopalatine fossa

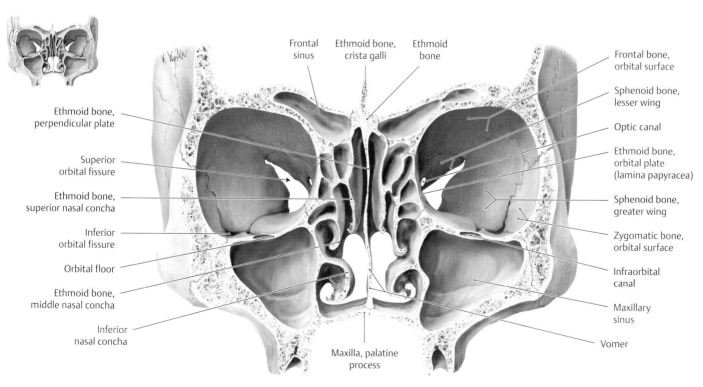

Ethmoid bone,
perpendicular plate

Frontal
sinus

Ethmoid bone,
crista galli

Ethmoid
bone

Frontal bone,
orbital surface

Sphenoid bone,
lesser wing

Superior
orbital fissure

Optic canal

Ethmoid bone,
superior nasal concha

Ethmoid bone,
orbital plate
(lamina papyracea)

Inferior
orbital fissure

Sphenoid bone,
greater wing

Orbital floor

Zygomatic bone,
orbital surface

Ethmoid bone,
middle nasal concha

Infraorbital
canal

Inferior
nasal concha

Maxillary
sinus

Maxilla, palatine
process

Vomer

D Coronal section, anterior view.

Muscles of the Orbit

Fig. 41.2 Extraocular muscles

The eyeball is moved by six extrinsic muscles: four rectus (superior, inferior, medial, and lateral) and two oblique (superior and inferior).

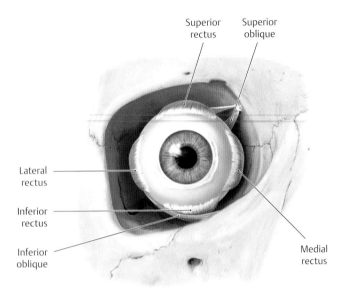

A Right eye, anterior view.

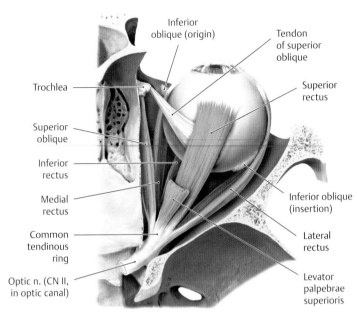

B Right eye, superior view of opened orbit.

Fig. 41.3 Actions of the extraocular muscles

Superior view of opened orbit. Vertical axis, red circle; horizontal axis, black; anteroposterior (visual/optical) axis, blue.

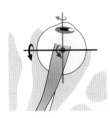 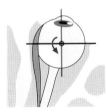 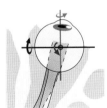 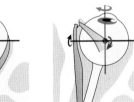 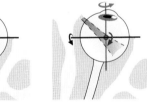

A Superior rectus. **B** Medial rectus. **C** Inferior rectus. **D** Lateral rectus. **E** Superior oblique. **F** Inferior oblique.

Table 41.3 Extraocular muscles

Muscle	Origin	Insertion	Vertical axis (red)	Horizontal axis (black)	Anteroposterior axis (blue)	Innervation
Superior rectus	Common tendinous ring (common annular tendon)	Sclera of the eye	Elevates	Adducts	Rotates medially	Oculomotor n. (CN III), superior branch
Medial rectus			—	Adducts	—	Oculomotor n. (CN III), inferior branch
Inferior rectus			Depresses	Adducts	Rotates laterally	
Lateral rectus			—	Abducts	—	Abducent n. (CN VI)
Superior oblique	Sphenoid bone[+]		Depresses	Abducts	Rotates medially	Trochlear n. (CN IV)
Inferior oblique	Medial orbital margin		Elevates	Abducts	Rotates laterally	Oculomotor n. (CN III), inferior branch

Action (see Fig. 41.3)[*]

* Starting from gaze directed anteriorly
+ The tendon of the superior oblique passes through a tendinous loop (trochlea) attached to the superomedial orbital margin.

Fig. 41.4 Testing the extraocular muscles

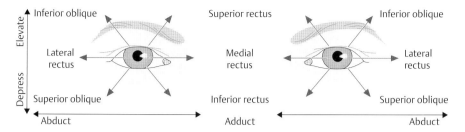

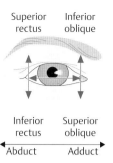

A Starting with the eyes directed anteriorly, movement to any of the cardinal directions of gaze (*arrows*) requires activation of two extraocular muscles, each of which is innervated by a different cranial nerve, thus testing the function of those pairs of muscles.

B Starting with the eyes adducted or abducted, elevating or lowering the eyes activates only the oblique or the rectus muscles, respectively, allowing for testing of the function of individual muscles.

Fig. 41.5 Innervation of the extraocular muscles
Right eye, lateral view with the temporal wall of the orbit removed.

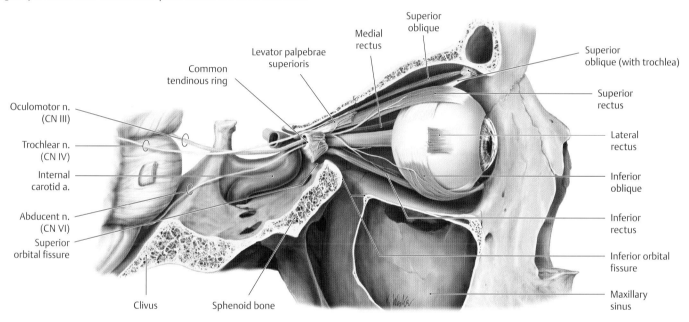

Clinical box 41.1

Oculomotor palsies
Oculomotor palsies may result from a lesion involving an eye muscle or its associated cranial nerve (at the nucleus or along the course of the nerve). If one extraocular muscle is weak or paralyzed, deviation of the eye will be noted.

Impairment of the coordinated actions of the extraocular muscles may cause the visual axis of one eye to deviate from its normal position. The patient will therefore perceive a double image (diplopia).

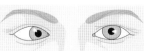

A Abducent nerve palsy. *Disabled:* Lateral rectus.

B Trochlear nerve palsy. *Disabled:* Superior oblique.

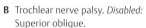

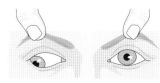

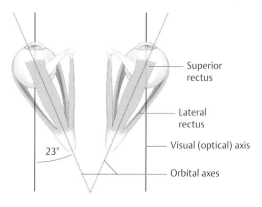

C Complete oculomotor palsy. *Disabled:* Superior, inferior, and medial recti and inferior oblique.

D Normal visual and orbital axes.

Neurovasculature of the Orbit

Fig. 41.6 Veins of the orbit
Lateral view of the right orbit. *Removed:* Lateral orbital wall. *Opened:* Maxillary sinus.

Supra-trochlear v.

Dorsal nasal v.

Superior ophthalmic v.

Lacrimal v.

Angular v.

Cavernous sinus

Ophthalmic v.

Inferior ophthalmic v.

Infraorbital v.

Facial v.

Fig. 41.7 Arteries of the orbit
Superior view of the right orbit. *Opened:* Optic canal and orbital roof.

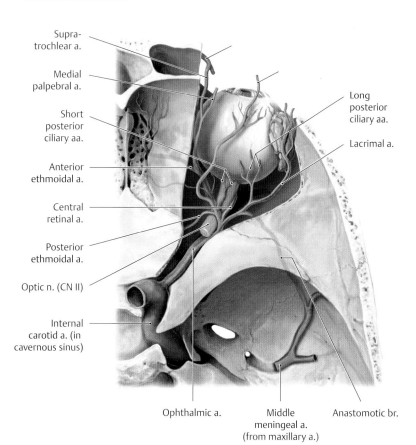

Supra-trochlear a.

Medial palpebral a.

Short posterior ciliary aa.

Anterior ethmoidal a.

Central retinal a.

Posterior ethmoidal a.

Optic n. (CN II)

Internal carotid a. (in cavernous sinus)

Long posterior ciliary aa.

Lacrimal a.

Ophthalmic a.

Middle meningeal a. (from maxillary a.)

Anastomotic br.

Clinical box 41.2

Cavernous sinus syndrome
Gravity allows venous blood from the danger triangle region of the face (see figure) to drain to the cavernous sinus via the valveless ophthalmic veins. Squeezing a pimple or boil in this facial region can result in infectious thrombi being forced into the venous system and passing back into the cavernous sinus. Cavernous sinus syndrome (CIS) is diagnosed by the loss of eyeball movement due to the various cranial nerves associated with the cavernous sinus becoming infected.

The abducent nerve (CN VI) is bathed in blood within the sinus, the first ocular movement to be affected is lateral deviation of the eyeball. The oculomotor (CN III) and trochlear (CN IV) nerves, embedded in the dural lateral wall of the sinus are also eventually affected as the infection penetrates the dura. The eyeball becomes frozen in the orbit as all nerves activating the extraocular mm. become infected. CN V_1 is also in the lateral dural wall so a tingling/parasthesia is felt in the sensory region covered (forehead). Occasionally CN V_2 may also be involved and this parasthesia may also extend to the skin of the face below the orbit. The intercavernous sinuses allow the infection to spread to the cavernous sinus on the opposite side. If left untreated, death can result however cavernous sinus septic thrombophlebitis mortality has decreased from 100% to 20% with the of improvements in diagnosis and treatment.

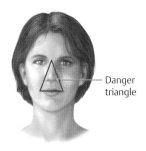

Danger triangle

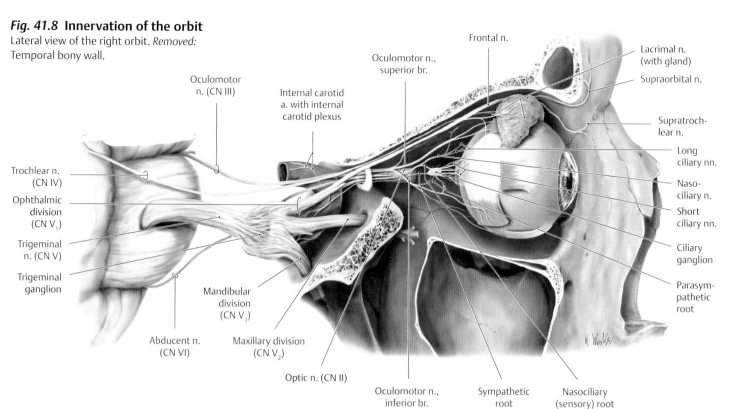

Fig. 41.8 Innervation of the orbit
Lateral view of the right orbit. *Removed:* Temporal bony wall.

Oculomotor n. (CN III)

Internal carotid a. with internal carotid plexus

Oculomotor n., superior br.

Frontal n.

Lacrimal n. (with gland)

Supraorbital n.

Supratroch-lear n.

Long ciliary nn.

Naso-ciliary n.

Short ciliary nn.

Ciliary ganglion

Parasym-pathetic root

Trochlear n. (CN IV)

Ophthalmic division (CN V₁)

Trigeminal n. (CN V)

Trigeminal ganglion

Abducent n. (CN VI)

Mandibular division (CN V₃)

Maxillary division (CN V₂)

Optic n. (CN II)

Oculomotor n., inferior br.

Sympathetic root

Nasociliary (sensory) root

Fig. 41.9 Cranial nerves in the orbit
Superior view of the anterior and middle cranial fossae. *Removed:* Cavernous sinus (lateral and superior walls), orbital roof, and periorbita (portions). The trigeminal ganglion has been retracted laterally.

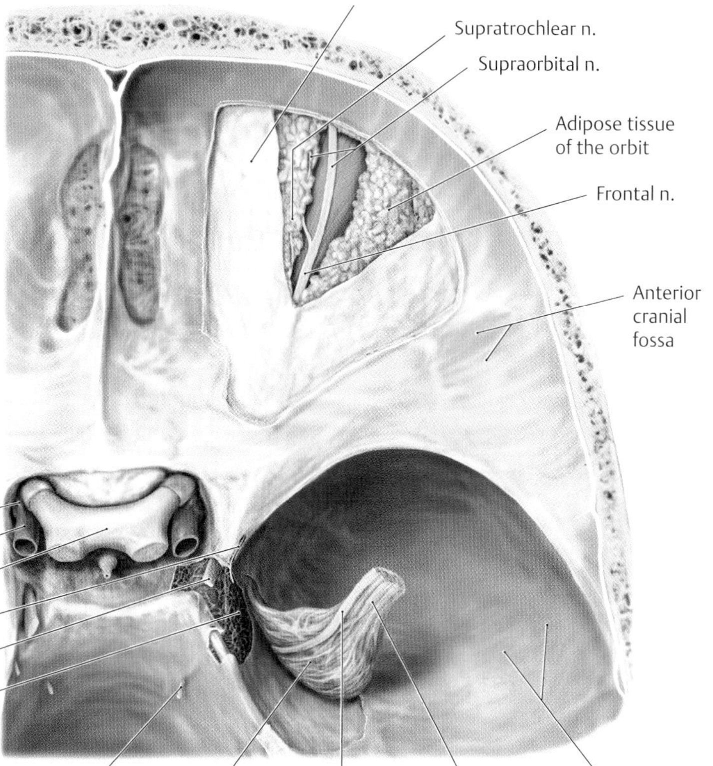

Periorbita (periosteum of the orbit)

Supratrochlear n.

Supraorbital n.

Adipose tissue of the orbit

Frontal n.

Anterior cranial fossa

Ophthalmic a.

Internal carotid a.

Optic chiasm (optic n., CN II)

Trochlear n. (CN IV)

Oculomotor n. (CN III)

Cavernous sinus

Abducent n. (CN VI)

Trigeminal ganglion

Motor root

Sensory root

Middle cranial fossa

Trigeminal n. (CN V)

Topography of the Orbit

Fig. 41.10 Neurovascular structures of the orbit

Anterior view. *Right side:* Orbicularis oculi removed. *Left side:* Orbital septum partially removed.

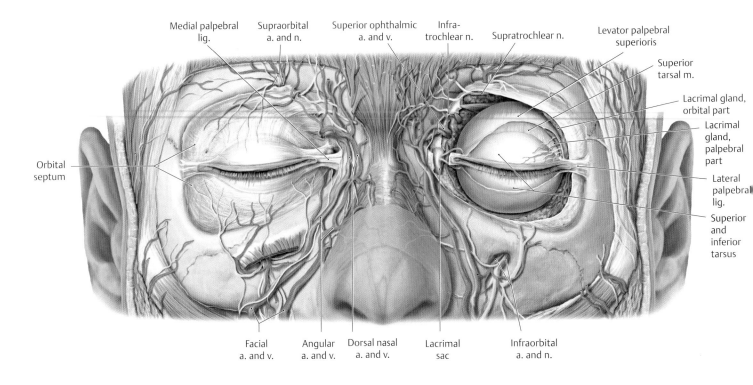

Medial palpebral lig.
Supraorbital a. and n.
Superior ophthalmic a. and v.
Infra-trochlear n.
Supratrochlear n.
Levator palpebral superioris
Superior tarsal m.
Lacrimal gland, orbital part
Lacrimal gland, palpebral part
Lateral palpebral lig.
Superior and inferior tarsus
Orbital septum
Facial a. and v.
Angular a. and v.
Dorsal nasal a. and v.
Lacrimal sac
Infraorbital a. and n.

Fig. 41.11 Passage of neurovascular structures through the orbit

Anterior view. *Removed:* Orbital contents. *Note:* The optic nerve and ophthalmic artery travel in the optic canal. The remaining structures pass through the superior orbital fissure.

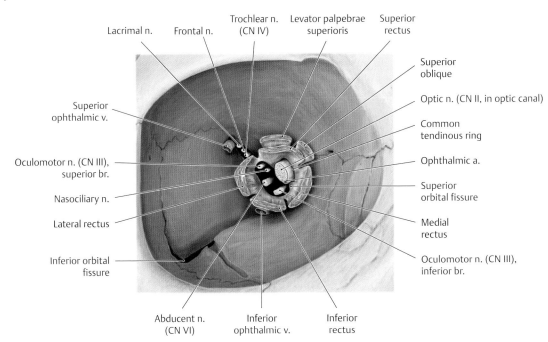

Lacrimal n.
Frontal n.
Trochlear n. (CN IV)
Levator palpebrae superioris
Superior rectus
Superior oblique
Optic n. (CN II, in optic canal)
Common tendinous ring
Ophthalmic a.
Superior orbital fissure
Medial rectus
Oculomotor n. (CN III), inferior br.
Superior ophthalmic v.
Oculomotor n. (CN III), superior br.
Nasociliary n.
Lateral rectus
Inferior orbital fissure
Abducent n. (CN VI)
Inferior ophthalmic v.
Inferior rectus

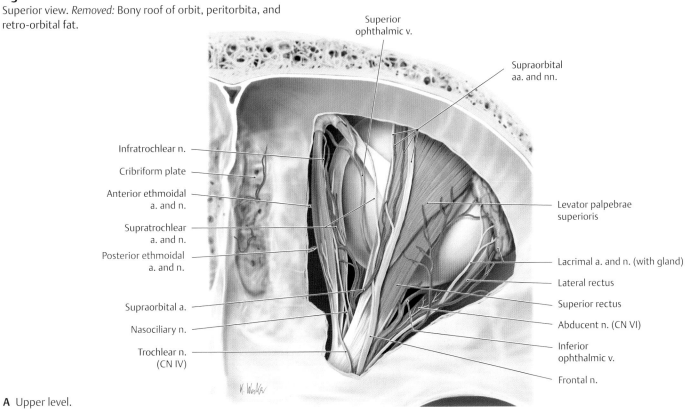

Fig. 41.12 **Neurovascular contents of the orbit**

Superior view. *Removed:* Bony roof of orbit, peritorbita, and retro-orbital fat.

Superior ophthalmic v.

Supraorbital aa. and nn.

Infratrochlear n.

Cribriform plate

Anterior ethmoidal a. and n.

Supratrochlear a. and n.

Posterior ethmoidal a. and n.

Supraorbital a.

Nasociliary n.

Trochlear n. (CN IV)

Levator palpebrae superioris

Lacrimal a. and n. (with gland)

Lateral rectus

Superior rectus

Abducent n. (CN VI)

Inferior ophthalmic v.

Frontal n.

A Upper level.

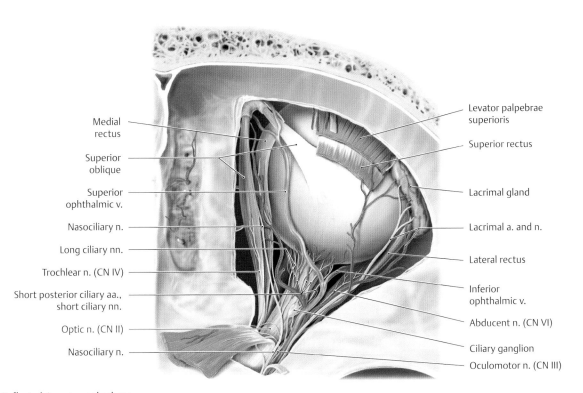

Medial rectus

Superior oblique

Superior ophthalmic v.

Nasociliary n.

Long ciliary nn.

Trochlear n. (CN IV)

Short posterior ciliary aa., short ciliary nn.

Optic n. (CN II)

Nasociliary n.

Levator palpebrae superioris

Superior rectus

Lacrimal gland

Lacrimal a. and n.

Lateral rectus

Inferior ophthalmic v.

Abducent n. (CN VI)

Ciliary ganglion

Oculomotor n. (CN III)

B Middle level. *Reflected:* Levator palpebrae superioris and superior rectus. *Revealed:* Optic nerve.

Orbit & Eyelid

Fig. 41.13 Topography of the orbit
Sagittal section through the right orbit, medial view.

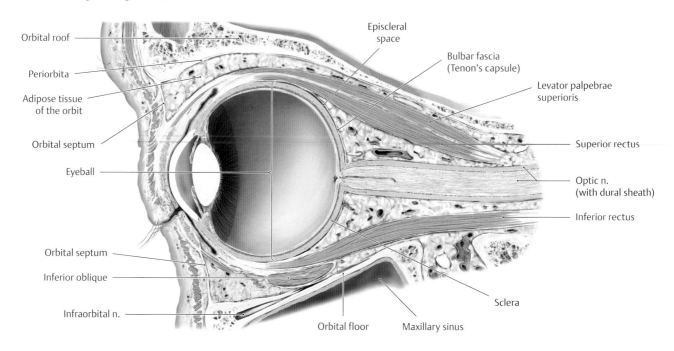

Fig. 41.14 Eyelids and conjuctiva
Sagittal section through the anterior orbital cavity.

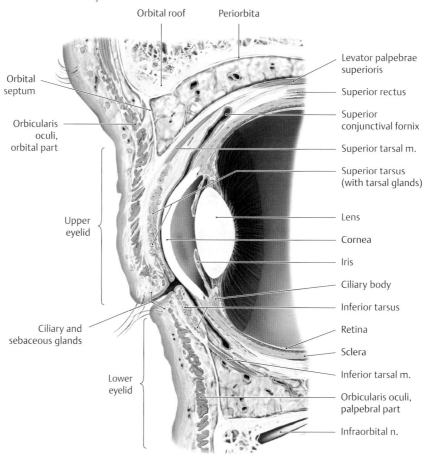

Fig. 41.15 Lacrimal apparatus

Right eye, anterior view. *Removed:* Orbital septum (partial). *Divided:*
Levator palpebrae superioris (tendon of insertion).

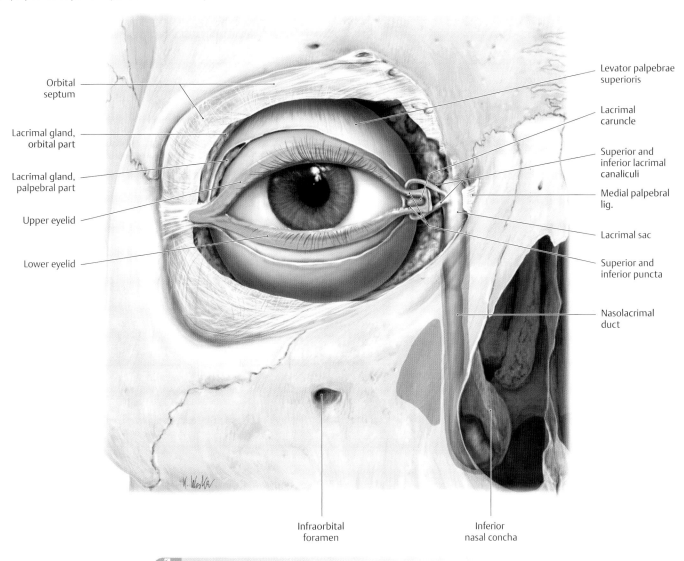

Orbital septum

Lacrimal gland, orbital part

Lacrimal gland, palpebral part

Upper eyelid

Lower eyelid

Levator palpebrae superioris

Lacrimal caruncle

Superior and inferior lacrimal canaliculi

Medial palpebral lig.

Lacrimal sac

Superior and inferior puncta

Nasolacrimal duct

Infraorbital foramen

Inferior nasal concha

Clinical box 41.3

Lacrimal drainage

Perimenopausal women are frequently subject to chronically dry eyes (*keratoconjunctivitis sicca*), due to insufficient tear production by the lacrimal gland. Acute inflammation of the lacrimal gland (due to bacteria) is less common and characterized by intense inflammation and extreme tenderness to palpation. The upper eyelid shows a characteristic S-curve.

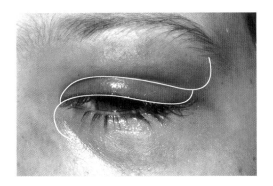

Eyeball

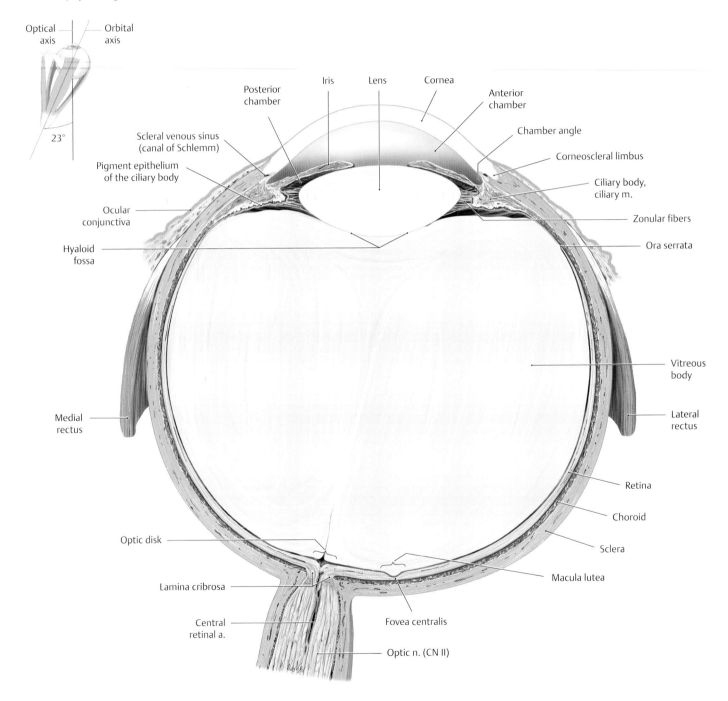

Fig. 41.16 Structure of the eyeball
Transverse section through right eyeball, superior view. *Note:* The orbital axis (running along the optic nerve through the optic disk) deviates from the optical axis (running through the center of the eye to the fovea centralis) by 23 degrees.

Optical axis

Orbital axis

23°

Iris

Lens

Cornea

Posterior chamber

Anterior chamber

Chamber angle

Scleral venous sinus (canal of Schlemm)

Corneoscleral limbus

Pigment epithelium of the ciliary body

Ciliary body, ciliary m.

Ocular conjunctiva

Zonular fibers

Hyaloid fossa

Ora serrata

Vitreous body

Medial rectus

Lateral rectus

Retina

Choroid

Optic disk

Sclera

Lamina cribrosa

Macula lutea

Central retinal a.

Fovea centralis

Optic n. (CN II)

Fig. 41.17 Blood vessels of the eyeball

Transverse section through the right eyeball at the level of the optic nerve, superior view. The arteries of the eye arise from the ophthalmic artery, a terminal branch of the internal carotid artery. Blood is drained by four to eight vorticose veins that open into the superior and inferior ophthalmic veins.

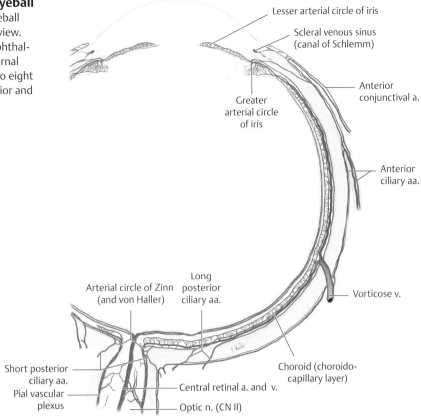

Lesser arterial circle of iris
Scleral venous sinus (canal of Schlemm)
Anterior conjunctival a.
Greater arterial circle of iris
Anterior ciliary aa.
Vorticose v.
Long posterior ciliary aa.
Arterial circle of Zinn (and von Haller)
Short posterior ciliary aa.
Pial vascular plexus
Central retinal a. and v.
Optic n. (CN II)
Choroid (choroido-capillary layer)

✳ Clinical box 41.4

Optic fundus

The optic fundus is the only place in the body where capillaries can be examined directly. Examination of the optic fundus permits observation of vascular changes that may be caused by high blood pressure or diabetes. Examination of the optic disk is important in determining intracranial pressure and diagnosing multiple sclerosis.

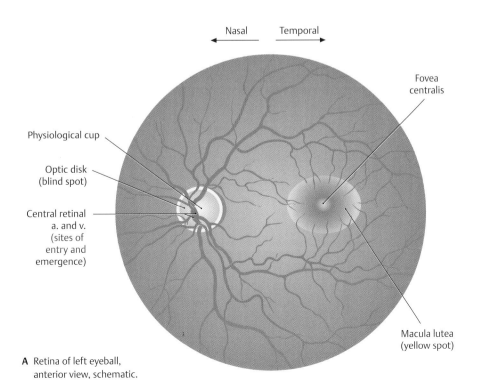

Nasal — Temporal

Physiological cup
Optic disk (blind spot)
Central retinal a. and v. (sites of entry and emergence)
Fovea centralis
Macula lutea (yellow spot)

A Retina of left eyeball, anterior view, schematic.

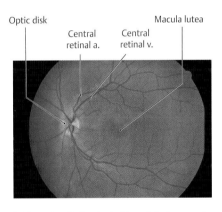

Optic disk
Central retinal a.
Central retinal v.
Macula lutea

B Normal optic fundus in the ophthalmoscopic examination.

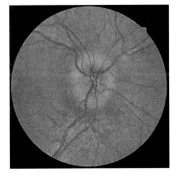

C High intracranial pressure; the edges of the optic disk appear less sharp.

Cornea, Iris & Lens

Fig. 41.18 Cornea, iris, and lens
Transverse section through the anterior segment of the eye. Anterosuperior view.

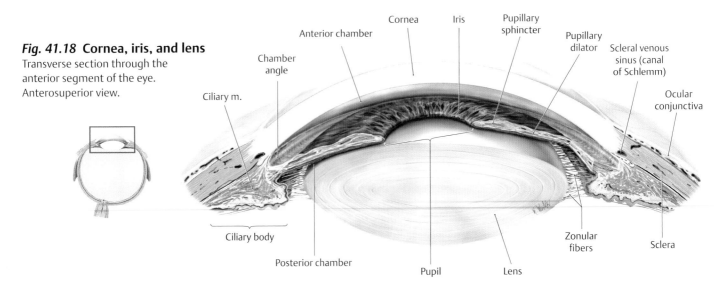

Fig. 41.19 Iris
Transverse section through the anterior segment of the eye. Anterosuperior view.

✚ *Clinical box 41.5*

Glaucoma

Aqueous humor produced in the posterior chamber passes through the pupil into the anterior chamber. It seeps through the spaces of the trabecular meshwork into the scleral venous sinus (canal of Schlemm) before passing into the episcleral veins. Obstruction of aqueous humor drainage causes an increase in intraocular pressure (glaucoma), which constricts the optic nerve in the lamina cribrosa. This constriction eventually leads to blindness. The most common glaucoma (approximately 90% of cases) is chronic (open-angle) glaucoma. The more rare acute glaucoma is characterized by red eye, strong headache and/or eye pain, nausea, dilated episcleral veins, and edema of the cornea.

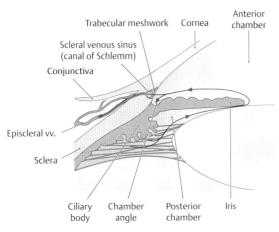

A Normal drainage.

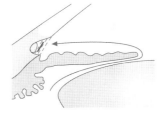

B Chronic (open-angle) glaucoma. Drainage through the trabecular meshwork is impaired.

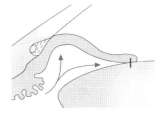

C Acute (angle-closure) glaucoma. The chamber angle is obstructed by iris tissue. Aqueous fluid cannot drain into the anterior chamber, which pushes portions of the iris upward, blocking the chamber angle.

Fig. 41.20 Pupil

Pupil size is regulated by two intraocular muscles of the iris: the pupillary sphincter, which narrows the pupil (parasympathetic innervation), and the pupillary dilator, which enlarges it (sympathetic innervation).

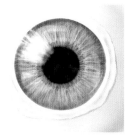
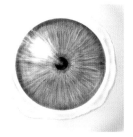
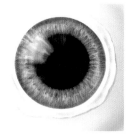

A Normal pupil size.

B Maximum constriction (miosis).

C Maximum dilation (mydriasis).

Fig. 41.21 **Lens and ciliary body**

Posterior view. The curvature of the lens is regulated by the muscle fibers of the annular ciliary body.

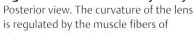

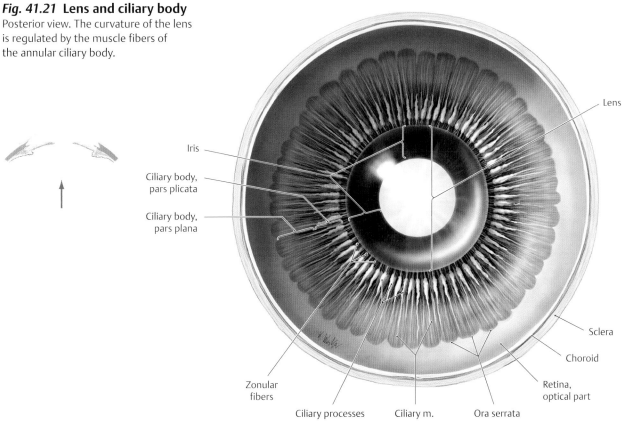

Iris
Ciliary body, pars plicata
Ciliary body, pars plana
Zonular fibers
Ciliary processes
Ciliary m.
Ora serrata
Lens
Sclera
Choroid
Retina, optical part

Fig. 41.22 **Light refraction by the lens**

Transverse section, superior view. In the normal (emmetropic) eye, light rays are refracted by the lens (and cornea) to a focal point on the retinal surface (fovea centralis). Tensing of the zonular fibers, with ciliary muscle relaxation, flattens the lens in response to parallel rays arriving from a distant source (far vision). Contraction of the ciliary muscle, with zonular fiber relaxation, causes the lens to assume a more rounded shape (near vision).

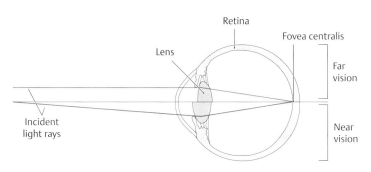

Retina
Lens
Fovea centralis
Far vision
Near vision
Incident light rays

A Normal dynamics of the lens.

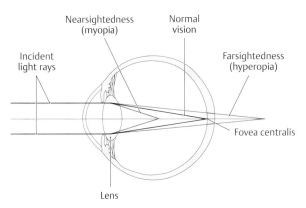

Nearsightedness (myopia)
Normal vision
Incident light rays
Farsightedness (hyperopia)
Fovea centralis
Lens

B Abnormal lens dynamics.

Bones of the Nasal Cavity

Fig. 42.1 Skeleton of the nose

The skeleton of the nose is composed of an upper bony portion and a lower cartilaginous portion. The proximal portions of the nostrils (alae) are composed of connective tissue with small embedded pieces of cartilage.

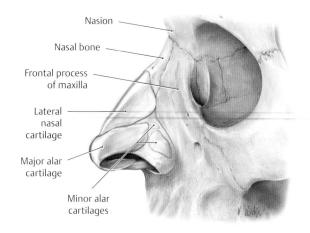

A Left lateral view.

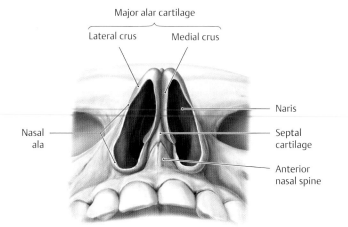

B Inferior view.

Fig. 42.2 Bones of the nasal cavity

The left and right nasal cavities are flanked by lateral walls and separated by the nasal septum. Air enters the nasal cavity through the anterior nasal aperture and travels through three passages: the superior, middle, and inferior meatuses (*arrows*). These passages are separated by the superior, middle, and inferior conchae. Air leaves the nose through the choanae, entering the nasopharynx.

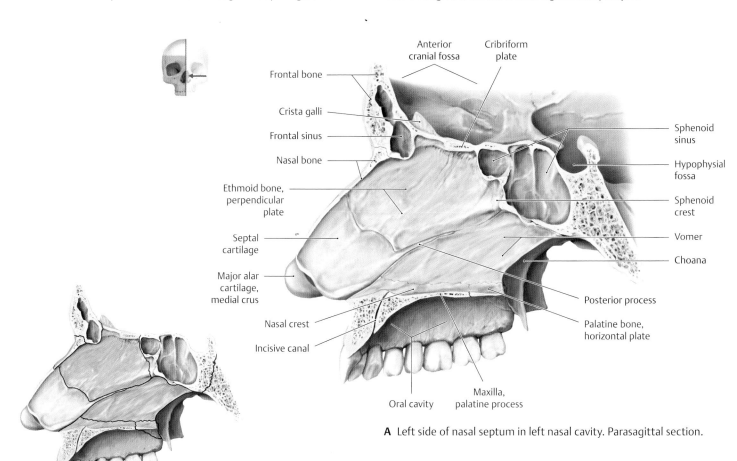

A Left side of nasal septum in left nasal cavity. Parasagittal section.

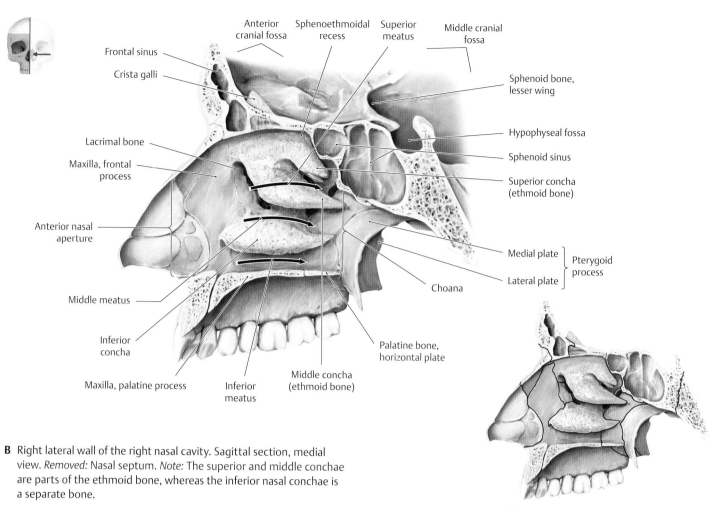

B Right lateral wall of the right nasal cavity. Sagittal section, medial view. *Removed:* Nasal septum. *Note:* The superior and middle conchae are parts of the ethmoid bone, whereas the inferior nasal conchae is a separate bone.

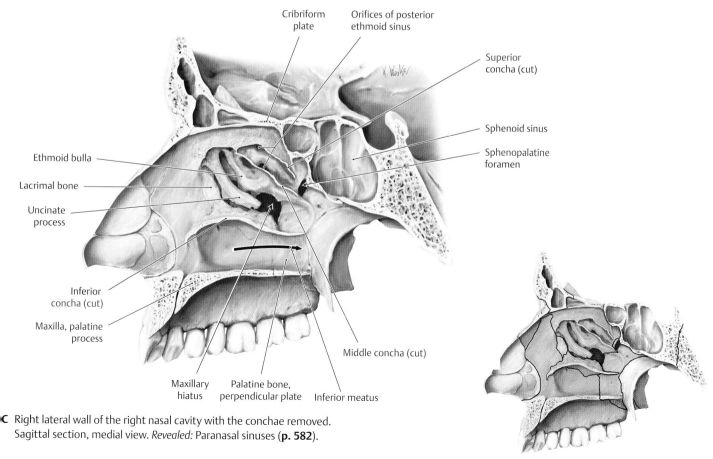

C Right lateral wall of the right nasal cavity with the conchae removed. Sagittal section, medial view. *Revealed:* Paranasal sinuses (**p. 582**).

Paranasal Air Sinuses

Fig. 42.3 Location of the paranasal sinuses

The paranasal sinuses (frontal, ethmoid, maxillary, and sphenoid) are air-filled cavities that reduce the weight of the skull.

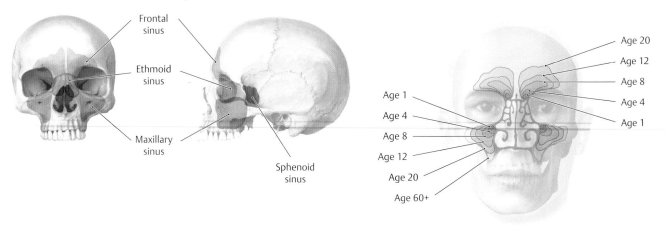

A Anterior view. **B** Left lateral view.

C Pneumatization (the formation of air-filled cells and cavities) of the sinuses with age. The frontal (yellow) and maxillary (orange) sinuses develop gradually over the course of cranial growth.

Fig. 42.4 Paranasal sinuses

Arrows indicate the flow of mucosal secretions from the sinuses and the nasolacrimal duct into the nasal cavity (see **Table 42.1**).

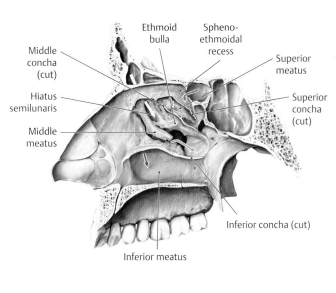

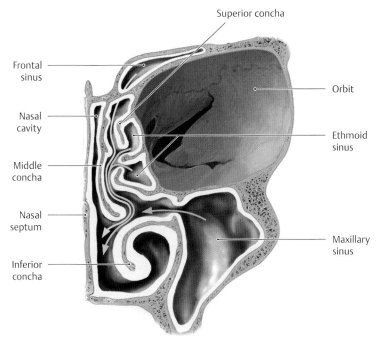

A Openings of the paranasal sinuses and nasolacrimal duct. Sagittal section, medial view of the right nasal cavity.

B Paranasal sinuses and osteomeatal unit in the left nasal cavity. Coronal section, anterior view.

Table 42.1	Nasal passages into which sinuses empty		
Sinuses/duct		**Nasal passage**	**Via**
Sphenoid sinus (blue)		Sphenoethmoidal recess	Direct
Ethmoid sinus (green)	Posterior cells	Superior meatus	Direct
	Anterior and middle cells	Middle meatus	Ethmoid bulla
Frontal sinus (yellow)		Middle meatus	Frontonasal duct into hiatus semilunaris
Maxillary sinus (orange)		Middle meatus	Hiatus semilunaris
Nasolacrimal duct (red)		Inferior meatus	Direct

Fig. 42.5 **Bony structure of the paranasal sinuses**
Coronal section, anterior view.

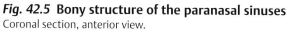

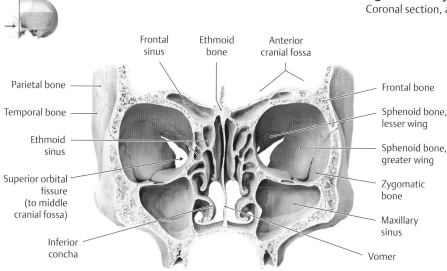

Parietal bone

Temporal bone

Ethmoid sinus

Superior orbital fissure (to middle cranial fossa)

Inferior concha

Frontal sinus

Ethmoid bone

Anterior cranial fossa

Frontal bone

Sphenoid bone, lesser wing

Sphenoid bone, greater wing

Zygomatic bone

Maxillary sinus

Vomer

A Bones of the paranasal sinuses.

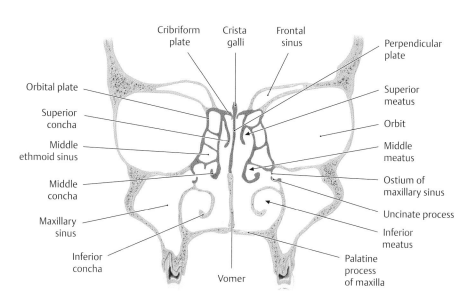

Cribriform plate

Crista galli

Frontal sinus

Perpendicular plate

Orbital plate

Superior concha

Middle ethmoid sinus

Middle concha

Maxillary sinus

Inferior concha

Vomer

Superior meatus

Orbit

Middle meatus

Ostium of maxillary sinus

Uncinate process

Inferior meatus

Palatine process of maxilla

B Ethmoid bone (red) in the paranasal sinuses.

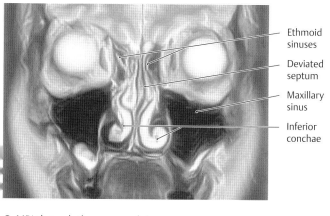

Ethmoid sinuses

Deviated septum

Maxillary sinus

Inferior conchae

C MRI through the paranasal sinuses.

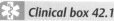

Clinical box 42.1

Deviated septum

The normal position of the nasal septum creates two roughly symmetrical nasal cavities. Extreme lateral deviation of the septum may result in obstruction of the nasal passages. This may be corrected by removing portions of the cartilage (septoplasty).

Sinusitis

When the mucosa in the ethmoid sinuses becomes swollen due to inflammation (*sinusitis*), it blocks the flow of secretions from the frontal and maxillary sinuses in the osteomeatal unit (see **Fig. 42.4**). This may cause microorganisms to become trapped, causing secondary inflammations. In patients with chronic sinusitis, the narrow sites can be surgically widened to establish more effective drainage routes.

Neurovasculature of the Nasal Cavity

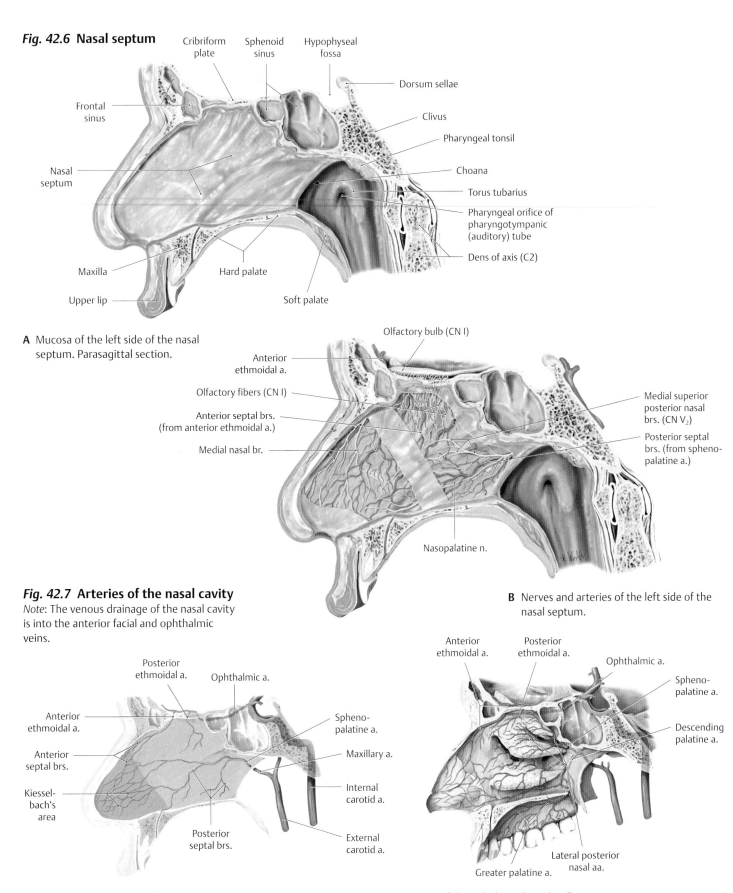

Fig. 42.6 Nasal septum

Cribriform plate · Sphenoid sinus · Hypophyseal fossa

Dorsum sellae

Frontal sinus

Clivus

Pharyngeal tonsil

Nasal septum

Choana

Torus tubarius

Pharyngeal orifice of pharyngotympanic (auditory) tube

Maxilla · Hard palate

Dens of axis (C2)

Upper lip · Soft palate

A Mucosa of the left side of the nasal septum. Parasagittal section.

Olfactory bulb (CN I)

Anterior ethmoidal a.

Olfactory fibers (CN I)

Medial superior posterior nasal brs. (CN V₂)

Anterior septal brs. (from anterior ethmoidal a.)

Posterior septal brs. (from sphenopalatine a.)

Medial nasal br.

Nasopalatine n.

B Nerves and arteries of the left side of the nasal septum.

Fig. 42.7 Arteries of the nasal cavity
Note: The venous drainage of the nasal cavity is into the anterior facial and ophthalmic veins.

Posterior ethmoidal a. · Ophthalmic a.

Anterior ethmoidal a.

Spheno-palatine a.

Anterior septal brs.

Maxillary a.

Kiesselbach's area

Internal carotid a.

Posterior septal brs.

External carotid a.

A Arteries of the left side of the nasal septum.

Anterior ethmoidal a. · Posterior ethmoidal a. · Ophthalmic a.

Spheno-palatine a.

Descending palatine a.

Lateral posterior nasal aa.

Greater palatine a.

B Arteries of the right lateral nasal wall.

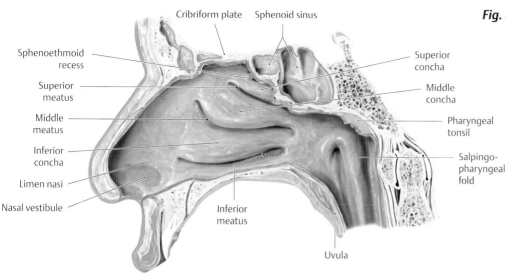

Fig. 42.8 Lateral nasal wall

Cribriform plate
Sphenoid sinus
Sphenoethmoid recess
Superior meatus
Middle meatus
Inferior concha
Limen nasi
Nasal vestibule
Inferior meatus
Uvula
Superior concha
Middle concha
Pharyngeal tonsil
Salpingo-pharyngeal fold

A Mucosa of the right lateral nasal wall. Sagittal section.

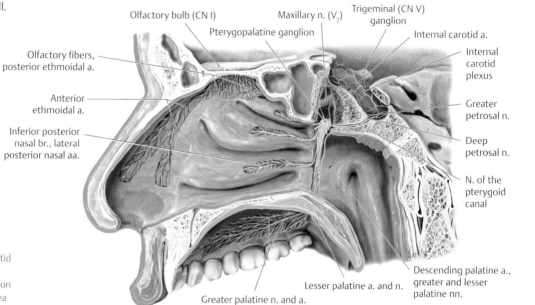

Olfactory bulb (CN I)
Maxillary n. (V₂)
Pterygopalatine ganglion
Trigeminal (CN V) ganglion
Internal carotid a.
Internal carotid plexus
Olfactory fibers, posterior ethmoidal a.
Anterior ethmoidal a.
Inferior posterior nasal br., lateral posterior nasal aa.
Greater petrosal n.
Deep petrosal n.
N. of the pterygoid canal
Descending palatine a., greater and lesser palatine nn.
Lesser palatine a. and n.
Greater palatine n. and a.

B Nerves and arteries of the right lateral nasal wall. Sagittal section. *Removed*: Sphenopalatine foramen.

Clinical box 42.2

Nosebleeds

Vascular supply to the nasal cavity arises from both the internal and external carotid arteries. The anterior part of the nasal septum contains a very vascularized region referred to as Kiesselbach's area. This area is the most common site of significant nosebleeds.

Fig. 42.9 Nerves of the nasal cavity

Left lateral view.

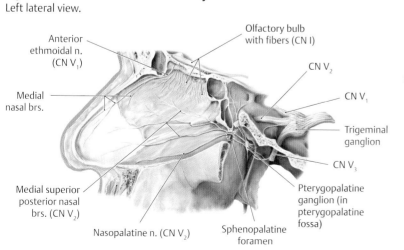

Anterior ethmoidal n. (CN V₁)
Olfactory bulb with fibers (CN I)
Medial nasal brs.
CN V₂
CN V₁
Trigeminal ganglion
CN V₃
Pterygopalatine ganglion (in pterygopalatine fossa)
Medial superior posterior nasal brs. (CN V₂)
Nasopalatine n. (CN V₂)
Sphenopalatine foramen

A Nerves of the left side of the nasal septum.

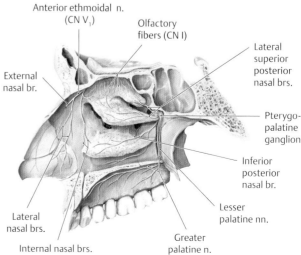

Anterior ethmoidal n. (CN V₁)
Olfactory fibers (CN I)
External nasal br.
Lateral superior posterior nasal brs.
Pterygo-palatine ganglion
Inferior posterior nasal br.
Lesser palatine nn.
Lateral nasal brs.
Internal nasal brs.
Greater palatine n.

B Nerves of the right lateral nasal wall.

585

Temporal Bone

Fig. 43.1 **Temporal bone**

Left bone. The temporal bone consists of three major parts: squamous, petrous, and tympanic (see **Fig. 43.2**).

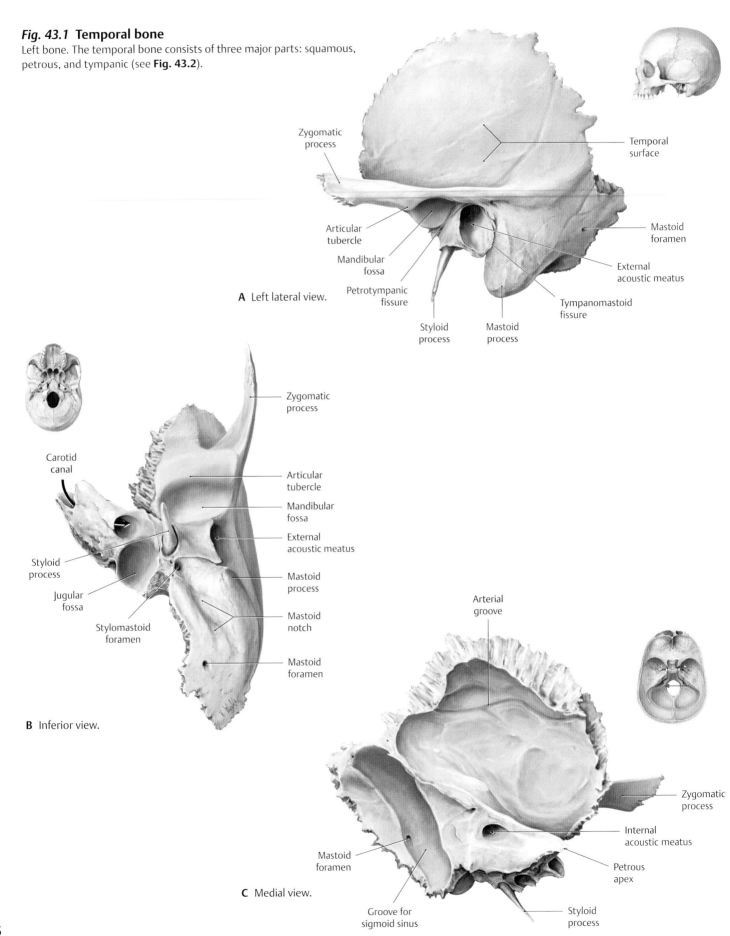

Zygomatic process

Temporal surface

Articular tubercle

Mandibular fossa

Petrotympanic fissure

Mastoid foramen

External acoustic meatus

Tympanomastoid fissure

Styloid process

Mastoid process

A Left lateral view.

Zygomatic process

Carotid canal

Articular tubercle

Mandibular fossa

External acoustic meatus

Styloid process

Jugular fossa

Mastoid process

Stylomastoid foramen

Mastoid notch

Mastoid foramen

B Inferior view.

Arterial groove

Zygomatic process

Internal acoustic meatus

Mastoid foramen

Petrous apex

Groove for sigmoid sinus

Styloid process

C Medial view.

Fig. 43.2 Parts of the temporal bone

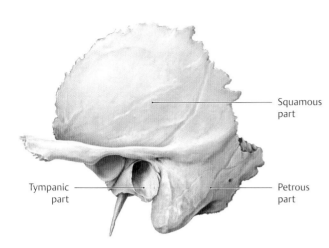

Squamous part

Tympanic part

Petrous part

A Left lateral view.

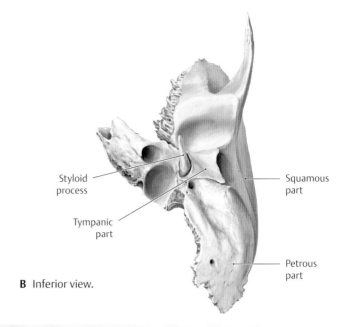

Styloid process

Tympanic part

Squamous part

Petrous part

B Inferior view.

 Clinical box 43.1

Structures in the temporal bone

The mastoid process contains mastoid air cells that communicate with the middle ear; the middle ear in turn communicates with the nasopharynx via the pharyngotympanic (auditory) tube (**A**). Bacteria may use this pathway to move from the nasopharynx into the middle ear. In severe cases, bacteria may pass from the mastoid air cells into the cranial cavity, causing meningitis.

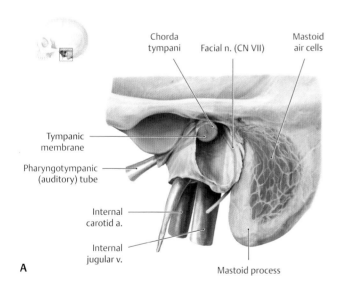

Chorda tympani

Facial n. (CN VII)

Mastoid air cells

Tympanic membrane

Pharyngotympanic (auditory) tube

Internal carotid a.

Internal jugular v.

Mastoid process

A

Irrigation of the auditory canal with warm (44°C) or cool (30°C) water can induce a thermal current in the endolymph of the semicircular canal, causing the patient to manifest vestibular nystagmus (jerky eye movements, vestibulo-ocular reflex). This caloric testing is important in the diagnosis of unexplained vertigo. The patient must be oriented so that the semicircular canal of interest lies in the vertical plane (**C**).

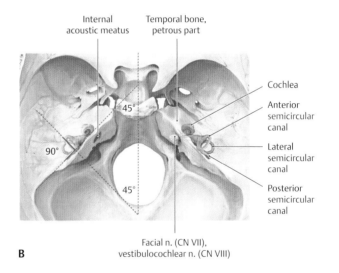

Internal acoustic meatus

Temporal bone, petrous part

Cochlea

Anterior semicircular canal

Lateral semicircular canal

Posterior semicircular canal

45°

90°

45°

Facial n. (CN VII), vestibulocochlear n. (CN VIII)

B

The petrous portion of the temporal bone contains the middle and inner ear as well as the tympanic membrane. The bony semicircular canals are oriented at an approximately 45-degree angle from the coronal, transverse, and sagittal planes (**B**).

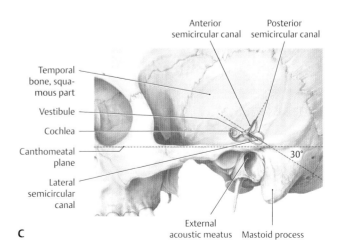

Anterior semicircular canal

Posterior semicircular canal

Temporal bone, squamous part

Vestibule

Cochlea

Canthomeatal plane

30°

Lateral semicircular canal

External acoustic meatus

Mastoid process

C

The auditory apparatus is divided into three main parts: external, middle, and inner ear. The external and middle ear are part of the sound conduction apparatus, and the inner ear is the actual organ of hearing (see **p. 596**). The inner ear also contains the vestibular apparatus, the organ of balance (see **p. 596**).

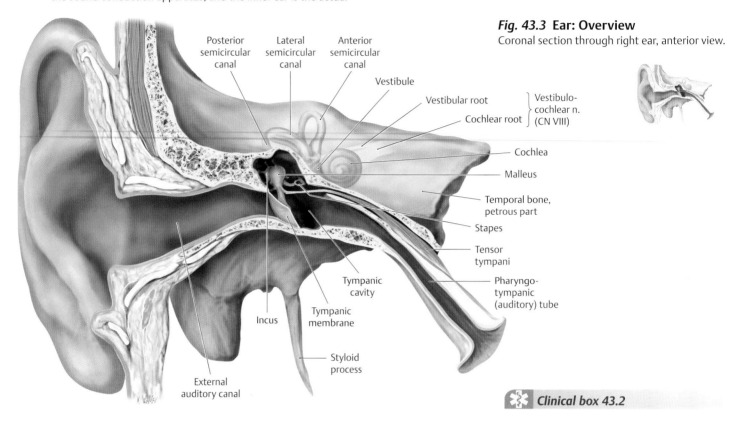

Fig. 43.3 Ear: Overview
Coronal section through right ear, anterior view.

Posterior semicircular canal • Lateral semicircular canal • Anterior semicircular canal • Vestibule • Vestibular root • Cochlear root • Vestibulo-cochlear n. (CN VIII) • Cochlea • Malleus • Temporal bone, petrous part • Stapes • Tensor tympani • Pharyngotympanic (auditory) tube • Tympanic cavity • Tympanic membrane • Incus • Styloid process • External auditory canal

Fig. 43.4 External auditory canal
Coronal section through right ear, anterior view. The tympanic membrane separates the external auditory canal from the tympanic cavity (middle ear). The outer third of the auditory canal is cartilaginous, and the inner two thirds are osseous (tympanic part of temporal bone).

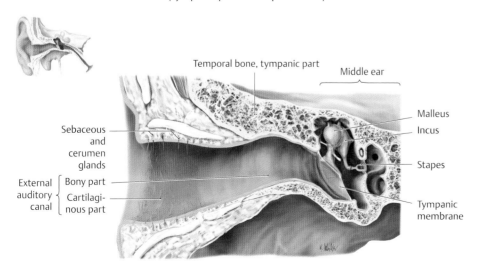

Temporal bone, tympanic part • Middle ear • Malleus • Incus • Stapes • Tympanic membrane • Sebaceous and cerumen glands • External auditory canal • Bony part • Cartilaginous part

Clinical box 43.2

Curvature of the external auditory canal
The external auditory canal is most curved in its cartilaginous portion. When an otoscope is being inserted, the auricle should be pulled backward and upward so the speculum can be introduced into a straightened canal.

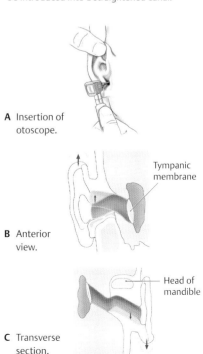

A Insertion of otoscope.
B Anterior view. Tympanic membrane
C Transverse section. Head of mandible

Fig. 43.5 Structure of the auricle

The auricle of the ear encloses a cartilaginous framework that forms a funnel-shaped receptor for acoustic vibrations. The muscles of the auricle are considered muscles of facial expression, although they are vestigial in humans.

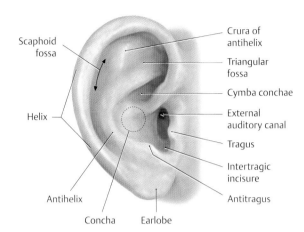

A Right auricle, right lateral view.

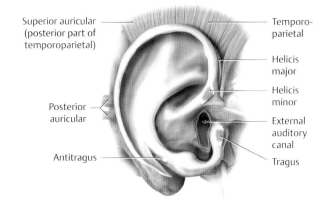

B Cartilage and muscles of the right auricle, right lateral view.

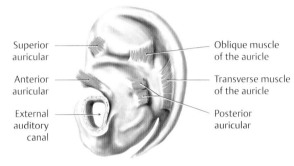

C Cartilage and muscles of the right auricle, medial view of posterior surface.

Fig. 43.6 Arteries of the auricle

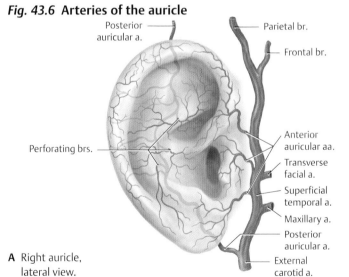

A Right auricle, lateral view.

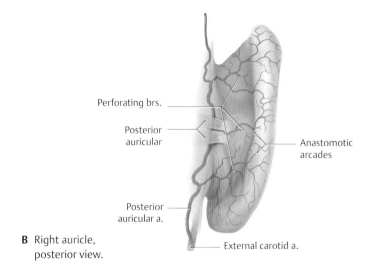

B Right auricle, posterior view.

Fig. 43.7 Innervation of the auricle

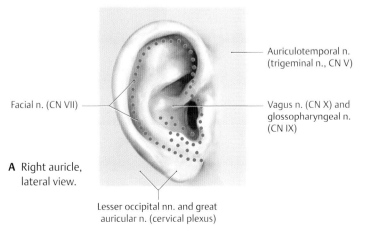

A Right auricle, lateral view.

Lesser occipital nn. and great auricular n. (cervical plexus)

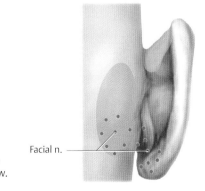

B Right auricle, posterior view.

Middle Ear: Tympanic Cavity

Fig. 43.8 Middle ear

Right petrous bone, superior view. The tympanic cavity of the middle ear communicates anteriorly with the pharynx via the pharyngotympanic (auditory) tube and posteriorly with the mastoid air cells.

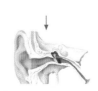

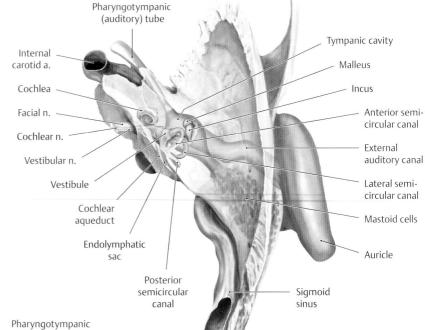

Fig. 43.9 Tympanic cavity and pharyngotympanic tube

Medial view of opened tympanic cavity.

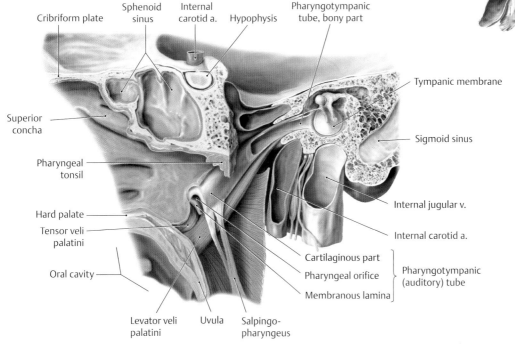

Table 43.1	Boundaries of the tympanic cavity			

During chronic suppurative otitis media (inflammation of the middle ear), pathogenic bacteria may spread to adjacent regions.

Direction	Wall	Anatomical boundary	Neighboring structures	Infection
Anterior	Carotid	Opening to pharyngotympanic tube	Carotid canal	
Lateral	Membranous	Tympanic membrane	External ear	
Superior	Tegmental	Tegmen tympani	Middle cranial fossa	Meningitis, cerebral abscess (especially of temporal lobe)
Medial	Labyrinthine	Promontory overlying basal turn of cochlea	Inner ear	
			CSF space (via petrous apex)	Abducent paralysis, trigeminal nerve irritation, visual disturbances (Gradenigo's syndrome)
Inferior	Jugular	Temporal bone, tympanic part	Bulb of jugular v.	
			Sigmoid sinus	Sinus thrombosis
Posterior	Mastoid	Aditus to mastoid antrum	Air cells of mastoid process	Mastoiditis
			Facial n. canal	Facial paralysis

CSF, cerebrospinal fluid.

Fig. 43.10 Tympanic cavity

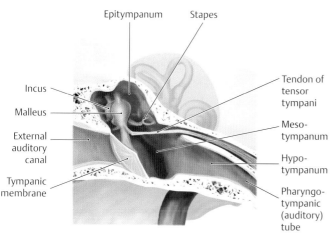

A Levels of the tympanic cavity. Anterior view. The tympanic cavity is divided into three levels: epi-, meso-, and hypotympanum.

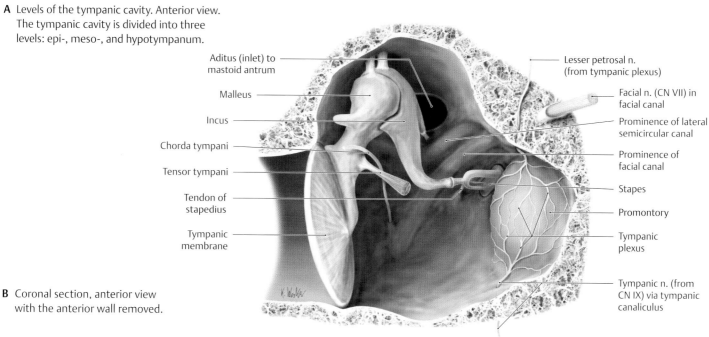

B Coronal section, anterior view with the anterior wall removed.

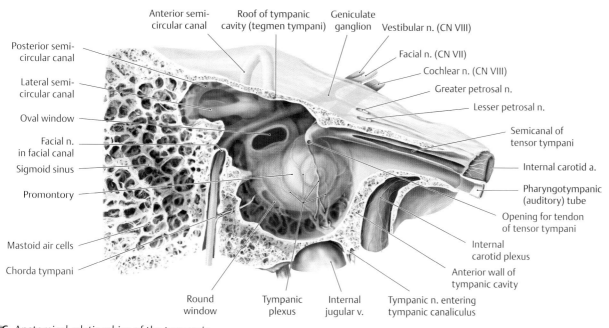

C Anatomical relationships of the tympanic cavity. Oblique sagittal section showing the medial wall.

Middle Ear: Ossicular Chain & Tympanic Membrane

Fig. 43.11 Auditory ossicles

Left ear. The ossicular chain consists of three small bones that establish an articular connection between the tympanic membrane and the oval window.

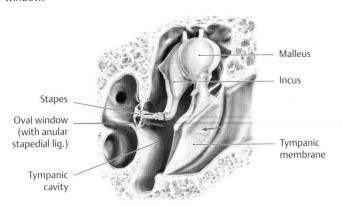

A Auditory ossicles in the middle ear. Anterior view.

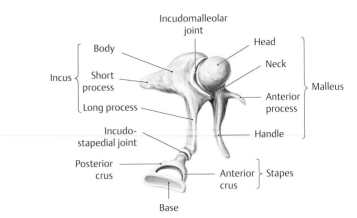

B Bones of the ossicular chain. Medial view of the left ossicular chain.

Fig. 43.12 Malleus ("hammer")

Left ear.

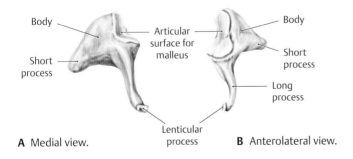

A Posterior view. **B** Anterior view.

Fig. 43.15 Tympanic membrane

Right tympanic membrane. The tympanic membrane is divided into four quadrantsquadrants (I–IV).

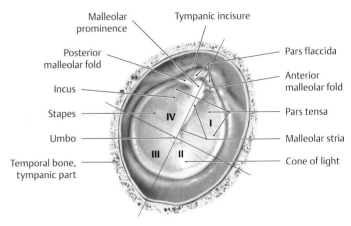

A Lateral view of the right tympanic membranewith quadrants indicated.

Fig. 43.13 Incus ("anvil")

Left ear.

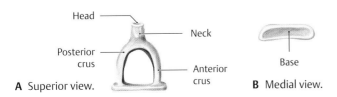

A Medial view. **B** Anterolateral view.

Fig. 43.14 Stapes ("stirrup")

Left ear.

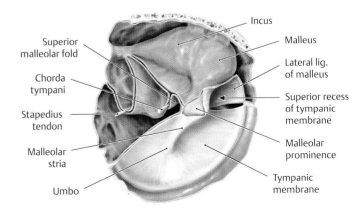

B Mucosal lining of the tympanic cavity. Posterolateral view with the tympanic membrane partially removed.

Fig. 43.16 **Ossicular chain in the tympanic cavity**

Lateral view of the right ear. *Revealed:* Ligaments of the ossicular chain and muscles of the middle ear (stapedius and tensor tympani).

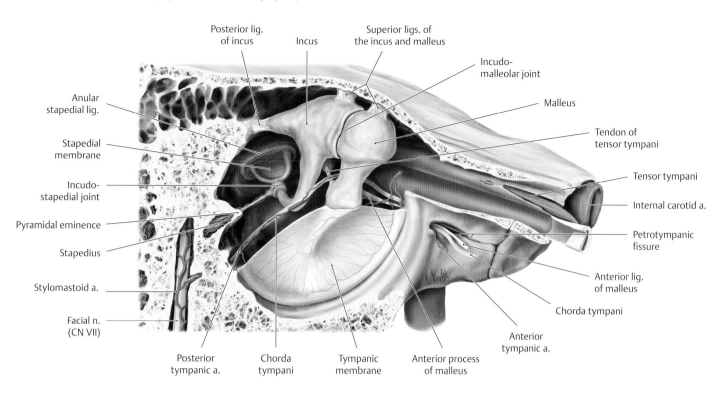

Clinical box 43.3

Ossicular chain in hearing

Sound waves funneled into the external auditory canal set the tympanic membrane into vibration. The ossicular chain transmits the vibrations to the oval window, which communicates them to the fluid column of the inner ear. Sound waves in fluid meet with higher impedance; they must therefore be amplified in the middle ear. The difference in surface area between the tympanic membrane and the oval window increases the sound pressure 17-fold. A total amplification factor of 22 is achieved through the lever action of the ossicular chain. If the ossicular chain fails to transform the sound pressure between the tympanic membrane and the footplate of the stapes, the patient will experience conductive hearing loss of magnitude 20 dB.

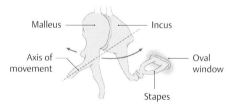

A Vibration of the tympanic membrane causes a rocking movement in the ossicular chain. The mechanical advantage of the lever action of the ossicular chain amplifies the sound waves by a factor of 1.3.

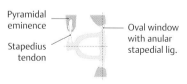

B The stapes in its normal position lies in the plane of the oval window.

C Rocking of the ossicular chain causes the stapes to tilt. The movement of the stapes base against the membrane of the oval window (stapedial membrane) induces corresponding waves in the fluid column of the inner ear.

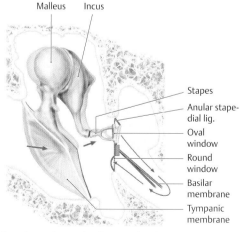

D Propagation of sound waves by the ossicular chain.

Arteries of the Middle Ear

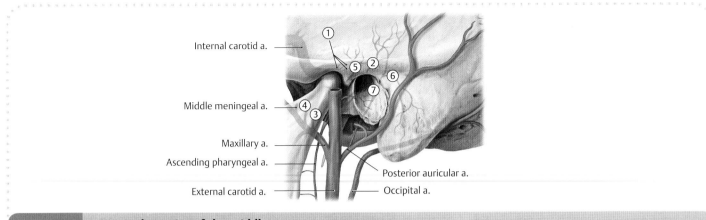

Table 43.2   Principal arteries of the middle ear

Origin	Artery		Distribution
Internal carotid a.	① Caroticotympanic aa.		Tympanic cavity (anterior wall), pharyngotympanic (auditory) tube
External carotid a.	Ascending pharyngeal a. (medial br.)	② Inferior tympanic a.	Tympanic cavity (floor), promontory
	Maxillary a. (terminal br.)	③ Deep auricular a.	Tympanic cavity (floor), tympanic membrane
		④ Anterior tympanic a.	Tympanic membrane, mastoid antrum, malleus, incus
	Middle meningeal a.	⑤ Superior tympanic a.	Tympanic cavity (roof), tensor tympani, stapes
	Posterior auricular a. (posterior br.)	Stylomastoid a.	⑥ Stylomastoid a.
			Tympanic cavity (posterior wall), mastoid air cells, stapedius m., stapes
		⑦ Posterior tympanic a.	Chorda tympani, tympanic membrane, malleus

Fig. 43.17 Arteries of the middle ear: Ossicular chain and tympanic membrane

Medial view of the right tympanic membrane. With inflammation, the arteries of the tympanic membrane may become so dilated that their course can be observed (as shown here).

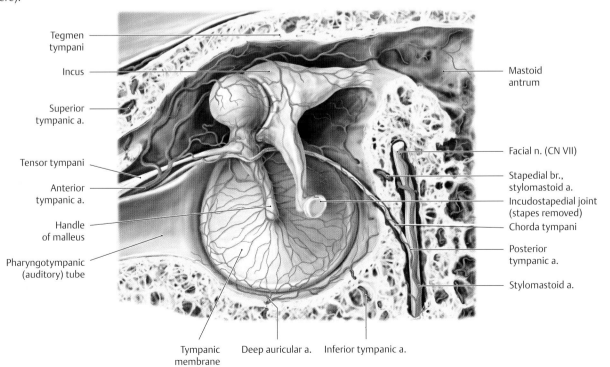

Fig. 43.18 **Arteries of the middle ear: Tympanic cavity**

Right petrous bone, anterior view. *Removed:* Malleus, incus, portions of chorda tympani, and anterior tympanic artery.

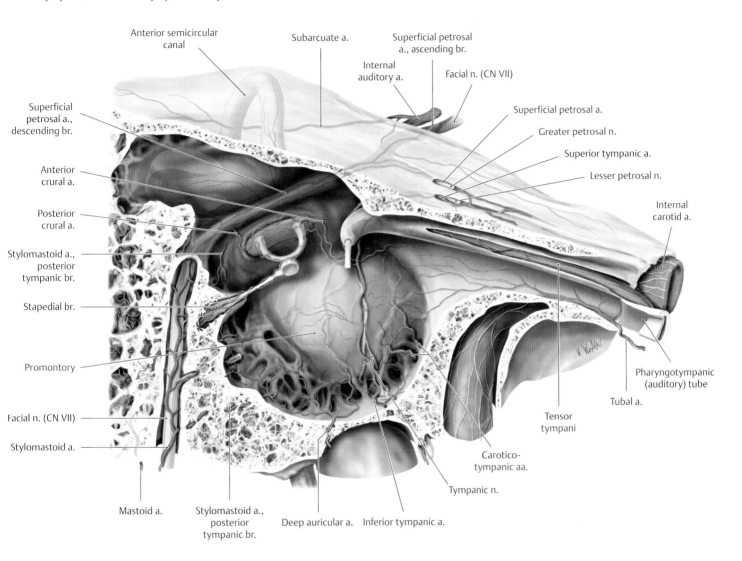

Labels (clockwise from top):
Anterior semicircular canal · Subarcuate a. · Superficial petrosal a., ascending br. · Internal auditory a. · Facial n. (CN VII) · Superficial petrosal a. · Greater petrosal n. · Superior tympanic a. · Lesser petrosal n. · Internal carotid a. · Pharyngotympanic (auditory) tube · Tubal a. · Tensor tympani · Carotico-tympanic aa. · Tympanic n. · Inferior tympanic a. · Deep auricular a. · Stylomastoid a., posterior tympanic br. · Mastoid a. · Stylomastoid a. · Facial n. (CN VII) · Promontory · Stapedial br. · Stylomastoid a., posterior tympanic br. · Posterior crural a. · Anterior crural a. · Superficial petrosal a., descending br.

Inner Ear

The inner ear consists of the vestibular apparatus (for balance) and the auditory apparatus (for hearing). Both are formed by a membranous labyrinth filled with endolymph floating within a bony labyrinth filled with perilymph and embedded in the petrous part of the temporal bone.

Fig. 43.19 **Vestibular apparatus**
Right lateral view.

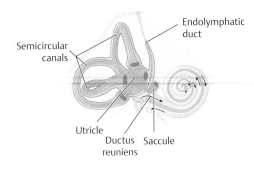

A Schematic. Ampullary crests and maculae of utricle and saccule shown in red.

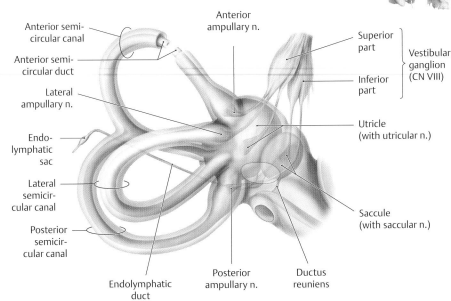

B Structure of the vestibular apparatus.

Fig. 43.20 **Auditory apparatus**
The cochlear labyrinth and its bony shell form the cochlea, which contains the sensory epithelium of the auditory apparatus (organ of Corti).

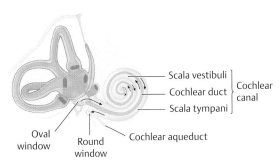

A Schematic.

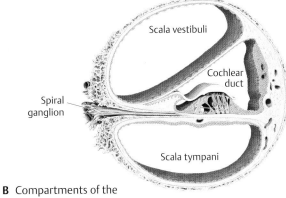

B Compartments of the cochlear canal, cross section.

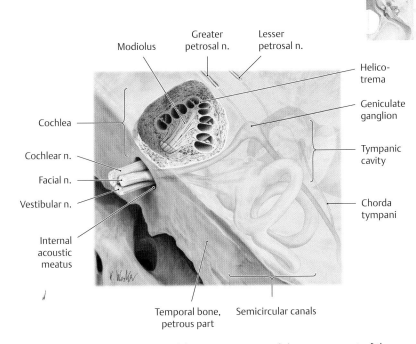

C Location of the cochlea. Superior view of the petrous part of the temporal bone with the cochlea sectioned transversely. The bony canal of the cochlea (spiral canal) makes 2.5 turns around its bony axis (modiolus).

Fig. 43.21 **Innervation of the membranous labyrinth**

Right ear, anterior view. The vestibulocochlear nerve (CN VIII; see **p. 536**) transmits afferent impulses from the inner ear to the brainstem through the internal acoustic meatus. The vestibulocochlear nerve is divided into the vestibular and cochlear nerves. *Note:* The sensory organs in the semicircular canals respond to angular acceleration, and the macular organs respond to horizontal and vertical linear acceleration.

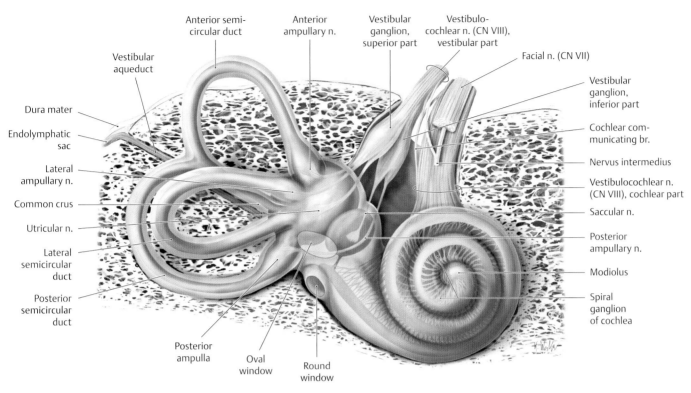

Fig. 43.22 **Blood vessels of the inner ear**

Right anterior view. The labyrinth receives its blood supply from the internal auditory artery, a branch of the anteroinferior cerebellar artery (see **p. 674**).

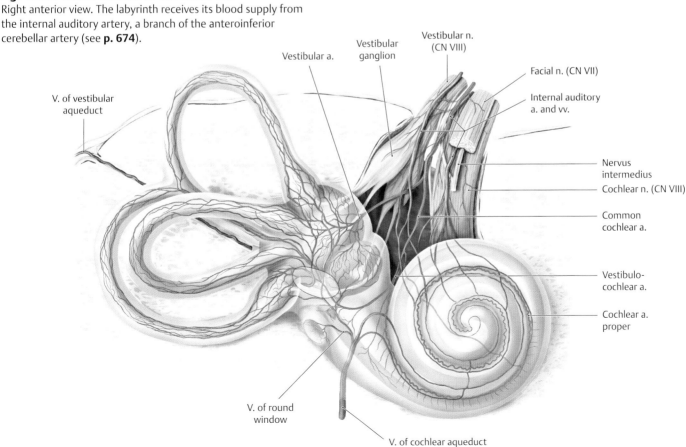

Bones of the Oral Cavity

The floor of the nasal cavity (the maxilla and palatine bone) forms the roof of the oral cavity, the hard palate. The two horizontal processes of the maxilla (the palatine processes) grow together during development, eventually fusing at the median palatine suture. Failure to fuse results in a cleft palate.

Fig. 44.1 **Hard palate**

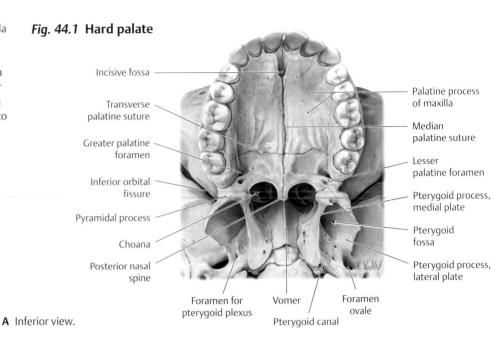

Incisive fossa
Transverse palatine suture
Greater palatine foramen
Inferior orbital fissure
Pyramidal process
Choana
Posterior nasal spine
Foramen for pterygoid plexus
Vomer
Pterygoid canal
Foramen ovale
Palatine process of maxilla
Median palatine suture
Lesser palatine foramen
Pterygoid process, medial plate
Pterygoid fossa
Pterygoid process, lateral plate

A Inferior view.

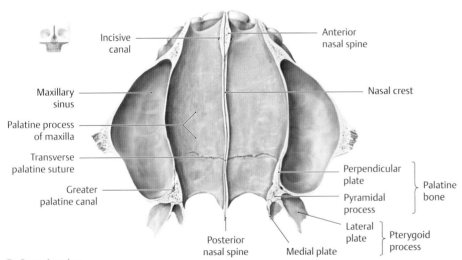

Incisive canal
Anterior nasal spine
Maxillary sinus
Nasal crest
Palatine process of maxilla
Transverse palatine suture
Greater palatine canal
Perpendicular plate
Pyramidal process
Palatine bone
Lateral plate
Pterygoid process
Posterior nasal spine
Medial plate

B Superior view.
Removed: Maxilla (upper part).

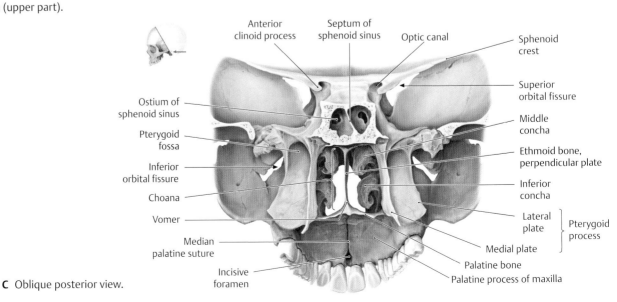

Anterior clinoid process
Septum of sphenoid sinus
Optic canal
Sphenoid crest
Ostium of sphenoid sinus
Pterygoid fossa
Inferior orbital fissure
Choana
Vomer
Median palatine suture
Incisive foramen
Superior orbital fissure
Middle concha
Ethmoid bone, perpendicular plate
Inferior concha
Lateral plate
Pterygoid process
Medial plate
Palatine bone
Palatine process of maxilla

C Oblique posterior view.

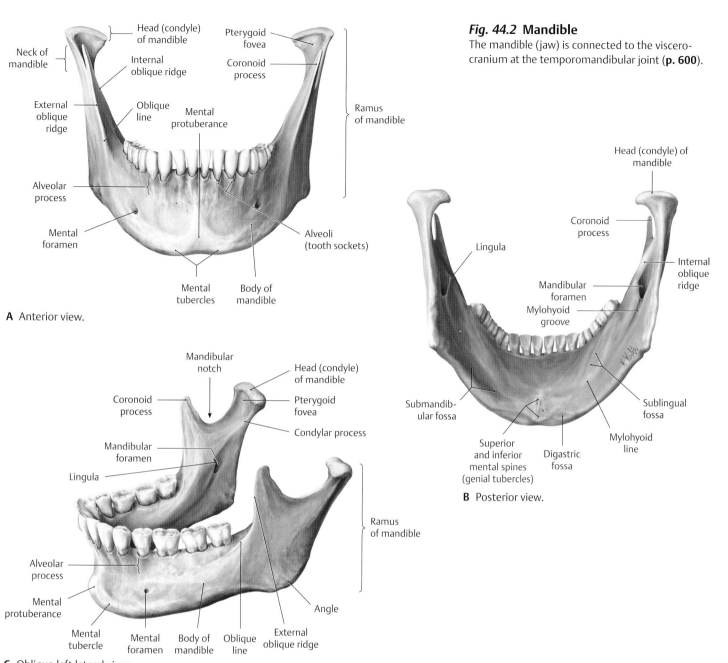

Fig. 44.2 Mandible

The mandible (jaw) is connected to the viscero-cranium at the temporomandibular joint (**p. 600**).

A Anterior view.

B Posterior view.

C Oblique left lateral view.

Fig. 44.3 Hyoid bone

The hyoid bone is suspended in the neck by muscles between the floor of the mouth and the larynx. Although not listed among the cranial bones, the hyoid bone gives attachment to the muscles of the oral floor. The greater horn and body of the hyoid are palpable in the neck.

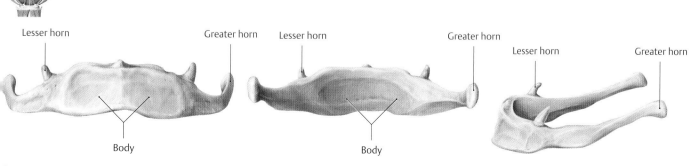

A Anterior view.

B Posterior view.

C Oblique left lateral view.

Temporomandibular Joint

Fig. 44.4 Temporomandibular joint

The head of the mandible articulates with the mandibular fossa in the temporomandibular joint.

Articular tubercle

Mandibular fossa

Articular disk

Head of mandible

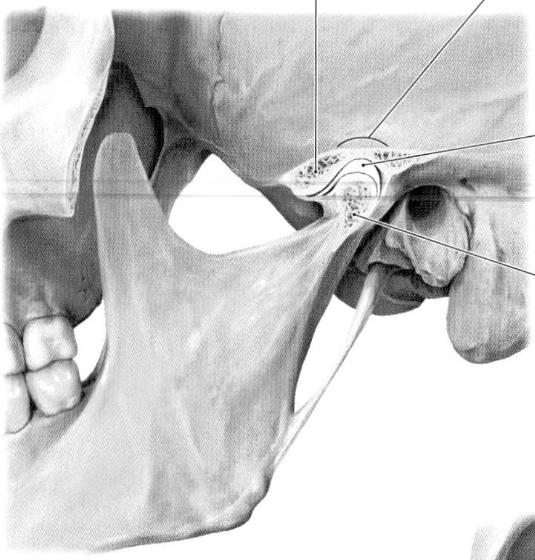

A Sagittally sectioned temporomandibular joint, left lateral view.

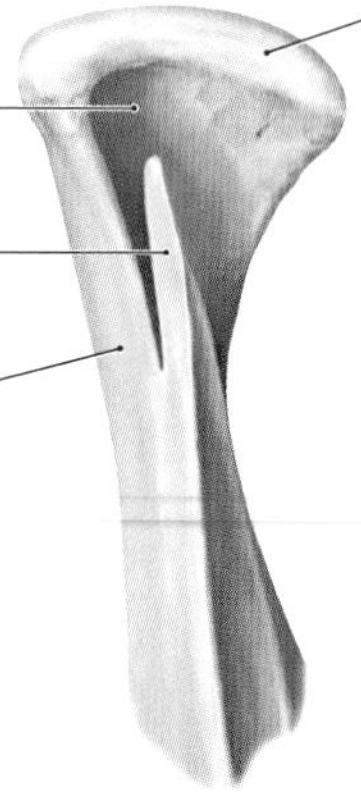

Head of
mandible

Pterygoid
fovea

Coronoid
process

Neck of
mandible

Neck of
mandible

Lingula

Mandibular
foramen

Mylohyoid
groove

B Head of mandible,
anterior view.

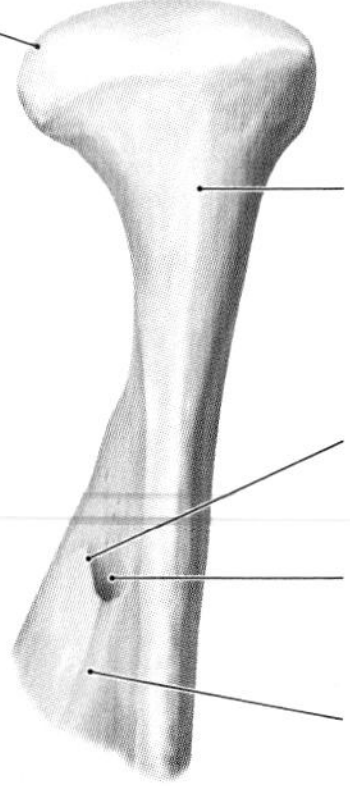

C Head of mandible,
posterior view.

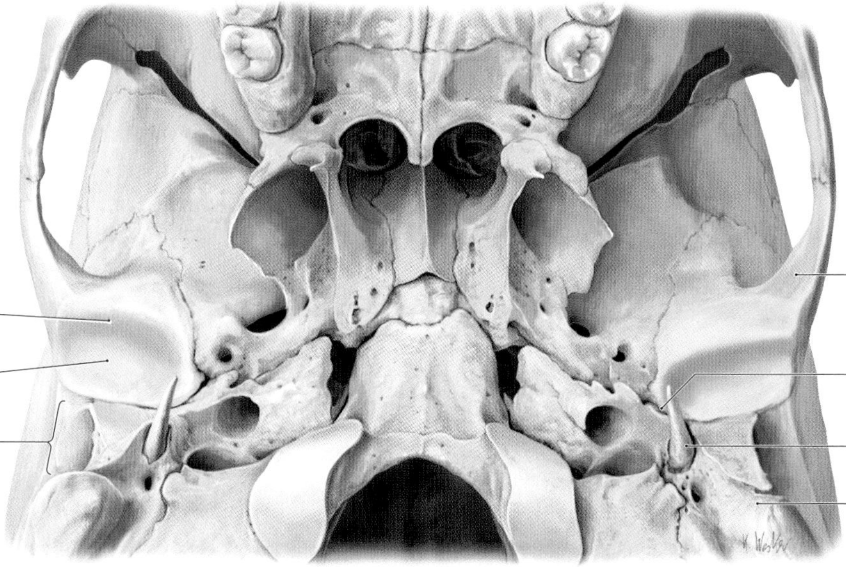

Articular
tubercle

Mandibular
fossa

External
acoustic
meatus
(to external
auditory
canal)

D Mandibular fossa
of the temporo-
mandibular joint,
inferior view.

Zygomatic process,
temporal bone

Petrotympanic
fissure

Styloid process,
temporal bone

Mastoid process,
temporal bone

Fig. 44.5 Ligaments of the temporomandibular joint

Joint
capsule

Lateral lig.

Stylomandibular lig.

Pterygoid process, lateral plate

Pterygospinous
lig.

Spheno-
mandibular lig.

Stylomandibular lig.

Pterygoid process,
medial plate

A Lateral view of the left temporomandibular joint.

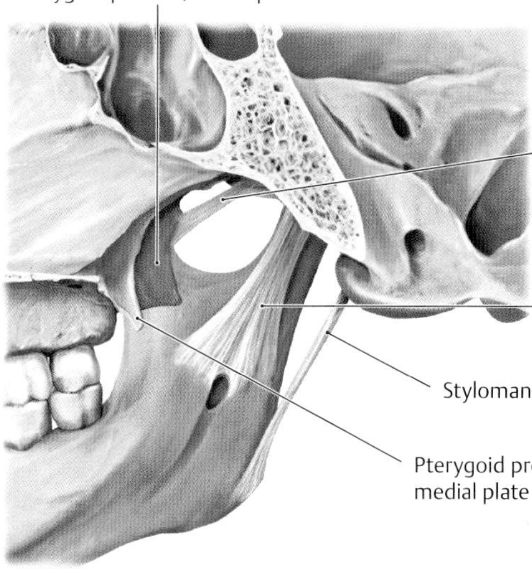

B Medial view of the right temporomandibular joint.

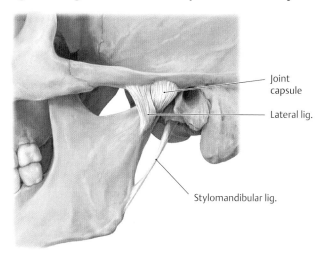

Fig. 44.6 Movement of the temporomandibular joint

Left lateral view. During the first 15 degrees of mandibular depression (opening of the mouth), the head of the mandible remains in the mandibular fossa. Past 15 degrees, the head of the mandible glides forward onto the articular tubercle.

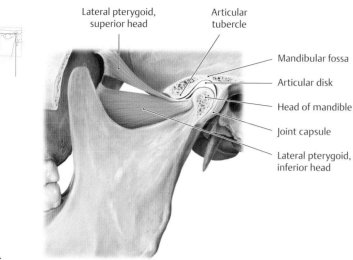

Lateral pterygoid, superior head
Articular tubercle
Mandibular fossa
Articular disk
Head of mandible
Joint capsule
Lateral pterygoid, inferior head

A Mouth closed.

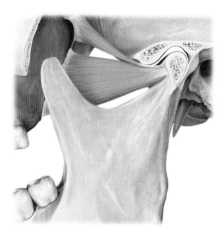

15°

B Mouth opened to 15 degrees.

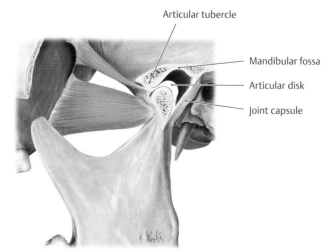
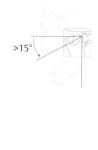

>15°

Articular tubercle
Mandibular fossa
Articular disk
Joint capsule

C Mouth opened past 15 degrees.

 Clinical box 44.1

Dislocation of the temporomandibular joint

Dislocation may occur if the head of the mandible slides past the articular tubercle. The mandible then becomes locked in a protruded position, a condition reduced by pressing on the mandibular row of teeth.

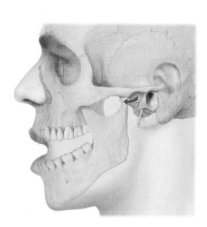

Fig. 44.7 Innervation of the temporomandibular joint capsule

Superior view.

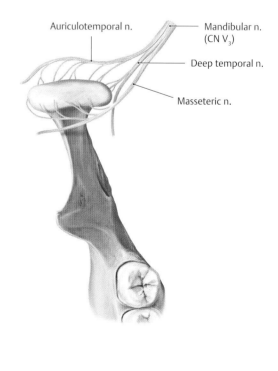

Auriculotemporal n.
Mandibular n. (CN V₃)
Deep temporal n.
Masseteric n.

Teeth

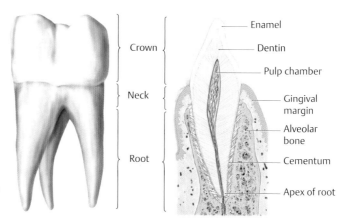

Fig. 44.8 Structure of a tooth

Each tooth consists of hard tissue (enamel, dentin, cementum) and soft tissue (dental pulp) arranged into a crown, neck (cervix), and root.

A Principal parts of a tooth (molar).

B Histology of a tooth (mandibular incisor).

Fig. 44.9 Permanent teeth

Each half of the maxilla and mandible contains a set of three anterior teeth (two incisors, one canine) and five posterior (postcanine) teeth (two premolars, three molars).

Fig. 44.10 Tooth surfaces

The top of the tooth is known as the occlusal surface.

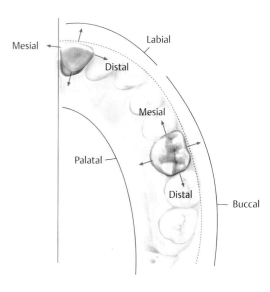

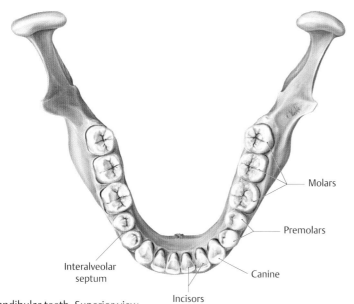

A Maxillary teeth. Inferior view of the maxilla.

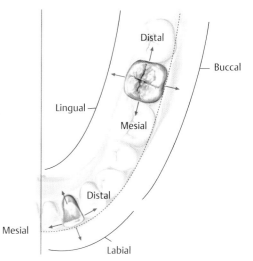

B Mandibular teeth. Superior view of the mandible.

Fig. 44.11 Coding of the teeth

In the United States, the 32 permanent teeth are numbered sequentially (not assigned to quadrants). *Note*: The 20 deciduous (baby) teeth are coded A to J (upper arch), and K to T in a similar clockwise fashion. The third upper right molar is 1; the second upper right premolar is A.

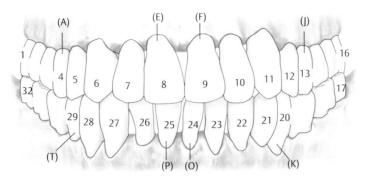

Fig. 44.12 Dental panoramic tomogram

The dental panoramic tomogram (DPT) is a survey radiograph that allows preliminary assessment of the temporomandibular joints, maxillary sinuses, maxillomandibular bone, and dental status (carious lesions, location of wisdom teeth, etc.). *DPT courtesy of Dr. U. J. Rother, Director of the Department of Diagnostic Radiology, Center for Dentistry and Oromaxillofacial Surgery, Eppendorf University Medical Center, Hamburg, Germany.*

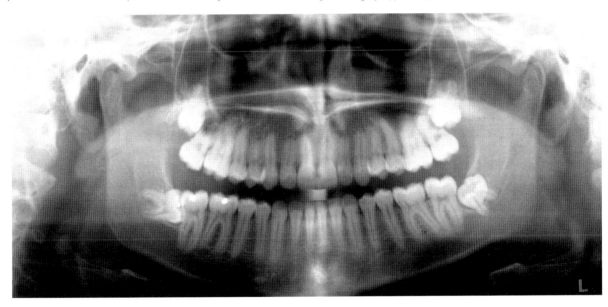

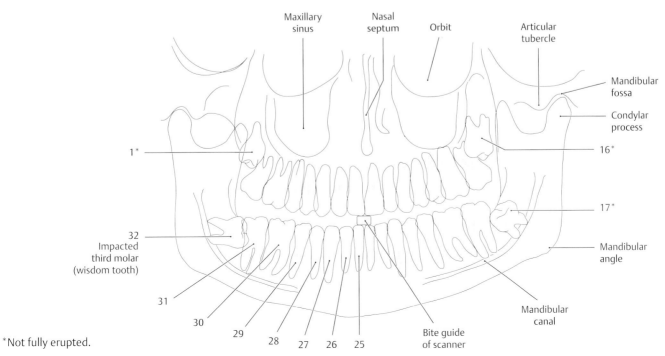

*Not fully erupted.

Oral Cavity Muscle Facts

Fig. 44.13 **Muscles of the oral floor**
See **pp. 620–621** for the infrahyoid muscles.

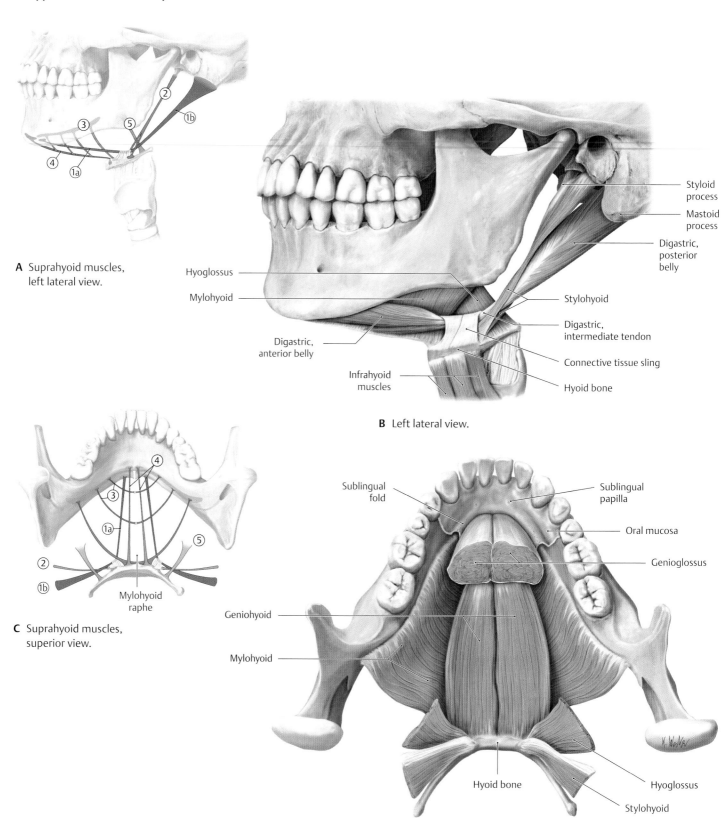

A Suprahyoid muscles, left lateral view.

Styloid process

Mastoid process

Digastric, posterior belly

Hyoglossus

Mylohyoid

Stylohyoid

Digastric, intermediate tendon

Connective tissue sling

Digastric, anterior belly

Infrahyoid muscles

Hyoid bone

B Left lateral view.

Mylohyoid raphe

C Suprahyoid muscles, superior view.

Sublingual fold

Sublingual papilla

Oral mucosa

Genioglossus

Geniohyoid

Mylohyoid

Hyoid bone

Hyoglossus

Stylohyoid

D Superior view of the mandible and hyoid bone.

Table 44.1   **Suprahyoid muscles**

Muscle		Origin	Insertion		Innervation	Action
① Digastric	①ⓐ Anterior belly	Mandible (digastric fossa)	Hyoid bone (body)	Via an intermediate tendon with a fibrous loop	Mylohyoid n. (from CN V₃)	Elevates hyoid bone (during swallowing), assists in opening mandible
	①ⓑ Posterior belly	Temporal bone (mastoid notch, medial to mastoid process)			Facial n. (CN VII)	
② Stylohyoid		Temporal bone (styloid process)		Via a split tendon		
③ Mylohyoid		Mandible (mylohyoid line)		Via median tendon of insertion (mylohyoid raphe)	Mylohyoid n. (from CN V₃)	Tightens and elevates oral floor, draws hyoid bone forward (during swallowing), assists in opening mandible and moving it side to side (mastication)
④ Geniohyoid		Mandible (inferior mental spine)	Body of hyoid bone		Anterior ramus of C1 via hypoglossal n. (CN XII)	Draws hyoid bone forward (during swallowing), assists in opening mandible
⑤ Hyoglossus		Hyoid bone (superior border of greater cornu)	Sides of tongue		Hypoglossal n. (CN XII)	Depresses the tongue

(Innervation column: Digastric anterior belly = Mylohyoid n. (from CN V₃); Digastric posterior belly and Stylohyoid = Facial n. (CN VII))

Fig. 44.14 Muscles of the soft palate

Inferior view. The soft palate forms the posterior boundary of the oral cavity, separating it from the oropharynx.

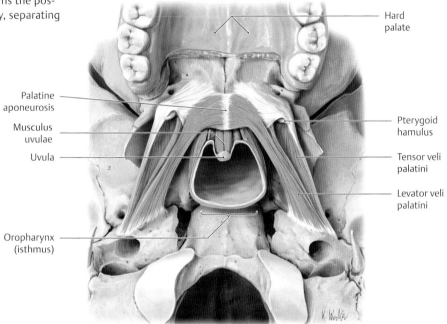

- Hard palate
- Palatine aponeurosis
- Musculus uvulae
- Uvula
- Pterygoid hamulus
- Tensor veli palatini
- Levator veli palatini
- Oropharynx (isthmus)

Table 44.2   **Muscles of the soft palate**

Muscle	Origin	Insertion	Innervation	Action
Tensor veli palatini	Medial pterygoid plate (scaphoid fossa); sphenoid bone (spine); cartilage of pharyngotympanic tube	Palatine aponeurosis	Medial pterygoid n. (CN V₃ via otic ganglion)	Tightens soft palate; opens inlet to pharyngotympanic (auditory) tube (during swallowing, yawning)
Levator veli palatini	Cartilage of pharyngotympanic tube; temporal bone (petrous part)		Vagus n. via pharyngeal plexus	Raises soft palate to horizontal position
Musculus uvulae	Uvula (mucosa)	Palatine aponeurosis; posterior nasal spine		Shortens and raises uvula
Palatoglossus*	Tongue (side)	Palatine aponeurosis		Elevates tongue (posterior portion); pulls soft palate onto tongue
Palatopharyngeus*				Tightens soft palate; during swallowing pulls pharyngeal walls superiorly, anteriorly, and medially

*For the palatoglossus, see **Figs. 44.18 and 44.19, p. 608**; and for the palatopharyngeus, see **Fig. 44.29C, p. 615.**

Innervation of the Oral Cavity

Fig. 44.15 Trigeminal nerve in the oral cavity

Right lateral view.

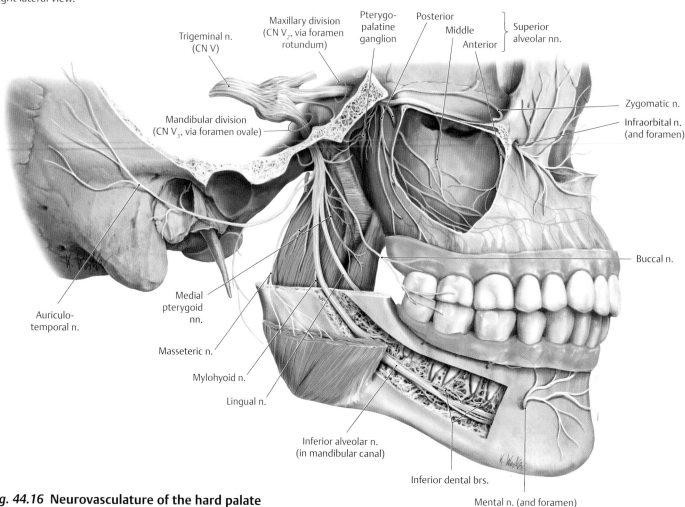

Fig. 44.16 Neurovasculature of the hard palate

Inferior view. The hard palate receives sensory innervation primarily from terminal branches of the maxillary division of the trigeminal nerve (CN V₂). The arteries of the hard palate arise from the maxillary artery.

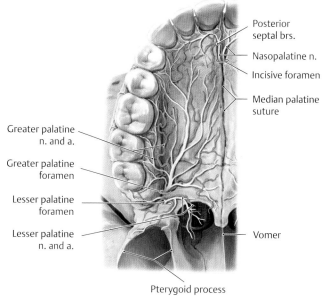

A Sensory innervation. *Note:* The buccal nerve is a branch of the mandibular division (CN V₃).

B Nerves and arteries.

The muscles of the oral floor have a complex nerve supply with contributions from the trigeminal nerve (CN V₃), facial nerve (CN VII), and C1 spinal nerve via the hypoglossal nerve (CN XII).

Fig. 44.17 **Innervation of the oral floor muscles**

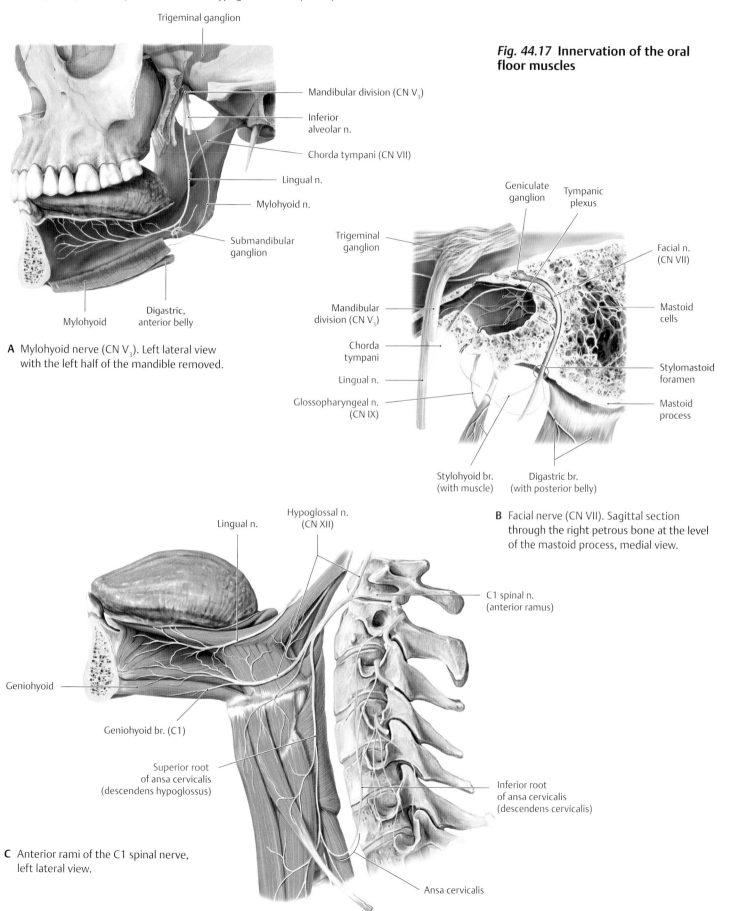

Trigeminal ganglion

Mandibular division (CN V₃)

Inferior alveolar n.

Chorda tympani (CN VII)

Lingual n.

Mylohyoid n.

Submandibular ganglion

Mylohyoid

Digastric, anterior belly

A Mylohyoid nerve (CN V₃). Left lateral view with the left half of the mandible removed.

Geniculate ganglion

Tympanic plexus

Trigeminal ganglion

Facial n. (CN VII)

Mandibular division (CN V₃)

Mastoid cells

Chorda tympani

Lingual n.

Stylomastoid foramen

Glossopharyngeal n. (CN IX)

Mastoid process

Stylohyoid br. (with muscle)

Digastric br. (with posterior belly)

B Facial nerve (CN VII). Sagittal section through the right petrous bone at the level of the mastoid process, medial view.

Lingual n.

Hypoglossal n. (CN XII)

C1 spinal n. (anterior ramus)

Geniohyoid

Geniohyoid br. (C1)

Superior root of ansa cervicalis (descendens hypoglossus)

Inferior root of ansa cervicalis (descendens cervicalis)

Ansa cervicalis

C Anterior rami of the C1 spinal nerve, left lateral view.

Tongue

 The dorsum of the tongue is covered by a highly specialized mucosa that supports its sensory functions (taste and fine tactile discrimination; see **p. 685**). The tongue is endowed with a very powerful muscular body to support its motor properties during mastication, swallowing, and speaking.

Fig. 44.18 Structure of the tongue

Superior view. The V-shaped sulcus terminalis divides the tongue into an anterior 2/3rds (oral, presulcal) and a posterior 1/3rd (pharyngeal, postsulcal).

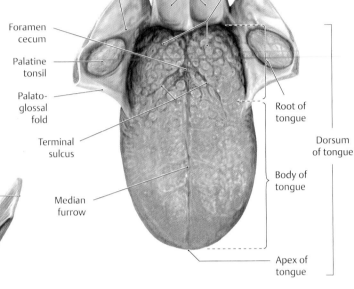

Fig. 44.19 Muscles of the tongue

The extrinsic lingual muscles (genioglossus, hyoglossus, palatoglossus, and styloglossus) have bony attachments and move the tongue as a whole. The intrinsic lingual muscles (superior and inferior longitudinal muscles, transverse muscle, and vertical muscle) have no bony attachments and alter the shape of the tongue.

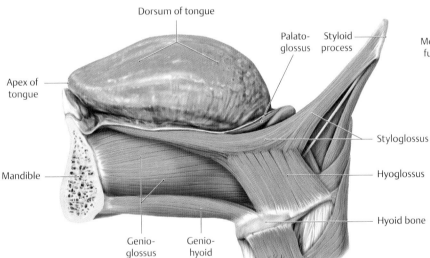

A Left lateral view.

Fig. 44.20 Somatosensory and taste innervation of the tongue

Superior view.

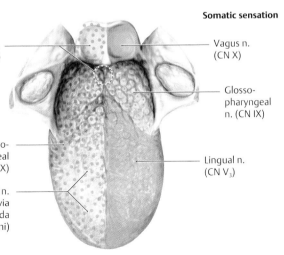

B Coronal section, anterior view.

Fig. 44.21 Neurovasculature of the tongue

The lingual muscles receive somatomotor innervation from the hypoglossal nerve (CN XII), with the exception of the palatoglossus (supplied by the vagus nerve, CN X).

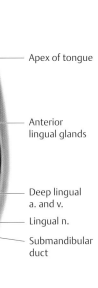

Apex of tongue

Anterior lingual glands

Frenulum

Sublingual fold

Sublingual papilla

Deep lingual a. and v.

Lingual n.

Submandibular duct

A Inferior surface of the tongue.

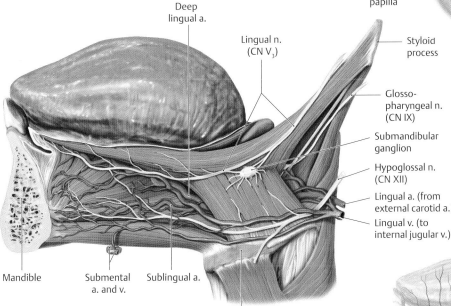

Deep lingual a.

Lingual n. (CN V₃)

Styloid process

Glosso-pharyngeal n. (CN IX)

Submandibular ganglion

Hypoglossal n. (CN XII)

Lingual a. (from external carotid a.)

Lingual v. (to internal jugular v.)

Mandible

Submental a. and v.

Sublingual a.

Hyoid bone

B Left lateral view.

Fig. 44.22 Lymphatic drainage of the tongue and oral floor

Left lateral view. Lymph flows to the submental and submandibular lymph nodes of the tongue and oral floor, which ultimately drain into the jugular lymph nodes along the internal jugular vein. Because these groups of lymph nodes receive drainage from the sides of the tongue, tumor cells may become widely disseminated in this region. Metastatic squamous cell carcinomas on the lateral border of the tongue frequently metastasize to the opposite side.

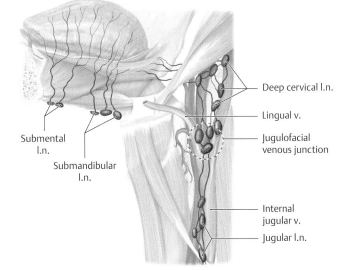

Deep cervical l.n.

Lingual v.

Jugulofacial venous junction

Submental l.n.

Submandibular l.n.

Internal jugular v.

Jugular l.n.

 Clinical box 44.2

Unilateral hypoglossal nerve palsy
Damage to the hypoglossal nerve causes paralysis of the genioglossus muscle on the affected side. The healthy (innervated) genioglossus on the unaffected side will therefore dominate. Upon protrusion, the tongue will deviate *toward* the paralyzed side.

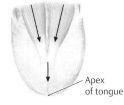

A Active protrusion with an intact hypoglossal nerve.

Apex of tongue

B Active protrusion with a unilateral hypoglossal nerve lesion.

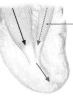

Paralyzed genioglossus on affected side

Topography of the Oral Cavity & Salivary Glands

 The oral cavity is located below the nasal cavity and anterior to the pharynx. It is bounded by the hard and soft palates, the tongue and muscles of the oral floor, and the uvula.

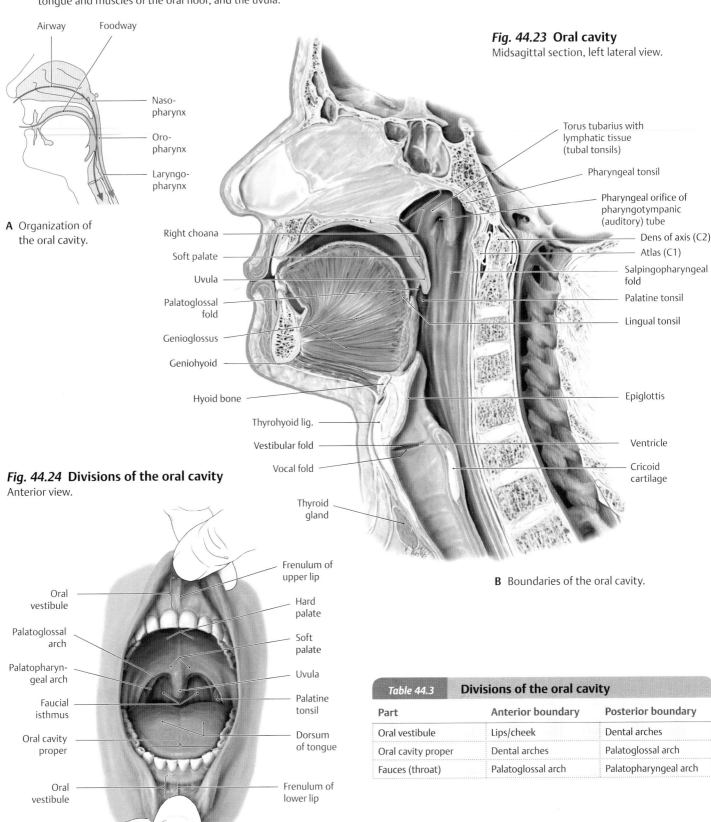

A Organization of the oral cavity.

Airway   Foodway

Naso-pharynx
Oro-pharynx
Laryngo-pharynx

Fig. 44.23 Oral cavity
Midsagittal section, left lateral view.

Torus tubarius with lymphatic tissue (tubal tonsils)
Pharyngeal tonsil
Pharyngeal orifice of pharyngotympanic (auditory) tube
Dens of axis (C2)
Atlas (C1)
Salpingopharyngeal fold
Palatine tonsil
Lingual tonsil

Right choana
Soft palate
Uvula
Palatoglossal fold
Genioglossus
Geniohyoid
Hyoid bone
Thyrohyoid lig.
Vestibular fold
Vocal fold
Thyroid gland

Epiglottis
Ventricle
Cricoid cartilage

B Boundaries of the oral cavity.

Fig. 44.24 Divisions of the oral cavity
Anterior view.

Oral vestibule
Palatoglossal arch
Palatopharyn-geal arch
Faucial isthmus
Oral cavity proper
Oral vestibule

Frenulum of upper lip
Hard palate
Soft palate
Uvula
Palatine tonsil
Dorsum of tongue
Frenulum of lower lip

Table 44.3	Divisions of the oral cavity	
Part	**Anterior boundary**	**Posterior boundary**
Oral vestibule	Lips/cheek	Dental arches
Oral cavity proper	Dental arches	Palatoglossal arch
Fauces (throat)	Palatoglossal arch	Palatopharyngeal arch

The three large, paired salivary glands are the parotid, submandibular, and sublingual glands. The parotid gland is a purely serous (watery) salivary gland. The sublingual gland is predominantly mucous; the submandibular gland is a mixed seromucous gland.

***Fig. 44.25* Salivary glands**

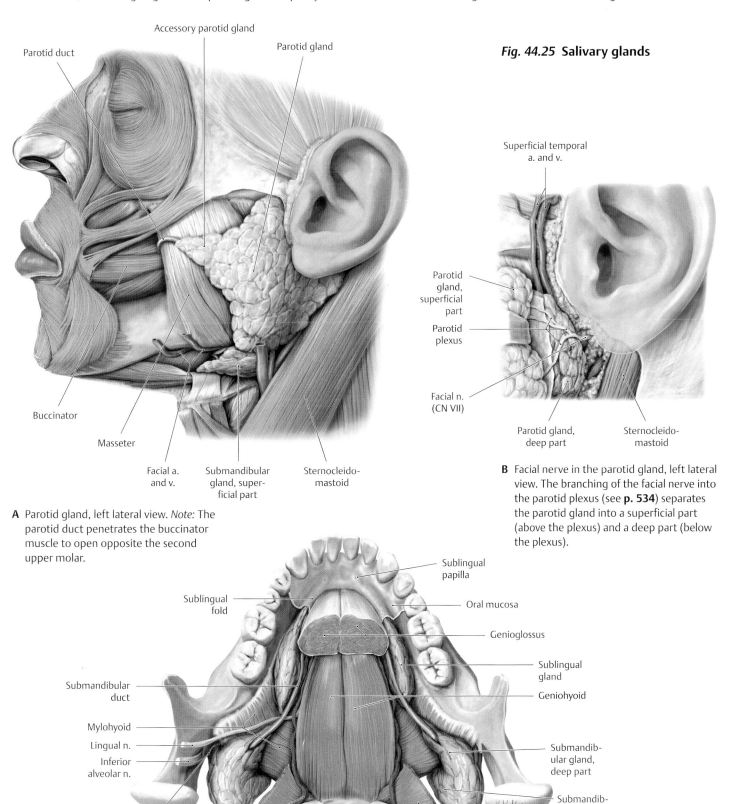

A Parotid gland, left lateral view. *Note:* The parotid duct penetrates the buccinator muscle to open opposite the second upper molar.

B Facial nerve in the parotid gland, left lateral view. The branching of the facial nerve into the parotid plexus (see **p. 534**) separates the parotid gland into a superficial part (above the plexus) and a deep part (below the plexus).

C Submandibular and sublingual glands, superior view with tongue removed.

Tonsils & Pharynx

Fig. 44.26 Tonsils

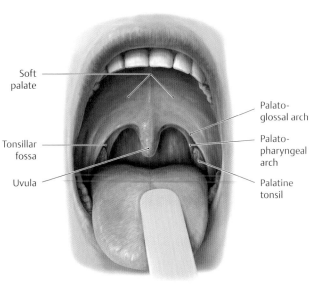

A Palatine tonsils, anterior view.

Soft palate
Tonsillar fossa
Uvula
Palato-glossal arch
Palato-pharyngeal arch
Palatine tonsil

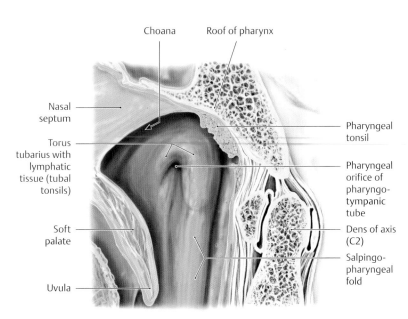

B Pharyngeal tonsils. Sagittal section through the roof of the pharynx.

Choana
Roof of pharynx
Nasal septum
Torus tubarius with lymphatic tissue (tubal tonsils)
Soft palate
Uvula
Pharyngeal tonsil
Pharyngeal orifice of pharyngo-tympanic tube
Dens of axis (C2)
Salpingo-pharyngeal fold

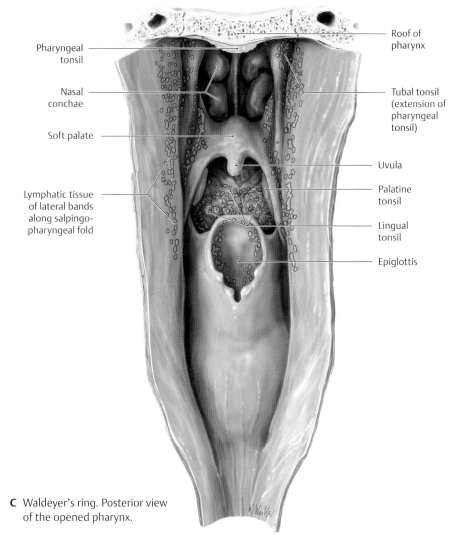

C Waldeyer's ring. Posterior view of the opened pharynx.

Pharyngeal tonsil
Nasal conchae
Soft palate
Lymphatic tissue of lateral bands along salpingo-pharyngeal fold
Roof of pharynx
Tubal tonsil (extension of pharyngeal tonsil)
Uvula
Palatine tonsil
Lingual tonsil
Epiglottis

Table 44.4	Structures in Waldeyer's ring	
Tonsil	**#**	
Pharyngeal tonsil	1	
Tubal tonsils	2	
Palatine tonsils	2	
Lingual tonsil	1	
Lateral bands	2	

Tonsil infections
Abnormal enlargement of the palatine tonsils due to severe viral or bacterial infection can result in obstruction of the oropharynx, causing difficulty swallowing.

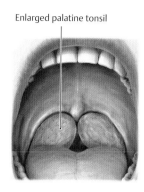

Enlarged palatine tonsil

Particularly well developed in young children, the pharyngeal tonsil begins to regress at 6 to 7 years of age. Abnormal enlargement is common, with the tonsil bulging into the nasopharynx and obstructing air passages, forcing the child to "mouth breathe."

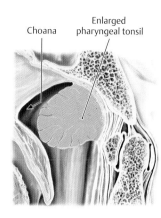

Choana   Enlarged pharyngeal tonsil

Fig. 44.27 **Pharyngeal mucosa**
Posterior view of the opened pharynx. The anterior portion of the muscular tube contains three openings: choanae (to the nasal cavity), faucial isthmus (to the oral cavity), and aditus (to the laryngeal inlet).

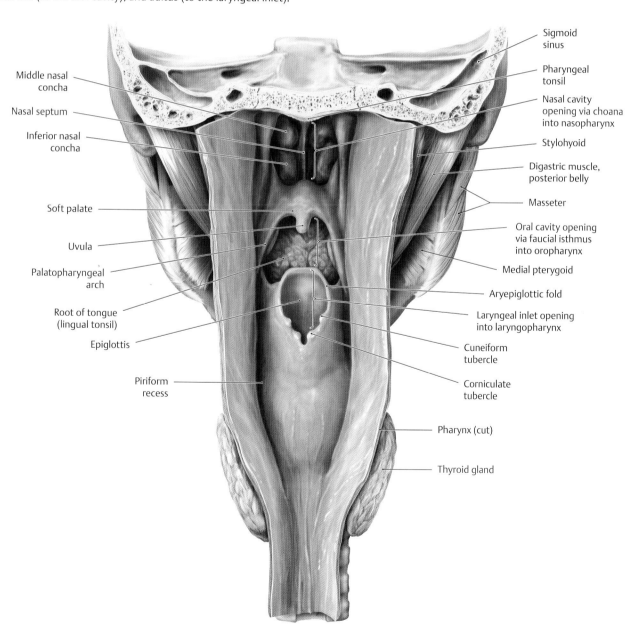

Labels (left side):
- Middle nasal concha
- Nasal septum
- Inferior nasal concha
- Soft palate
- Uvula
- Palatopharyngeal arch
- Root of tongue (lingual tonsil)
- Epiglottis
- Piriform recess

Labels (right side):
- Sigmoid sinus
- Pharyngeal tonsil
- Nasal cavity opening via choana into nasopharynx
- Stylohyoid
- Digastric muscle, posterior belly
- Masseter
- Oral cavity opening via faucial isthmus into oropharynx
- Medial pterygoid
- Aryepiglottic fold
- Laryngeal inlet opening into laryngopharynx
- Cuneiform tubercle
- Corniculate tubercle
- Pharynx (cut)
- Thyroid gland

Pharyngeal Muscles

Fig. 44.28 **Pharyngeal muscles: Left lateral view**

Fig. 44.28 **Pharyngeal muscles: Left lateral view**

The pharyngeal musculature consists of the pharyngeal constrictors and the relatively weak pharyngeal elevators.

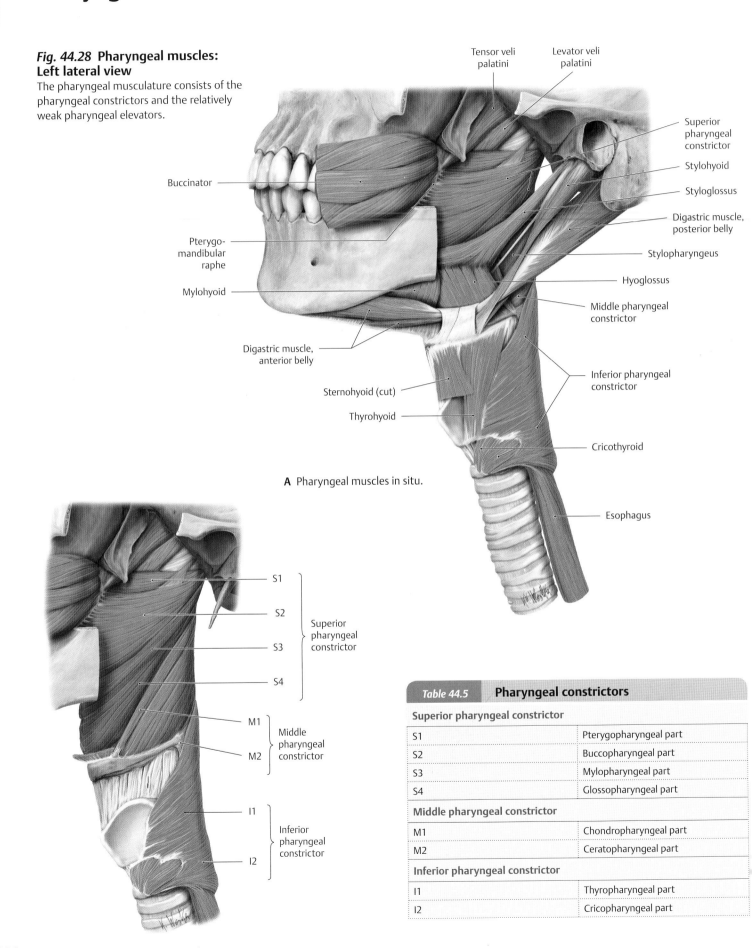

A Pharyngeal muscles in situ.

B Subdivisions of the pharyngeal constrictors.

Table 44.5	Pharyngeal constrictors
Superior pharyngeal constrictor	
S1	Pterygopharyngeal part
S2	Buccopharyngeal part
S3	Mylopharyngeal part
S4	Glossopharyngeal part
Middle pharyngeal constrictor	
M1	Chondropharyngeal part
M2	Ceratopharyngeal part
Inferior pharyngeal constrictor	
I1	Thyropharyngeal part
I2	Cricopharyngeal part

Fig. 44.29 **Pharyngeal muscles: Posterior view**

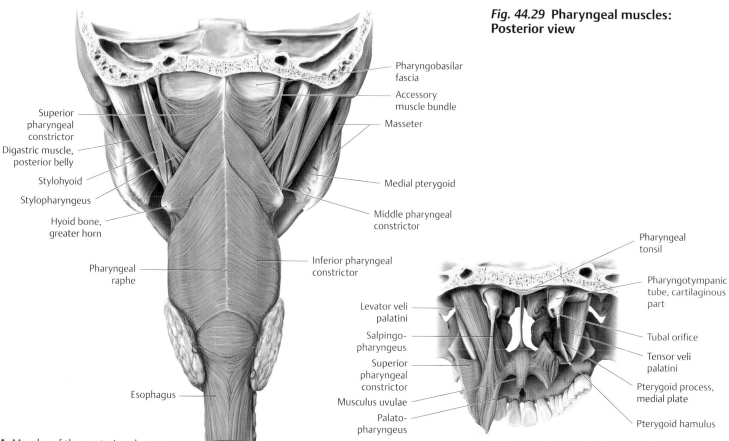

Pharyngobasilar fascia

Accessory muscle bundle

Masseter

Superior pharyngeal constrictor

Digastric muscle, posterior belly

Stylohyoid

Stylopharyngeus

Medial pterygoid

Hyoid bone, greater horn

Middle pharyngeal constrictor

Pharyngeal raphe

Inferior pharyngeal constrictor

Esophagus

A Muscles of the posterior pharynx.

Pharyngeal tonsil

Pharyngotympanic tube, cartilaginous part

Levator veli palatini

Salpingo-pharyngeus

Tubal orifice

Superior pharyngeal constrictor

Tensor veli palatini

Musculus uvulae

Pterygoid process, medial plate

Palato-pharyngeus

Pterygoid hamulus

B Muscles of the soft palate and pharyngo-tympanic tube. The muscles of the fauces form the posterior boundary of the oral cavity. *Cut on right side:* Levator veli palatini and salpingopharyngeus.

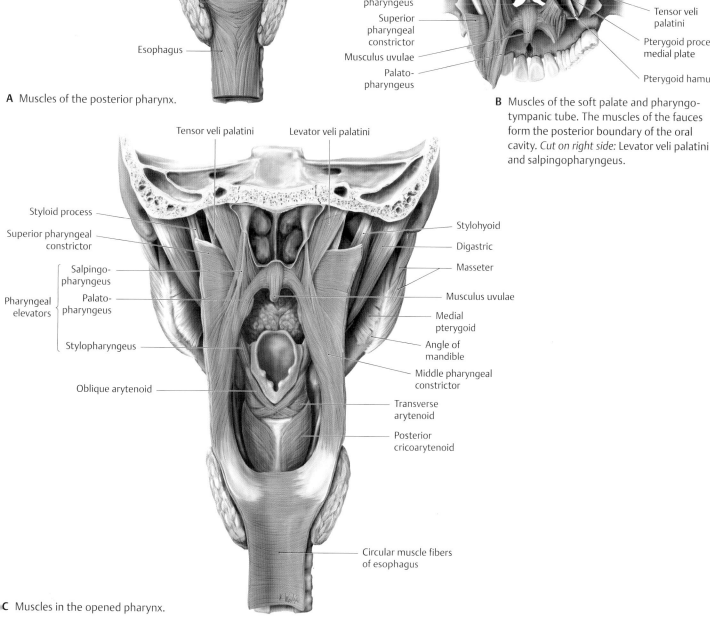

Tensor veli palatini

Levator veli palatini

Styloid process

Superior pharyngeal constrictor

Stylohyoid

Digastric

Pharyngeal elevators

Salpingo-pharyngeus

Masseter

Palato-pharyngeus

Musculus uvulae

Medial pterygoid

Stylopharyngeus

Angle of mandible

Oblique arytenoid

Middle pharyngeal constrictor

Transverse arytenoid

Posterior cricoarytenoid

Circular muscle fibers of esophagus

C Muscles in the opened pharynx.

615

Neurovasculature of the Pharynx

***Fig. 44.30* Neurovasculature in the parapharyngeal space**
Posterior view. *Removed:* Vertebral column and posterior structures.

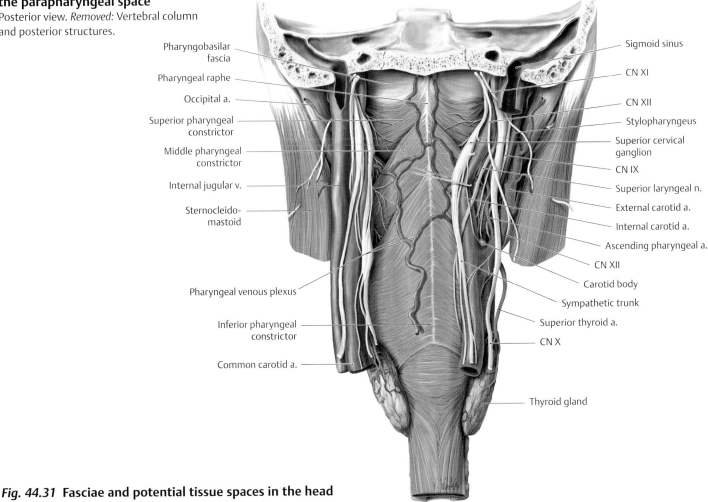

- Pharyngobasilar fascia
- Pharyngeal raphe
- Occipital a.
- Superior pharyngeal constrictor
- Middle pharyngeal constrictor
- Internal jugular v.
- Sternocleido-mastoid
- Pharyngeal venous plexus
- Inferior pharyngeal constrictor
- Common carotid a.

- Sigmoid sinus
- CN XI
- CN XII
- Stylopharyngeus
- Superior cervical ganglion
- CN IX
- Superior laryngeal n.
- External carotid a.
- Internal carotid a.
- Ascending pharyngeal a.
- CN XII
- Carotid body
- Sympathetic trunk
- Superior thyroid a.
- CN X
- Thyroid gland

***Fig. 44.31* Fasciae and potential tissue spaces in the head**
Transverse section at the level of the tongue, superior view.

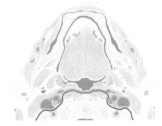

A Fascial boundaries are key to outlining pathways for the spread of infection. The prevertebral fascia (red) is the outermost layer. A space (retropharyngeal) exists between this layer and the alar fascia (green). Potential spaces in the head become true spaces when they are infiltrated by products of infection. These spaces seen on **Fig. 44.31B** are defined by bones, muscles and fascia and initially confine an infection but eventually allow it to spread through communications between spaces.

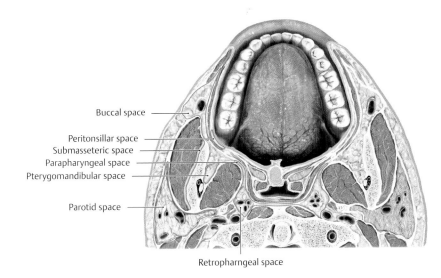

- Buccal space
- Peritonsillar space
- Submasseteric space
- Parapharyngeal space
- Pterygomandibular space
- Parotid space
- Retropharngeal space

B Transverse section at the level of the tonsillar fossa, superior view.

Fig. 44.32 **Neurovasculature of the opened pharynx**
Posterior view.

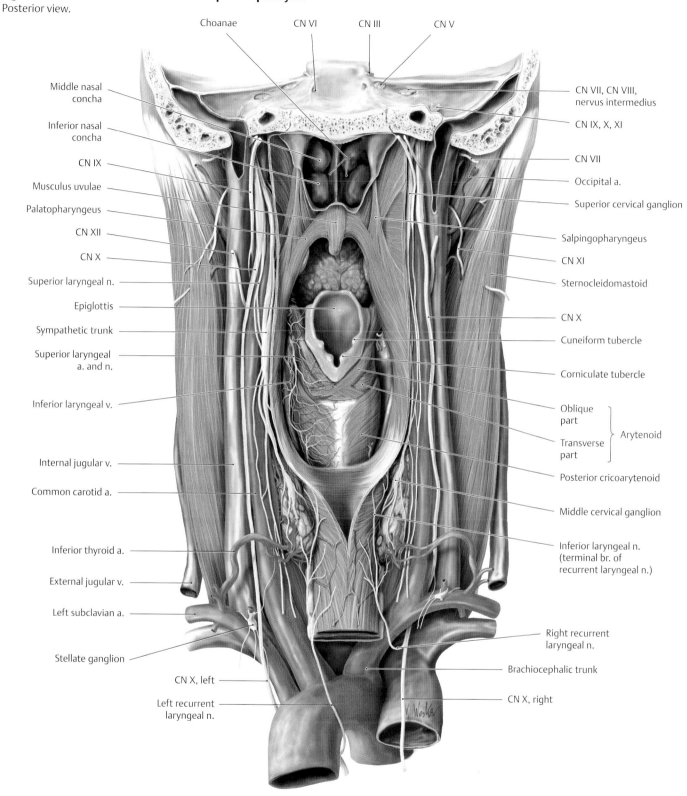

Choanae

CN VI

CN III

CN V

Middle nasal concha

Inferior nasal concha

CN IX

Musculus uvulae

Palatopharyngeus

CN XII

CN X

Superior laryngeal n.

Epiglottis

Sympathetic trunk

Superior laryngeal a. and n.

Inferior laryngeal v.

Internal jugular v.

Common carotid a.

Inferior thyroid a.

External jugular v.

Left subclavian a.

Stellate ganglion

CN X, left

Left recurrent laryngeal n.

CN VII, CN VIII, nervus intermedius

CN IX, X, XI

CN VII

Occipital a.

Superior cervical ganglion

Salpingopharyngeus

CN XI

Sternocleidomastoid

CN X

Cuneiform tubercle

Corniculate tubercle

Oblique part

Transverse part

Arytenoid

Posterior cricoarytenoid

Middle cervical ganglion

Inferior laryngeal n. (terminal br. of recurrent laryngeal n.)

Right recurrent laryngeal n.

Brachiocephalic trunk

CN X, right

CN III, oculomotor n.; CN V, trigeminal n.; CN VI, abducent n.;
CN VII, facial n.; CN VIII, vestibulocochlear n.; CN IX, glossopharyngeal n.;
CN X, vagus n.; CN XI, accessory n.; CN XII, hypoglossal n..
See Chapter 39 for the cranial nerves.

Muscle Facts (I)

The bones, joints, and ligaments of the neck and the six topographic classes of neck muscles are covered in this or the Back unit (see **Table 45.1**). However, some muscles in the same topographic class belong in different functional classes; for example, the platysma belongs to the muscles of facial expression; the trapezius, to the muscles of the shoulder girdle; and the nuchal muscles, to the intrinsic back muscles. Note that the suboccipital muscles (short nuchal and craniovertebral joint muscles) are covered with the lateral (deep) muscles of the neck.

Table 45.1	Bones, joints, ligaments, and muscles of the neck			
Bones, joints, and ligaments				
Bones of the cervical spine	See **pp. 8-9**	Joints & ligaments of the craniovertebral junction		See **pp. 18-19**
Joints & ligaments of the cervical spine	See **pp. 16-17, 20-21**	Hyoid bone & larynx		**Fig. 44.3, Fig. 45.18**
Muscles				
I	**Superficial neck muscles**	**III**	**Suprahyoid muscles**	
	Platysma, ①, ② sternocleidomastoid, ③, ④, ⑤ trapezius	**Fig. 45.3**	Digastric, geniohyoid, mylohyoid, stylohyoid	**Fig. 45.4A**
II	**Nuchal muscles (intrinsic back muscles)**	**IV**	**Infrahyoid muscles**	
	⑥ Semispinalis capitis ⑦ Semispinalis cervicis	See **p. 34**	Sternohyoid, sternothyroid, thyrohyoid, omohyoid	**Fig. 45.4B**
	⑧ Splenius capitis ⑨ Splenius cervicis		**V**	**Prevertebral muscles**
	⑩ Longissimus capitis ⑪ Longissimus cervicis	See **p. 32**	Longus capitis, longus coli, rectus capitis anterior and lateralis	See **p. 31** **Fig. 45.6A**
	⑫ Iliocostalis cervicis		**VI**	**Lateral (deep) neck muscles**
	Suboccipital muscles (short nuchal and craniovertebral joint muscles)	**Fig. 45.6C**	Anterior, middle, and posterior scalenes	**Fig. 45.6B**

Fig. 45.1 Superficial neck muscles schematic

See **Table 45.2** for details.

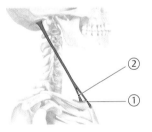

A Sternocleidomastoid.

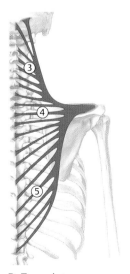

B Trapezius.

Fig. 45.2 Nuchal muscles schematic

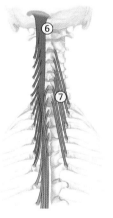

A Semispinalis.

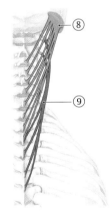

B Splenius.

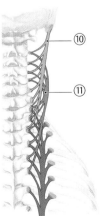

C Longissimus.

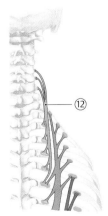

D Iliocostalis.

Fig. 45.3 **Superficial neck muscles**

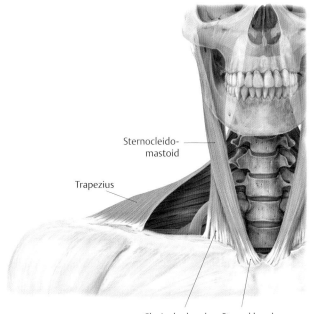

A Anterior view.

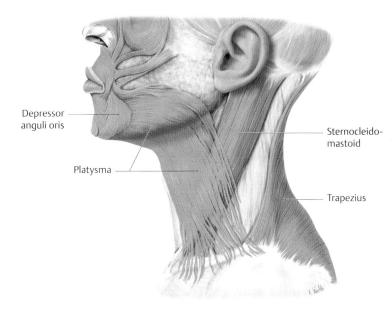

B Left lateral view.

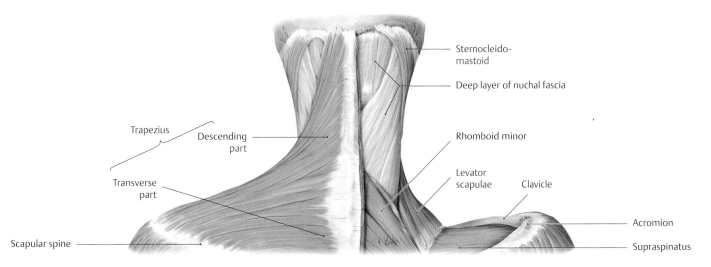

C Posterior view. *Removed:* Trapezius (right side).

Table 45.2	**Superficial neck muscles**				
Muscle		**Origin**	**Insertion**	**Innervation**	**Action**
Platysma		Skin over lower neck and upper lateral thorax	Mandible (inferior border), skin over lower face and angle of mouth	Cervical branch of facial n. (CN VII)	Depresses and wrinkles skin of lower face and mouth, tenses skin of neck, aids forced depression of mandible
Sternocleido-mastoid	① Sternal head	Sternum (manubrium)	Temporal bone (mastoid process), occipital bone (superior nuchal line)	*Motor:* Accessory n. (CN XI) *Pain and proprioception:* Cervical plexus (C3, C4)	*Unilateral:* Tilts head to same side, rotates head to opposite side *Bilateral:* Extends head, aids in respiration when head is fixed
	② Clavicular head	Clavicle (medial one third)			
Trapezius	③ Descending part*	Occipital bone, spinous processes of C1–C7	Clavicle (lateral one third)		Draws scapula obliquely upward, rotates glenoid cavity superiorly

* The transverse ④ and ascending ⑤ parts are described on **p. 316**.

Muscle Facts (II)

| Table 45.3 | | Suprahyoid muscles | | | | |

The suprahyoid muscles are also considered accessory muscles of mastication.

Muscle		Origin	Insertion		Innervation	Action
Digastric	① Anterior belly	Mandible (digastric fossa)	Via an intermediate tendon with a fibrous loop	Hyoid bone (body)	Mylohyoid n. (from CN V₃)	Elevates hyoid bone (during swallowing), assists in opening mandible
	①ᵇ Posterior belly	Temporal bone (mastoid notch, medial to mastoid process)			Facial n. (CN VII)	
② Stylohyoid		Temporal bone (styloid process)	Via a split tendon			
③ Mylohyoid		Mandible (mylohyoid line)	Via median tendon of insertion (mylohyoid raphe)		Mylohyoid n. (from CN V₃)	Tightens and elevates oral floor, draws hyoid bone forward (during swallowing), assists in opening mandible and moving it side to side (during mastication)
④ Geniohyoid		Mandible (inferior mental spine)	Directly		Anterior ramus of C1 via hypoglossal n. (CN XII)	Draws hyoid bone forward (during swallowing), assists in opening mandible

Fig. 45.4 **Suprahyoid and infrahyoid muscles**

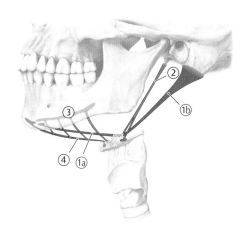

A Suprahyoid muscles, left lateral view.

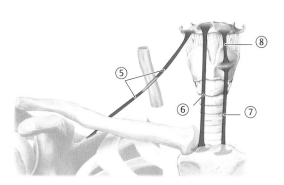

B Infrahyoid muscles, anterior view.

| Table 45.4 | Infrahyoid muscles | | | |

Muscle	Origin	Insertion	Innervation	Action
⑤ Omohyoid	Scapula (superior border) – inferior belly	Hyoid bone (body) – superior belly	Ansa cervicalis (C1–C3) of cervical plexus	Depresses (fixes) hyoid, draws larynx and hyoid down for phonation and terminal phases of swallowing*
⑥ Sternohyoid	Manubrium and sternoclavicular joint (posterior surface)			
⑦ Sternothyroid	Manubrium (posterior surface)	Thyroid cartilage (oblique line)	Ansa cervicalis (C2–C3) of cervical plexus	
⑧ Thyrohyoid	Thyroid cartilage (oblique line)	Hyoid bone (body)	Anterior ramus of C1 via hypoglossal n. (CN XII)	Depresses and fixes hyoid, raises the larynx during swallowing

* The omohyoid also tenses the cervical fascia (via its intermediate tendon).

Fig. 45.5 **Suprahyoid and infrahyoid muscles**

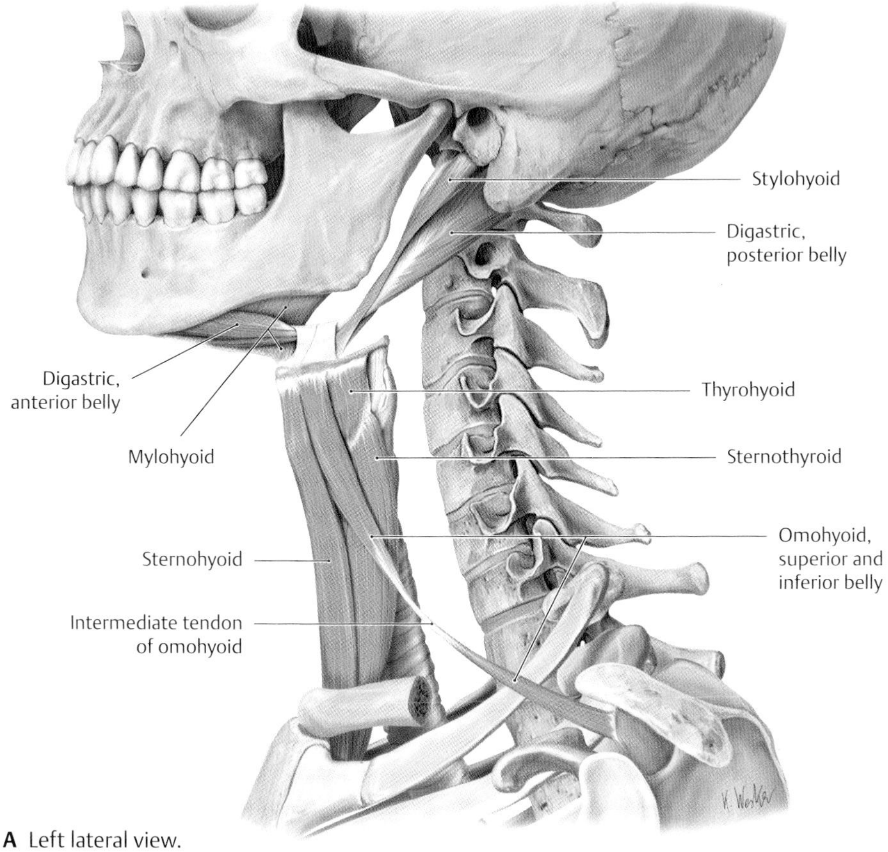

Stylohyoid

Digastric, posterior belly

Thyrohyoid

Sternothyroid

Omohyoid, superior and inferior belly

Digastric, anterior belly

Mylohyoid

Sternohyoid

Intermediate tendon of omohyoid

A Left lateral view.

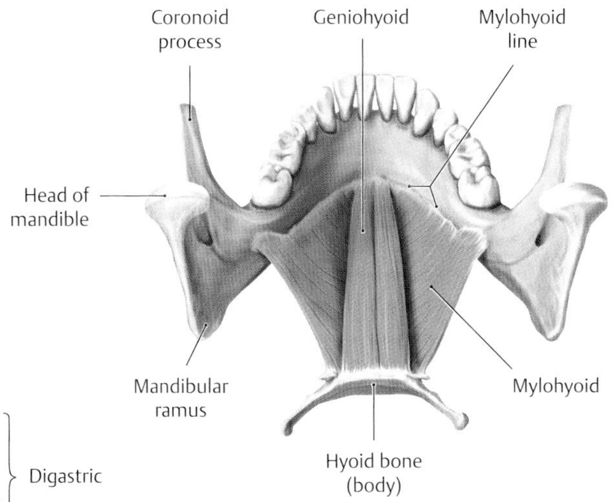

Coronoid process

Geniohyoid

Mylohyoid line

Head of mandible

Mandibular ramus

Mylohyoid

Hyoid bone (body)

B Mylohyoid and geniohyoid (oral floor), posterosuperior view.

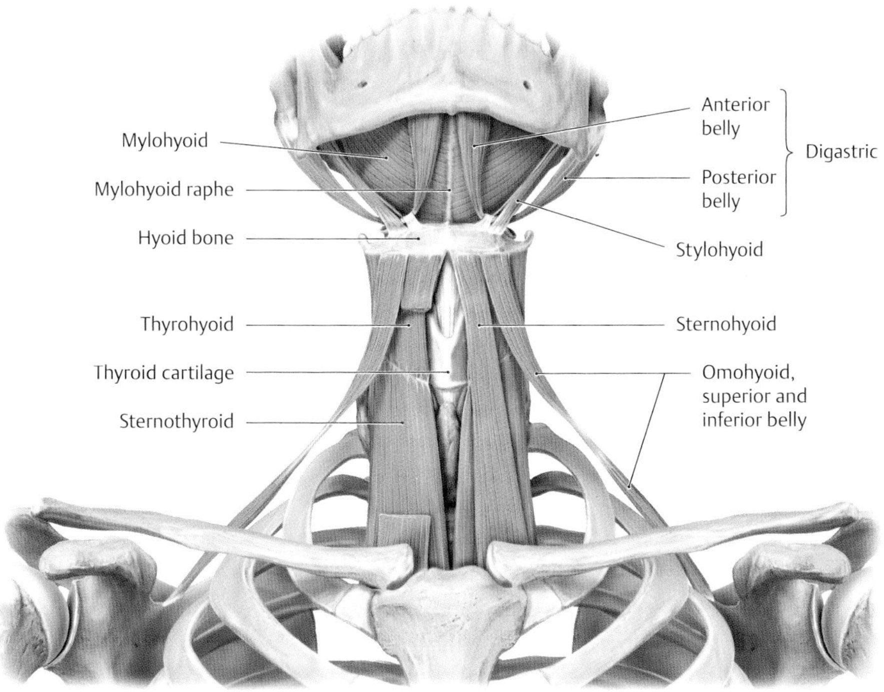

Mylohyoid

Mylohyoid raphe

Hyoid bone

Thyrohyoid

Thyroid cartilage

Sternothyroid

Anterior belly

Posterior belly

Digastric

Stylohyoid

Sternohyoid

Omohyoid, superior and inferior belly

C Anterior view. The sternohyoid has been cut (right).

Muscle Facts (III)

Fig. 45.6 Deep muscles of the neck

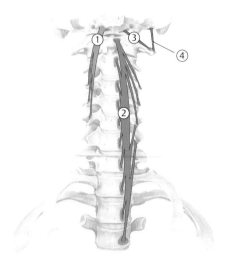

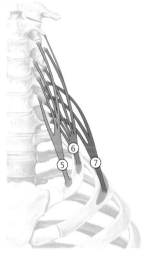

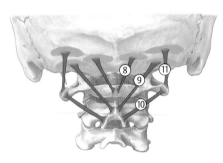

C Suboccipital muscles, posterior view.

A Prevertebral muscles, anterior view.

B Scalene muscles, anterior view.

Table 45.5		Deep muscles of the neck			
Muscle		**Origin**	**Insertion**	**Innervation**	**Action**
Prevertebral muscles					
① Longus capitis		C3–C6 (anterior tubercles of transverse processes)	Occipital bone (basilar part)	Anterior rami of C1–C3	Flexion of head at atlanto-occipital joints
② Longus colli	Vertical (intermediate) part	C5–T3 (anterior surfaces of vertebral bodies)	C2–C4 (anterior surfaces)	Anterior rami of C1–C6	*Unilateral:* Tilts and rotates cervical spine to opposite side *Bilateral:* Forward flexion of cervical spine
	Superior oblique part	C3–C5 (anterior tubercles of transverse processes)	Atlas (anterior tubercle)		
	Inferior oblique part	T1–T3 (anterior surfaces of vertebral bodies)	C5–C6 (anterior tubercles of transverse processes)		
③ Rectus capitis anterior		C1 (lateral mass)	Occipital bone (basilar part)	Anterior rami of C1 and C2	*Unilateral:* Lateral flexion of the head at the atlanto-occipital joint *Bilateral:* Flexion of the head at the atlanto-occipital joint
④ Rectus capitis lateralis		C1 (transverse process)	Occipital bone (basilar part, lateral to occipital condyles)		
Scalene muscles					
⑤ Anterior scalene		C3–C6 (anterior tubercles of transverse processes)	1st rib (scalene tubercle)	Anterior rami of C4–C6	*With ribs mobile:* Elevates upper ribs (during forced inspiration) *With ribs fixed:* Bends cervical spine to same side (unilateral), flexes neck (bilateral)
⑥ Middle scalene		C1–C2 (transverse processes), C3–C7 (posterior tubercles of transverse processes)	1st rib (posterior to groove for subclavian a.)	Anterior rami of C3–C8	
⑦ Posterior scalene		C5–C7 (posterior tubercles of transverse processes)	2nd rib (outer surface)	Anterior rami of C6–C8	
Suboccipital muscles (short nuchal and craniovertebral joint muscles)					
⑧ Rectus capitis posterior minor		C1 (posterior tubercle)	Occipital bone (inner third of inferior nuchal line)	Posterior ramus of C1 (suboccipital n.)	*Unilateral:* Rotates head to same side *Bilateral:* Extends head
⑨ Rectus capitis posterior major		C2 (spinous process)	Occipital bone (middle third of inferior nuchal line)		
⑩ Obliquus capitis inferior			C1 (transverse process)		
⑪ Obliquus capitis superior		C1 (transverse process)	Occipital bone (above insertion of rectus capitis posterior major)		*Unilateral:* Tilts head to same side, rotates it to opposite side *Bilateral:* Extends head

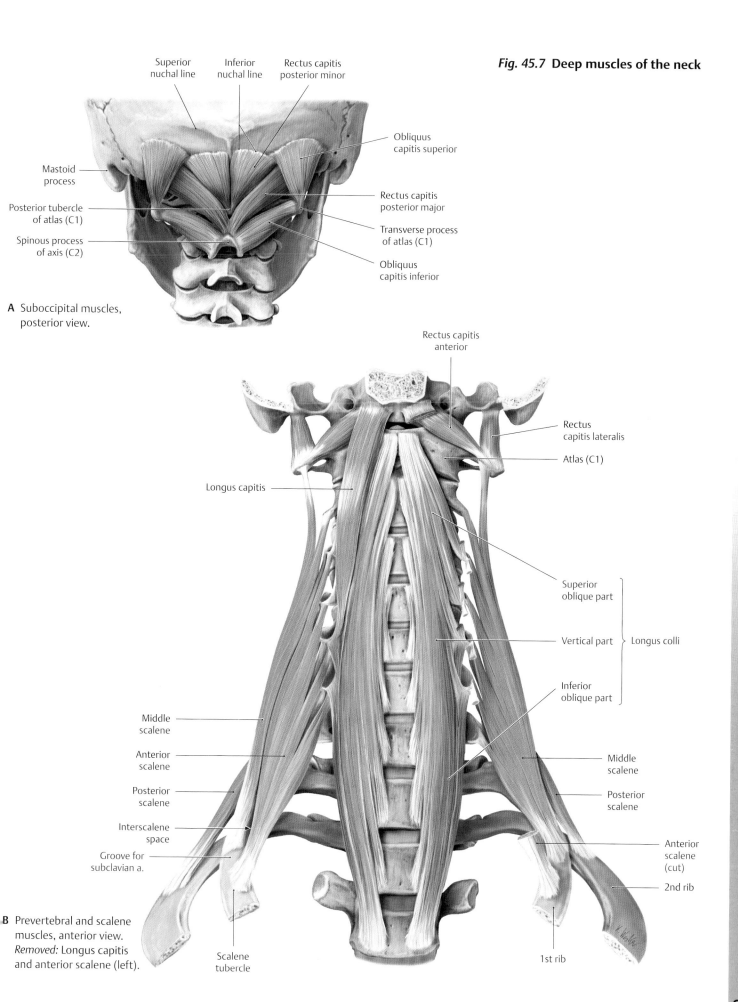

Fig. 45.7 **Deep muscles of the neck**

Superior nuchal line

Inferior nuchal line

Rectus capitis posterior minor

Obliquus capitis superior

Mastoid process

Posterior tubercle of atlas (C1)

Spinous process of axis (C2)

Rectus capitis posterior major

Transverse process of atlas (C1)

Obliquus capitis inferior

A Suboccipital muscles, posterior view.

Rectus capitis anterior

Rectus capitis lateralis

Atlas (C1)

Longus capitis

Superior oblique part

Vertical part

Inferior oblique part

⎫
⎬ Longus colli
⎭

Middle scalene

Anterior scalene

Posterior scalene

Interscalene space

Groove for subclavian a.

Middle scalene

Posterior scalene

Anterior scalene (cut)

2nd rib

B Prevertebral and scalene muscles, anterior view. *Removed:* Longus capitis and anterior scalene (left).

Scalene tubercle

1st rib

Arteries & Veins of the Neck

Fig. 45.8 Arteries of the neck

Left lateral view. The structures of the neck are primarily supplied by
the external carotid artery (anterior branches) and the subclavian artery
(vertebral artery, thyrocervical trunk, and costocervical trunk).

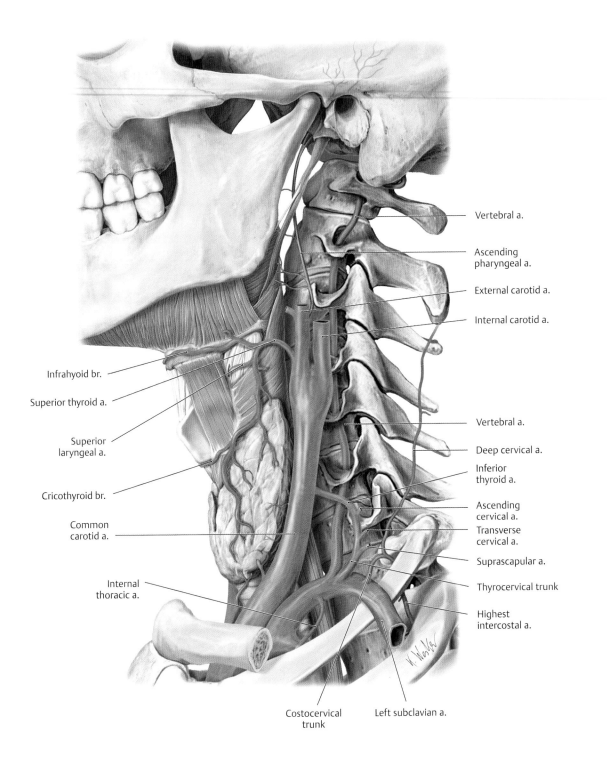

Vertebral a.

Ascending
pharyngeal a.

External carotid a.

Internal carotid a.

Infrahyoid br.

Superior thyroid a.

Superior
laryngeal a.

Vertebral a.

Deep cervical a.

Inferior
thyroid a.

Cricothyroid br.

Ascending
cervical a.

Transverse
cervical a.

Common
carotid a.

Suprascapular a.

Thyrocervical trunk

Internal
thoracic a.

Highest
intercostal a.

Costocervical
trunk

Left subclavian a.

Fig. 45.9 **Veins of the neck**

Left lateral view. The principal veins of the neck are the internal, external, and anterior jugular veins.

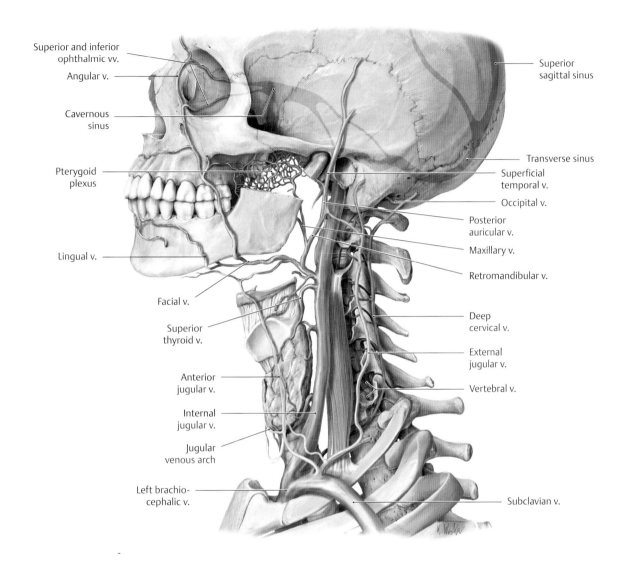

- Superior and inferior ophthalmic vv.
- Angular v.
- Cavernous sinus
- Pterygoid plexus
- Lingual v.
- Facial v.
- Superior thyroid v.
- Anterior jugular v.
- Internal jugular v.
- Jugular venous arch
- Left brachio-cephalic v.
- Superior sagittal sinus
- Transverse sinus
- Superficial temporal v.
- Occipital v.
- Posterior auricular v.
- Maxillary v.
- Retromandibular v.
- Deep cervical v.
- External jugular v.
- Vertebral v.
- Subclavian v.

 Clinical box 45.1

Impeded blood flow and veins of the neck

When clinical factors (e.g., chronic lung disease, mediastinal tumors, or infections) impede the flow of blood to the right heart, blood dams up in the superior vena cava and, consequently, the jugular veins (**A**). This causes conspicuous swelling in the jugular (and sometimes more minor) veins (**B**).

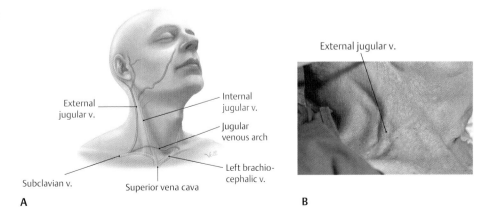

- External jugular v.
- Subclavian v.
- Superior vena cava
- Internal jugular v.
- Jugular venous arch
- Left brachio-cephalic v.
- External jugular v.

A

B

Lymphatics of the Neck

***Fig. 45.10* Lymphatic drainage regions**
Right lateral view.

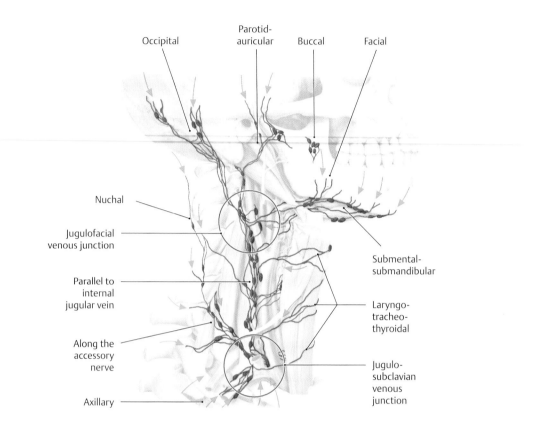

Tumor metastasis
Lymph from the entire body is channeled to the left and right jugulosubclavian junctions (red circles). Gastric carcinoma may metastasize to the left supraclavicular group of lymph nodes, producing an enlarged *sentinel node* (see **p. 77**). Systemic lymphomas may also spread to the cervical lymph nodes by this pathway.

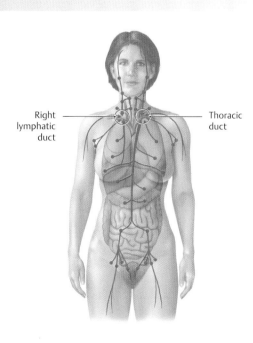

Fig. 45.11 Superficial cervical lymph nodes
Right lateral view.

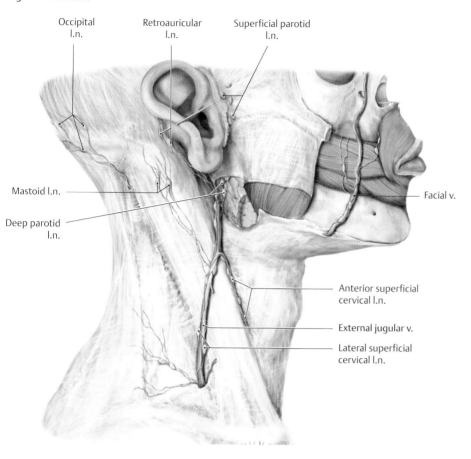

Occipital l.n. Retroauricular l.n. Superficial parotid l.n.

Mastoid l.n.

Deep parotid l.n.

Facial v.

Anterior superficial cervical l.n.

External jugular v.

Lateral superficial cervical l.n.

Table 45.6	Superficial cervical lymph nodes	
Lymph nodes (l.n.)	**Drainage region**	
Retroauricular l.n.	Occiput	
Occipital l.n.		
Mastoid l.n.		
Superficial parotid l.n.	Parotid-auricular region	
Deep parotid l.n.		
Anterior superficial cervical l.n.	Sternocleidomastoid region	
Lateral superficial cervical l.n.		

Fig. 45.12 Deep cervical lymph nodes
Right lateral view.

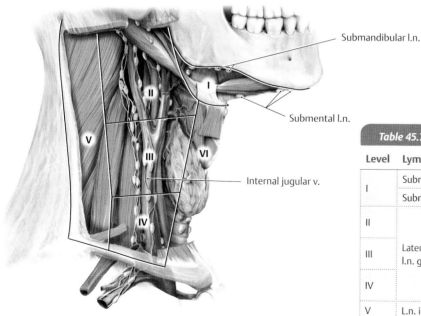

Submandibular l.n.

Submental l.n.

Internal jugular v.

Table 45.7	Deep cervical lymph nodes		
Level	**Lymph nodes (l.n.)**		**Drainage region**
I	Submental l.n.		Face
	Submandibular l.n.		
II	Lateral jugular l.n. group	Upper lateral group	Nuchal region, laryngo-tracheo-thyroidal region
III		Middle lateral group	
IV		Lower lateral group	
V	L.n. in posterior cervical triangle		Nuchal region
VI	Anterior cervical l.n.		Laryngo-tracheo-thyroidal region

Innervation of the Neck

Table 45.8   **Branches of the spinal nerves in the neck**

Posterior (dorsal) ramus

	Nerve	Sensory function	Motor function
C1	Suboccipital n.	No C1 dermatome	Innervate intrinsic nuchal muscles
C2	Greater occipital n.	Innervate C2 dermatome	
C3	3rd occipital n.	Innervate C3 dermatome	

Anterior (ventral) ramus

	Sensory branches	Sensory function	Motor branches	Motor function
C1	—	—	Form ansa cervicalis (motor part of cervical plexus)	Innervate infrahyoid muscles (except thyrohyoid)
C2	Lesser occipital n.	Form sensory part of cervical plexus, innervate anterior and lateral neck		
C2–C3	Great auricular n.			
	Transverse cervical n.			
C3–C4	Supraclavicular nn.		Contribute to phrenic n.*	Innervate diaphragm and pericardium*

* The anterior roots of C3–C5 combine to form the phrenic nerve (see **p. 66**).

Branching of the cervical plexus.

Fig. 45.13 Sensory innervation of the nuchal region
Posterior view.

A Dermatomes.

B Cutaneous nerve territories.

C Spinal nerve branches.

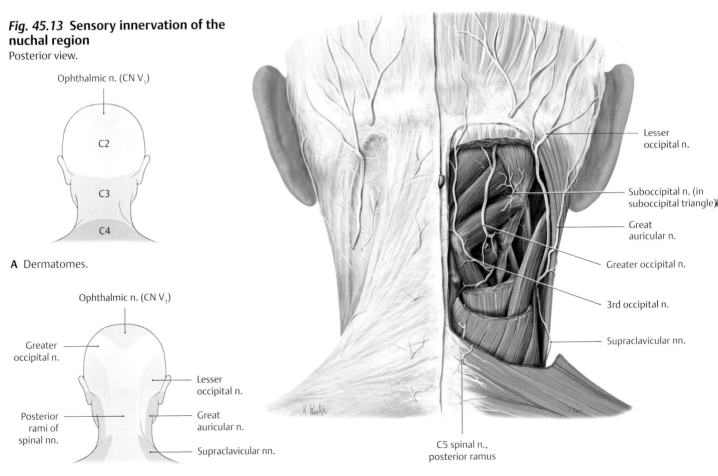

Fig. 45.14 Sensory innervation of the anterolateral neck
Left lateral view.

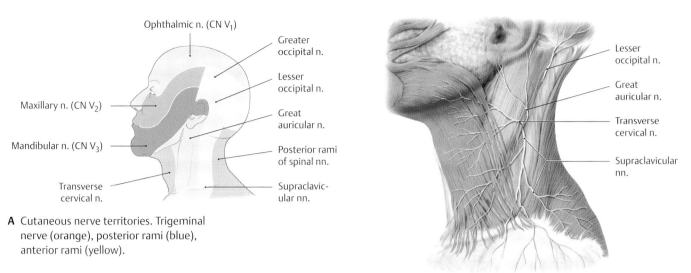

A Cutaneous nerve territories. Trigeminal nerve (orange), posterior rami (blue), anterior rami (yellow).

Ophthalmic n. (CN V₁)

Maxillary n. (CN V₂)

Mandibular n. (CN V₃)

Transverse cervical n.

Greater occipital n.

Lesser occipital n.

Great auricular n.

Posterior rami of spinal nn.

Supraclavicular nn.

Lesser occipital n.

Great auricular n.

Transverse cervical n.

Supraclavicular nn.

B Sensory branches of the cervical plexus.

Fig. 45.15 Motor innervation of the anterolateral neck
Left lateral view.

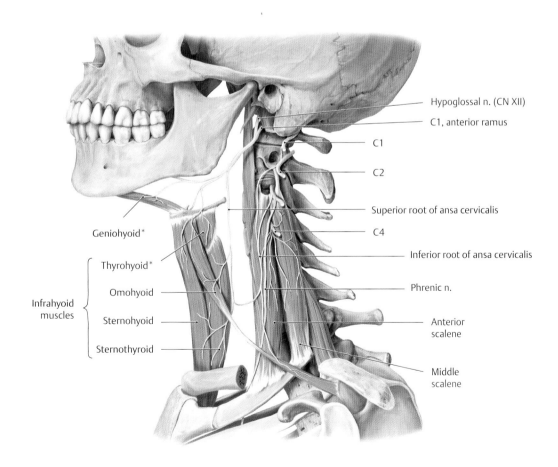

Geniohyoid*

Thyrohyoid*

Omohyoid

Sternohyoid

Sternothyroid

Infrahyoid muscles

Hypoglossal n. (CN XII)

C1, anterior ramus

C1

C2

Superior root of ansa cervicalis

C4

Inferior root of ansa cervicalis

Phrenic n.

Anterior scalene

Middle scalene

* Innervated by the anterior ramus of C1 (distributed by the hypoglossal n.).

Larynx: Cartilage & Structure

Fig. 45.16 Laryngeal cartilages

Left lateral view. The larynx consists of five laryngeal cartilages: epiglottic, thyroid, cricoid, and the paired arytenoid and corniculate cartilages. They are connected to each other, the trachea, and the hyoid bone by elastic ligaments.

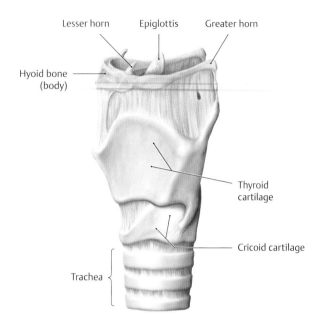

Lesser horn | Epiglottis | Greater horn

Hyoid bone (body)

Thyroid cartilage

Cricoid cartilage

Trachea

Fig. 45.17 Epiglottic cartilage

The elastic epiglottic cartilage comprises the internal skeleton of the epiglottis, providing resilience to return it to its initial position after swallowing.

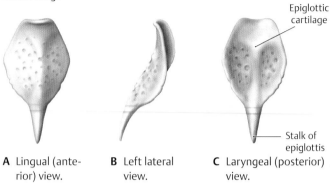

Epiglottic cartilage

Stalk of epiglottis

A Lingual (anterior) view. **B** Left lateral view. **C** Laryngeal (posterior) view.

Fig. 45.18 Thyroid cartilage

Left oblique view.

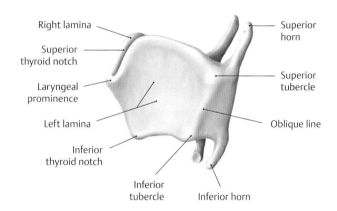

Right lamina | Superior horn

Superior thyroid notch

Laryngeal prominence | Superior tubercle

Left lamina | Oblique line

Inferior thyroid notch

Inferior tubercle | Inferior horn

Fig. 45.19 Cricoid cartilage

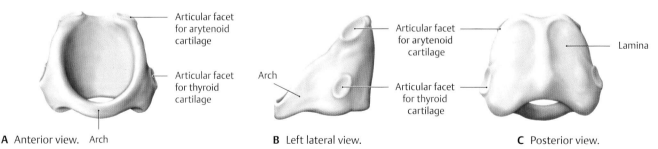

Articular facet for arytenoid cartilage

Articular facet for thyroid cartilage

Articular facet for arytenoid cartilage

Arch

Articular facet for thyroid cartilage

Lamina

A Anterior view. Arch

B Left lateral view.

C Posterior view.

Fig. 45.20 Arytenoid and corniculate cartilages

Right cartilages.

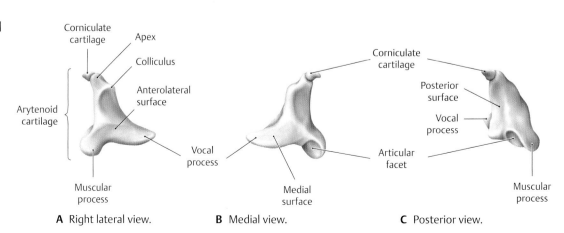

Corniculate cartilage | Apex

Colliculus

Anterolateral surface

Arytenoid cartilage

Vocal process

Muscular process

Corniculate cartilage

Posterior surface

Vocal process

Articular facet

Medial surface

Muscular process

A Right lateral view. **B** Medial view. **C** Posterior view.

Fig. 45.21 **Structure of the larynx**

The larynx is suspended from the hyoid bone, primarily by the thyro-hyoid membrane. The hyoid bone provides the sites for attachment of the suprahyoid and infrahyoid muscles.

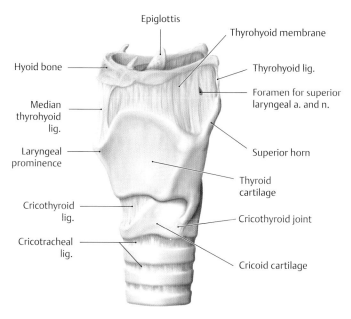

A Left anterior oblique view.

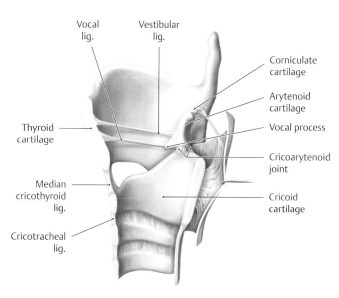

B Sagittal section, viewed from the left medial aspect. The arytenoid cartilage alters the position of the vocal folds during phonation.

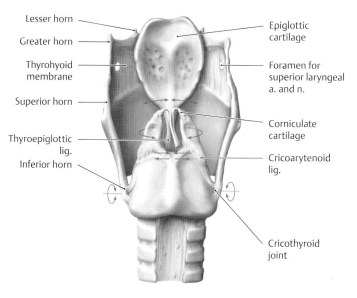

C Posterior view. Arrows indicate the directions of movement in the various joints.

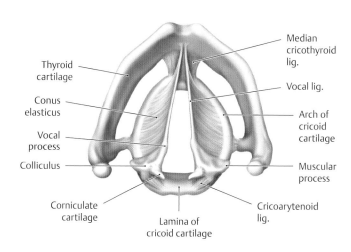

D Superior view.

Larynx: Muscles & Levels

Fig. 45.22 Laryngeal muscles

The laryngeal muscles move the laryngeal cartilages relative to one another, affecting the tension and/or position of the vocal folds. Muscles that move the larynx as a whole (infra- and suprahyoid muscles) are described on **p. 620**.

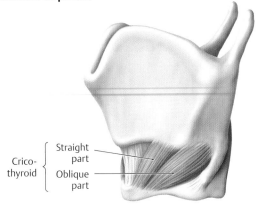

A Intrinsic laryngeal muscles, left lateral oblique view.

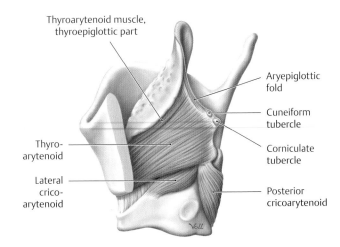

B Intrinsic laryngeal muscles, left lateral view. *Removed:* Thyroid cartilage (left half). *Revealed:* Epiglottis and external thyroarytenoid muscle.

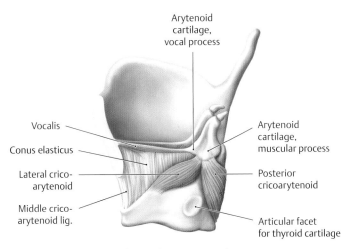

C Left lateral view with the epiglottis removed.

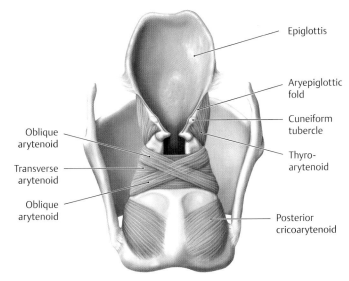

D Posterior view.

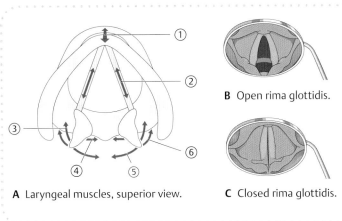

A Laryngeal muscles, superior view.

B Open rima glottidis.

C Closed rima glottidis.

Table 45.9	Actions of the laryngeal muscles	
Muscle	**Action**	**Effect on rima glottidis**
① Cricothyroid m.*	Tightens the vocal folds	None
② Vocalis m.		
③ Thyroarytenoid m.	Adducts the vocal folds	Closes
④ Transverse arytenoid m.		
⑤ Posterior cricoarytenoid m.	Abducts the vocal folds	Opens
⑥ Lateral cricoarytenoid m.	Adducts the vocal folds	Closes

* The cricothyroid is innervated by the external laryngeal n. All other intrinsic laryngeal mm. are innervated by the recurrent laryngeal n.

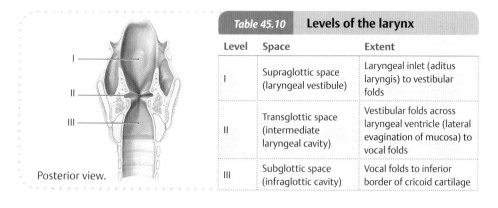

Table 45.10	Levels of the larynx	
Level	Space	Extent
I	Supraglottic space (laryngeal vestibule)	Laryngeal inlet (aditus laryngis) to vestibular folds
II	Transglottic space (intermediate laryngeal cavity)	Vestibular folds across laryngeal ventricle (lateral evagination of mucosa) to vocal folds
III	Subglottic space (infraglottic cavity)	Vocal folds to inferior border of cricoid cartilage

Posterior view.

Fig. 45.23 **Cavity of the larynx**

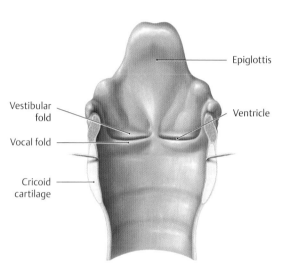

A Posterior view with the larynx splayed open.

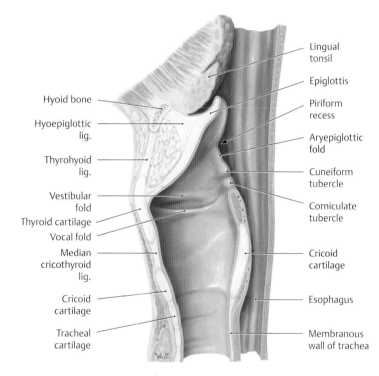

B Midsagittal section viewed from the left side.

Fig. 45.24 **Vestibular and vocal folds**
Coronal section, superior view.

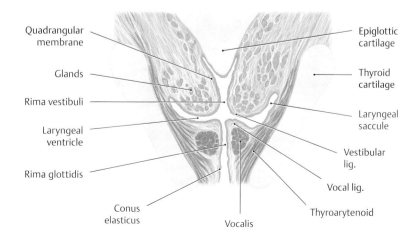

Neurovasculature of the Larynx, Thyroid & Parathyroids

Fig. 45.25 **Thyroid and parathyroid glands**

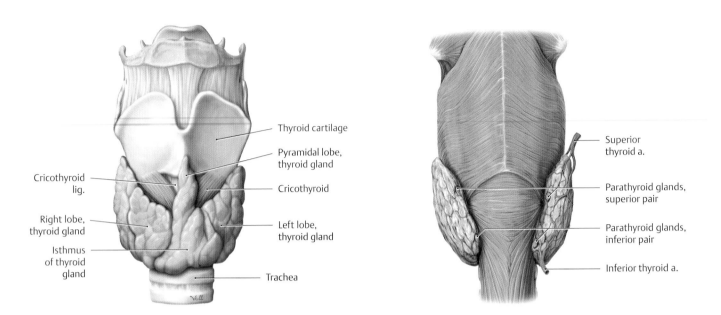

A Thyroid gland, anterior view.

Thyroid cartilage

Pyramidal lobe, thyroid gland

Cricothyroid

Left lobe, thyroid gland

Trachea

Cricothyroid lig.

Right lobe, thyroid gland

Isthmus of thyroid gland

B Thyroid and parathyroid glands, posterior view.

Superior thyroid a.

Parathyroid glands, superior pair

Parathyroid glands, inferior pair

Inferior thyroid a.

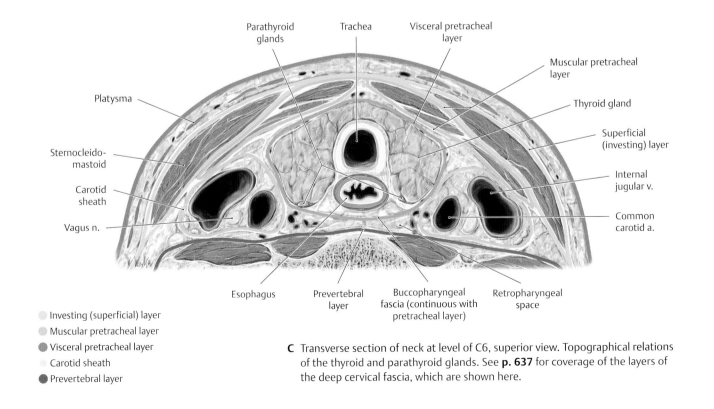

Parathyroid glands

Trachea

Visceral pretracheal layer

Muscular pretracheal layer

Thyroid gland

Superficial (investing) layer

Internal jugular v.

Common carotid a.

Platysma

Sternocleido-mastoid

Carotid sheath

Vagus n.

Esophagus

Prevertebral layer

Buccopharyngeal fascia (continuous with pretracheal layer)

Retropharyngeal space

- Investing (superficial) layer
- Muscular pretracheal layer
- Visceral pretracheal layer
- Carotid sheath
- Prevertebral layer

C Transverse section of neck at level of C6, superior view. Topographical relations of the thyroid and parathyroid glands. See **p. 637** for coverage of the layers of the deep cervical fascia, which are shown here.

Fig. 45.26 Arteries and nerves of the larynx

Anterior view. *Removed:* Thyroid gland (right half).

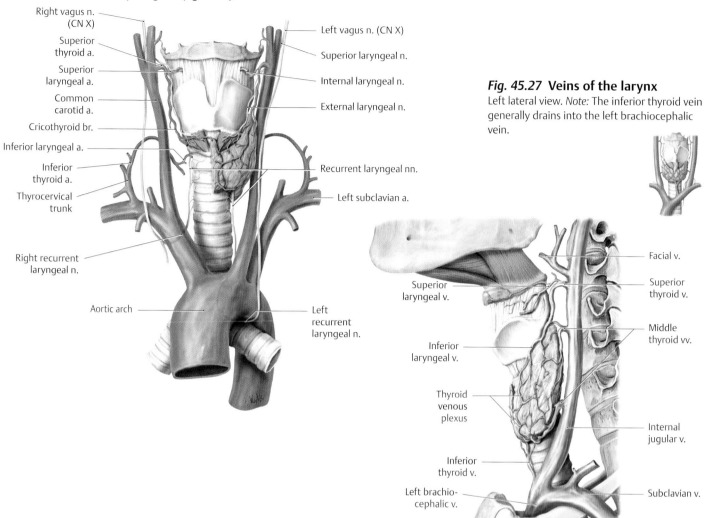

Right vagus n. (CN X)
Superior thyroid a.
Superior laryngeal a.
Common carotid a.
Cricothyroid br.
Inferior laryngeal a.
Inferior thyroid a.
Thyrocervical trunk
Right recurrent laryngeal n.
Aortic arch

Left vagus n. (CN X)
Superior laryngeal n.
Internal laryngeal n.
External laryngeal n.
Recurrent laryngeal nn.
Left subclavian a.
Left recurrent laryngeal n.

Fig. 45.27 Veins of the larynx

Left lateral view. *Note:* The inferior thyroid vein generally drains into the left brachiocephalic vein.

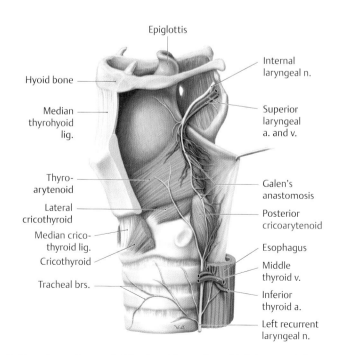

Superior laryngeal v.
Inferior laryngeal v.
Thyroid venous plexus
Inferior thyroid v.
Left brachiocephalic v.

Facial v.
Superior thyroid v.
Middle thyroid vv.
Internal jugular v.
Subclavian v.

Fig. 45.28 Neurovasculature of the larynx

Left lateral view.

Hyoid bone
Thyrohyoid membrane
Thyrohyoid
Median cricothyroid lig.
Cricothyroid
Thyroid gland

Superior laryngeal n.
Internal laryngeal n.
Superior laryngeal a. and v.
Inferior pharyngeal constrictor
External laryngeal n.
Middle thyroid v.
Inferior thyroid a.
Esophagus

Left recurrent laryngeal n.

A Superficial layer.

Epiglottis

Hyoid bone
Median thyrohyoid lig.
Thyro-arytenoid
Lateral cricothyroid
Median cricothyroid lig.
Cricothyroid
Tracheal brs.

Internal laryngeal n.
Superior laryngeal a. and v.
Galen's anastomosis
Posterior cricoarytenoid
Esophagus
Middle thyroid v.
Inferior thyroid a.
Left recurrent laryngeal n.

B Deep layer. *Removed:* Cricothyroid muscle and left lamina of thyroid cartilage. *Retracted:* Pharyngeal mucosa.

Topography of the Neck: Regions & Fascia

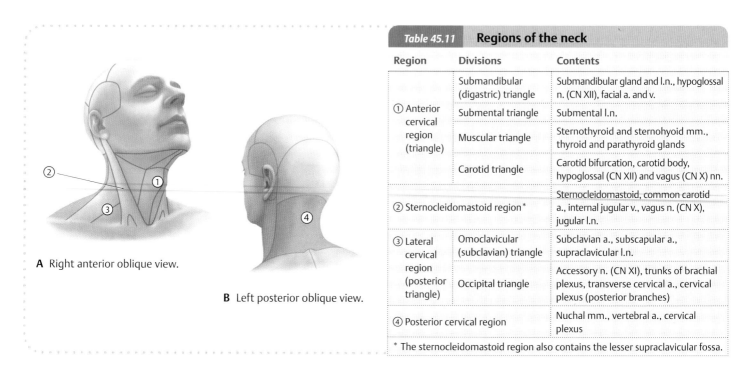

A Right anterior oblique view.

B Left posterior oblique view.

Table 45.11	Regions of the neck	
Region	**Divisions**	**Contents**
① Anterior cervical region (triangle)	Submandibular (digastric) triangle	Submandibular gland and l.n., hypoglossal n. (CN XII), facial a. and v.
	Submental triangle	Submental l.n.
	Muscular triangle	Sternothyroid and sternohyoid mm., thyroid and parathyroid glands
	Carotid triangle	Carotid bifurcation, carotid body, hypoglossal (CN XII) and vagus (CN X) nn.
② Sternocleidomastoid region*		Sternocleidomastoid, common carotid a., internal jugular v., vagus n. (CN X), jugular l.n.
③ Lateral cervical region (posterior triangle)	Omoclavicular (subclavian) triangle	Subclavian a., subscapular a., supraclavicular l.n.
	Occipital triangle	Accessory n. (CN XI), trunks of brachial plexus, transverse cervical a., cervical plexus (posterior branches)
④ Posterior cervical region		Nuchal mm., vertebral a., cervical plexus

* The sternocleidomastoid region also contains the lesser supraclavicular fossa.

Fig. 45.29 **Cervical regions**

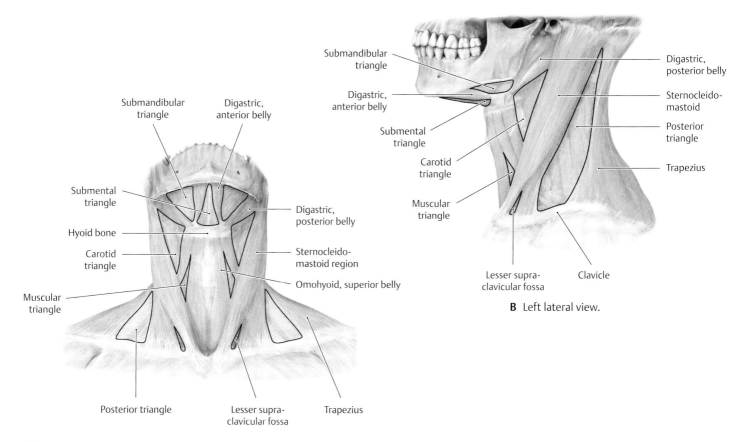

A Anterior view.

B Left lateral view.

Table 45.12   **Deep cervical fascia**

The deep cervical fascia is divided into four layers that enclose the structures of the neck.

Layer	Type of fascia	Description
① Investing (superficial) layer	Muscular	Envelopes entire neck; splits to enclose sternocleidomastoid and trapezius muscles
Pretracheal layer	② Muscular	Encloses infrahyoid muscles
	③ Visceral	Surrounds thyroid gland, larynx, trachea, pharynx, and esophagus
④ Prevertebral layer	Muscular	Surrounds cervical vertebral column and associated muscles
⑤ Carotid sheath	Neurovascular	Encloses common carotid artery, internal jugular vein, and vagus nerve

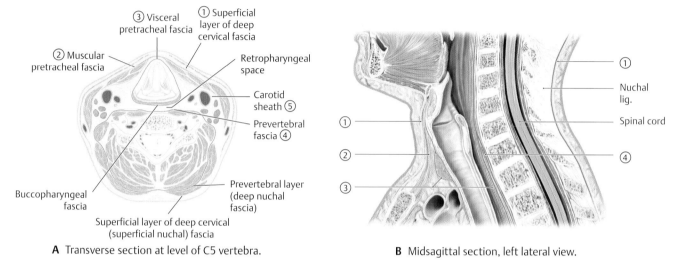

A Transverse section at level of C5 vertebra.

B Midsagittal section, left lateral view.

Fig. 45.30 Deep cervical fascial layers

Anterior view.

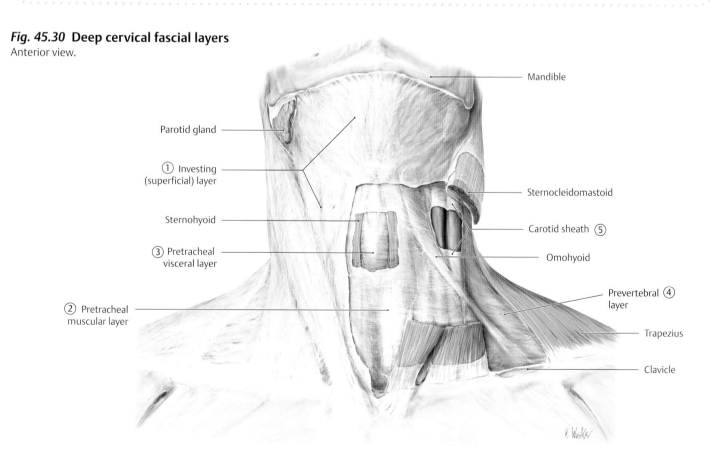

Topography of the Anterior Cervical Region

***Fig. 45.31* Anterior cervical triangle**
Anterior view.

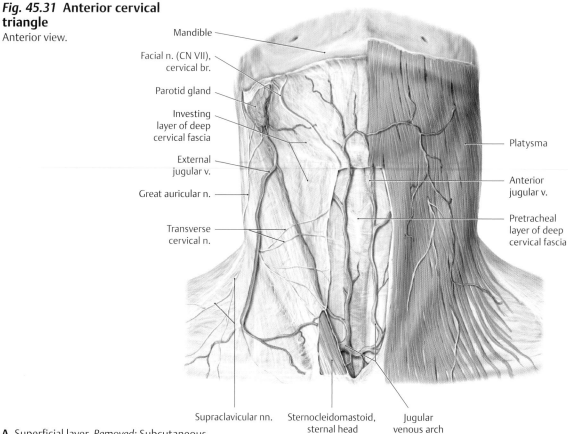

Mandible

Facial n. (CN VII), cervical br.

Parotid gland

Investing layer of deep cervical fascia

External jugular v.

Great auricular n.

Transverse cervical n.

Platysma

Anterior jugular v.

Pretracheal layer of deep cervical fascia

Supraclavicular nn.

Sternocleidomastoid, sternal head

Jugular venous arch

A Superficial layer. *Removed:* Subcutaneous platysma (right side) and investing layer of deep cervical fascia (center).

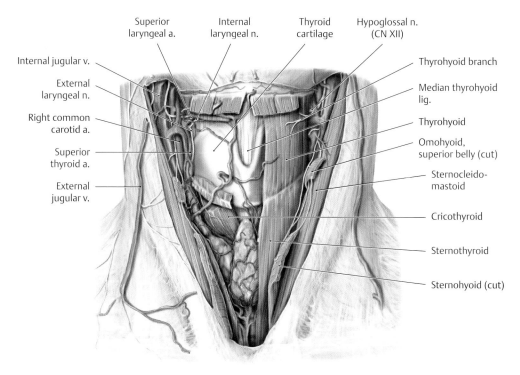

Superior laryngeal a.

Internal laryngeal n.

Thyroid cartilage

Hypoglossal n. (CN XII)

Internal jugular v.

External laryngeal n.

Right common carotid a.

Superior thyroid a.

External jugular v.

Thyrohyoid branch

Median thyrohyoid lig.

Thyrohyoid

Omohyoid, superior belly (cut)

Sternocleido-mastoid

Cricothyroid

Sternothyroid

Sternohyoid (cut)

B Deep layer. *Removed:* Pretracheal lamina (middle layer of cervical fascia). *Cuts:* Sternohyoid, sternothyroid, and thyrohyoid (right side); sternohyoid (left side).

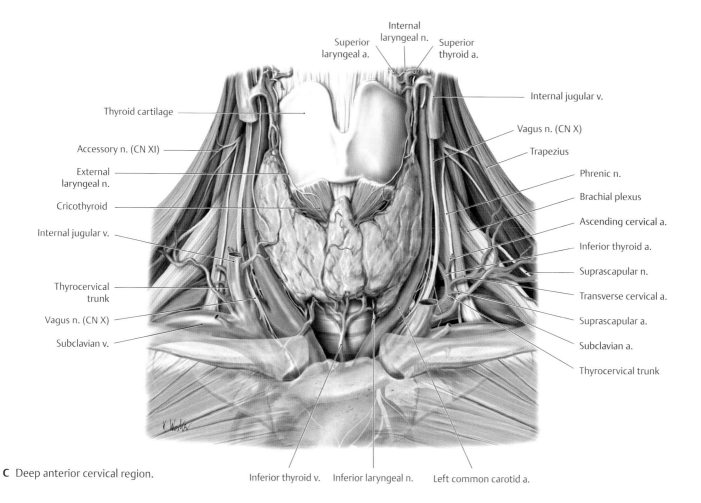

Superior laryngeal a.

Internal laryngeal n.

Superior thyroid a.

Thyroid cartilage

Internal jugular v.

Accessory n. (CN XI)

Vagus n. (CN X)

External laryngeal n.

Trapezius

Cricothyroid

Phrenic n.

Internal jugular v.

Brachial plexus

Ascending cervical a.

Inferior thyroid a.

Thyrocervical trunk

Suprascapular n.

Vagus n. (CN X)

Transverse cervical a.

Subclavian v.

Suprascapular a.

Subclavian a.

Thyrocervical trunk

C Deep anterior cervical region.

Inferior thyroid v.   Inferior laryngeal n.   Left common carotid a.

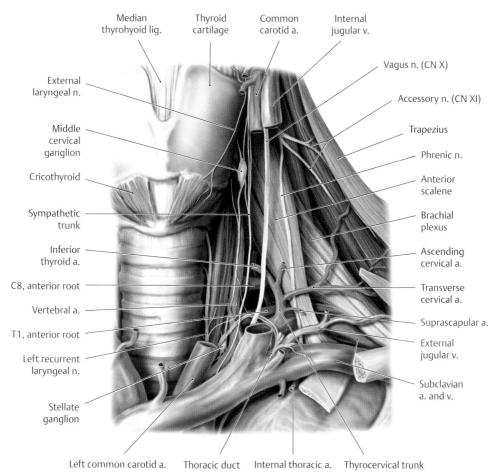

Median thyrohyoid lig.

Thyroid cartilage

Common carotid a.

Internal jugular v.

External laryngeal n.

Vagus n. (CN X)

Accessory n. (CN XI)

Middle cervical ganglion

Trapezius

Cricothyroid

Phrenic n.

Sympathetic trunk

Anterior scalene

Inferior thyroid a.

Brachial plexus

C8, anterior root

Ascending cervical a.

Vertebral a.

Transverse cervical a.

T1, anterior root

Suprascapular a.

Left recurrent laryngeal n.

External jugular v.

Stellate ganglion

Subclavian a. and v.

D Root of the neck.

Left common carotid a.   Thoracic duct   Internal thoracic a.   Thyrocervical trunk

Topography of the Anterior & Lateral Cervical Regions

Fig. 45.32 Deep anterior cervical region
The deep midline viscera of the anterior cervical region are the larynx and thyroid gland. The two lateral neurovascular pathways primarily supply these organs.

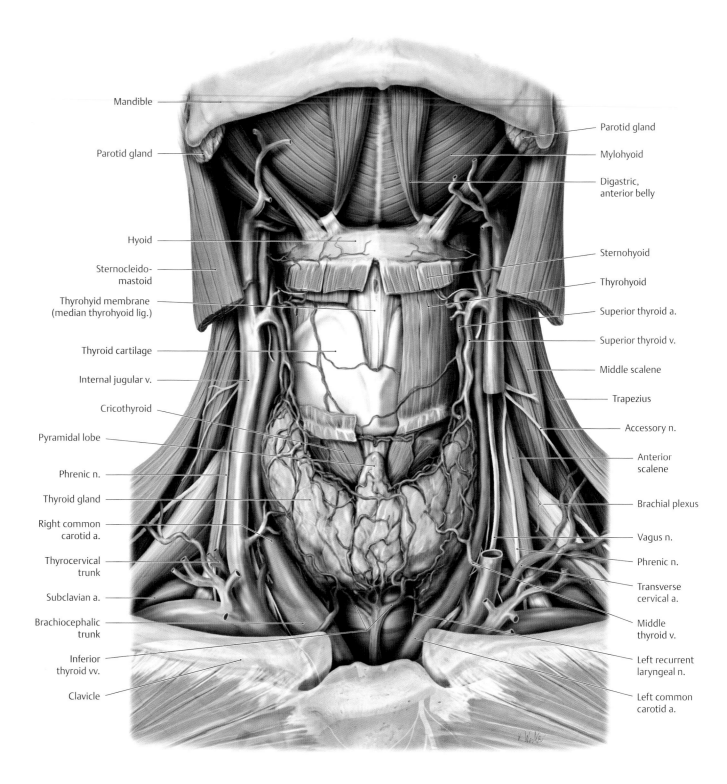

Mandible

Parotid gland

Hyoid

Sternocleido-mastoid

Thyrohyid membrane (median thyrohyoid lig.)

Thyroid cartilage

Internal jugular v.

Cricothyroid

Pyramidal lobe

Phrenic n.

Thyroid gland

Right common carotid a.

Thyrocervical trunk

Subclavian a.

Brachiocephalic trunk

Inferior thyroid vv.

Clavicle

Parotid gland

Mylohyoid

Digastric, anterior belly

Sternohyoid

Thyrohyoid

Superior thyroid a.

Superior thyroid v.

Middle scalene

Trapezius

Accessory n.

Anterior scalene

Brachial plexus

Vagus n.

Phrenic n.

Transverse cervical a.

Middle thyroid v.

Left recurrent laryngeal n.

Left common carotid a.

Fig. 45.33 **Carotid triangle**
Right lateral view.

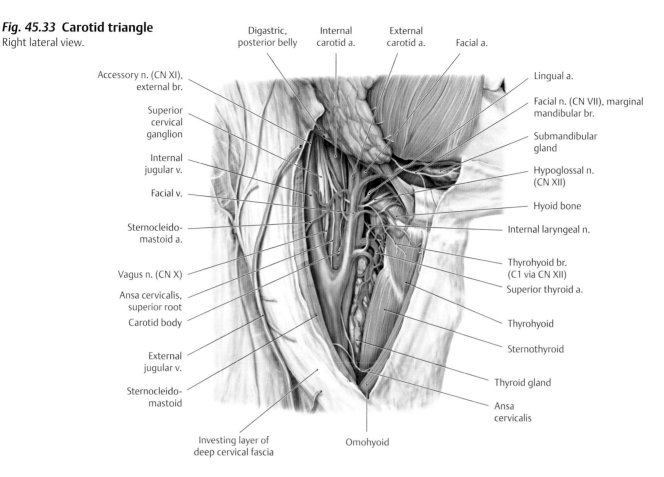

Digastric, posterior belly
Internal carotid a.
External carotid a.
Facial a.

Accessory n. (CN XI), external br.
Superior cervical ganglion
Internal jugular v.
Facial v.
Sternocleido-mastoid a.
Vagus n. (CN X)
Ansa cervicalis, superior root
Carotid body
External jugular v.
Sternocleido-mastoid

Lingual a.
Facial n. (CN VII), marginal mandibular br.
Submandibular gland
Hypoglossal n. (CN XII)
Hyoid bone
Internal laryngeal n.
Thyrohyoid br. (C1 via CN XII)
Superior thyroid a.
Thyrohyoid
Sternothyroid
Thyroid gland
Ansa cervicalis

Investing layer of deep cervical fascia
Omohyoid

Fig. 45.34 **Deep lateral cervical region**
Right lateral view with sternocleidomastoid windowed.

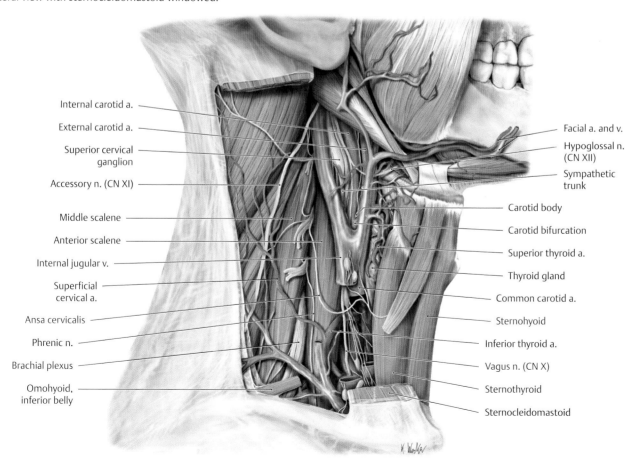

Internal carotid a.
External carotid a.
Superior cervical ganglion
Accessory n. (CN XI)
Middle scalene
Anterior scalene
Internal jugular v.
Superficial cervical a.
Ansa cervicalis
Phrenic n.
Brachial plexus
Omohyoid, inferior belly

Facial a. and v.
Hypoglossal n. (CN XII)
Sympathetic trunk
Carotid body
Carotid bifurcation
Superior thyroid a.
Thyroid gland
Common carotid a.
Sternohyoid
Inferior thyroid a.
Vagus n. (CN X)
Sternothyroid
Sternocleidomastoid

Topography of the Lateral Cervical Region

***Fig. 45.35* Lateral cervical region**
Right lateral view. The contents of the deep lateral cervical region are found in **Fig. 45.34.**

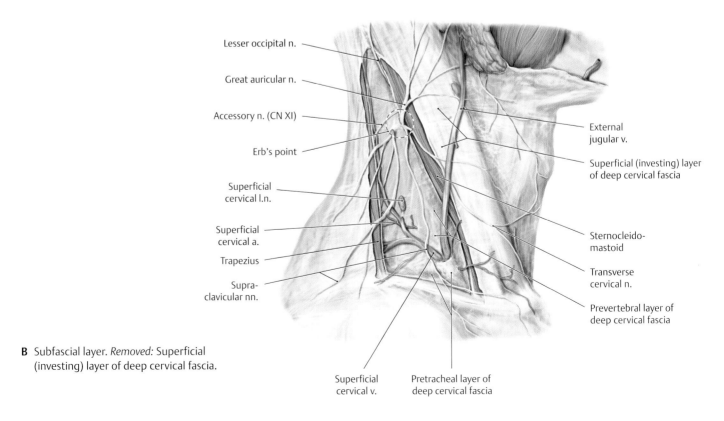

A Subcutaneous layer.

Labels for panel A:
- Parotid gland
- Facial n. (CN VII), cervical br.
- Masseter
- Lesser occipital n.
- Great auricular n.
- Erb's point
- Lateral supra-clavicular nn.
- Trapezius, anterior border
- External jugular v.
- Sternocleido-mastoid, posterior border
- Transverse cervical and CN VII anastomosis
- Superficial (investing) layer of deep cervical fascia
- Transverse cervical n.
- Clavicle
- Intermediate supra-clavicular nn.
- Medial supra-clavicular nn.

B Subfascial layer. *Removed:* Superficial (investing) layer of deep cervical fascia.

Labels for panel B:
- Lesser occipital n.
- Great auricular n.
- Accessory n. (CN XI)
- Erb's point
- Superficial cervical l.n.
- Superficial cervical a.
- Trapezius
- Supra-clavicular nn.
- External jugular v.
- Superficial (investing) layer of deep cervical fascia
- Sternocleido-mastoid
- Transverse cervical n.
- Prevertebral layer of deep cervical fascia
- Superficial cervical v.
- Pretracheal layer of deep cervical fascia

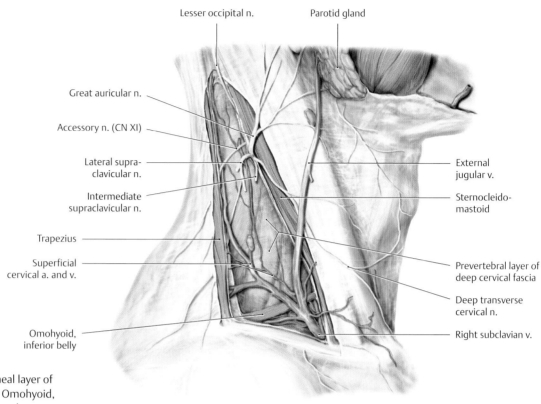

Lesser occipital n.

Parotid gland

Great auricular n.

Accessory n. (CN XI)

Lateral supra-
clavicular n.

Intermediate
supraclavicular n.

Trapezius

Superficial
cervical a. and v.

Omohyoid,
inferior belly

External
jugular v.

Sternocleido-
mastoid

Prevertebral layer of
deep cervical fascia

Deep transverse
cervical n.

Right subclavian v.

C Deep layer. *Removed:* Pretracheal layer of
deep cervical fascia. *Revealed:* Omohyoid,
omoclavicular (subclavian) triangle.

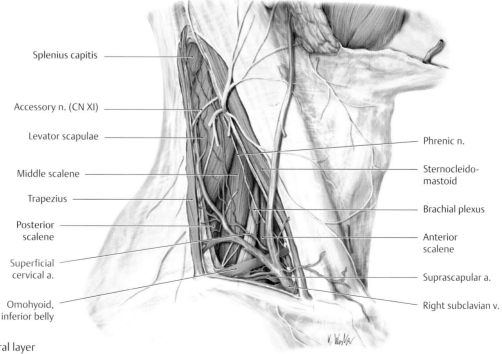

Splenius capitis

Accessory n. (CN XI)

Levator scapulae

Middle scalene

Trapezius

Posterior
scalene

Superficial
cervical a.

Omohyoid,
inferior belly

Phrenic n.

Sternocleido-
mastoid

Brachial plexus

Anterior
scalene

Suprascapular a.

Right subclavian v.

D Deepest layer. *Removed:* Prevertebral layer
of deep cervical fascia. *Revealed:* Muscular
floor of posterior triangle, brachial plexus,
and phrenic nerve.

643

Topography of the Posterior Cervical Region

Fig. 45.36 Occipital and posterior cervical regions

Posterior view. Subcutaneous layer (left), subfascial layer (right). The occiput is technically a region of the head, but it is included here due to the continuity of the vessels and nerves from the neck. *Removed on right side:* Investing layer of deep cervical fascia.

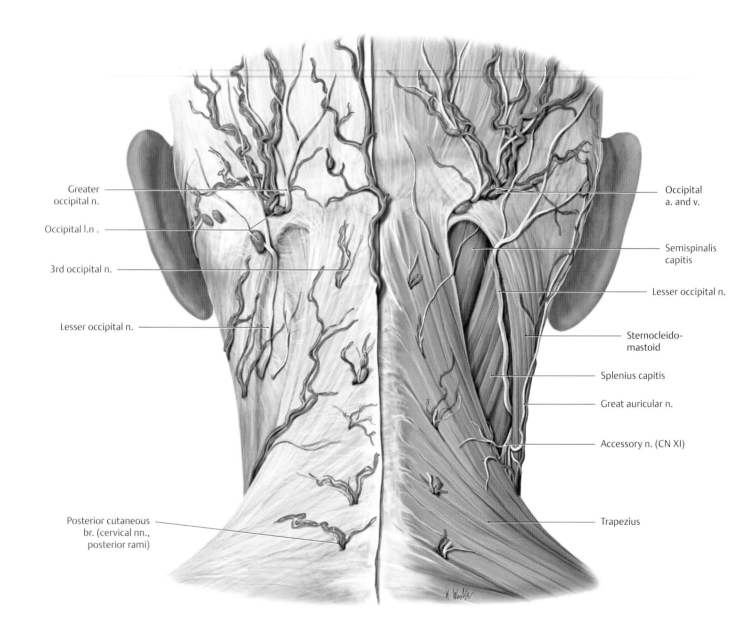

Greater occipital n.

Occipital l.n .

3rd occipital n.

Lesser occipital n.

Posterior cutaneous br. (cervical nn., posterior rami)

Occipital a. and v.

Semispinalis capitis

Lesser occipital n.

Sternocleido- mastoid

Splenius capitis

Great auricular n.

Accessory n. (CN XI)

Trapezius

Fig. 45.37 Suboccipital triangle

Right side, posterior view, windowed. The suboccipital triangle is bounded by the suboccipital muscles (rectus capitis posterior major and obliquus capitis superior and inferior) and contains the vertebral artery. The left and right vertebral arteries pass through the atlanto-occipital membrane and combine to form the basilar artery.

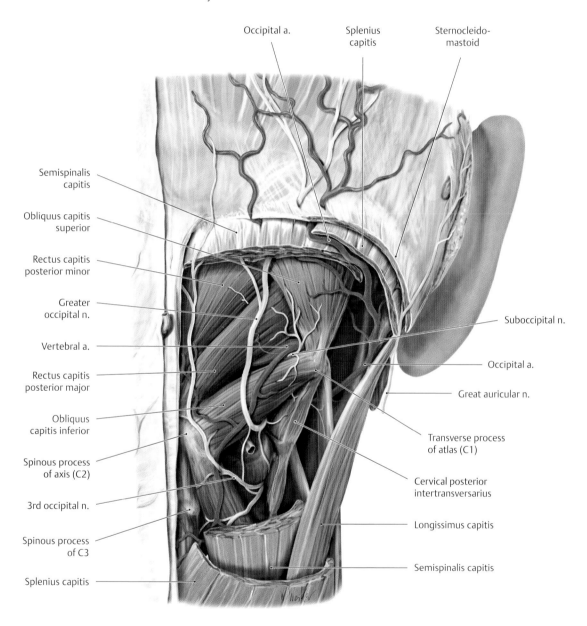

Occipital a.

Splenius capitis

Sternocleido-mastoid

Semispinalis capitis

Obliquus capitis superior

Rectus capitis posterior minor

Greater occipital n.

Vertebral a.

Rectus capitis posterior major

Obliquus capitis inferior

Spinous process of axis (C2)

3rd occipital n.

Spinous process of C3

Splenius capitis

Suboccipital n.

Occipital a.

Great auricular n.

Transverse process of atlas (C1)

Cervical posterior intertransversarius

Longissimus capitis

Semispinalis capitis

Sectional Anatomy of the Head & Neck (I)

Fig. 46.1 Coronal section through the anterior orbital margin

Anterior view. This section shows four regions of the head: the oral cavity, the nasal cavity and sinuses, the orbit, and the anterior cranial fossa. Muscles of the oral floor, the apex of the tongue, the hard palate, the neurovascular structures in the mandibular canal, and the first molar are all seen in the region of the oral cavity. This section reinforces the clinical implications of the relationship of the maxillary sinus with the maxillary teeth and the floor of the orbit and with the maxillary nerve in the infraorbital groove. The medial wall of the orbit shares a thin bony wall (orbital plate) with the ethmoid air cells (sinus). The section is enough anterior so that the lateral bony walls of the orbit are not included due to the lateral curvature of the skull.

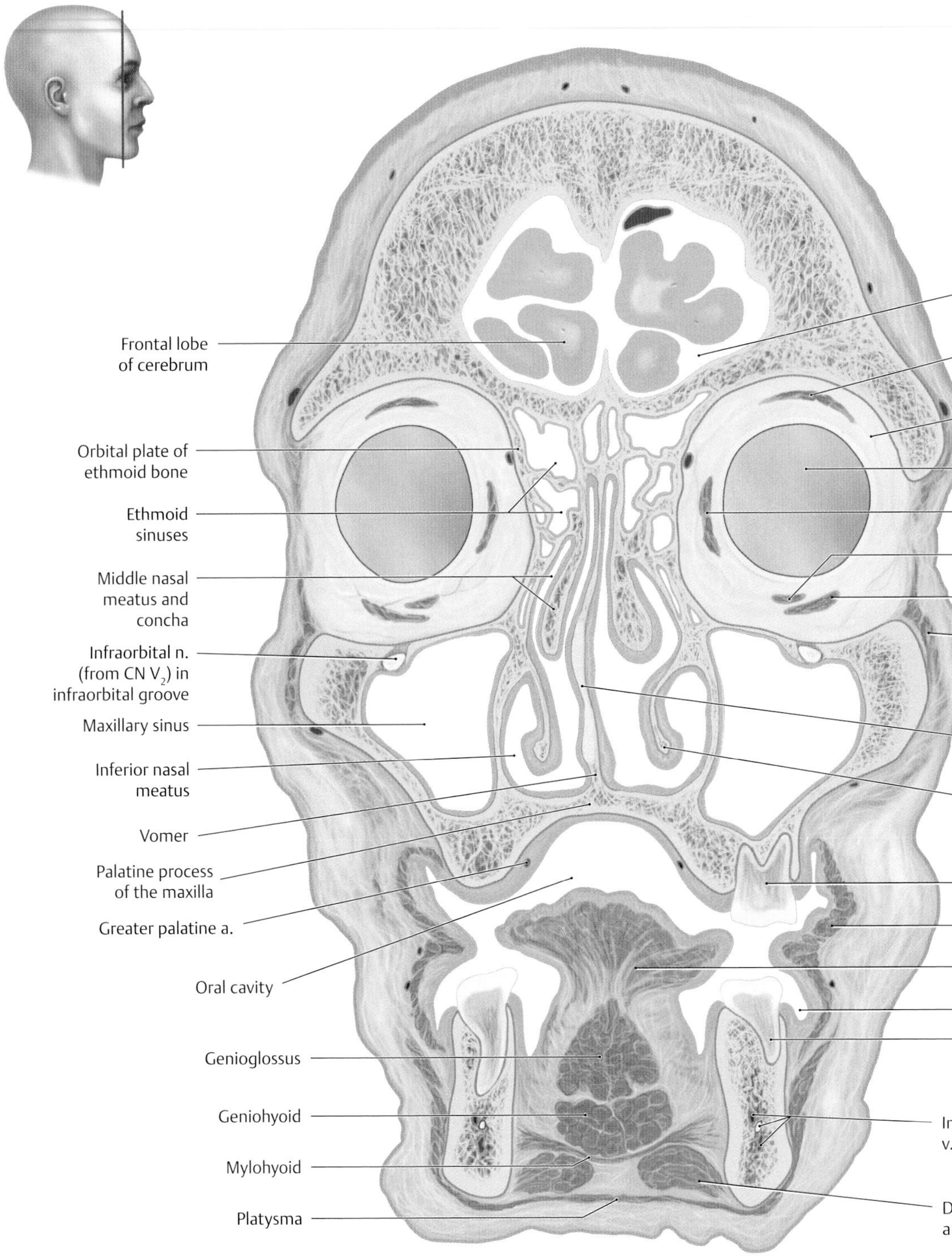

Frontal lobe of cerebrum
Orbital plate of ethmoid bone
Ethmoid sinuses
Middle nasal meatus and concha
Infraorbital n. (from CN V_2) in infraorbital groove
Maxillary sinus
Inferior nasal meatus
Vomer
Palatine process of the maxilla
Greater palatine a.
Oral cavity
Genioglossus
Geniohyoid
Mylohyoid
Platysma
Anterior cranial fossa
Levator palpebrae superioris
Periorbital fat
Vitreous body
Medial rectus
Inferior rectus
Inferior oblique
Orbicularis oculi
Cartilaginous nasal septum
Inferior nasal concha
First upper molar
Buccinator
Tongue
Oral vestibule
First lower molar
Inferior alveolar a., n., and v. in mandibular canal
Digastric, anterior belly

Fig. 46.2 Coronal section through the orbital apex

Anterior view. In this more posterior section than that of **Fig. 46.1**, the soft palate now separates the oral and nasal cavities. The buccal fat pad is also visible. The section is slightly angled, producing an apparent discontinuity in the mandibular ramus on the left side.

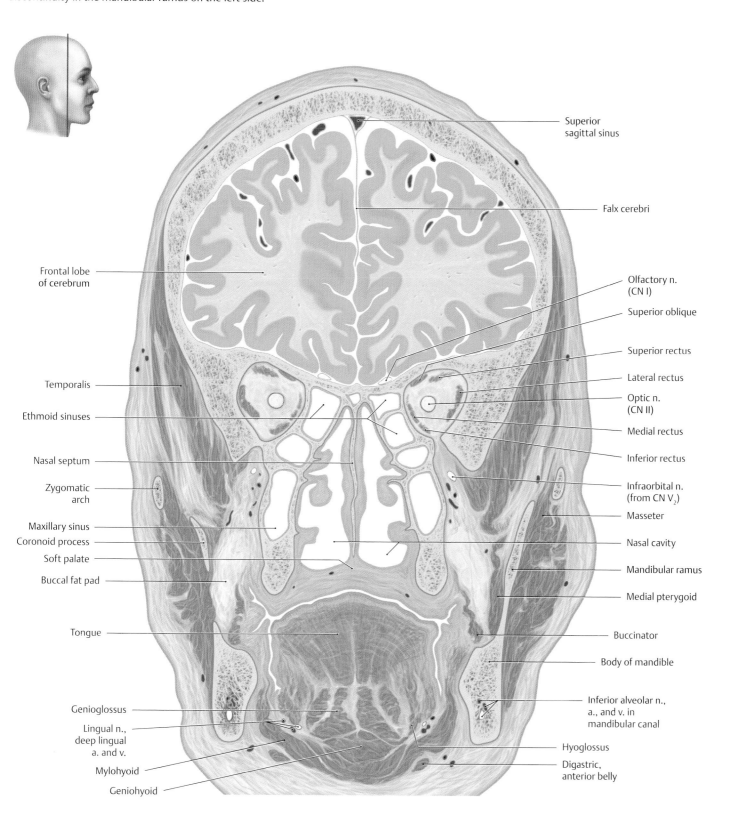

Superior sagittal sinus

Falx cerebri

Frontal lobe of cerebrum

Olfactory n. (CN I)

Superior oblique

Superior rectus

Lateral rectus

Temporalis

Optic n. (CN II)

Ethmoid sinuses

Medial rectus

Inferior rectus

Nasal septum

Infraorbital n. (from CN V$_2$)

Zygomatic arch

Masseter

Maxillary sinus

Nasal cavity

Coronoid process

Soft palate

Mandibular ramus

Buccal fat pad

Medial pterygoid

Tongue

Buccinator

Body of mandible

Genioglossus

Inferior alveolar n., a., and v. in mandibular canal

Lingual n., deep lingual a. and v.

Hyoglossus

Digastric, anterior belly

Mylohyoid

Geniohyoid

Sectional Anatomy of the Head & Neck (II)

Fig. 46.3 Coronal section through the pituitary
Anterior view.

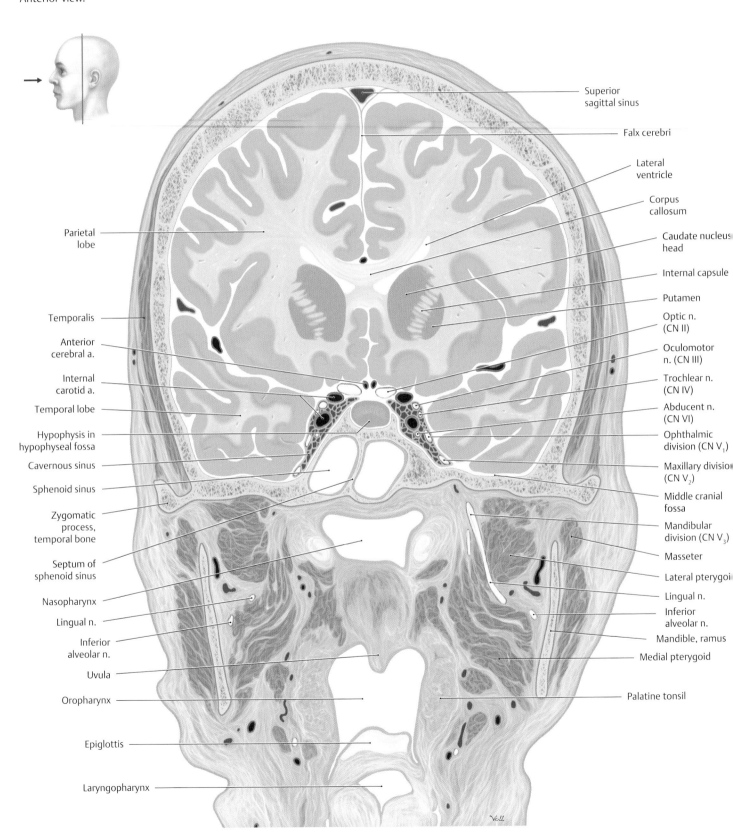

Superior sagittal sinus

Falx cerebri

Lateral ventricle

Corpus callosum

Caudate nucleus head

Internal capsule

Putamen

Optic n. (CN II)

Oculomotor n. (CN III)

Trochlear n. (CN IV)

Abducent n. (CN VI)

Ophthalmic division (CN V₁)

Maxillary division (CN V₂)

Middle cranial fossa

Mandibular division (CN V₃)

Masseter

Lateral pterygoid

Lingual n.

Inferior alveolar n.

Mandible, ramus

Medial pterygoid

Palatine tonsil

Parietal lobe

Temporalis

Anterior cerebral a.

Internal carotid a.

Temporal lobe

Hypophysis in hypophyseal fossa

Cavernous sinus

Sphenoid sinus

Zygomatic process, temporal bone

Septum of sphenoid sinus

Nasopharynx

Lingual n.

Inferior alveolar n.

Uvula

Oropharynx

Epiglottis

Laryngopharynx

***Fig. 46.4* Midsagittal section through the nasal septum**
Left lateral view.

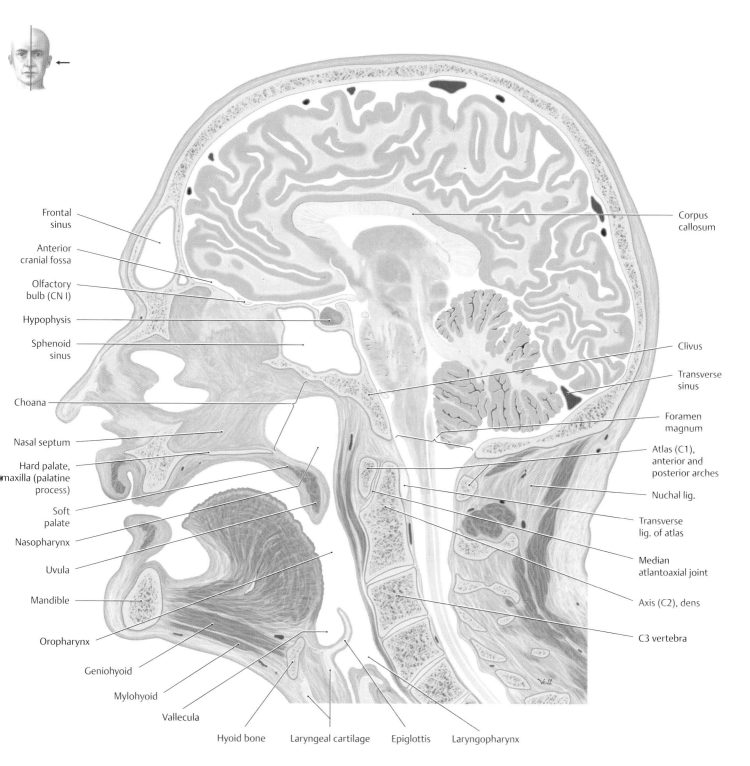

Frontal sinus

Anterior cranial fossa

Olfactory bulb (CN I)

Hypophysis

Sphenoid sinus

Choana

Nasal septum

Hard palate, maxilla (palatine process)

Soft palate

Nasopharynx

Uvula

Mandible

Oropharynx

Geniohyoid

Mylohyoid

Vallecula

Hyoid bone

Laryngeal cartilage

Epiglottis

Laryngopharynx

Corpus callosum

Clivus

Transverse sinus

Foramen magnum

Atlas (C1), anterior and posterior arches

Nuchal lig.

Transverse lig. of atlas

Median atlantoaxial joint

Axis (C2), dens

C3 vertebra

Sectional Anatomy of the Head & Neck (III)

***Fig. 46.5* Sagittal section through the medial orbital wall**

Left lateral view. This section passes through the inferior and middle conchae of the lateral nasal wall. Three of the four paranasal air sinuses (ethmoid, sphenoid, and frontal) are seen in this section and in relation to the nasal cavity into which they drain. In the region of the cervical spine, the vertebral artery is cut at multiple levels. The spinal nerves have been cut just prior to their lateral exit through the intervertebral foramina.

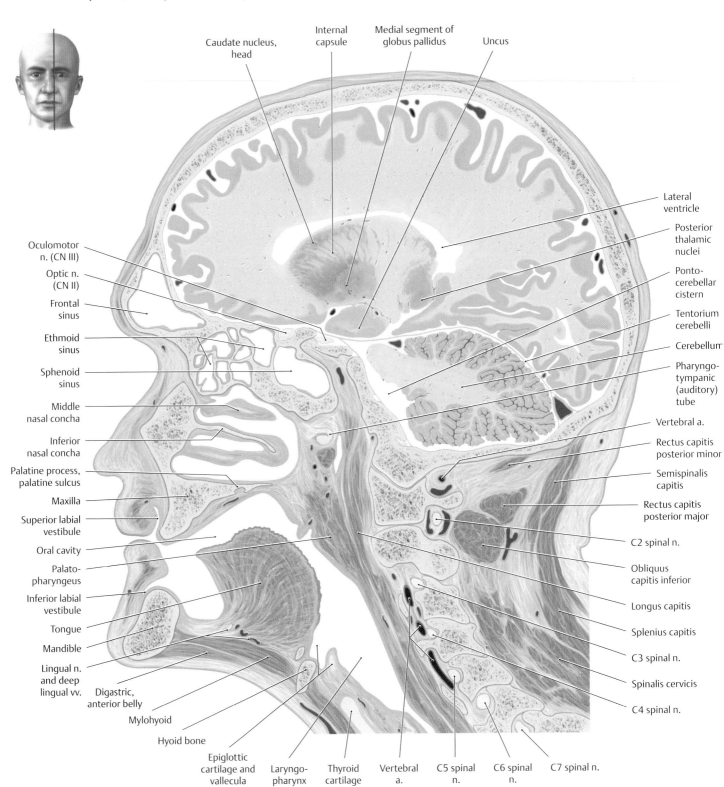

Fig. 46.6 Sagittal section through the inner third of the orbit

Left lateral view. This section passes through the maxillary, frontal, and sphenoid sinuses and a single ethmoidal air cell. The pharyngeal and masticatory muscles are revealed grouped around the cartilaginous part of the pharyngotympanic (auditory) tube. The palatine tonsil of the oral cavity and medial portion of the submandibular gland below the floor of the mouth are also seen in this section.

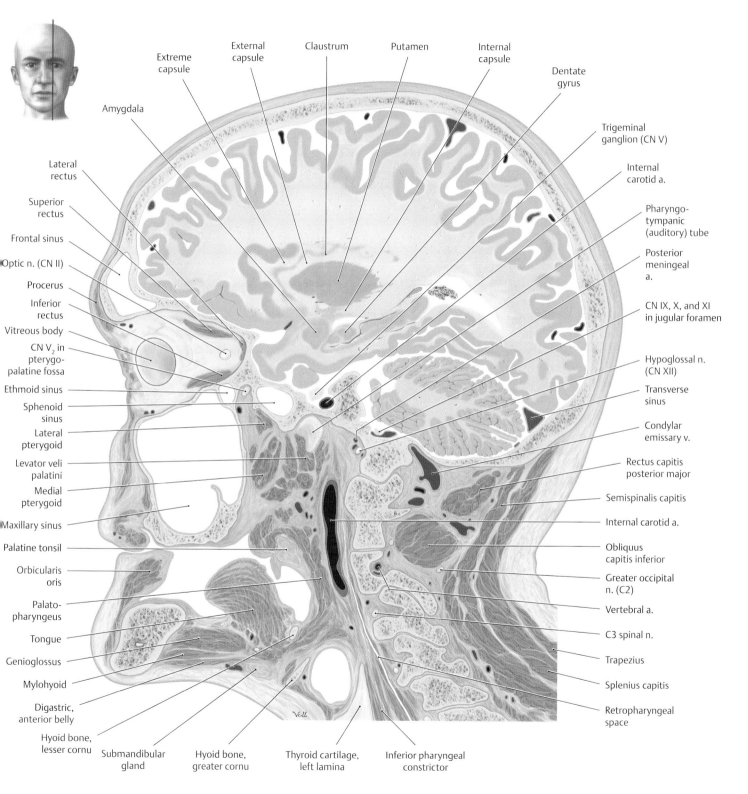

Extreme capsule

External capsule

Claustrum

Putamen

Internal capsule

Dentate gyrus

Amygdala

Trigeminal ganglion (CN V)

Internal carotid a.

Lateral rectus

Pharyngo-tympanic (auditory) tube

Superior rectus

Posterior meningeal a.

Frontal sinus

Optic n. (CN II)

CN IX, X, and XI in jugular foramen

Procerus

Inferior rectus

Hypoglossal n. (CN XII)

Vitreous body

CN V₂ in pterygo-palatine fossa

Transverse sinus

Ethmoid sinus

Condylar emissary v.

Sphenoid sinus

Rectus capitis posterior major

Lateral pterygoid

Semispinalis capitis

Levator veli palatini

Internal carotid a.

Medial pterygoid

Obliquus capitis inferior

Maxillary sinus

Greater occipital n. (C2)

Palatine tonsil

Vertebral a.

Orbicularis oris

C3 spinal n.

Palato-pharyngeus

Trapezius

Tongue

Splenius capitis

Genioglossus

Retropharyngeal space

Mylohyoid

Digastric, anterior belly

Hyoid bone, lesser cornu

Submandibular gland

Hyoid bone, greater cornu

Thyroid cartilage, left lamina

Inferior pharyngeal constrictor

Sectional Anatomy of the Head & Neck (IV)

***Fig. 46.7* Transverse section through the optic nerve and pituitary**
Inferior view.

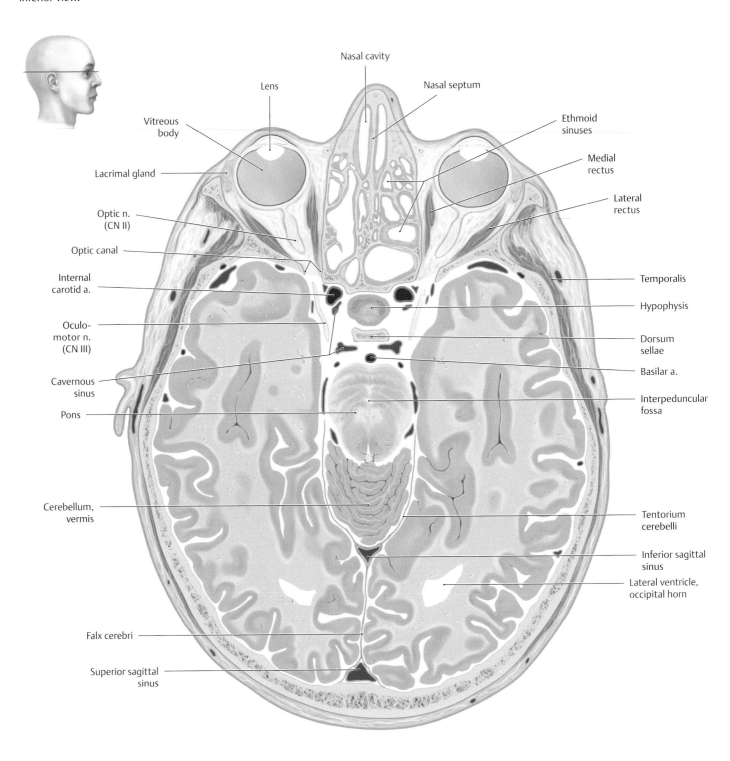

Nasal cavity

Lens

Nasal septum

Vitreous body

Ethmoid sinuses

Lacrimal gland

Medial rectus

Lateral rectus

Optic n. (CN II)

Optic canal

Temporalis

Internal carotid a.

Hypophysis

Oculo-motor n. (CN III)

Dorsum sellae

Basilar a.

Cavernous sinus

Interpeduncular fossa

Pons

Cerebellum, vermis

Tentorium cerebelli

Inferior sagittal sinus

Lateral ventricle, occipital horn

Falx cerebri

Superior sagittal sinus

***Fig. 46.8* Transverse section of head through the median atlantoaxial joint**

Superior view. This section passes through the soft palate and mucoperiosteum of the hard palate. The articulation of the odontoid process (dens of C2) with the axis (C1) at the median atlantoaxial joint is shown, as well as the carotid sheath, containing the vertical neuro-

vascular elements of the neck. The vertebral artery is sectioned as it prepares to enter the foramen magnum and fuse with its opposite to form the basilar artery.

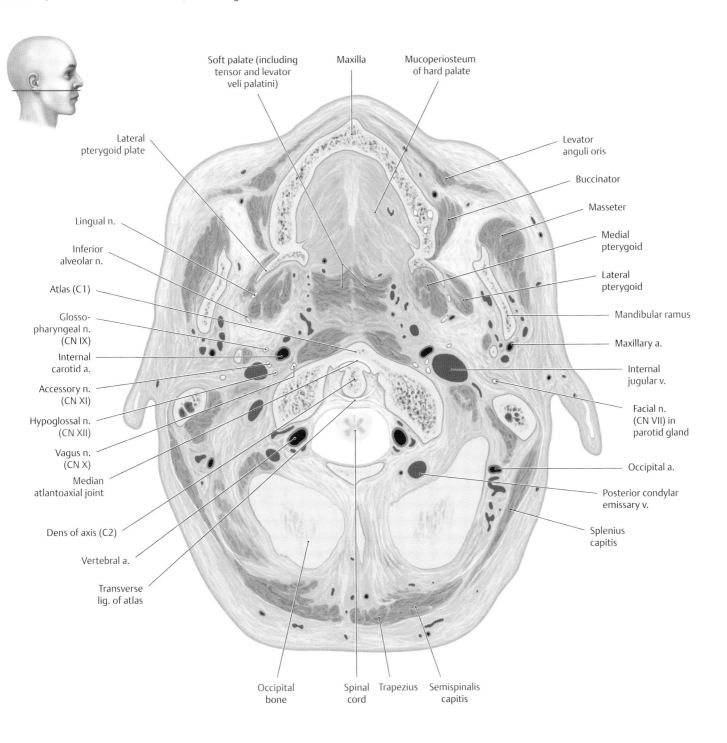

Sectional Anatomy of the Head & Neck (V)

Fig. 46.9 Transverse section of the neck

Transverse section at the level of the C5 vertebral body. Inferior view. The internal and external jugular veins are separated by the sternocleidomastoid. The accessory nerve (CN XI) is just medial to this muscle as it prepares to innervate it from behind. The elongated spinous process of the C7 vertebra (vertebra prominens) is also visible in the section due to the lordotic curvature of the neck.

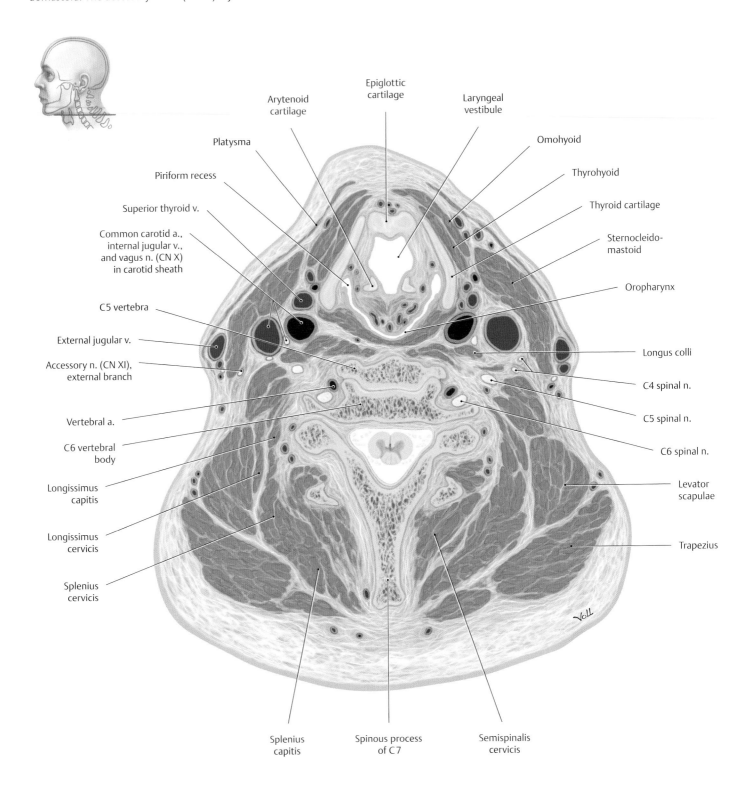

Fig. 46.10 Transverse section at the level of the C6 vertebral body

Inferior view.

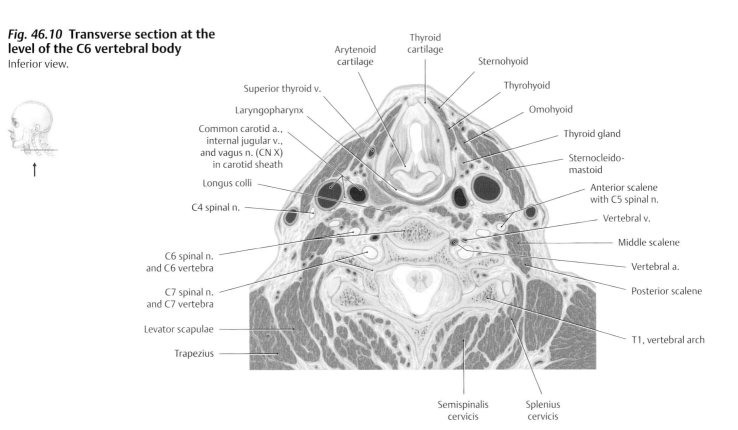

Arytenoid cartilage

Thyroid cartilage

Sternohyoid

Superior thyroid v.

Thyrohyoid

Laryngopharynx

Omohyoid

Common carotid a., internal jugular v., and vagus n. (CN X) in carotid sheath

Thyroid gland

Sternocleido-mastoid

Longus colli

Anterior scalene with C5 spinal n.

C4 spinal n.

Vertebral v.

Middle scalene

C6 spinal n. and C6 vertebra

Vertebral a.

C7 spinal n. and C7 vertebra

Posterior scalene

Levator scapulae

T1, vertebral arch

Trapezius

Semispinalis cervicis

Splenius cervicis

Fig. 46.11 Transverse section of the neck

Transverse section at the level of the C7/T1 vertebral junction. Inferior view. This section reveals the roots of spinal nerves C6 to C8 of the brachial plexus passing between the anterior and middle scalene muscles. The phrenic nerve is on the anterior surface of the anterior scalene and the components of the carotid sheath (internal jugular vein, common carotid artery, and vagus nerve) lie in the interval between this muscle, the sternocleidomastoid, and the thyroid gland.

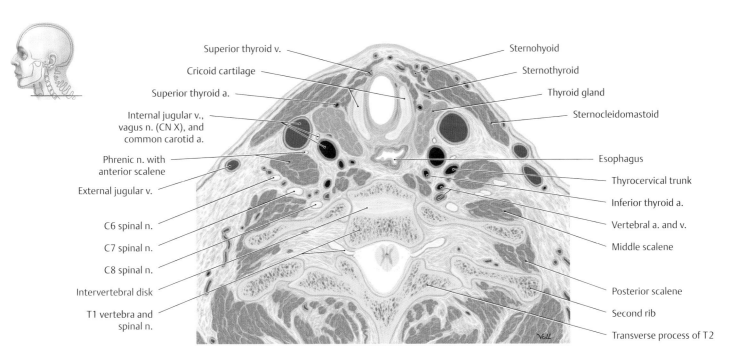

Superior thyroid v.

Sternohyoid

Cricoid cartilage

Sternothyroid

Superior thyroid a.

Thyroid gland

Internal jugular v., vagus n. (CN X), and common carotid a.

Sternocleidomastoid

Phrenic n. with anterior scalene

Esophagus

External jugular v.

Thyrocervical trunk

Inferior thyroid a.

C6 spinal n.

Vertebral a. and v.

C7 spinal n.

Middle scalene

C8 spinal n.

Intervertebral disk

Posterior scalene

T1 vertebra and spinal n.

Second rib

Transverse process of T 2

Radiographic Anatomy of the Head & Neck (I)

Fig. 46.12 Radiograph of the skull
Anteroposterior view.

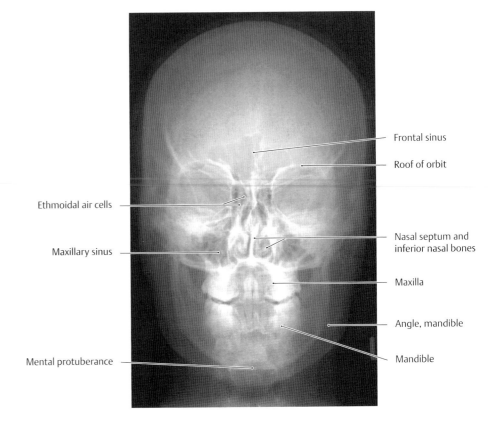

Frontal sinus

Roof of orbit

Ethmoidal air cells

Nasal septum and inferior nasal bones

Maxillary sinus

Maxilla

Angle, mandible

Mental protuberance

Mandible

Fig. 46.13 Coronal MRI through the eyeball
Anterior view.

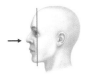

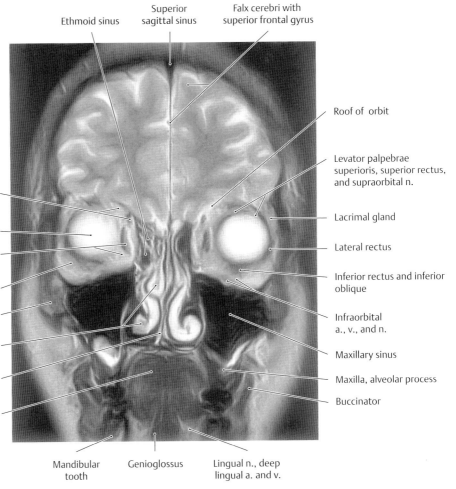

Ethmoid sinus

Superior sagittal sinus

Falx cerebri with superior frontal gyrus

Roof of orbit

Levator palpebrae superioris, superior rectus, and supraorbital n.

Superior oblique with superior ophthalmic v.

Lacrimal gland

Eyeball

Lateral rectus

Medial rectus with ophthalmic a.

Inferior rectus and inferior oblique

Periorbital fat

Zygomatic bone

Infraorbital a., v., and n.

Middle and inferior nasal conchae

Maxillary sinus

Nasal septum

Maxilla, alveolar process

Tongue

Buccinator

Mandibular tooth

Genioglossus

Lingual n., deep lingual a. and v.

Fig. 46.14 Radiograph of the skull
Left lateral view.

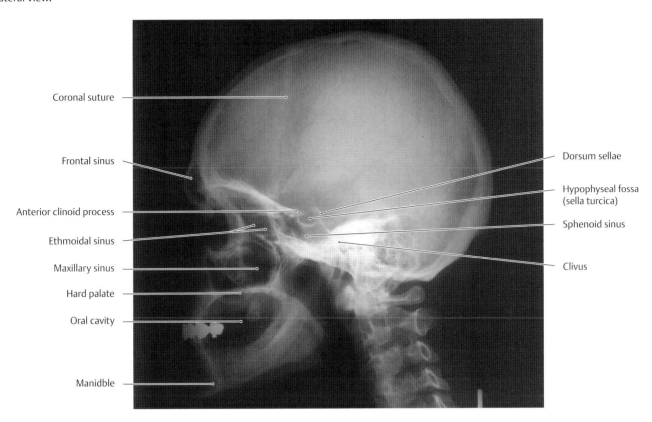

Coronal suture

Frontal sinus

Anterior clinoid process

Ethmoidal sinus

Maxillary sinus

Hard palate

Oral cavity

Manidble

Dorsum sellae

Hypophyseal fossa
(sella turcica)

Sphenoid sinus

Clivus

Fig. 46.15 Midsagittal MRI through the nasal septum

Left lateral view. Boxed area represents the location of the ventricular system, thalamus, and pons. A more detail labeled version of this area can be seen in **Fig. 51.5, p.688.**

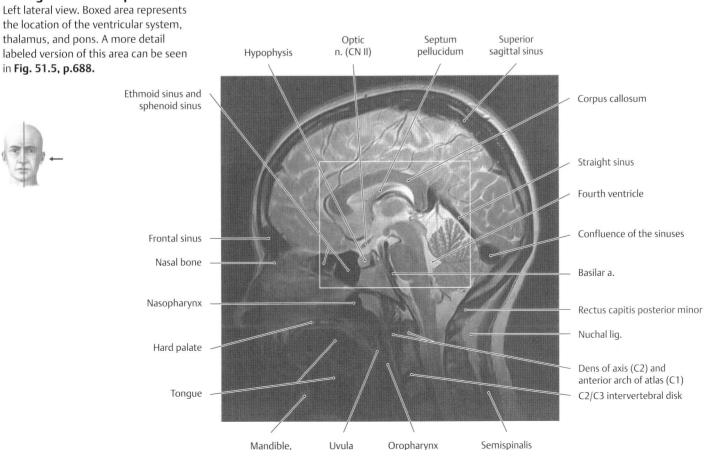

Hypophysis

Optic
n. (CN II)

Septum
pellucidum

Superior
sagittal sinus

Ethmoid sinus and
sphenoid sinus

Corpus callosum

Straight sinus

Fourth ventricle

Confluence of the sinuses

Frontal sinus

Nasal bone

Basilar a.

Rectus capitis posterior minor

Nasopharynx

Nuchal lig.

Hard palate

Dens of axis (C2) and
anterior arch of atlas (C1)

Tongue

C2/C3 intervertebral disk

Mandible,
body

Uvula

Oropharynx

Semispinalis
capitis

Radiographic Anatomy of the Head & Neck (II)

Fig. 46.16 **Radiograph of the skull**
Inferosuperior oblique view (Waters view).

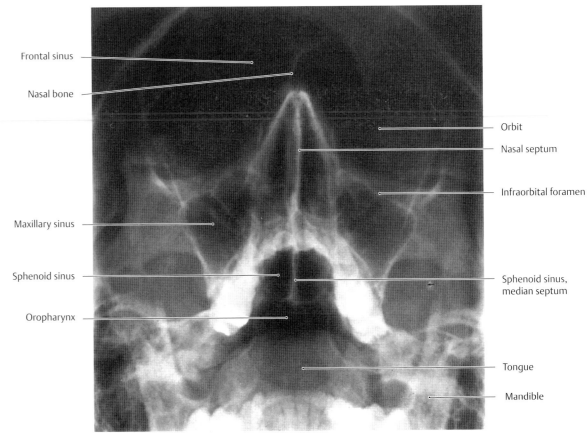

Frontal sinus

Nasal bone

Orbit

Nasal septum

Infraorbital foramen

Maxillary sinus

Sphenoid sinus

Sphenoid sinus, median septum

Oropharynx

Tongue

Mandible

Fig. 46.17 **Radiograph of the mandible**
Left lateral view.

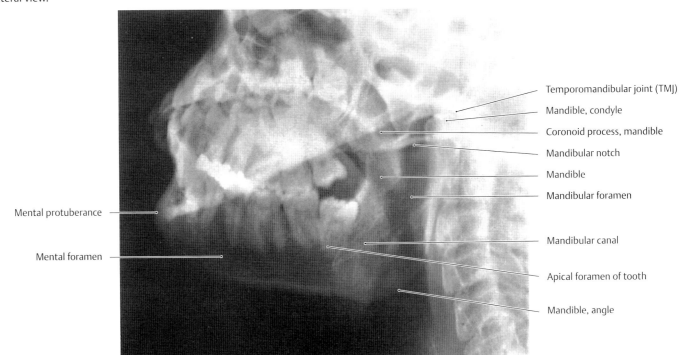

Temporomandibular joint (TMJ)

Mandible, condyle

Coronoid process, mandible

Mandibular notch

Mandible

Mandibular foramen

Mental protuberance

Mandibular canal

Mental foramen

Apical foramen of tooth

Mandible, angle

Fig. 46.18 Transverse MRI through the orbit and nasolacrimal duct
Inferior view.

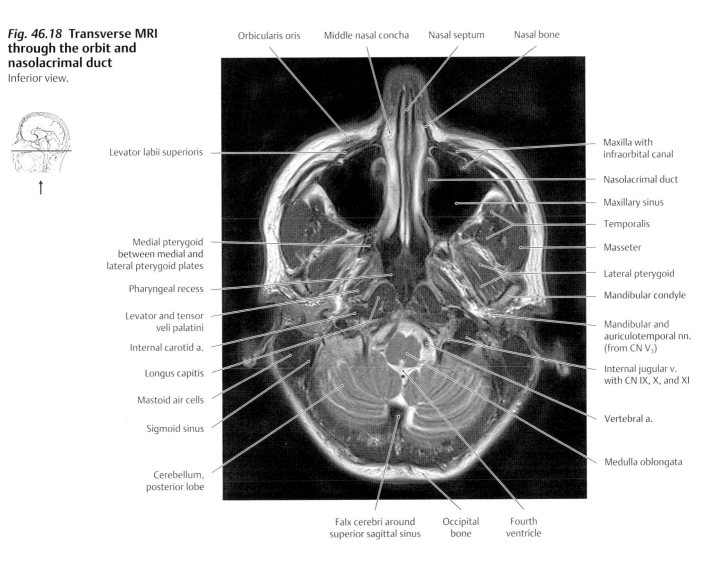

Orbicularis oris
Middle nasal concha
Nasal septum
Nasal bone

Levator labii superioris

Medial pterygoid between medial and lateral pterygoid plates
Pharyngeal recess
Levator and tensor veli palatini
Internal carotid a.
Longus capitis
Mastoid air cells
Sigmoid sinus
Cerebellum, posterior lobe

Maxilla with infraorbital canal
Nasolacrimal duct
Maxillary sinus
Temporalis
Masseter
Lateral pterygoid
Mandibular condyle
Mandibular and auriculotemporal nn. (from CN V₃)
Internal jugular v. with CN IX, X, and XI
Vertebral a.
Medulla oblongata

Falx cerebri around superior sagittal sinus
Occipital bone
Fourth ventricle

Fig. 46.19 Transverse MRI through the neck
Inferior view

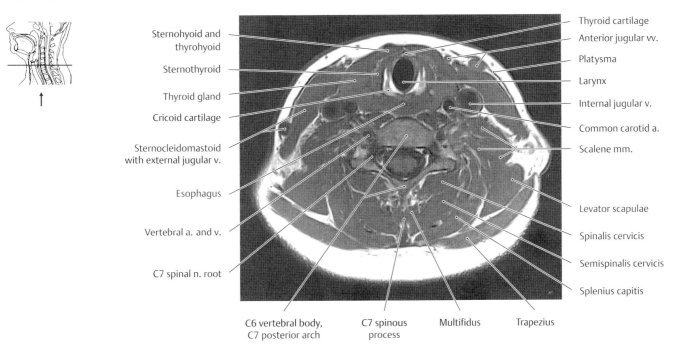

Sternohyoid and thyrohyoid
Sternothyroid
Thyroid gland
Cricoid cartilage
Sternocleidomastoid with external jugular v.
Esophagus
Vertebral a. and v.
C7 spinal n. root

Thyroid cartilage
Anterior jugular vv.
Platysma
Larynx
Internal jugular v.
Common carotid a.
Scalene mm.
Levator scapulae
Spinalis cervicis
Semispinalis cervicis
Splenius capitis

C6 vertebral body, C7 posterior arch
C7 spinous process
Multifidus
Trapezius

Radiographic Anatomy of the Head & Neck (III)

***Fig. 46.20* Temporomandibular joint (TMJ)**
Coronal section.

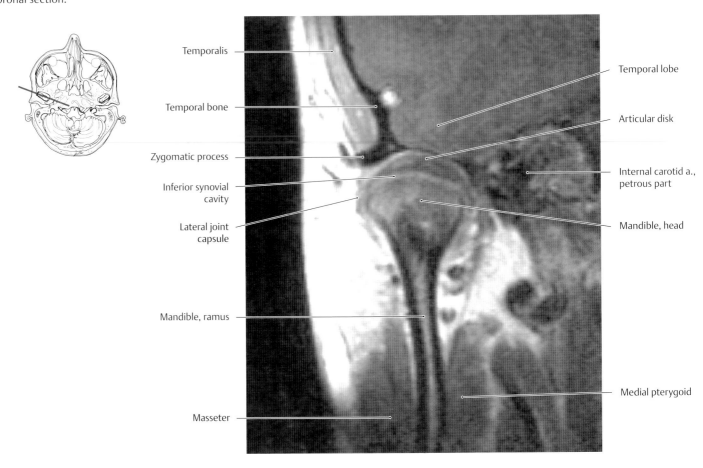

- Temporalis
- Temporal bone
- Zygomatic process
- Inferior synovial cavity
- Lateral joint capsule
- Mandible, ramus
- Masseter
- Temporal lobe
- Articular disk
- Internal carotid a., petrous part
- Mandible, head
- Medial pterygoid

***Fig. 46.21* Temporomandibular joint (TMJ)**
Sagittal section, mouth closed.

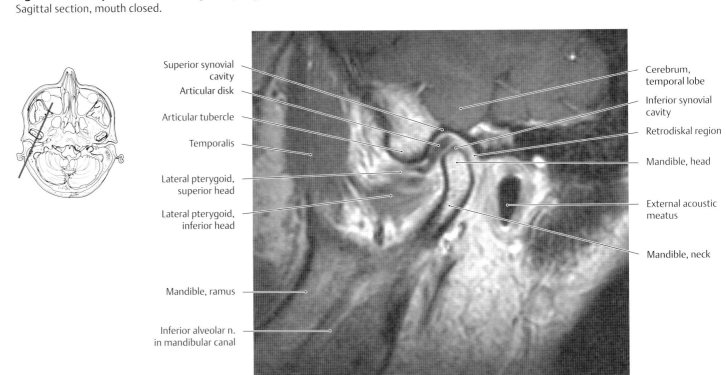

- Superior synovial cavity
- Articular disk
- Articular tubercle
- Temporalis
- Lateral pterygoid, superior head
- Lateral pterygoid, inferior head
- Mandible, ramus
- Inferior alveolar n. in mandibular canal
- Cerebrum, temporal lobe
- Inferior synovial cavity
- Retrodiskal region
- Mandible, head
- External acoustic meatus
- Mandible, neck

Fig. 46.22 Cranial MR angiography

Cranial view. In this angiogram note that the right posterior cerebral a. arises from the internal carotid artery instead of the basilar artery—a variant. The normal configuration is seen on the left side.

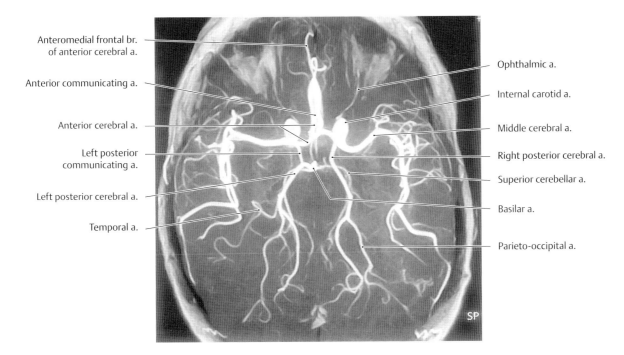

Anteromedial frontal br. of anterior cerebral a.

Anterior communicating a.

Anterior cerebral a.

Left posterior communicating a.

Left posterior cerebral a.

Temporal a.

Ophthalmic a.

Internal carotid a.

Middle cerebral a.

Right posterior cerebral a.

Superior cerebellar a.

Basilar a.

Parieto-occipital a.

Fig. 46.23 Dural venous sinus system of the head

Right lateral view.

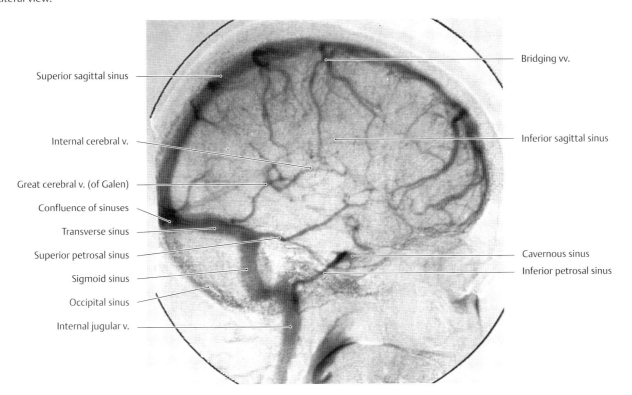

Superior sagittal sinus

Internal cerebral v.

Great cerebral v. (of Galen)

Confluence of sinuses

Transverse sinus

Superior petrosal sinus

Sigmoid sinus

Occipital sinus

Internal jugular v.

Bridging vv.

Inferior sagittal sinus

Cavernous sinus

Inferior petrosal sinus

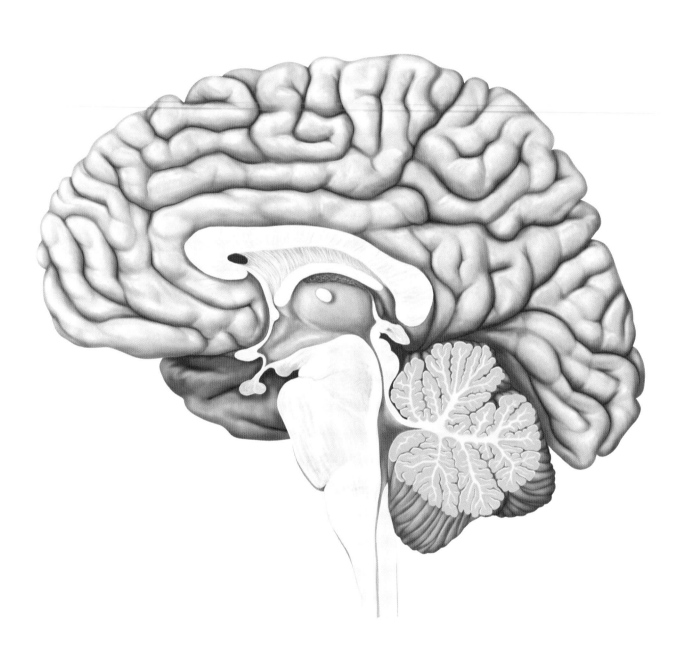

Brain & Nervous System

Nervous System: Overview

Fig. 47.1 Central and peripheral nervous systems

The nervous system is divided into the central (CNS) and peripheral (PNS) nervous systems. The CNS consists of the brain and spinal cord, which constitute a functional unit. The PNS consists of the nerves emerging from the brain and spinal cord (cranial and spinal nerves, respectively).

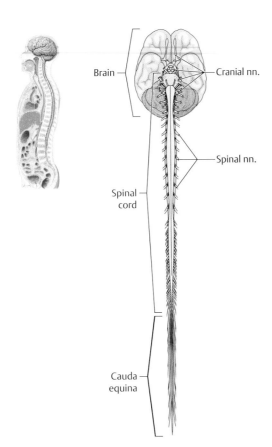

Fig. 47.2 Gray and white matter in the CNS

Nerve cell bodies appear gray in gross inspection, whereas nerve cell processes (axons) and their insulating myelin sheaths appear white.

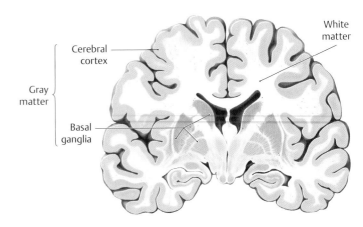

A Coronal section through the brain.

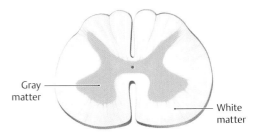

B Transverse section through the spinal cord.

Table 47.1	Development of the brain			
	Primary vesicle	**Region**		**Structure**
Neural tube	Prosencephalon (forebrain)	Telencephalon (cerebrum)		Cerebral cortex, white matter, and basal ganglia
		Diencephalon		Epithalamus (pineal), dorsal thalamus, subthalamus, and hypothalamus
	Mesencephalon (midbrain)*			Tectum, tegmentum, and cerebral peduncles
	Rhombencephalon (hindbrain)	Metencephalon	Cerebellum	Cerebellar cortex, nuclei, and peduncles
			Pons*	Nuclei and fiber tracts
		Myelencephalon	Medulla oblongata*	

* The mesencephalon, pons, and medulla oblongata are collectively known as the brainstem.

Fig. 47.3 Embryonic development of the brain
Left lateral view.

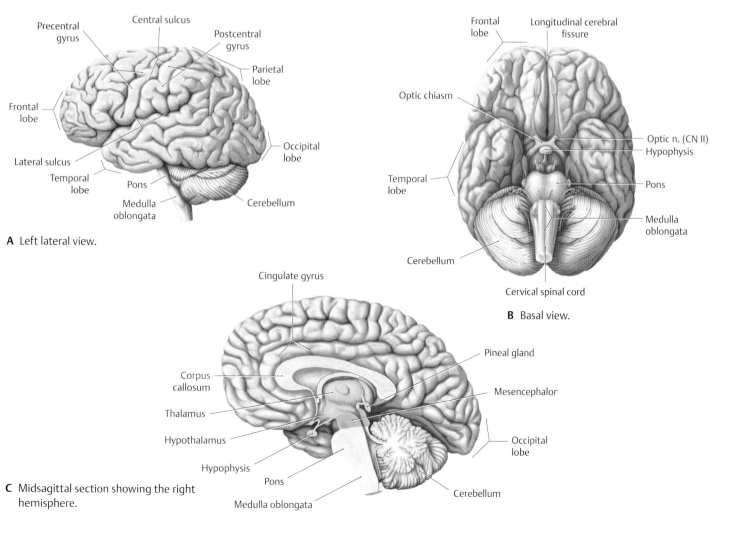

Cervical flexure
Medulla oblongata
Cranial flexure
Pons
Optic cup

A Start of 2nd month.

Insula
Pons
Medulla oblongata

C 3rd month of development.

Telodien-cephalic sulcus
Hypophysis primordium
Olfactory bulb
Mammillary tubercle

B End of 2nd month.

Insula
Eye
Pons
Medulla oblongata

D 7th month.

Fig. 47.4 Adult brain
See **Fig. 47.7** for lobes of the cerebrum. CN, cranial nerve.

Precentral gyrus
Central sulcus
Postcentral gyrus
Parietal lobe
Frontal lobe
Occipital lobe
Lateral sulcus
Temporal lobe
Pons
Medulla oblongata
Cerebellum

A Left lateral view.

Frontal lobe
Longitudinal cerebral fissure
Optic chiasm
Optic n. (CN II)
Hypophysis
Temporal lobe
Pons
Medulla oblongata
Cerebellum
Cervical spinal cord

B Basal view.

Cingulate gyrus
Pineal gland
Corpus callosum
Mesencephalor
Thalamus
Hypothalamus
Hypophysis
Occipital lobe
Pons
Medulla oblongata
Cerebellum

C Midsagittal section showing the right hemisphere.

Brain, Macroscopic Organization

Fig. 47.5 Cerebrum

Left lateral view. The cerebrum is part of the anterior subdivision of the embryonic forebrain (telencephalon)—the part of the adult forebrain that includes the cerebral hemispheres and associated structures. The surface anatomy of the cerebrum can be divided macroscopically into 4 lobes: frontal, parietal, temporal, and occipital. The surface contours of the cerebrum are defined by convolutions (gyri) and depressions (sulci).

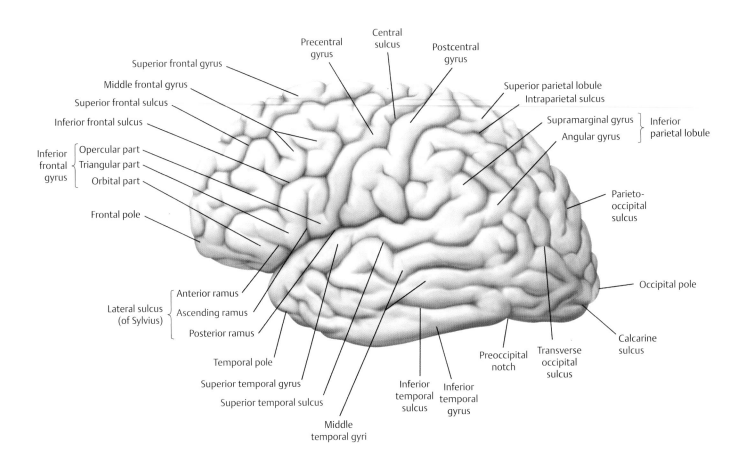

Fig. 47.6 Insular lobe

Lateral view of the retracted left cerebral hemisphere. Part of the cerebral cortex sinks below the surface during development forming the insula (or insular lobe). Those portions of the cerebral cortex that overlie this deeper cortical region are called opercula ("little lids").

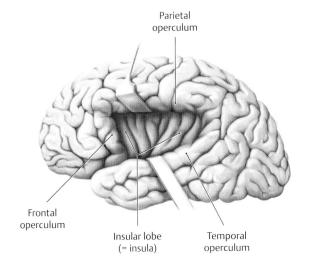

Fig. 47.7 Lobes in the cerebral hemispheres

The isocortex also may be functionally divided into association areas (lobes).

Frontal lobe
Parietal lobe
Temporal lobe
Occipital lobe
Insular lobe (insula)
Limbic lobe (limbus)

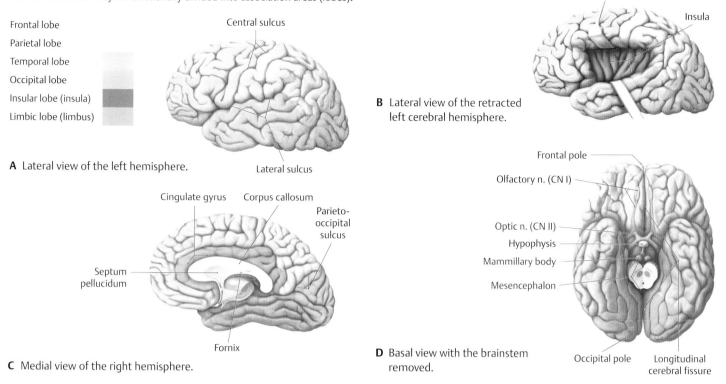

A Lateral view of the left hemisphere.

Central sulcus

Lateral sulcus

B Lateral view of the retracted left cerebral hemisphere.

Insula

Cingulate gyrus   Corpus callosum
Parieto-occipital sulcus

Septum pellucidum

Fornix

C Medial view of the right hemisphere.

Frontal pole
Olfactory n. (CN I)
Optic n. (CN II)
Hypophysis
Mammillary body
Mesencephalon

D Basal view with the brainstem removed.

Occipital pole   Longitudinal cerebral fissure

Fig. 47.8 Midsagittal section of the brain showing the medial surface of the right hemisphere

The brain has been split along the longitudinal cerebral fissure.

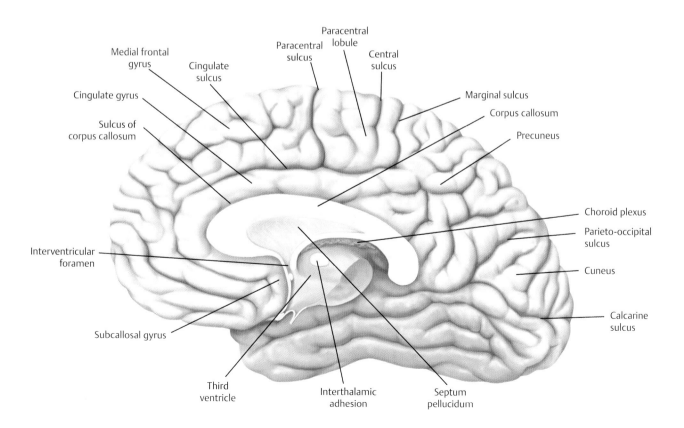

Medial frontal gyrus
Cingulate gyrus
Sulcus of corpus callosum
Cingulate sulcus
Paracentral sulcus
Paracentral lobule
Central sulcus
Marginal sulcus
Corpus callosum
Precuneus
Choroid plexus
Parieto-occipital sulcus
Cuneus
Calcarine sulcus
Interventricular foramen
Subcallosal gyrus
Third ventricle
Interthalamic adhesion
Septum pellucidum

Diencephalon

 The diencephalon is the posterior subdivision of the forebrain—the part of the adult forebrain that includes the thalamus and associated structures.

Fig. 47.9 Diencephalon

Midsagittal section, medial view of the right hemisphere. The major components of the diencephalon are the thalamus, hypothalamus, and hypophysis (anterior lobe). The diencephalon is located below the corpus callosum, part of the cerebrum, and above the midbrain. The thalamus makes up four-fifths of the diencephalon but the only parts that can be seen externally are the hypothalamus (seen on the basal aspect of the brain) and portions of the epithalamus. In the adult brain the diencephalon is involved in endocrine functioning and autonomic coordination of the pineal, neurohypophysis, and hypothalamus. It also acts as a relay station for sensory information and somatic motor control via the thalamus.

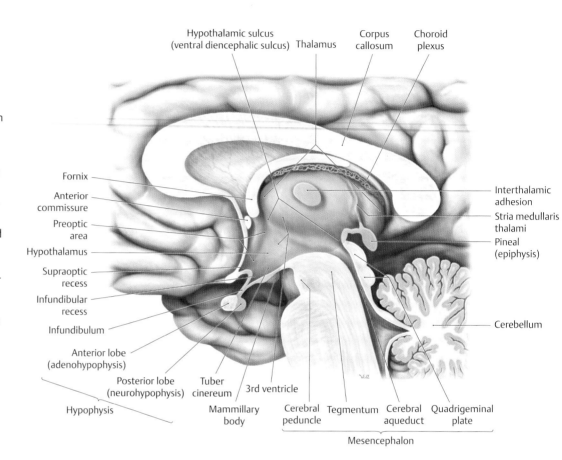

Fig. 47.10 Arrangement of the diencephalon around the third ventricle

Posterior view of an oblique transverse section through the telecephalon with the corpus callosum, fornix, and choroid plexus removed. This figure clearly illustrates that the lateral wall of the third ventricle forms the medial boundary of the diencephalon.

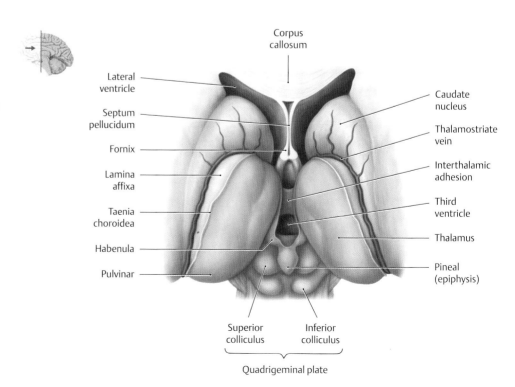

Brain & Nervous System

Fig. 47.11 **The diencephalon and brainstem**

Left lateral view. The cerebral hemispheres have been removed from around the thalamus. The cerebellum has also been removed. The parts of the diencephalon visible in this dissection are the thalamus, the lateral geniculate body, and the optic tract. The latter two are components of the visual pathway. This dissection illustrates the role the diencephalon plays in linking the underlying brainstem to the overlying cerebral hemispheres.

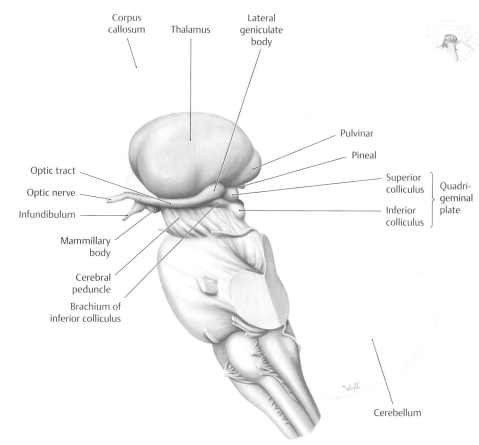

Fig. 47.12 **Location of the diencephalon in the adult brain**

Basal view of the brain (brainstem has been sectioned at the level of the pons). The structures that can be identified in this view represent those parts of the diencephalon situated on the basal surface of the brain. This view also demonstrates how the optic tract winds around the cerebral peduncles. The expansion of the telencephalon during development limits the number of structures of the diencephalon visible on the undersurface of the brain. They are:

- Optic nerve
- Optic chiasm
- Optic tract
- Tuber cinerum with the infundibulum
- Mammilary bodies
- Lateral geniculate body
- Neurohypophysis

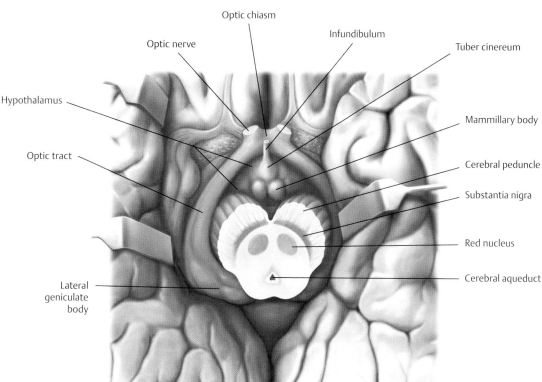

Brainstem & Cerebellum

The stalk-like region of the brain connecting the cerebral hemispheres to the cerebellum and spinal cord consists of the diencephalon (thalamus and associated structures) and the brainstem— composed of the mesencephalon or midbrain, pons and medulla oblongata moving sequentially caudal. Fiber bundles pass through this region from the spinal cord on their way to and from the cerebrum; thick fiber bundles pass contralaterally from the cerebrum into the cerebellar hemispheres; and 10 of the 12 cranial nerves are associated with the brainstem.

Fig. 47.13 Diencephalon, brainstem, and cerebellum
Left lateral view.

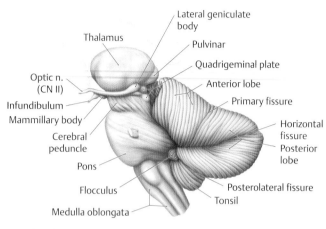

A Isolated structures.

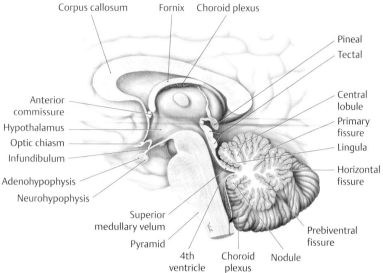

B Midsagittal section.

Fig. 47.14 Cerebellum

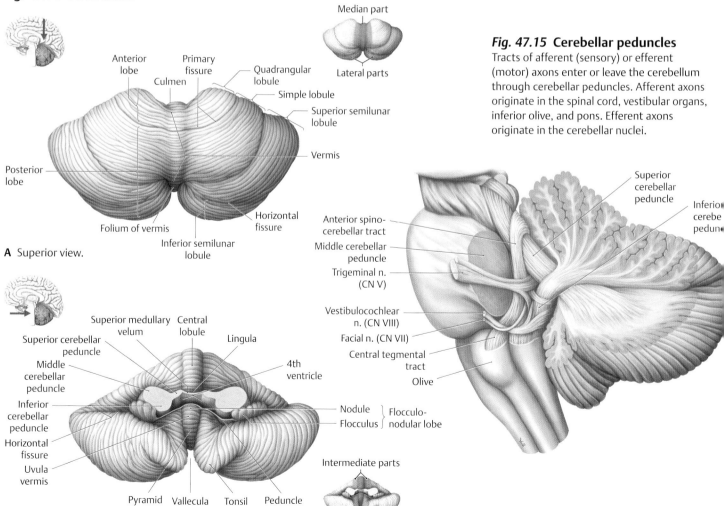

A Superior view.

Fig. 47.15 Cerebellar peduncles
Tracts of afferent (sensory) or efferent (motor) axons enter or leave the cerebellum through cerebellar peduncles. Afferent axons originate in the spinal cord, vestibular organs, inferior olive, and pons. Efferent axons originate in the cerebellar nuclei.

B Anterior view.

Fig. 47.16 **Brainstem**

The brainstem is the site of emergence and entry of the 10 pairs of true cranial nerves (CN III–XII). See **p. 526** for an overview of the cranial nerves and their nuclei.

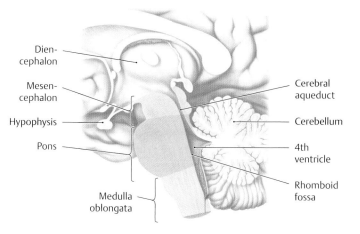

Dien-
cephalon
Mesen-
cephalon
Hypophysis
Pons

Cerebral
aqueduct
Cerebellum
4th
ventricle
Rhomboid
fossa

Medulla
oblongata

A Levels of the brainstem.

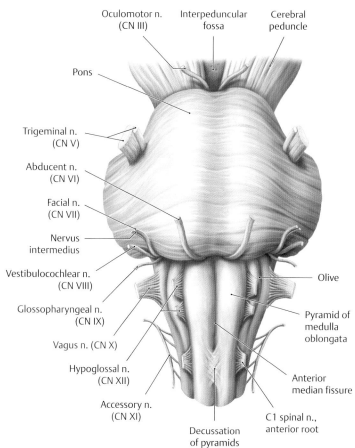

Oculomotor n.
(CN III) Interpeduncular
fossa Cerebral
peduncle

Pons

Trigeminal n.
(CN V)

Abducent n.
(CN VI)

Facial n.
(CN VII)

Nervus
intermedius

Vestibulocochlear n.
(CN VIII)

Glossopharyngeal n.
(CN IX)

Vagus n. (CN X)

Hypoglossal n.
(CN XII)

Accessory n.
(CN XI)

Decussation
of pyramids

Olive

Pyramid of
medulla
oblongata

Anterior
median fissure

C1 spinal n.,
anterior root

B Anterior view.

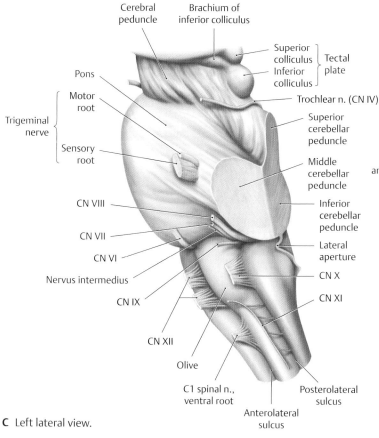

Cerebral
peduncle Brachium of
inferior colliculus

Superior
colliculus ⎫
            ⎬ Tectal
Inferior   ⎪ plate
colliculus ⎭

Pons

Motor
root

Trigeminal
nerve

Sensory
root

Trochlear n. (CN IV)

Superior
cerebellar
peduncle

Middle
cerebellar
peduncle

CN VIII

CN VII

CN VI

Nervus intermedius

CN IX

CN XII

Olive

C1 spinal n.,
ventral root

Anterolateral
sulcus

Inferior
cerebellar
peduncle

Lateral
aperture

CN X

CN XI

Posterolateral
sulcus

C Left lateral view.

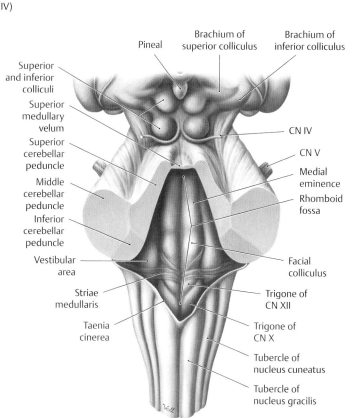

Pineal Brachium of
superior colliculus Brachium of
inferior colliculus

Superior
and inferior
colliculi

Superior
medullary
velum

Superior
cerebellar
peduncle

Middle
cerebellar
peduncle

Inferior
cerebellar
peduncle

Vestibular
area

Striae
medullaris

Taenia
cinerea

CN IV

CN V

Medial
eminence

Rhomboid
fossa

Facial
colliculus

Trigone of
CN XII

Trigone of
CN X

Tubercle of
nucleus cuneatus

Tubercle of
nucleus gracilis

D Posterior view.

Ventricles & CSF Spaces

Fig. 47.17 Circulation of cerebrospinal fluid (CSF)

The brain and spinal cord are suspended in CSF. Produced continually in the choroid plexus, CSF occupies the subarachnoid space and ventricles of the brain and drains through arachnoid granulations into the dural venous sinus system (primarily the superior sagittal sinus) of the cranial cavity. Smaller amounts drain along proximal portions of the spinal nerves into venous plexuses or lymphatic pathways.

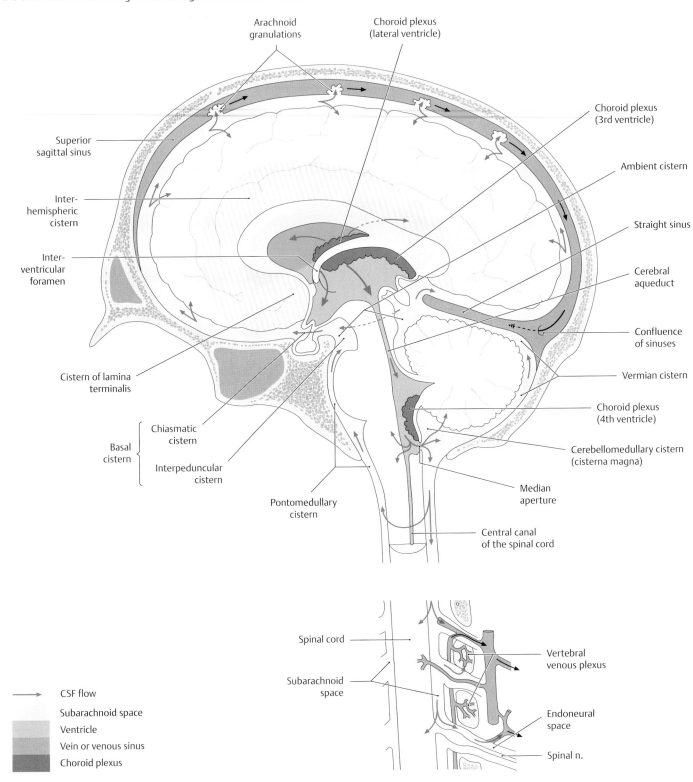

Fig. 47.18 Ventricular system

The ventricular system is a continuation of the central spinal canal into the brain. Cast specimens are used to demonstrate the connections between the four ventricular cavities.

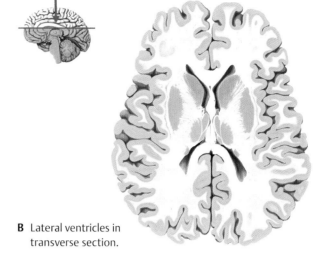

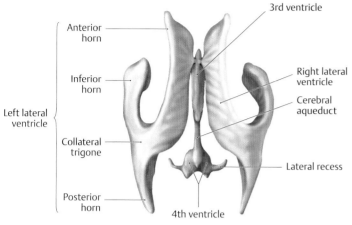

A Superior view.

B Lateral ventricles in transverse section.

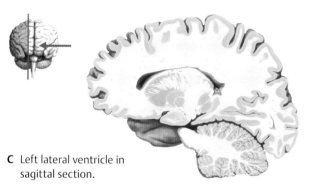

C Left lateral ventricle in sagittal section.

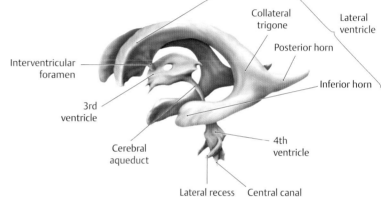

D Left lateral view.

Fig. 47.19 Ventricular system in situ

Left lateral view.

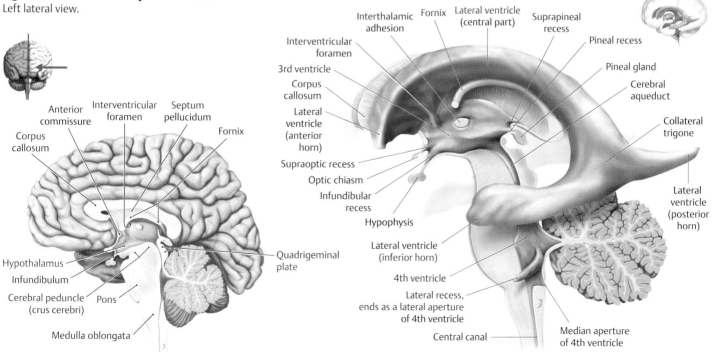

A 3rd and 4th ventricles in the midsagittal section.

B Ventricular system with neighboring structures.

Veins and Venous Sinuses of the Brain

 Additional information on the venous sinus system and dural folds of the cranial cavity can be found on **pp. 554–557.**

***Fig. 48.1* Superficial cerebral veins**

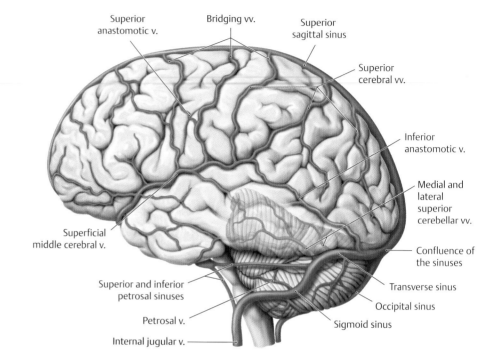

A Lateral view of the left hemisphere.

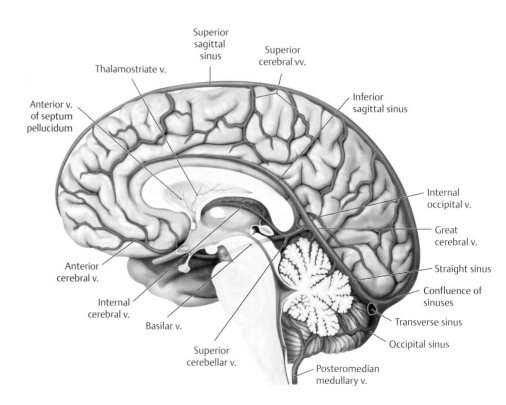

B Medial view of the right hemisphere.

Fig. 48.2 Basal cerebral venous system
Basal view.

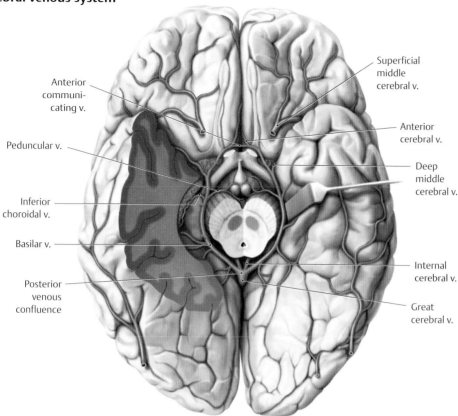

Anterior communicating v.

Peduncular v.

Inferior choroidal v.

Basilar v.

Posterior venous confluence

Superficial middle cerebral v.

Anterior cerebral v.

Deep middle cerebral v.

Internal cerebral v.

Great cerebral v.

Fig. 48.3 Veins of the brainstem
Basal view.

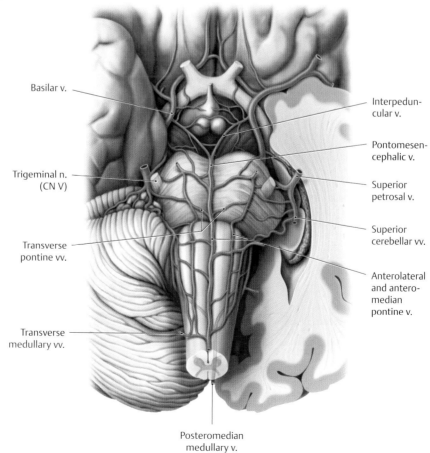

Basilar v.

Trigeminal n. (CN V)

Transverse pontine vv.

Transverse medullary vv.

Posteromedian medullary v.

Interpeduncular v.

Pontomesencephalic v.

Superior petrosal v.

Superior cerebellar vv.

Anterolateral and anteromedian pontine v.

Arteries of the Brain

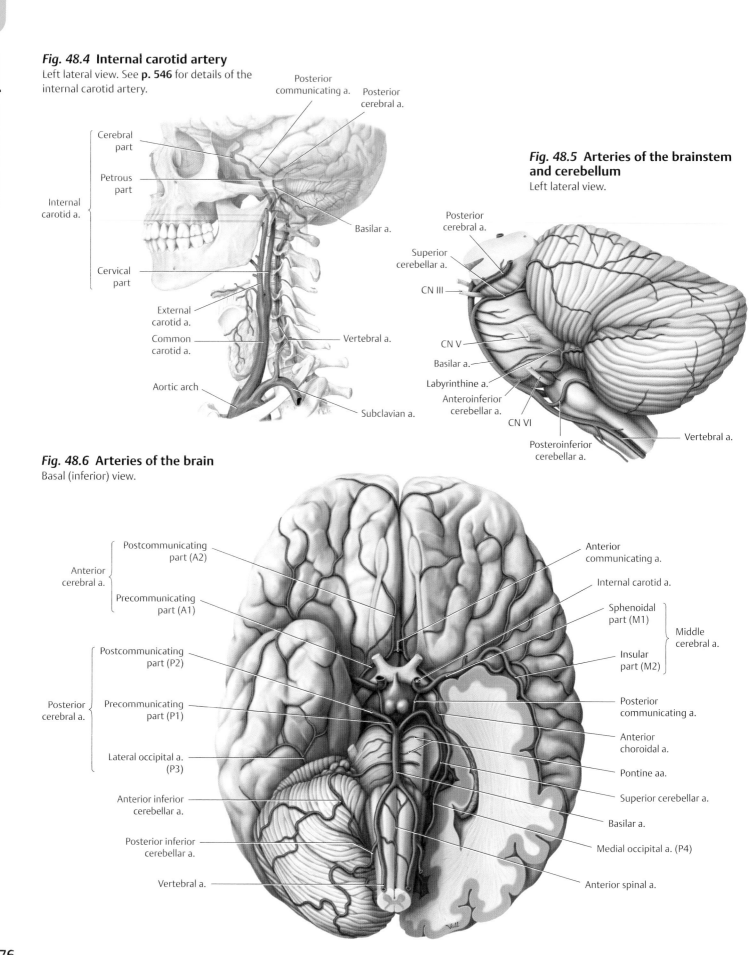

Fig. 48.4 Internal carotid artery

Left lateral view. See **p. 546** for details of the internal carotid artery.

Cerebral part
Petrous part
Internal carotid a.
Cervical part
External carotid a.
Common carotid a.
Aortic arch
Posterior communicating a.
Posterior cerebral a.
Basilar a.
Vertebral a.
Subclavian a.

Fig. 48.5 Arteries of the brainstem and cerebellum

Left lateral view.

Posterior cerebral a.
Superior cerebellar a.
CN III
CN V
Basilar a.
Labyrinthine a.
Anteroinferior cerebellar a.
CN VI
Posteroinferior cerebellar a.
Vertebral a.

Fig. 48.6 Arteries of the brain

Basal (inferior) view.

Anterior cerebral a.
Postcommunicating part (A2)
Precommunicating part (A1)
Posterior cerebral a.
Postcommunicating part (P2)
Precommunicating part (P1)
Lateral occipital a. (P3)
Anterior inferior cerebellar a.
Posterior inferior cerebellar a.
Vertebral a.
Anterior communicating a.
Internal carotid a.
Sphenoidal part (M1)
Insular part (M2)
Middle cerebral a.
Posterior communicating a.
Anterior choroidal a.
Pontine aa.
Superior cerebellar a.
Basilar a.
Medial occipital a. (P4)
Anterior spinal a.

Fig. 48.7 **Cerebral arteries**

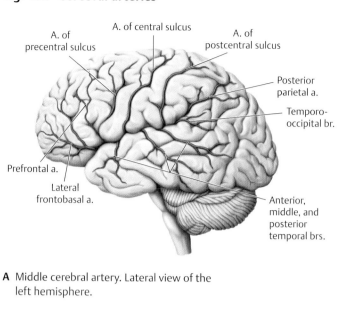

A **Middle cerebral artery. Lateral view of the left hemisphere.**

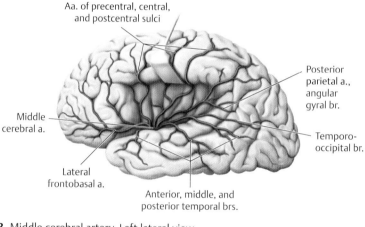

B **Middle cerebral artery. Left lateral view with the lateral sulcus retracted.**

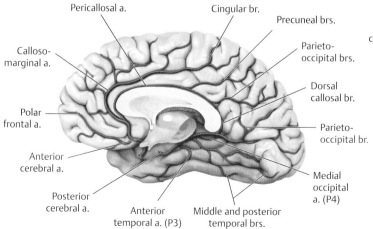

C **Anterior and posterior cerebral arteries. Medial view of the right hemisphere.**

Fig. 48.8 **Cerebral arteries: Distribution areas**
The central gray and white matter have a complex blood supply (yellow) that includes the anterior choroidal artery.

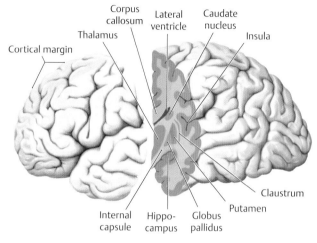

☐ Anterior cerebral a.
☐ Middle cerebral a.
☐ Posterior cerebral a.

A **Lateral view of the left hemisphere.**

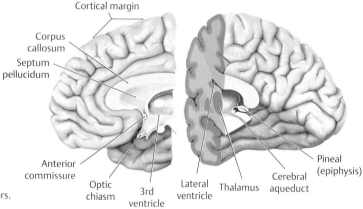

B **Medial view of the right hemisphere.**

Anatomy & Organization of the Spinal Cord

Fig. 49.1 Anatomy of a spinal cord segment

Three dimensional representation, oblique anterior view from upper left. The gray matter of the spinal cord is found internally, surrounding the central canal in an H-shaped, or butterfly-like, configuration. This is the reverse of what was seen in the brain where the gray matter was on the external aspect in a cortical configuration. The primary function of the spinal cord is to conduct impulses to and from the brain and to facilitate this, both gray and white matter are organized into longitudinal groupings.

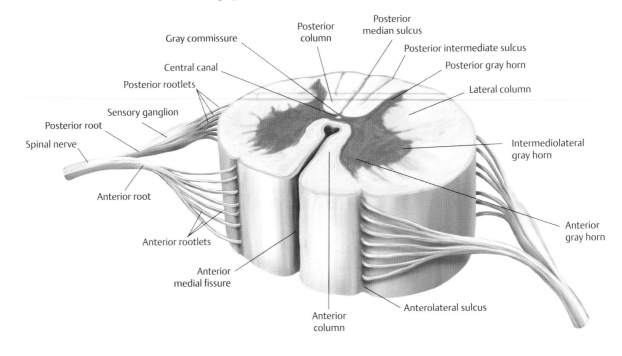

Fig. 49.2 Organization of the gray matter

Left oblique anterosuperior view. The gray matter of the spinal cord is divided into three columns (horns).

- Anterior column (horn): contains motor neurons
- Lateral column (horn): contains sympathetic or parasympathetic (visceromotor) neurons in selected regions
- Posterior column (horn): contains sensory neurons

Afferent (blue) and efferent (red) neurons within these columns are clustered in nuclei according to function.

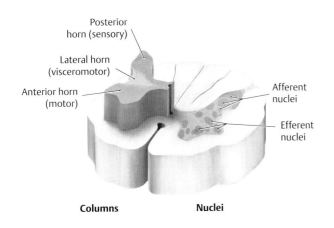

Fig. 49.3 Innervation of muscles

Motor neurons that innervate specific muscles are arranged into vertical columns in the anterior horn of gray matter, the columns themselves can be called nuclei, in a fashion similar to that seen in brainstem motor nuclei. Most muscles (intersegmental muscles) receive innervation from numerous motor nuclei spanning several spinal cord segments. Monosegmental (or indicator) muscles have their motor neurons located entirely within a single spinal cord segment.

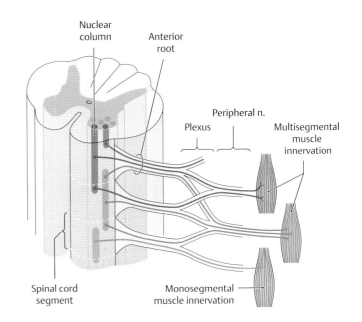

Fig. 49.4A Organization of the white matter

Left oblique anterosuperior view. The gray matter columns partition the white matter analogously into anterior, lateral, and posterior columns or funiculi. The white matter of the spinal cord contains ascending and descending tracts which are the CNS equivalent of peripheral nerves.

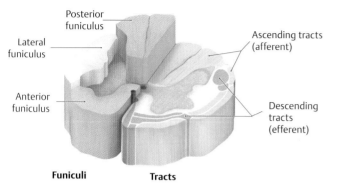

Posterior funiculus

Lateral funiculus

Anterior funiculus

Ascending tracts (afferent)

Descending tracts (efferent)

Funiculi   **Tracts**

Fig. 49.4B Overview of sensorimotor integration

Schematic illustrates the pathway of incoming primary afferent (sensory) neuron impulses, the axon of which ascends to synapse with the secondary and tertiary afferent (sensory) neurons in the brainstem and cerebrum ending in a synapse on a neuron in the sensory cortex. An interneuron links this with an upper motor neuron in the motor cortex which then descends through the white matter funiculi of the spinal cord to a motor neuron, which then synapses with a lower motor neuron, the axon of which passes out the spinal nerve to the effector organ.

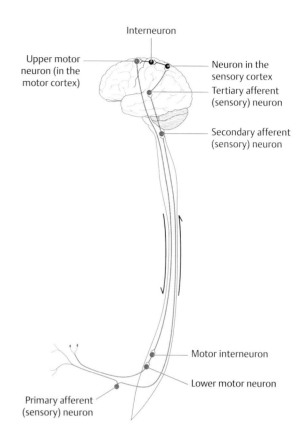

Interneuron

Upper motor neuron (in the motor cortex)

Neuron in the sensory cortex

Tertiary afferent (sensory) neuron

Secondary afferent (sensory) neuron

Motor interneuron

Lower motor neuron

Primary afferent (sensory) neuron

Fig. 49.5A Principle intrinsic fascicles of the spinal cord (shaded yellow)

Left oblique anterosuperior view. The majority of muscles have a multi-segmental mode of innervaton that necessitates axons to ascend/descend multiple spinal cord segments to coordinate spinal reflexes. The neurons of these axons originate from interneurons in the gray matter forming intrinsic reflex pathways of the spinal cord. These axons are collected into intrinsic fascicles which are arranged chiefly around the gray matter. These bundles make up the intrinsic circuits of the spinal cord.

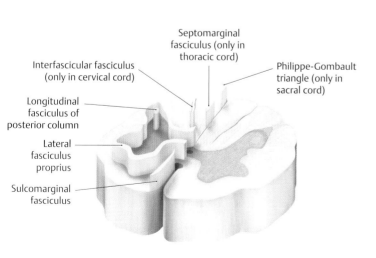

Interfascicular fasciculus (only in cervical cord)

Septomarginal fasciculus (only in thoracic cord)

Philippe-Gombault triangle (only in sacral cord)

Longitudinal fasciculus of posterior column

Lateral fasciculus proprius

Sulcomarginal fasciculus

Fig. 49.5B Intrinsic circuits of the spinal cord

Afferent neurons are shown in blue, efferent neurons in red. The neurons of the spinal reflex circuits are in black. These chains of interneurons, which are entirely contained within the spinal cord, comprise the intrinsic circuits of the cord. The axons of these intrinsic circuits pass to adjacent segments in intrinsic fascicles located along the edge of the gray matter.

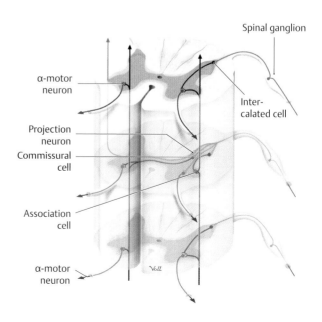

Spinal ganglion

α-motor neuron

Inter-calated cell

Projection neuron

Commissural cell

Association cell

α-motor neuron

Sensory & Motor Pathways

Fig. 49.6 Sensory pathways (ascending tracts)

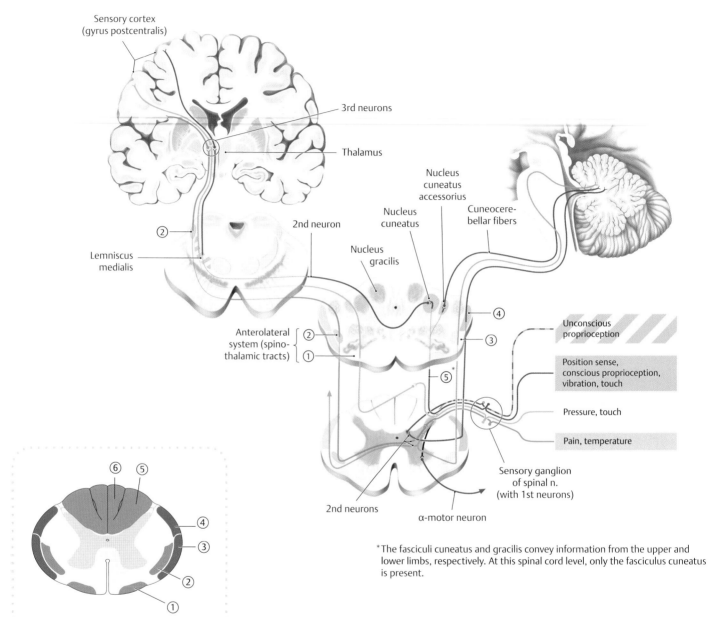

Sensory cortex (gyrus postcentralis)

3rd neurons

Thalamus

Nucleus cuneatus accessorius

Nucleus cuneatus

Cuneocere-bellar fibers

2nd neuron

Nucleus gracilis

Lemniscus medialis

Unconscious proprioception

Anterolateral system (spino-thalamic tracts) ② ①

Position sense, conscious proprioception, vibration, touch

Pressure, touch

Pain, temperature

Sensory ganglion of spinal n. (with 1st neurons)

2nd neurons

α-motor neuron

*The fasciculi cuneatus and gracilis convey information from the upper and lower limbs, respectively. At this spinal cord level, only the fasciculus cuneatus is present.

Table 49.1	**Sensory pathways (ascending tracts) of the spinal cord**			
Tract	**Location**	**Function**		**Neurons**
① Anterior spino-thalamic tract	Anterior funiculus	Pathway for crude touch and pressure sensation		1st afferent neurons located in spinal ganglia; contain 2nd neurons and cross in the anterior commissure
② Lateral spino-thalamic tract	Anterior and lateral funiculi	Pathway for pain, temperature, tickle, itch, and sexual sensation		
③ Anterior spino-cerebellar tract	Lateral funiculus	Pathway for unconscious coordination of motor activities (unconscious proprioception, automatic processes, e.g., jogging, riding a bike) to the cerebellum		Projection (2nd) neurons receive proprioceptive signals from 1st afferent fibers originating at the 1st neurons of spinal ganglia
④ Posterior spino-cerebellar tract				
⑤ Fasciculus cuneatus	Posterior funiculus	Pathway for position sense (conscious proprioception) and fine cutaneous sensation (touch, vibration, fine pressure sense, two-point discrimination)	Conveys information from *upper* limb (not present below T3)	Cell bodies of 1st neuron located in spinal ganglion; pass uncrossed to the dorsal column nuclei
⑥ Fasciculus gracilis			Conveys information from *lower* limb	

**Corticospinal tracts
(pyramidal tract)**

**Descending tracts from brainstem
(extrapyramidal motor system)**

Fig. 49.7 **Motor pathways
(descending tracts)**

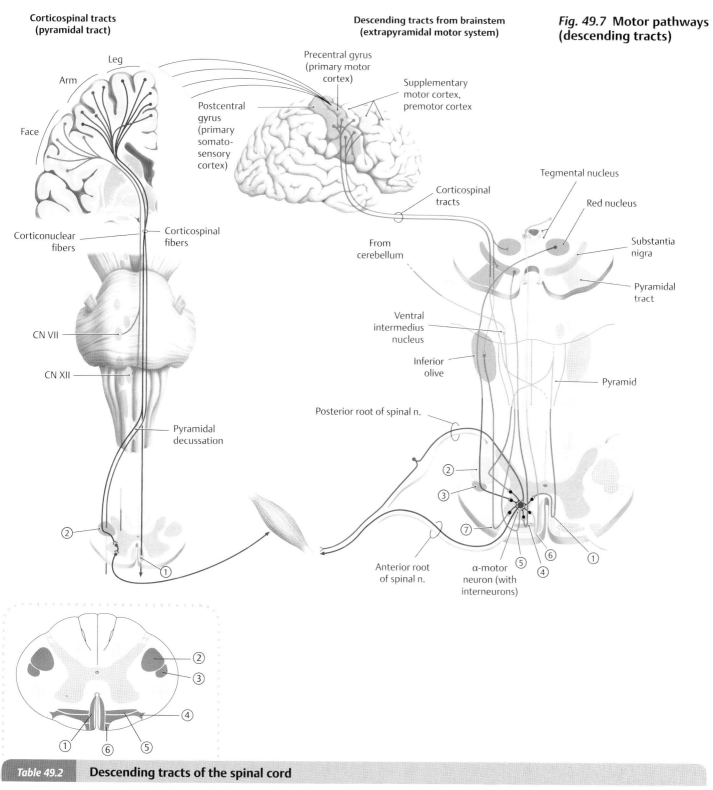

Table 49.2		Descending tracts of the spinal cord		
Tract			**Function**	
Corticospinal tract (pyramidal tract)	①	Anterior corticospinal tract	Most important pathway for voluntary motor function	Originates in the motor cortex *Corticonuclear* fibers to motor nuclei of cranial nerves *Corticospinal* fibers to motor cells in anterior horn of the spinal cord *Corticoreticular* fibers to nuclei of the reticular formation
	②	Lateral corticospinal tract		
Descending tracts from the brainstem (Extrapyramidal motor system)	③	Rubrospinal tract	Pathway for automatic and learned motor processes (e.g., walking, running, cycling)	
	④	Reticulospinal tract		
	⑤	Vestibulospinal tract		
	⑥	Tectospinal tract		
	⑦	Olivospinal tract		

Autonomic Nervous System (I): Overview

Fig. 50.1 Autonomic nervous system

The autonomic nervous system is the part of the peripheral nervous system that innervates smooth muscle, cardiac muscle, and glands. It is subdivided into the sympathetic (red) and the parasympathetic (blue) nervous systems, which often act in antagonistic fashion to regulate blood flow, secretions, and organ function.

Both the sympathetic and parasympathetic nervous systems have a two-neuron pathway, which is under central nervous system control via an upper motor neuron with its cell body in the hypothalamus.

In the sympathetic system, the preganglionic neuron synapses within the ganglia of the sympathetic trunk (paired, one on each side of vertebral column) or on one of the unpaired prevertebral ganglia located at the base of the artery for which the ganglion was named (celiac, superior and inferior mesenteric). Sympathetic postganglionic neurons then either reenter spinal nerves via gray rami communicantes and are distributed to their target structure or they reach their target structure by travelling with arteries. Except in the head, parasympathetic preganglionic neurons synapse in ganglia in the wall of the target organ. Short postganglioinc parasympathetic neurons then innervate the organ. In the head there are four parasympathetic ganglia: ciliary, pterygopalatine, submandibular, and otic, which are associated with cranial nerves III, VII, and IX, respectively. These four ganglia are responsible for distributing fibers to smooth muscle within the eye and to the salivary glands and glands of the nasal cavity, paranasal sinuses, hard and soft palate, and pharynx.

Both sympathetic and parasympathetic preganglionic neurons secrete acetylcholine, which acts upon nicotinic receptors in the ganglia. Sympathetic postganglionic neurons secrete norepinephrine, which acts upon adrenoceptors (α or β) in target tissues. Parasympathetic postganglionic neurons secrete acetylcholine, which acts upon muscarinic receptors in target tissues.

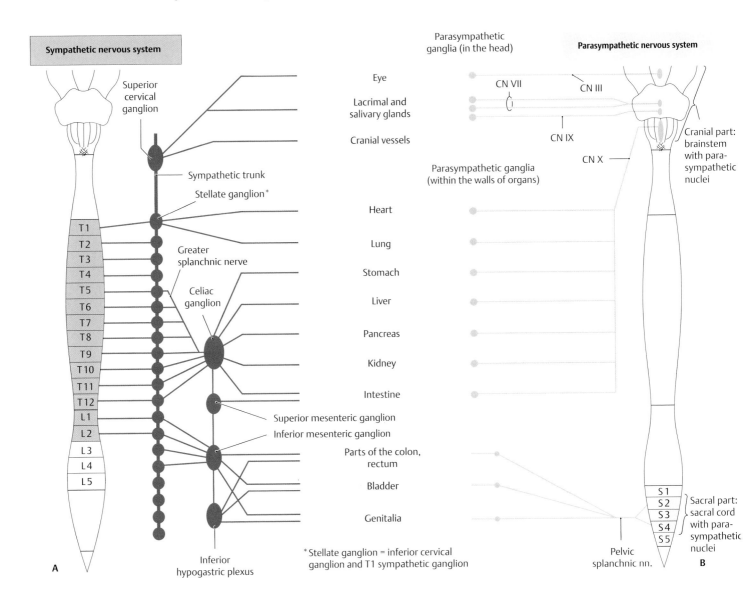

* Stellate ganglion = inferior cervical ganglion and T1 sympathetic ganglion

Table 50.1	Parasympathetic pathways
Neuron	**Location of cell body**
Upper motor neuron	**Hypothalamus:** The cell bodies of parasympathetic upper motor neurons are located in the hypothalamus. Their axons descend via white matter tracts to synapse with the lower motor neuron in the brainstem and sacral spinal cord (S2–S4).
Preganglionic neuron (lower motor neuron)	The parasympathetic nervous system is divided into two parts (cranial and sacral), based on the location of the preganglionic parasympathetic neurons.
	Brainstem cranial nerve nuclei: The axons of these secondary neurons leave the CNS as the motor root of cranial nn. III, VII, IX, and X. **Spinal cord (S2–S4):** The axons of these secondary neurons leave the CNS (S2–S4) as the pelvic splanchnic nn. These nerves travel in the posterior rami of the S2–S4 spinal nn. and are distributed via the sympathetic plexuses to the pelvic viscera.
Postganglionic neuron	**Cranial nerve parasympathetic ganglia:** The parasympathetic cranial nn. of the head each have at least one ganglion: • CN III: Ciliary ganglion • CN VII: Pterygopalatine ganglion and submandibular ganglion • CN IX: Otic ganglion • CN X: Small unnamed ganglia close to target structures
Distribution of postganglionic fibers	Parasympathetic fibers course with other fiber types to their targets. In the head, the postganglionic fibers from the pterygopalatine ganglion (CN VII) and otic ganglion (CN IX) are distributed via branches of the trigeminal n. (CN V). Postganglionic fibers from the ciliary ganglion (CN III) course with sympathetic and sensory fibers in the short ciliary nn. (preganglionic fibers travel with the somatomotor fibers of CN III). In the thorax, abdomen, and pelvis, preganglionic parasympathetic fibers from CN X and the pelvic splanchnic nn. combine with postganglionic sympathetic fibers to form plexuses (e.g., cardiac, pulmonary, esophageal).

Table 50.2	Sympathetic pathways
Neuron	**Location of cell body**
Upper motor neuron	**Hypothalamus:** The cell bodies of parasympathetic upper motor neurons are located in the hypothalamus. Their axons descend via white matter tracts to synapse with the lower motor neuron in the lateral horn of the spinal cord (T1–L2).
Preganglionic neuron (lower motor neuron)	**Lateral horn of spinal cord (T1–L2):** The lateral horn is the middle portion of the gray matter of the spinal cord, situated between the anterior and posterior horns. It contains exclusively autonomic (sympathetic) neurons. The axons of these neurons leave the CNS as the motor root of the spinal nn. and enter the paravertebral ganglia via the white rami communicantes (myelinated).
Preganglionic neurons in paravertebral ganglia	All preganglionic sympathetic neurons enter the sympathetic chain. There they may synapse in a chain ganglion or ascend or descend to synapse. Preganglionic sympathetic neurons synapse in one of two places, yielding two types of sympathetic ganglia.
	Synapse in the paravertebral ganglia Pass without synapsing through the parasympathetic ganglia. These fibers travel in the thoracic, lumbar, and sacral splanchnic nn. to synapse in the prevertebral ganglia.
Postganglionic neuron	**Paravertebral ganglia:** These ganglia form the sympathetic nerve trunks that flank the spinal cord. Postganglionic axons leave the sympathetic trunk via the gray rami communicantes (unmyelinated). **Prevertebral ganglia:** Associated with peripheral plexuses, which spread along the abdominal aorta. There are three primary prevertebral ganglia: • Celiac ganglion • Superior mesenteric ganglion • Inferior mesenteric ganglion
Distribution of postganglionic fibers	Postganglionic fibers are distributed in two ways: 1. Spinal nerves: Postganglionic neurons may re-enter the spinal nn. via the gray rami communicantes. These sympathetic neurons induce constriction of blood vessels, sweat glands, and arrector pili (muscle fibers attached to hair follicles, "goose bumps"). 2. Arteries and ducts: Nerve plexuses may form along existing structures. Postganglionic sympathetic fibers may travel with arteries to target structures. Viscera are innervated by this method (e.g., sympathetic innervation concerning vasoconstriction, bronchial dilatation, glandular secretions, pupillary dilatation, smooth muscle contraction).

Autonomic Nervous System (II)

Fig. 50.2 Typical spinal nerve

All spinal nerves arising from the spinal cord contain somatic sensory (or afferent, from body wall) and somatic motor (or efferent, to body wall) fibers. Sensory fibers come from the posterior (back) region via the posterior ramus and anterolateral regions of the body wall via the anterior ramus of the spinal nerve. The somatic afferent fibers approach the spinal cord via the posterior root. The cell bodies for these fibers lie in the sensory (spinal/dorsal root) ganglion. They synapse with sensory neurons in the posterior horn of gray matter within the spinal cord sending the majority to the brain for interpretation. Somatic motor fibers have their neurons in the anterior horn of gray matter and send their fibers to the spinal n. via the anterior root. This pattern of somatic innervation occurs in all spinal nerves from C1 through S5, whether they are involved in a plexus or not.

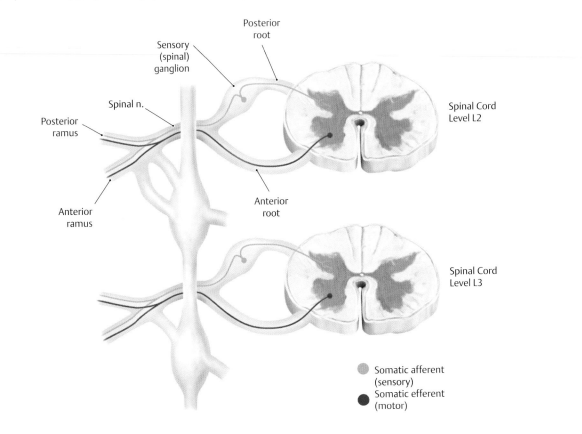

Posterior root

Sensory (spinal) ganglion

Spinal n.

Posterior ramus

Anterior ramus

Anterior root

Spinal Cord Level L2

Spinal Cord Level L3

⬤ Somatic afferent (sensory)
● Somatic efferent (motor)

Fig. 50.3 ANS Circuitry

Body wall dermatomes also require sympathetic fibers to contract smooth muscle and cause glands in the dermatome to secrete. Preganglionic sympathetic fibers (purple) arise from cell bodies in the intermediolateral gray horn of the spinal cord. They exit the spinal cord via the outgoing/efferent (anterior) root—along with the somatic motor (efferent) fibers—and enter the spinal nerve. The smooth muscle of the body wall requires innervation by postganglionic sympathetic fibers so the preganglionic fiber looks for the closest synapse site—the paravertebral sympathetic ganglia—found in a chain-like arrangement on either side of the vertebral column. Each ganglion is connected to the spinal n. by communicating branches—the rami communicantes. The white ramus communicans is found furthest out and conveys the preganglionic (myelinated = white) sympathetic fiber to the ganglion. Once in the paravertebral ganglion one of two things can happen:

a) The preganglionic sympathetic fiber can synapse in the ganglion and the postganglionic sympathetic fiber (orange) passes along the gray ramus communicans (unmyelinated) back to the spinal n. Now postganglionic sympathetic fibers can be distributed to structures in the dermatome via the anterior and posterior rami—along with somatic motor and sensory fibers.

b) The preganglionic fiber can run up or down the sympathetic trunk to synapse in an upper or lower paravertebral ganglion. This is especially important as the source of sympathetic innervation is limited to spinal cord levels T1 to L2. This figure depicts sympathetic innervation from the last spinal cord segment to contain it (L2) descending along the sympathetic trunk to the paravertebral ganglion at L3. It synapses here and the postganglionic sympathetic fiber exits into the spinal nerve of L3. Note that there is only a gray ramus communicans at this level as white rami communicans are input fibers (T1–L2), while the gray are output fibers above and below T1 and L2. Therefore, there are more gray rami than white rami. Both anterior and posterior rami now contain postganglionic sympathetic fibers distributed to the dermatome of L3 along with the typical somatic sensory and motor fibers of each vertebral level.

Now that the body wall has been supplied with postganglionic sympathetic innervation, we'll turn our attention to the viscera. The third option for preganglionic sympathetic fibers entering a prevertebral ganglion has the fibers passing through the paravertebral ganglion at that level without synapsing and passing into a splanchnic n. to synapse in one of 3 prevertebral (or collateral) ganglia found in the abdomen along the anterior surface of the aorta at the base of one of the three main visceral branches (celiac a., superior mesenteric a., and inferior mesenteric a.). The postganglionic sympathetic fibers (orange) are distributed by following arterial branches to the viscera where they control smooth muscle contraction in the wall of the organ, as well as being secretomotor to glands in the wall of the organ.

The body wall does not receive any parasympathetic innervation. Dilation of the blood vessel walls occurs as the postganglionic sympathetics stop firing to cause vasoconstriction. However, the intricate control of movement of the wall of the intestine, or secretion of the glands within its wall, does require the antagonistic input of the parasympathetic division. Parasympathetic innervation to the viscera of the thorax and much of the abdomen (to the mid transverse colon) is supplied by the vagus n. (dark blue). The vagus sends branches to the various sympathetic prevertebral ganglia of the abdomen but they do not synapse here. They pass through, following the branches of the blood vessel to the wall of the organs supplied. Here they synapse in tiny parasympathetic (intramural) ganglion within the wall of the organ.

The postganglionic parasympathetic fibers (light blue) are therefore extremely short. The remainder of the abdominal and pelvic viscera receive their parasympathetic supply in a similar fashion but from preganglionic parasympathetic fibers from spinal cord levels S2-4. Viscera also exhibit pain, relayed back to the CNS as visceral afferents (dark green). Note that the visceral afferent fibers follow the pathway of the sympathetic pre- and postganglionic fibers back from the viscera. They pass through the prevertebral ganglion without synapsing, back along the splanchnic n., do not synapse in the paravertebral ganglion, pass back through the white ramus communicans (as visceral afferent fibers are also myelinated) and follow the posterior root back to the sensory ganglion where the cell body is found interspersed amongst those for the body wall. They finally synapse in the posterior horn of gray matter in the spinal cord amongst the somatic afferents also synapsing there. This is the basis for referred pain as the brain finds it difficult to distinguish visceral pain from somatic pain as the latter outnumber the former very significantly. Therefore, pain from internal organs is often referred to sites on the body wall.

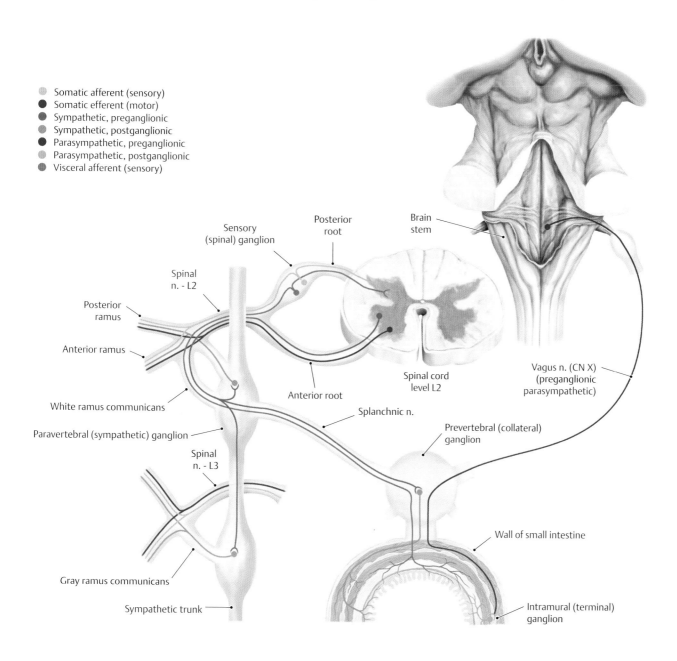

- Somatic afferent (sensory)
- Somatic efferent (motor)
- Sympathetic, preganglionic
- Sympathetic, postganglionic
- Parasympathetic, preganglionic
- Parasympathetic, postganglionic
- Visceral afferent (sensory)

Sectional Anatomy of the Nervous System

Fig. 51.1 Sagittal section through the midline of the brain

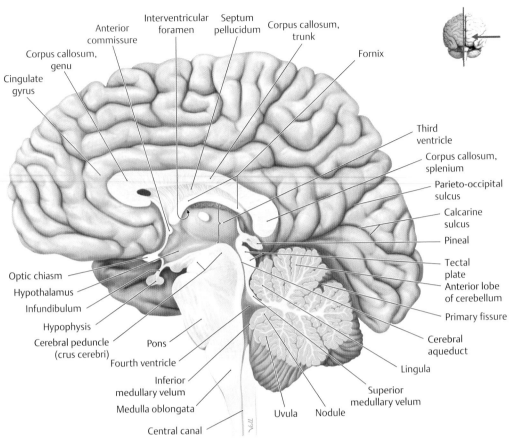

Anterior commissure
Interventricular foramen
Septum pellucidum
Corpus callosum, trunk
Corpus callosum, genu
Fornix
Cingulate gyrus
Third ventricle
Corpus callosum, splenium
Parieto-occipital sulcus
Calcarine sulcus
Pineal
Tectal plate
Optic chiasm
Anterior lobe of cerebellum
Hypothalamus
Infundibulum
Primary fissure
Hypophysis
Cerebral aqueduct
Cerebral peduncle (crus cerebri)
Pons
Fourth ventricle
Lingula
Inferior medullary velum
Superior medullary velum
Medulla oblongata
Uvula
Nodule
Central canal

Fig. 51.2 Frontal section through the brain I

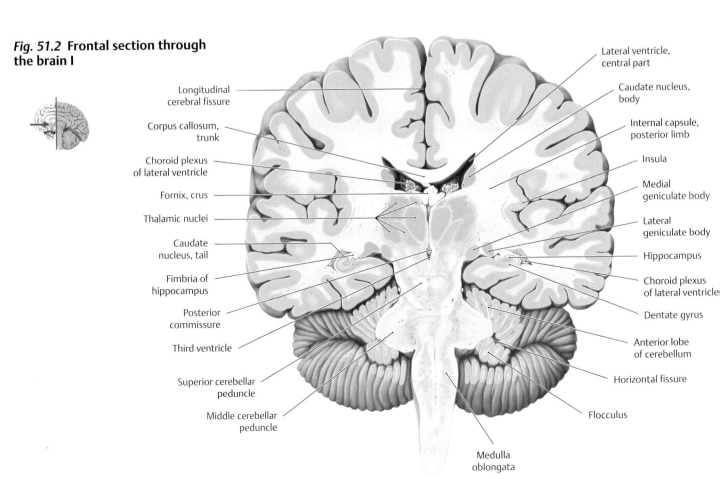

Longitudinal cerebral fissure
Lateral ventricle, central part
Caudate nucleus, body
Corpus callosum, trunk
Internal capsule, posterior limb
Choroid plexus of lateral ventricle
Insula
Fornix, crus
Medial geniculate body
Thalamic nuclei
Lateral geniculate body
Caudate nucleus, tail
Hippocampus
Fimbria of hippocampus
Choroid plexus of lateral ventricle
Posterior commissure
Dentate gyrus
Third ventricle
Anterior lobe of cerebellum
Superior cerebellar peduncle
Horizontal fissure
Middle cerebellar peduncle
Flocculus
Medulla oblongata

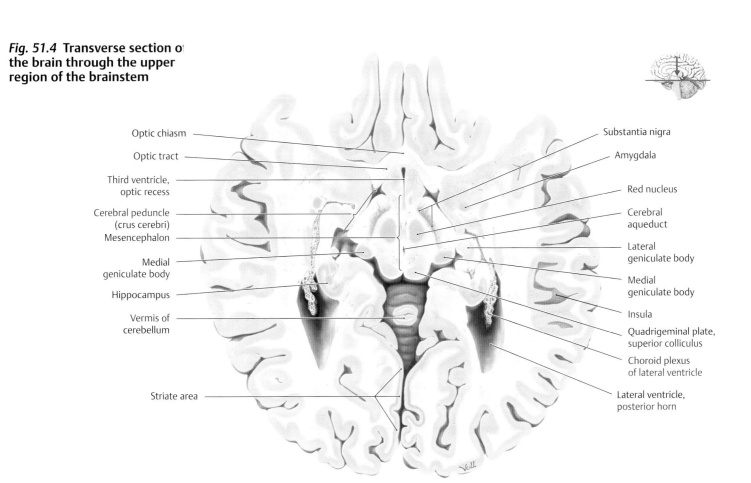

Fig. 51.3 Frontal section through the brain II

Longitudinal cerebral fissure

Corpus callosum, trunk

Choroid plexus of lateral ventricle

Fornix, crus

Thalamus, pulvinar

Caudate nucleus, tail

Quadrigeminal plate, superior colliculus

Central gray matter

Middle cerebellar peduncle

Rhomboid fossa

Lateral ventricle, central part

Caudate nucleus, body

Insula

Internal cerebral veins

Pineal

Hippocampus

Choroid plexus of lateral ventricle

Cerebral aqueduct

Anterior lobe of cerebellum

Posterior lobe of cerebellum

Choroid plexus of fourth ventricle

Cerebellar tonsil

Fig. 51.4 Transverse section of the brain through the upper region of the brainstem

Optic chiasm

Optic tract

Third ventricle, optic recess

Cerebral peduncle (crus cerebri)

Mesencephalon

Medial geniculate body

Hippocampus

Vermis of cerebellum

Striate area

Substantia nigra

Amygdala

Red nucleus

Cerebral aqueduct

Lateral geniculate body

Medial geniculate body

Insula

Quadrigeminal plate, superior colliculus

Choroid plexus of lateral ventricle

Lateral ventricle, posterior horn

Radiographic Anatomy of the Nervous System

 Additional radiological images of the blood supply to the brain can be found on **p. 661.**

Fig. 51.5 **MRI of the brain**
Midsagittal section, left lateral view.

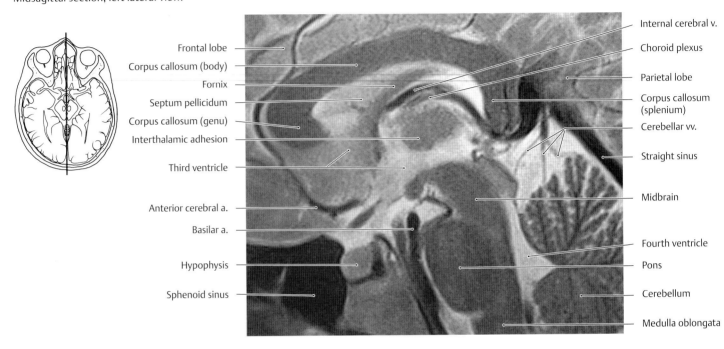

Frontal lobe
Corpus callosum (body)
Fornix
Septum pellicidum
Corpus callosum (genu)
Interthalamic adhesion
Third ventricle
Anterior cerebral a.
Basilar a.
Hypophysis
Sphenoid sinus

Internal cerebral v.
Choroid plexus
Parietal lobe
Corpus callosum (splenium)
Cerebellar vv.
Straight sinus
Midbrain
Fourth ventricle
Pons
Cerebellum
Medulla oblongata

Fig. 51.6 **MRI of the brain**
Transverse (axial) section through the cerebral hemispheres. Inferior view.

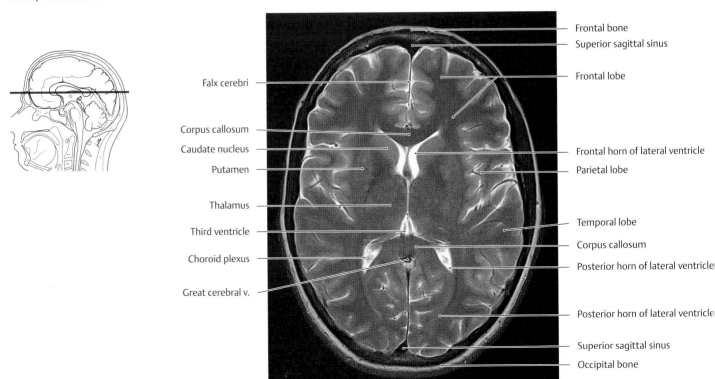

Falx cerebri
Corpus callosum
Caudate nucleus
Putamen
Thalamus
Third ventricle
Choroid plexus
Great cerebral v.

Frontal bone
Superior sagittal sinus
Frontal lobe
Frontal horn of lateral ventricle
Parietal lobe
Temporal lobe
Corpus callosum
Posterior horn of lateral ventricle
Posterior horn of lateral ventricle
Superior sagittal sinus
Occipital bone

Fig. 51.7 MRI of the brain

Coronal section through the ventricular system.

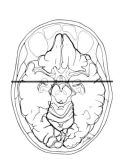

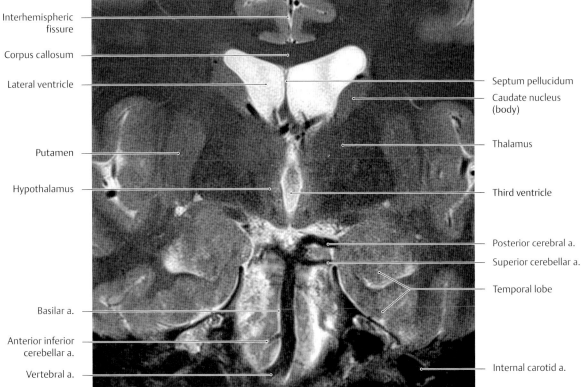

Interhemispheric fissure

Corpus callosum

Lateral ventricle

Putamen

Hypothalamus

Basilar a.

Anterior inferior cerebellar a.

Vertebral a.

Septum pellucidum

Caudate nucleus (body)

Thalamus

Third ventricle

Posterior cerebral a.

Superior cerebellar a.

Temporal lobe

Internal carotid a.

Fig. 51.8 MRI of the neck

Coronal section through the cervical spinal cord. Anterior view.

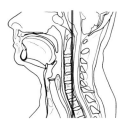

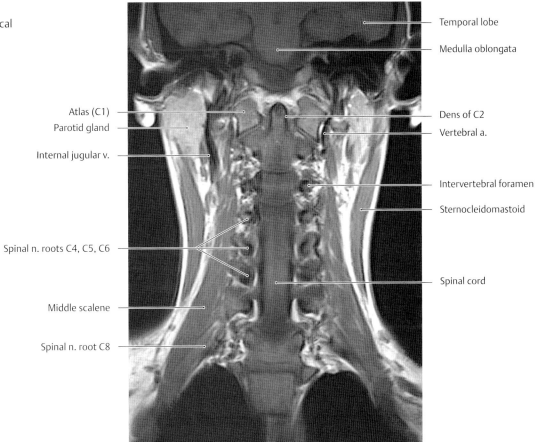

Atlas (C1)

Parotid gland

Internal jugular v.

Spinal n. roots C4, C5, C6

Middle scalene

Spinal n. root C8

Temporal lobe

Medulla oblongata

Dens of C2

Vertebral a.

Intervertebral foramen

Sternocleidomastoid

Spinal cord

Index

Index

colic
 intermediate, 207
 left, 201, 206, 207
 middle, 201, 206
 right, 201, 206
cubital, 76, 363
cystic, 201, 204, 205
epicolic, 207
facial, 626
foraminal, 201, 205
gastric
 left, 201, 204, 205
 right, 201, 205
gastro-omental
 left, 201, 204, 205
 right, 201, 204, 205
gluteal
 inferior, 203, 273
 superior, 203, 273
hepatic, 201, 204, 205
ileocolic, 201, 206, 207
iliac
 common, 200t, 202, 203, 270, 271t, 272, 273, 469
 external, 202, 203, 271, 271t, 272, 273, 469, 482
 internal, 271, 271t, 273, 469
inguinal
 deep, 155, 202, 203, 271, 272, 273, 469, 482
 inferior, 482
 superficial, 202, 203, 271, 271t, 273, 469, 482
  horizontal group, 271t, 272, 273
  vertical group, 271t, 272, 273
 superolateral, 482
 superomedial, 482
intercostal, 84, 110, 128
interiliac, 203, 273
intrapulmonary, 85, 128, 129
jugular, 609
 lateral group, 627t
juxta-intestinal, 201, 206
lacunar
 intermediate, 202, 203, 273
 lateral, 203, 273
 medial, 203, 273
laryngotracheothyroidal, 626
lumbar, 200t, 218, 270t, 272, 273, 469
 intermediate, 202, 203, 218, 272, 273
 lateral, 218
 lateral aortic, 201, 203, 206
 lateral caval, 203, 273
 left, 201, 203, 206
  lateral, 203
  lateral aortic, 202
  preaortic. See Lymph nodes, preaortic
  retroaortic. See Lymph nodes, retroaortic
 right lateral aortic (caval), 202
mastoid, 627, 627t

mesenteric
 inferior, 200t, 201, 202, 207, 270t, 271t, 272, 273
 intermediate, 206
 superior, 200t, 201, 202, 205, 206, 207, 270t, 271t
mesocolic, 201, 206
nuchal, 626
obturator, 203, 273
occipital, 626, 627, 627t, 644
pancreatic, 205
 inferior, 201, 205
 superior, 201, 205
pancreaticoduodenal, 205
 inferior, 201
 superior, 201
paracolic, 207
paraesophageal, 85, 111
paramammary, 85
pararectal, 273
parasternal, 76, 85, 128
paratracheal, 85, 110, 111, 129
parauterine, 273
paravaginal, 273
paravertebral, 85
parietal, 202
parotid, deep, 627, 627t
parotidauricular, 626
pericardial, lateral, 85, 91
phrenic
 inferior, 111, 128, 200t, 202, 203, 204, 270t
 superior, 85, 87, 88, 91, 95, 110, 204
popliteal
 deep, 469, 489
 superficial, 469
preaortic, 200t, 201, 203, 206, 270t, 271t, 273
precaval, 273
prececal, 201, 206, 207
prepericardial, 85
prevertebral, 110
prevesical, 273
promontory, 203, 272, 273
pyloric, 201, 204
rectal, 271
 superior, 201, 206, 207
retroaortic, 200t, 202, 203, 270t
retroauricular, 627, 627t
retrocaval, 202, 203, 273
retrocecal, 201
retrocolic, 206
retropreaortic, 273
retropyloric, 201, 205
retrovesical, 273
Rosenmüller's, 482, 483
sacral, 202, 203, 271, 272, 273
sigmoid, 201, 206, 207
splenic, 201, 204, 205
subaortic, 203, 273
submandibular, 609, 626, 627, 627t

submental, 609, 627, 627t
subpyloric, 201, 204, 205
superolateral, 469
superomedial, 469
supraclavicular, 76
suprapyloric, 201, 204, 205
supratrochlear, 76
thoracic, 85
tracheobronchial, 85, 87, 88, 110, 111, 128
 inferior, 110, 111, 128, 129
 superior, 129
vesical, lateral, 273
visceral pelvic, 273
Lymph nodes (of region or organ)
 of abdomen, 200–207, 200t
 of breast, 76, 76t
 of genitalia
  in female, 273
  in male, 272
 of hand, 363
 of ileum, 206
 of inguinal region, 482
 of jejunum, 296
 of large intestine, 207
 of liver, 204
 of mediastinum, 85, 87t, 110–111
 of pleural cavity, 128–129
 of rectum, 271
 of spleen, 205
 of stomach, 204
 of thoracic cavity, 84–85
 of thoracic wall, 85
 of tongue, 609
 of upper limb, 363
 of urethra, 271
 of urinary bladder, 271
Lymphatic drainage
 of abdomen, 200–207, 270, 270t
 of bladder, 271
 of breast, 76, 76t
 of genitalia
  in female, 271, 273
  in male, 271, 272
 of heart, 110
 of intestines, 206
 of liver, 201, 204, 205
 of lower limb, 469
 of neck
  deep, 627t
  superficial, 627t
 of oral cavity, 609
 of pancreas, 201, 205
 of pelvis, 271t
 of pleural cavity, 128–128
 by quadrants, 85
 of rectum, 201, 271
 of spleen, 201, 205
 of stomach, 201, 204, 205
 of thoracic cavity, 84–85
 of tongue, 609